# Clinical Research in OCCUPATIONAL THERAPY

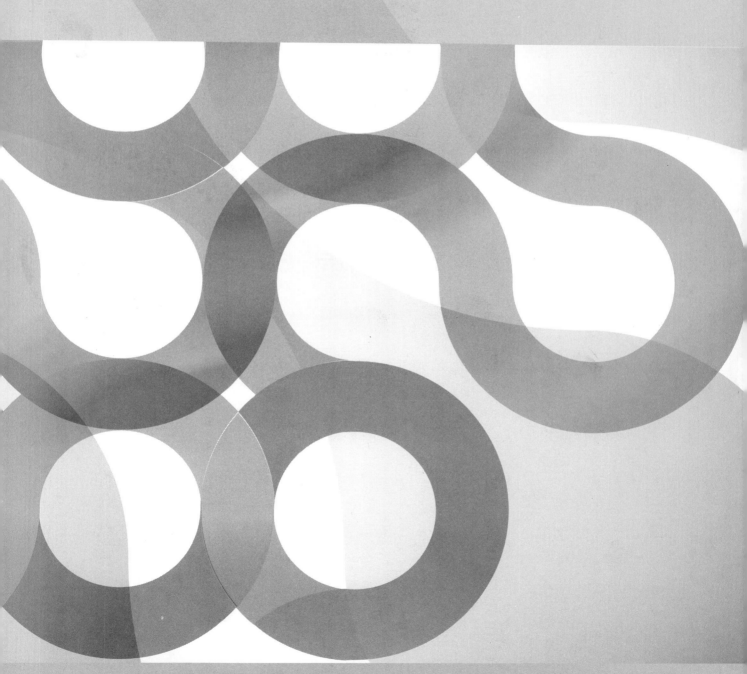

# Clinical Research in OCCUPATIONAL THERAPY

## Fifth Edition

**Franklin Stein, Ph.D., OTR/L, FAOTA**

Professor Emeritus, Occupational Therapy,
The University of South Dakota
Vermillion, South Dakota

**Martin S. Rice, PhD., OTR/L**

Professor, Occupational Therapy,
The University of Toledo
Toledo, Ohio

**Susan K. Cutler, Ph.D., NCSP, ABSNP**

School Psychologist
Bemidji, Minnesota

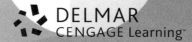

DELMAR
CENGAGE Learning™

Australia • Canada • Mexico • Singapore • Spain • United Kingdom • United States

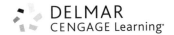

**Clinical Research in Occupational Therapy**
**Fifth Edition**
Franklin Stein, Ph.D., OTR/L, FAOTA
Martin S. Rice, PhD., OTR/L
Susan K. Cutler, Ph.D., NCSP, ABSNP

Vice President, Careers & Computing: Dave Garza

Director of Learning Solutions: Matthew Kane

Associate Acquisitions Editor: Christina Gifford

Managing Editor: Marah Bellegarde

Senior Product Manager: Laura J. Wood

Editorial Assistant: Anthony Souza

Vice President, Marketing: Jennifer Ann Baker

Marketing Director: Wendy E. Mapstone

Senior Marketing Manager: Nancy Bradshaw

Associate Marketing Manager: Erica Ropitzky

Senior Director, Education Production:
    Wendy A. Troeger

Production Manager: Andrew Crouth

Senior Content Project Manager:
    Kara A. DiCaterino

Senior Art Director: David Arsenault

For product information and technology assistance, contact us at
**Cengage Learning Customer & Sales Support, 1-800-354-9706**
For permission to use material from this text or product,
submit all requests online at **www.cengage.com/permissions**.
Further permissions questions can be e-mailed to
**permissionrequest@cengage.com**

Library of Congress Control Number: 2011933698

ISBN-13: 978-1-111-64331-7

ISBN-10: 1-111-64331-8

**Delmar**
5 Maxwell Drive
Clifton Park, NY 12065-2919
USA

Cengage Learning is a leading provider of customized learning solutions with office locations around the globe, including Singapore, the United Kingdom, Australia, Mexico, Brazil, and Japan. Locate your local office at:
**international.cengage.com/region**

Cengage Learning products are represented in Canada by Nelson Education, Ltd.

To learn more about Delmar, visit **www.cengage.com/delmar**
Purchase any of our products at your local college store or at our preferred online store **www.cengagebrain.com**

**Notice to the Reader**
Publisher does not warrant or guarantee any of the products described herein or perform any independent analysis in connection with any of the product information contained herein. Publisher does not assume, and expressly disclaims, any obligation to obtain and include information other than that provided to it by the manufacturer. The reader is expressly warned to consider and adopt all safety precautions that might be indicated by the activities described herein and to avoid all potential hazards. By following the instructions contained herein, the reader willingly assumes all risks in connection with such instructions. The publisher makes no representations or warranties of any kind, including but not limited to, the warranties of fitness for particular purpose or merchantability, nor are any such representations implied with respect to the material set forth herein, and the publisher takes no responsibility with respect to such material. The publisher shall not be liable for any special, consequential, or exemplary damages resulting, in whole or part, from the readers' use of, or reliance upon, this material.

Printed in the United States of America
1 2 3 4 5 6 7 16 15 14 13 12

# Contents

## CHAPTER 1

### A Short History of the Scientific Method in Medicine, Rehabilitation, and Habilitation . . . . . . . . . . . . . . . . . . . . . . . . . . . . . . . . . . . . . . 1

## CHAPTER 2

**The Scientific Method and Research Models** . . . . . . . . . . . . . . . . . . . . . . . . **51**

## CHAPTER 3

## CHAPTER 4

## CHAPTER 5

## CHAPTER 6

## CHAPTER 7

## CHAPTER 8

## Data Analysis and Statistics . . . . . . . . . . . . . . . . . . . . . . . . . . . . . . . . . . . **307**

## CHAPTER 9

## CHAPTER 10

# Preface to the Fifth Edition

The first edition of this book, *Anatomy of Research in Allied Health*, was published by Schenkman Publishing Company in Cambridge, Massachusetts, and John Wiley and Sons in 1976. The book was a result of a sabbatical in Cambridge, England, in 1974 when I was a professor at Sargent College, Boston University. It was the first textbook by an occupational therapist on research methodology. At that time, the purpose for writing a text on research was to demonstrate how the allied health professions, including occupational therapy, was part of the evolution of the medical progress throughout the world. I felt that occupational therapy as a health care profession was very much tied to the knowledge base of scientific medicine. It is important for occupational therapists to know the history of medicine and rehabilitation as the foundation for understanding occupational therapy's development as a profession. In the first edition, I wrote: "The overall purposes of the book are two-fold. One is to assist clinicians and students in the health fields to become effective evaluators and consumers of published research and two is to facilitate research skills by communicating the process of research and the abilities needed to plan and implement a research project" (Stein, F.,1976, p. viii). These goals are still relevant and appropriate today. However, the terminology that best characterizes the application of research results to practice is the concept of evidence-based practice (EBP).

Evidence-based practice is the standard for the health professions in the twenty-first century. The main purpose of EBP is to apply the results of research and scientific evidence to clinical practice in assessing and treating clients. Clinical reasoning is an important aspect of EBP because the clinician has to evaluate whether the research is appropriate, relevant, and valid. If EBP is to be applied efficiently in the clinical setting, then the health care provider must be able to judge the effectiveness of the research. In other words, the clinician has to critically digest the research studies published in journals and to critically evaluate evidence and then apply the results to practice.

In this new edition, I am very pleased that Dr. Martin Rice has joined us as the second author of the Fifth Edition. Martin is a professor of occupational therapy at the University of Toledo. Besides being a personal friend, Martin is an occupational therapy scholar and researcher with direct experience in teaching research design, as well as carrying out research studies in occupational learning with an exceptional population. The third author is Dr. Sue Cutler, who I first met in 1993 when we were both professors at the University of South Dakota. We "clicked" as colleagues, and Sue has worked in tandem with me on two other texts, *Psychosocial Occupational Therapy: A Holistic Approach* (2nd ed.; 2002) and *Occupational Therapy and Ergonomics* (2006). Sue has wide experience as a special educator, school psychologist with emphasis in neuropsychology, and college professor. Working on this text has been a labor of love. I am working with capable people who also enjoy what they do.

How is the text organized and what changes have been made since the Fourth Edition was published in 2000? First, the text has been updated with recent research studies coming out of universities throughout the world. As editor of *Occupational Therapy International*, I have had the unique opportunity of reading many published research studies in occupational therapy. In organizing the new edition, we went through the Fourth Edition line by line to identify where corrections needed to be made, tables replaced, and research studies replaced. Martin, Sue, and I divided the work according to our expertise in the areas of research design. Essentially the table of contents has not changed. What have been the major changes is in the inclusion of recent research in occupational therapy and rehabilitation throughout the chapters. Graduate students from the University of Toledo have helped in updating the material in Chapter 10 on scientific writing and thesis preparation. An example from a student's actual thesis proposal is included. The chapter on statistics has been reviewed by a statistician to include any new information that would benefit graduate students in analyzing data.

## Specific Revisions to the Fifth Edition

1. The addition of Dr. Martin Rice, as the second author, a noted researcher, and scholar in the Occupational Therapy Department at the University of Toledo.
2. A thorough update of the published research in occupational therapy and health care.
3. Major revisions in all the chapters especially the Review of the Literature, Selecting a Test Instrument, and Qualitative and Quantitative Research.
4. New and current examples of quantitative and qualitative research studies organized into Research Boxes.
5. A new example of a research proposal from the Occupational Therapy Department at the University of Toledo.
6. An update of the tests and evaluations used by occupational therapists in research studies as outcome instruments and for clinical assessments.
7. Update of web addresses for health care organizations and health consumer groups.
8. Revision and additions to the glossary of terms in research and statistics.
9. Updated example of an informed consent form from the University of Toledo that is currently used to obtain approval from the Institutional Review Board (IRB).
10. Update of the Landmarks in the History of Occupational Therapy.
11. Addition of statistical tests for analyzing and interpreting data with the most up-to-date statistical software programs.
12. Update from the American Psychological Association (APA) Sixth edition, 2010, *Style Manual*.
13. In general the Fifth Edition enables the graduate student and clinical researcher to carry out a research study from the formulation of a research hypothesis to collecting data in user-friendly step-by-step procedures.
14. The text's contents were reviewed by the University of Toledo graduate students in occupational therapy for usefulness in completing graduate research projects.

Stein, F. (1976). *Anatomy of research in allied health*. Cambridge, MA: Schenkman Publishing Co.

## ALSO AVAILABLE: INSTRUCTOR COMPANION WEBSITE

ISBN-13: 978-1-13378-901-7

The Instructor Companion Website to accompany *Clinical Research in Occupational Therapy* includes slides created in Microsoft PowerPoint® to accompany each chapter along with a research syllabus, teaching tips, and various worksheets that can be utilized with students.

To access these resources, contact your sales representative or log on to http://login.cengage.com.

# Acknowledgements

The Fifth Edition is the result of a cumulative effort over the years from the feedback of students and colleagues who in many cases provided specific examples of their research studies. I would also like to thank the University of South Dakota where I am Professor Emeritus. The University facilities are still available to me, however at a distance because I live in Madison, Wisconsin. I would also like to thank my friends and former colleagues in the universities and colleges that I have gotten to know through AOTA conferences and the World Federation of Occupational Therapists.

—Frank Stein, August, 2010, Madison, Wisconsin

**Martin Rice** would like to thank his family, colleagues, and students who have supported him in this endeavor. In particular, Martin is grateful for occupational therapy doctoral students Mallory Schroeder, Katelin Rudolf, and Stacey Niemeyer who helped with preliminary readings and made suggestions for this manuscript. In addition, a special thanks to Mallory for helping with the compilation of several of the boxes for Chapter 3. Lastly, Martin would like to thank his daughter Ashley for her tabulation skills and his son Clayton for his proofreading skills.

**Sue Cutler** acknowledges her many graduate advisees at Bemidji State University. Their struggles in writing research papers have enabled her to identify pitfalls in the process and to incorporate solutions for avoiding those pitfalls. She also acknowledges the opportunities provided by Bemidji State University for gaining additional experience at national and international presentations. Examples from those experiences have been incorporated into this text. The past year spent in a post-doc program has given her new insight into assessment and evaluation. That information has been used in revising the chapter on testing. Finally, she acknowledges colleagues who have supported her in this endeavor.

## Reviewers

Dr. Tamara Avi-Itzhak, D.Sc.
Associate Professor
Department of Occupational Therapy,
    York College, CUNY
Jamaica, NY

Karen Ann V. Cameron, Ph.D., OTD, OTR/L
Associate Professor of Occupational Therapy and
    Graduate Program Coordinator
Alvernia University
Reading, PA

Catherine Emery, MS, OTR/L
Assistant Professor
Alvernia University
Reading, PA

Tammy R. Gipson, MS, OTR/L
OTA Program Director
Wallace State Community College
Hanceville, AL

John P. Jackson, Ed.D., OTR
Assistant Professor
TTUHSC
Lubbock, TX

# About the Authors

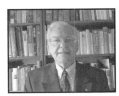

**Franklin Stein,** Ph.D., OTR/L, FAOTA is professor emeritus of Occupational Therapy at the University of South Dakota and founding editor of *Occupational Therapy International.* Prior to coming to the University of South Dakota, he was director of the School of Medical Rehabilitation at the University of Manitoba in Winnipeg, Canada, director of the Occupational Therapy Program at the University of Wisconsin, Milwaukee and associate professor, Graduate Division at Sargent College, Boston University. He is the author with Susan Cutler of the textbooks *Psychosocial Occupational Therapy: A Holistic Approach 2nd ed.* (2001), *Clinical Research in Occupational Therapy 4th edition* (2000), *Occupational Therapy and Ergonomics* (2006) and *Pocketguide to Treatment in Occupational Therapy* (2000) with Becky Roose, *Stress Management Questionnaire* with associates (2003) and over 50 articles in journals and books related to rehabilitation and psychosocial research. He has presented more than a hundred seminars, workshops, institutes, short courses, and research papers at national and international conferences.

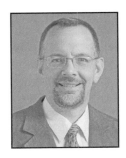

**Martin Rice,** Ph.D., OTR/L is currently a professor at The University of Toledo. Dr. Rice received his Ph.D. in 1996 in Motor Learning and Control and his B.S. in 1984 in Rehabilitation Education from the Pennsylvania State University. In 1987, he received his M.S. in Occupational Therapy from the Western Michigan University. Dr. Rice has served on the editorial boards of AJOT and OTI, and has served as a reviewer for several other peer-reviewed journals. He has published over three dozen research papers and has given over one hundred presentations nationally and internationally. He completed a sabbatical at the Sheffield Hallam University where he studied safe patient handling practices within the United Kingdom.

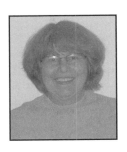

**Susan K. Cutler,** NCSP, ABSNP, received a Ph.D. in special education with a minor in neuropsychology from the University of New Mexico. She has recently completed a post-doctorate program in school neuropsychology. Although she has retired from teaching at the university, she continues to work in private practice as a school psychologist. At present, she assesses students in an Ojibwe tribal school and in charter schools in Northern Minnesota. She holds national certification in school psychology and is a diplomate in school neuropsychology. Dr. Cutler is a national and international conference speaker in the field of special education and assessment. Her focus is on helping parents and teachers use formal and informal assessment to develop appropriate educational programs and interventions for students who struggle in school. She has co-authored three books with Frank Stein.

# Introduction

The First Edition of this text was published in 1976. At that time, it was the first textbook on clinical research in the allied health professions. Since then, numerous texts have been published about research from the perspective of clinical practice in occupational therapy, physical therapy, and speech-language pathology and audiology. The current edition, the Fifth, is a collaborative effort where the three authors combine their expertise as professors, researchers, and clinicians. In preparing this edition, we raised the question: What characterizes a good textbook in clinical research? In reviewing other textbooks and re-examining the strengths and weaknesses of this text, we proposed the following points:

1. The textbook should be practical, well-written, and easily understood by researchers, clinicians, and graduate and undergraduate students. Complex concepts should be explained carefully and presented in a logical step-by-step sequence so that the textbook can serve as a "tutorial mentor."

2. There should be a historical perspective in the text that connects the reader to other researchers who laid the foundation for evidence-based practice. The evolution of the profession of occupational therapy is a continuation of the scientific and medical revolutions that created the health professions. As health care clinicians, we are dependent on the early research in anatomy and physiology, testing and measurement, medical instrumentation, clinical medi-

cine, and environmental health. The knowledge gained in the basic sciences impact strongly on the clinical professions. As scholars, we know that current practice stands on the shoulders of the past and current researchers in basic and clinical science.

3. Within the context of the text, there should be many examples from the current scientific literature, as well as hypothetical examples explaining theoretical concepts and research principles. The text should come from a pragmatic perspective that presents feasible ideas for best practice.

4. The text should be a resource for further study in related areas. References and addresses should be liberally found throughout the text so that the researcher can readily locate resources in designing and implementing a research study.

5. Statistical procedures and tests should be clearly explained in a stepwise procedure. The concept underlying the statistical technique should be emphasized. Although there are a number of software programs and statistical packages available, it is important for the student to understand how the statistical results are derived. The student should have a strong background in descriptive statistics before learning inferential statistics.

6. In the textbook, there should be an example of a research proposal that can serve as a model for the researcher. The research proposal should be clearly described and realistically implemented.

7. The textbook should be comprehensive and include a number of different research models that are appropriate for research in occupational therapy

8. Qualitative, as well as quantitative, research models should be described with examples from the literature. Both models are appropriate and relevant. The research design is judged on its own merits as far as validity and application to clinical practice.

9. An important emphasis in research is in raising relevant, significant, and feasible research questions. The researcher should be encouraged to ask questions that generate intellectual interest and curiosity. The processes of doing research and searching the research literature are as important as reporting results. Research should be a process of discovery and intellectual excitement.

10. The individual who is designing and carrying out a research study should see the relationship between one's research study and one's professional role, whether it be a clinician, administrator, educator, or researcher. In other words, research does not exist in a vacuum. Basic research and applied research are equally important in leading to effective interventions. However, collecting data alone without purpose is not appropriate.

11. The research text should help the student to develop a critical view of research. The student should be able to read the literature with a critical eye and carry over this knowledge to clinical practice, especially in applying clinical reasoning. The researcher should also be able to critique the research methodology and to evaluate the validity and limitations of the results.

12. The researcher should have a strong appreciation of the ethical issues involved with human investigation. Researchers should be able to design an informed consent form and be able to safeguard the research subject from unnecessary psychological or physical risks.

One of the major purposes of this textbook is to link research to clinical practice. It is important within this context that the researcher raises many questions relating to clinical practice in developing a research proposal. As the student or clinical researcher works on the preparation of a research design, he or she should keep in mind the practical implications of the research study. The content of the chapters in this textbook are organized comprehensively to include all the components in research, from generating a significant research question, carrying out a literature review, designing a research study, selecting a measuring instrument, outlining a statistical analysis of data, and writing a scientific paper. The textbook is organized to enable a student to write a research proposal, critically evaluate a published study, and prepare a manuscript for a refereed journal. In writing this Fifth Edition, the authors developed a conceptual model that serves as a rationale for the text.

1. Although the medical model is an essential component of the healthcare systems throughout the world in the twenty-first century, it is important to note that in practice other interventions exist that are effective and deserve research consideration. For example, alternative medicine has become a significant area of practice outside the medical model. Historically, the medical model includes arriving at a diagnosis that serves as the basis of treatment. Understanding of the medical model and its historical perspective is important for occupational therapists because they work closely with physicians in a team approach in hospitals and clinics. The consideration of educational, psychological, and sociological factors in treatment does not negate the medical model. Effective rehabilitation and habilitation depends on a holistic approach to the patient that includes the medical model alongside a biopsychosocial approach.

2. Conceptually, we emphasize the strengths of individuals with disabilities as the basis of good treatment. In planning interventions, the occupational therapist evaluates both the strengths and weaknesses in the client and then develops with the client a goal-directed plan for achieving functional independence.

3. Good treatment means fitting the treatment procedure to the patient or client and not fitting the patient to a treatment method. The clinician should avoid a "Procrustean bed" where treatment methods are advocated and generalized to all patients. Good treatment is based on the individual needs of the patient and the consideration of multiple approaches.

4. The goal of clinical research is to discover, through objective and systematic inquiry, the most effective interventions that can be applied to the client with a disability. Research should be driven by theory and rational explanation.

5. The relationship between clinical research and clinical practice is based on the premise that good treatment depends on multiple factors, including the occupational therapist's skill, the effectiveness of a treatment methodology, the appropriateness of the client, and environmental factors that affect treatment. Clinical research strives to understand the relationship between these factors in clinical treatment.

6. Doing research and critically evaluating the findings help the student to become an effective clinician. Because clinical practice is dependent on clinical reasoning and decision making, the effective clinician applies the scientific method in practice. The research-oriented practitioner is able to evaluate the literature and to incorporate current research findings into clinical practice.

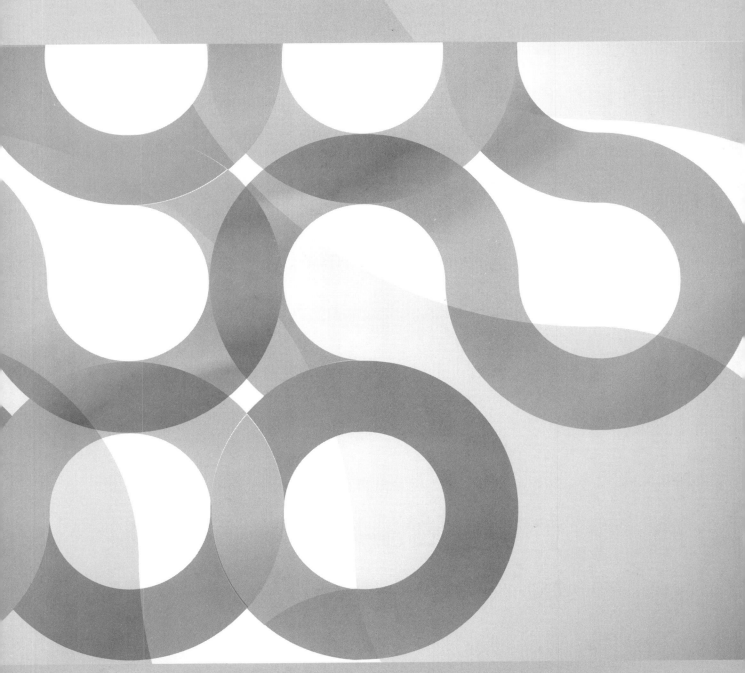

# Clinical Research in
# OCCUPATIONAL THERAPY

## CHAPTER 1

# A Short History of the Scientific Method in Medicine, Rehabilitation, and Habilitation

*Medical research on the scale to which it is developed today is a modern invention. A hundred years ago it was limited to the part-time activities of a few dozen individuals working in their private rooms (one could hardly call them laboratories) at home or in a university. Today it provides a life-time's career for thousands of medical scientists working in specially built laboratories in universities and research institutes financed by government or the pharmaceutical industry.*

—N. Poynter, 1971, *Medicine and Man*, p. 6

## Operational Learning Objectives

By the end of this chapter, the learner will:

- Define *research* and explore the primary purposes and its application to occupational therapy.
- Describe seven stages in the history of medicine.
- Explain the cyclical nature of medical progress into the twenty-first century.
- Recognize the important contributions of medical researchers toward eliminating disease and improving the health of individuals.
- Understand the importance of methodological discoveries in diagnosis, assessment, prevention, and intervention.
- Describe the growth of the allied health professions and its relationship to the rehabilitation movement.
- Detail occupational therapy's role in special education.
- Identify trends in rehabilitation research.

## 1.1 Definition and Purposes of Research in Occupational Therapy

What is research? **Research** is a systematic and objective investigation using the scientific method of identifying a problem, stating a hypothesis or guiding question, and collecting primary data. The emerging methods of research have generated qualitative and quantitative designs. Action research, the application of research to a site-specific environment, is an outgrowth of both qualitative and quantitative research.

Research in occupational therapy has many purposes, some of which are listed in the following examples:

- **Measure effectiveness of treatment methods, interventions, and teaching techniques.** For example, one might want to determine the effectiveness of sensory integration therapy on the academic achievement of students with a learning disability or the effectiveness of relaxation therapy on alleviating symptoms of depression.
- **Promote accountability in communicating the effectiveness of treatment methods, interventions, and teaching procedures to government agencies and funding sources.** For example, the researcher decides to publish the results of several research studies that demonstrate the effectiveness of occupational therapy for consumers with disabilities or for students in a special education program.
- **Explore and compare different strategies for treatment and intervention.** For example, therapists might compare the effectiveness of constraint movement interventions for individuals with strokes or for social skills training for persons with schizophrenia.
- **Help clinicians to plan action research in site-specific environment.** For example, occupational therapists may wish to collect data on how to decrease the number of Medicare rejections in a specific hospital. Another study using action research might examine the effectiveness of small group intervention versus individual therapy for treating children with learning disabilities in a specific school system.

- **Enable clinicians to be better consumers of research.** For example, a clinician doing a research study in splinting can evaluate other studies in the same area. The availability and access to information in the twenty-first century has led researchers to use online research sites. Researchers rely on PubMed.com (http://www.ncbi.nlm.nih.gov/pubmed/) for the latest research that is published online. Throughout this text, Internet sources are identified.
- **Develop interventions, treatment protocols, educational strategies, assessment procedures and tools, or software products that will later be evaluated for effectiveness.** For example, an occupational therapist may be interested in developing a treatment protocol to reduce anxiety in individuals with depression or to apply research techniques to evaluate programs and facilities in meeting standards of practice. For example, The Rehabilitation Accreditation Commission (CARF) applies research methods to evaluate a rehabilitation facility.
- **Reconstruct historical events to understand the basis for a current treatment.** For example, an occupational therapist may want to examine the historical basis for treating individuals with spinal cord injuries in the United States in the twentieth century.
- **Examine reasons for improvement or failure of a specific intervention through a retrospective case study.** For example, a client with a diagnosis of multiple sclerosis showed remission of symptoms after a three-month intervention. The researcher seeks to examine the variables that led to improvement.
- **Explore relationships between associated variables.** A clinician might want to examine the relationship between perceptual motor skills and self-care abilities or perceptual motor skills and writing achievement in children with Asperger Syndrome.
- **Examine the characteristics of a homogeneous population.** For example, one might want to explore the leisure interests of individuals with disabilities.

Research in rehabilitation and habilitation is a direct result of the methodology of scientific medicine. The rehabilitation professions emerged from the scientific findings in medicine that began in the nineteenth and twentieth centuries. In the rehabilitation professions, such as occupational therapy, physical therapy, speech pathology, and audiology, the results of these findings have led to direct application. In this chapter, we review the eight stages in scientific medicine that are the forerunners of scientific inquiry in the rehabilitation professions.

---

### BOX 1-1

### Selected International Landmarks in the History of Occupational Therapy as a Profession

| | |
|---|---|
| 1752 | Pennsylvania Hospital in Philadelphia was established. Psychiatric patients were prescribed manual labor to counteract disease process. |
| 1780 | Clement-Joseph Tissot, a French physician in the cavalry, published a book prescribing the use of crafts and recreational activities for individuals with muscle and joint injuries. |
| 1786 | Philippe Pinel, a French psychiatrist in the Bicetre Asylum for the insane, prescribed humane treatment in the care of those with mental illness, including physical exercises, manual occupation, and music. |
| 1803 | Johanann Christian Reil, a German psychiatrist, advocated that activities such as swimming, dancing, gymnastics, arts and crafts, music, and theater be part of the everyday routine for patients. |
| 1812 | Benjamin Rush, the father of American psychiatry, prescribed work, leisure activities, chess and other board games, exercise, and theatre for treatment of mental illness. |
| 1813 | Samuel Tuke, an English Quaker, founded the Retreat Asylum for the Insane in York, England. Tuke introduced the term *moral treatment*, which was the application of humane practices—including exercise, recreation, arts and crafts, gardening, and regular employment—in the maintenance of the hospital. |
| 1833 | Samuel Woodard, a physician at the Worcester State Lunatic Hospital in Massachusetts, introduced the term *occupational therapy* as a therapeutic method to keep inmates active in varied tasks and leisure activities in regular routines. The therapeutic program was observed to be clinically effective and produced a significant recovery rate. |
| 1838 | Jean Étienne Esquirol, a French psychiatrist, described the importance of corporal exercise, horseback riding, tennis, fencing, swimming, and travel for the treatment of depression. |

*continues*

BOX 1-1

## Selected International Landmarks in the History of Occupational Therapy as a Profession *continued*

| | |
|---|---|
| 1840 | Francois Leuret, a French psychiatrist, advanced that moral treatment, including arts and crafts and work, is effective in treating individuals with mental illness and intellectual disabilities. |
| 1843 | Dorothea Dix, a social reformer, worked diligently in the United States for humanistic care for individuals with mental illness, which included the use of therapeutic activities. |
| 1854 | Thomas Kirkbride, one of the founders of the American Psychiatric Association, advocated a highly structured regimen for patients that included exercise, lectures, music, arts and crafts, and entertainment. |
| 1895 | William Rush Dunton, a psychiatrist and innovator in applying occupational therapy, used arts and crafts activities at Sheppard and Pratt Asylum in Baltimore. |
| 1895/1922 | Adolph Meyer, a strong advocate of occupation, believed in a holistic approach to treatment centering on sleep habits, nutrition, work, play, and socialization. |
| 1895 | Mary Potter Meyer, a social worker and wife of Adolph Meyer, used arts and crafts activities in the State Hospital in Worcester, Massachusetts. |
| 1904 | Herbert Hall, a physician, prescribed occupation as a medicine to regulate the life and direct interests of the patient. He called this the "work cure." |
| 1905 | Susan Tracy, a nurse, applied occupational therapy activities in working with individuals with mental illness while she was director of the Training School for Nurses at the Adams Nervine Asylum in Boston. |
| 1906 | Herbert Hall was awarded a grant of $1,000 by Harvard University to study the application of activities and graded manual occupation in the treatment of psychiatric disorders. |
| 1908 | Training courses in occupations for hospital attendants were initiated at Chicago School of Civics and Philanthropy. |
| 1909 | Clifford Beers, founder of the National Committee for Mental Hygiene, described his emotional illness in the book, *A Mind that Found Itself* (1908). Beers reinforced the application of therapeutic activities in treating individuals with mental illness. |
| 1910 | Susan Tracy authored the first book on occupation studies, *Invalid Occupations: A Manual for Nurses and Attendants*. |

| | |
|---|---|
| 1911 | Susan Tracy initiated the first course on occupation at Massachusetts General Hospital in Boston. |
| 1911 | Eleanor Clark Slagle, a social worker, established an occupation department at Phipps Psychiatric Clinic at Johns Hopkins University in Baltimore. |
| 1914 | George Edward Barton, an architect who had contracted tuberculosis, introduced the term *occupational therapy* at a meeting in Boston of hospital workers. |
| 1917 | The National Society for the Promotion of Occupational Therapy was founded in Consolation House in Clifton Springs, New York. The charter members included George Barton, an architect; Eleanor Clark Slagle, a social worker at Hull House, Chicago; Thomas Kidner, vocational specialist from Canada; William Rush Dunton, a psychiatrist at Sheppard and Pratt Hospital in Baltimore; Susan Cox Johnson, an arts and crafts instructor from New York City; Isabel Newton; and Susan B. Tracy, a nurse at the Adams Nervine Asylum in Boston. This meeting led to the occupational therapy profession in the United States. |
| 1917 | Reconstruction aides were recruited to serve in U.S. army hospitals during World War I, applying arts and crafts and exercises in the treatment of physical and mental disorders. |
| 1918 | Formal educational training programs in occupational therapy were established at the Henry B. Favil School in Chicago, Teachers College of Columbia University, and the Boston School of Occupational Therapy. |
| 1919 | Bird T. Baldwin authored the U.S. *Army Manual on Occupational Therapy* that included information on evaluation and treatment procedures for the restoration of physical function. |
| 1919 | George Barton wrote the book *Teaching the Sick, A Manual of Occupational Therapy as Reeducation*. |
| 1922 | The *Archives of Occupational Therapy* was published and became the official journal of the American Association of Occupational Therapy. |
| 1925 | *Occupational Therapy and Rehabilitation* was first published. |
| 1928 | Six programs became available to prepare occupational therapists: Boston School; Philadelphia School; St. Louis School; Milwaukee-Downer College; University of Minnesota; and the University of Toronto. |
| 1931 | National registry for the American Occupational Therapy Association was established. |
| 1933 | The American Medical Association (AMA) began the accreditation of occupational therapy educational programs. |
| 1934 | Essentials of an acceptable education curriculum in occupational therapy were adopted by the American Medical Education Council on Medical Education and Hospitals. |

*continues*

BOX 1-1

**Selected International Landmarks in the History of Occupational Therapy as a Profession** *continued*

| | |
|---|---|
| 1939 | Among all AMA-approved hospitals, 13 percent employed occupational therapists. |
| 1943 | The Barden-LaFollette Vocational Rehabilitation Act was passed by Congress, providing coverage of medical services, including occupational therapy for individuals in vocational rehabilitation programs. |
| 1945 | Eighteen programs in occupational therapy were approved in the United States compared with five in 1940. |
| 1947 | First national registration examination for U.S. occupational therapists was given. |
| 1947 | Advanced master's degree in occupational therapy was offered at the University of Southern California and New York University. |
| 1947 | Helen Willard and Clare S. Spackman, occupational therapy educators, authored the first textbook in occupational therapy. |
| 1952 | The World Federation of Occupational Therapists was established. The 10 founding member countries included Australia, Canada, Denmark, Great Britain, India, Israel, New Zealand, South Africa, Sweden, and the United States. |
| 1958 | Essentials and Guidelines were adopted for an approved Educational Program for Occupational Therapy Assistants in the United States. |
| 1964 | Certified occupational therapists assistants (COTAs) were certified in the United States. |
| 1964 | The first entry-level master's program in occupational therapy was established at the University of Southern California. Shortly thereafter, basic master's programs were begun at Boston University and Virginia Commonwealth University. |
| 1965 | The American Occupational Therapy Foundation (AOTF) was established as a philanthropic organization for advancing the science of occupational therapy. |
| 1973 | The Rehabilitation Act was passed by Congress, protecting the rights of persons with disabilities. Section 504 of the Rehabilitation Act of 1973 prohibits discrimination based on disability in programs or activities receiving federal financial assistance. (See http://www.access.gpo.gov/nara/cfr/waisidx_99/34cfr104_99.html and http://www2.ed.gov/policy/speced/reg/narrative.html.) |
| 1974 | New York University developed the first doctoral program in occupational therapy. |
| 1975 | *Education for All Handicapped Children Act* (EHA; PL 94–142) facilitated free appropriate public education services for students with disabilities at all levels and |

provided funding for these services. The concept of least restrictive environment (LRE), inherent in the law, specifies that students with disabilities are educated with typical students "to the maximum extent possible."

1976    Support was given to students in occupational therapy for development of their organization on a national level, which was later named the American Student Occupational Therapy Alliance.

1979    "Uniform Terminology System for Reporting Occupational Therapy Services" was developed and adopted by the Representative Assembly (RA).

1980    AOTF published the *Occupational Therapy Journal of Research.*

1981    Entry-level Role Delineation for OTRs and COTAs was adopted by RA.

1981    *Occupational Therapy Journal of Research* was published.

1986    Medicare amendments expanded coverage for occupational therapy services under Part B in the United States.

1990    *The Americans with Disabilities Act* (ADA; PL 101–336; [42 USC 12101]) was passed by Congress and signed by President Bush. The ADA guarantees equal opportunity for individuals with disabilities in employment, public accommodations, transportation, governmental services, and telecommunications (FCTD, 2010). (See also http://www.usdoj.gov/crt/ada/cguide.htm#anchor62335 and http://www.ada.gov.)

1990    PL 94–142 reauthorized and renamed the *Individuals with Disabilities Education Act* (IDEA). This law continued federal funding from 94–142 and increased services by adding related services, transition from school to work, and parental involvement. Under this act, occupational therapy is considered a related service in helping students with disabilities in public schools.

1991    The AOTA Representative Assembly (RA) approved a physical agent modalities (PAMS) position paper that recommended the use of PAMS as an adjunct to purposeful activity to enhance occupational performance.

1994    *Occupational Therapy International* was founded as the first refereed journal publishing manuscripts by occupational therapists throughout the world.

1997    *The Balanced Budget Act* PL 105–33 (BBA) significantly changed the procedures for payment of services for rehabilitation personnel affecting the quality of care, especially in home health.

1999    The AOTA Representative Assembly passed a resolution to mandate that entry-level education in occupational therapy should be at the master's level.

1998    The *Assistive Technology Act* (PL105–394 [29 USC 2201]) was passed. This legislation provides funds to the states to support the establishment of assistive technology (AT) demonstration centers, information centers, facilities, referral services, and advocacy services to help people with disabilities to access AT services.

*continues*

BOX 1-1

### Selected International Landmarks in the
### History of Occupational Therapy as a Profession *continued*

| | |
|---|---|
| | The act also provides low-interest loans to purchase AT (FCTD, 2010). (See also http://www.ataporg.org/atap/index.php and http://www.assistivetech.net/webresources/stateTechActProjects.php for information regarding state projects.) |
| 1998 | Carl D. Perkins Vocational and Technical Education Act Amendments of 1998 (PL105–332 Section 1 (b) [20 USC 2302]) was passed. This act required schools to integrate academic, vocational, and technical training; increase technology use; provide professional development opportunities; develop, implement, and expand quality programs; and link secondary and post-secondary vocational education (FCTD, 2010). (See also http://www.ed.gov/offices/OVAE/CTE/legis.html) |
| 2001 | *The International Classification of Functioning, Disability and Health*, known more commonly as ICF, is a classification of health and health-related domains. These domains are classified from body, individual, and societal perspectives by means of two lists: a list of body functions and structure and a list of domains of activity and participation. Because an individual's functioning and disability occurs in a context, the ICF also includes a list of environmental factors. The ICF is WHO's framework for measuring health and disability at both individual and population levels. |
| 2002 | *No Child Left Behind* (NCLB; PL 107–110; http://www2.ed.gov/policy/elsec/leg/esea02/index.html) was enacted. As part of the need to improve education, the law focused on requiring each state to develop and implement a statewide accountability system that insured adequate yearly gain for all schools in reading and math. It is based on the concept that setting standards and measurable educational goals can improve academic performance in the classroom. |
| 2002 | The *Occupational Therapy Practice Framework: Domain and Process (Framework)* was developed in response to current practice needs, intended to "more clearly affirm and articulate occupational therapy's unique focus on occupation and daily life activities and the application of an intervention process that facilitates engagement in occupation to support participation in life" (AOTA, 2002, p. 609). |
| 2004 | The *Individuals with Disabilities Education Improvement Act of 2004* (IDEIA; PL108–556; http://idea.ed.gov/) is the reauthorization of PL 94-142 enacted in 1975. The law ensures that services are provided to eligible infants, toddlers, children, and youth with disabilities throughout the nation. With this reauthorization, |

IDEA-2000 was aligned with NCLB. In addition to funding, IDEIA governs how states and public agencies provide early intervention, special education, and related services.

2005     The fourth edition of the *Canadian Occupational Performance Measure* (COPM; Law et al., 2005) was published. It is an individualized, client-centred measure designed for use by occupational therapists to detect change in a client's self-perception of occupational performance over time. It is designed to be used as an outcome measure. The COPM is designed for use with clients with a variety of disabilities and across all developmental stages. The COPM has been used in more than 35 countries and has been translated into more than 20 languages.

2008     *Occupational Therapy Practice Framework (2nd) edition* was published (AOTA, 2008; Roley, et al., 2008).

2009     New emerging areas of occupational therapy practice in the United States were identified by AOTA: psychosocial needs of children and youth, health and wellness, driver rehabilitation, low vision services, ergonomics, community health, welfare to work and technology and assistive device development and consulting.

2009     *Americans with Disabilities Act Amendment* (PL 110–325; http://www.judiciary.state.nj.us/legis/110-325_Law.pdf), was signed on September 25, 2008, by President Bush and went into effect on January 1, 2009. The definition of disability was broadened to include individuals who have or are perceived as having an impairment, without regard to whether it substantially limits a major life activity. The Amendment also expanded the term "major life activities" as "caring for oneself, performing manual tasks, seeing, hearing, eating, sleeping, walking, standing, lifting, bending, speaking, breathing, learning, reading, concentrating, thinking, communicating, and working" (Sec. 12102(2)(A)). Another important change required that impairments that are episodic or in remission qualify as a disability if they would qualify in their active stage.

2010     On March 23, President Obama signed the *Affordable Health Care for America Act* (PL 111–148; http://democrats.senate.gov/reform/patient-protection-affordable-care-act-as-passed.pdf). The general principle is to ensure that all Americans have access to quality, affordable health care. It is projected that the Bill will provide health care coverage to 95 percent of Americans. (See http://www.aota.org/Practitioners/Advocacy/Federal/Highlights/Reform.aspx, for the impact of the Act on occupational therapy.)

2010     World Federation of Occupational Therapy (WFOT) convened in Santiago, Chile, for its 15th Congress. There are 70 member countries of WFOT.

## 1.2 Historical Review of Research in Medicine, Rehabilitation, and Habilitation

Before the beginnings of modern science in the latter half of the nineteenth century, relationships between causes and effects still retained explanations that bordered on the supernatural. Vitalism, a recurrent movement in medicine, was typified by the eighteenth-century physician who ascribed mysterious substances in the blood to life functions. This theory was an outcome of the prescientific thinking that gave way to the systematic and orderly explanations that we now associate with modern scientific research. The breakthrough in understanding the disease process began with the laboratory experimentation of Louis Pasteur (1822–1895), who served as a model for the medical scientist. The impact of scientific technology in the treatment and rehabilitation of the sick and of those with disabilities has been a remarkable record in human progress. In only a few other areas of knowledge has humanity made greater strides.

The analysis of the progress in medical science, and in rehabilitation, is divided into seven stages identified in Figure 1–1. These seven stages are progressive, interactive, and dynamic. For example, basic research in biological and chemical processes in Stage I continues to be important as evidenced by the investigations of DNA and RNA as the building blocks in protoplasm. Similarly, methodological research is in the forefront by virtue of the integration of high technology with clinical practice as demonstrated in the areas of robotics, prosthetics, transplant operations, kidney dialysis techniques, and artificial replacement of bodily organs. Medical scientists are constantly refining treatment and preventive methodologies. Immunologists who formerly sought chemicals to destroy harmful bacteria and viruses have led the way for present-day investigators searching for vaccines to prevent cancerous growths and life-threatening diseases, such as Acquired Immune Deficiency Syndrome (AIDS).

Progress in science is cyclical and cumulative. As knowledge grows, medical scientists refine their methods of research. Stages of development in medicine point to the cumulative process of obtaining knowledge and to the evolutionary process of scientific methodology and its impact on clinical practice.

## 1.3 Biological Description—Stage I

### 1.3.1 The Growth of Scientific Anatomy and Physiology

The earliest medical research started with the discovery of the physiological processes and anatomical systems of the body. Biological description: Stage I, the evolution of medical research, is outlined in Table 1–1. Knowledge of the anatomical structure of animals during the Middle Ages and the Renaissance was greatly influenced by Galen (AD 138–201), who experimented on lower mammals; by Leonardo Da Vinci (1452–1519), who made precise drawings of human anatomy; and later by Vesalius (1514–1564), who, through careful dissection, described human anatomy. Identifying and describing the anatomical structures of the body led to increased knowledge about relationships between systems and the interrelationships of cardiovascular, respiratory, and genitourinary functions. Harvey's (1578–1657) concept of the circulation of blood, for example, led the way to an understanding of the internal environment of the body. Galen, Da Vinci, and Harvey were among the first scholars to accurately describe the human body; however, the ancient Greeks initially brought rational thought to an evaluation of health and disease. The Hippocratic writings reflect the depth of Greek thought.

### 1.3.2 The Hippocratic Writings

The first stage in the history of medicine was essentially clinical observation. The healer applying Hippocratic methods used himself as a measuring instrument, carefully noting what he saw, felt, smelled, and heard. He used rational thought regarding the causes and treatments of diseases based on these observations. In the ancient Greek civilization, scholars were allowed the freedom to speculate on all aspects of human life. Thus, the model for the Western physician emerged.

Hippocrates, who is traditionally called the Father of Medicine, was probably representative of a number of individuals. It is more accurate to speak of the "Hippocratic writings" than to attribute all of ancient Greek medicine to one individual. The Hippocratic writings cover many areas of medicine, including ethics, disease etiology, anatomy, physiology, and treatment. These writings are not a consistent work linking theory to practice, but a compendium of clinical histories and a description of Hellenistic medicine.

We know little about Hippocrates' life, except that he lived during the fifth century BC in Cos, an island off the Greek mainland, and that he was a famous practitioner and teacher of medicine. The

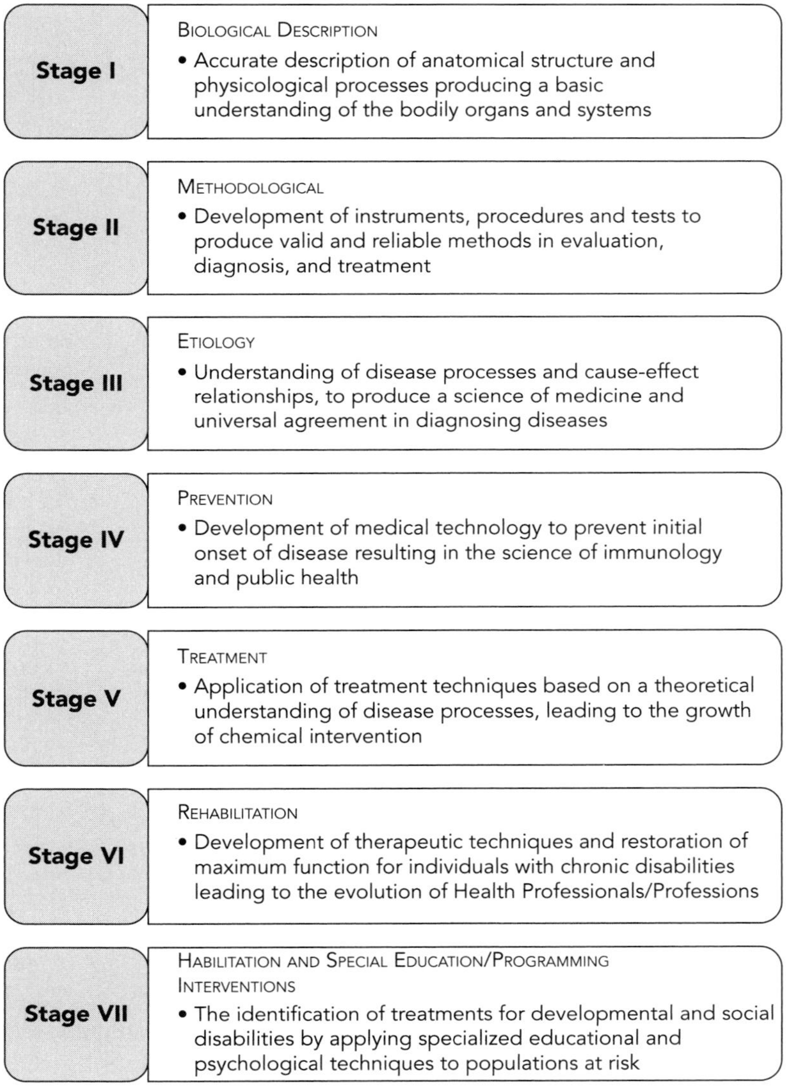

**Stage I**
BIOLOGICAL DESCRIPTION
• Accurate description of anatomical structure and physicological processes producing a basic understanding of the bodily organs and systems

**Stage II**
METHODOLOGICAL
• Development of instruments, procedures and tests to produce valid and reliable methods in evaluation, diagnosis, and treatment

**Stage III**
ETIOLOGY
• Understanding of disease processes and cause-effect relationships, to produce a science of medicine and universal agreement in diagnosing diseases

**Stage IV**
PREVENTION
• Development of medical technology to prevent initial onset of disease resulting in the science of immunology and public health

**Stage V**
TREATMENT
• Application of treatment techniques based on a theoretical understanding of disease processes, leading to the growth of chemical intervention

**Stage VI**
REHABILITATION
• Development of therapeutic techniques and restoration of maximum function for individuals with chronic disabilities leading to the evolution of Health Professionals/Professions

**Stage VII**
HABILITATION AND SPECIAL EDUCATION/PROGRAMMING INTERVENTIONS
• The identification of treatments for developmental and social disabilities by applying specialized educational and psychological techniques to populations at risk

© Cengage Learning 2013

**FIGURE 1-1**  Seven Stages in the History of Medicine, Health, and Rehabilitation: The seven stages are progressive, interactive, and dynamic.

TABLE 1-1

**The Emergence of the Medical Scientist—Stage I**

| Medical Events | Discovery Dates | Scientists | Implications |
|---|---|---|---|
| Hippocratic writings | 400–500 BC | Hippocrates (500 BC) | Provided a model for medical practitioners based on ethical and humane treatment |
| Systematic study of bodily processes | AD 169–180 | Claudius Galen (AD 129–199) | Influenced medical practice for 1,300 years, presenting an eclectic synthesis of prior knowledge |
| "The Canon of Medicine" | translated 1187 | Avicenna (980–1037) | Significant figure of Arabic medicine whose work was dogma during the Middle Ages |
| "Paragranum": The four pillars of medicine: philosophy, astronomy, chemistry, and virtue | 1530 | Paracelsus (1493–1541) | Created the foundation for general medical practice based on a knowledge of pharmaceutical chemistry |
| Atlas of Anatomy "De humani corporis fabrica" | 1543 | Andreas Vesalius (1514–1564) | Made descriptive anatomy the basis of medicine and replaced aspects of Galen's work |
| Manual of Surgery | 1543 | Ambroise Pare (1510–1590) | Generated surgical innovations based on accurate anatomical knowledge |
| Discovery of the circulation of the blood "Exercitatio" | 1628 | William Harvey (1578–1657) | Integrated anatomy with physiological knowledge of blood circulation |
| Digestive system "Experiments and Observations of Gastric Juice and the Physiology of Digestion" | 1833 | William Beaumont (1785–1853) | Used objective observation in discovering the process of digestion |

following excerpt from the Hippocratic writings, *On the Articulations* (ca. 400 BC/1952) translated by Francis Adams, demonstrates the method of clinical observation used to diagnose a dislocation of the shoulder joint and the importance of individual differences in human anatomy:

A dislocation may be recognized by the following symptoms: Since the parts of a man's body are proportionate to one another, as the arms and the legs, the sound should always be compared with the unsound, the unsound with the sound, not paying regard to the joints of other individuals (for one person's joints are more prominent than another's), but looking to those of the patient, to ascertain whether the sound joint be unlike the unsound. This is a proper rule, and yet it may lead to much error; and on this account it is not sufficient to know this art in theory, but also by actual practice; for many persons from pain, or from any other cause, when their joints are not dislocated, cannot put the parts into the same positions as the sound body can be put into; one ought therefore to know and be acquainted beforehand with such an attitude. But in a dislocated joint the head of the humerus appears lying much more in the armpit than it is in the sound joint; and also, above, at the top of the shoulder, the part appears hollow, and the acromion is prominent, owing to the bone of the joint having sunk into the part below; there is a source of error in this case also, as will be described and also, the elbow of the dislocated arm is farther removed from the ribs than that of the other; but by using force it may be approximated, though with considerable pain; and also they cannot with the elbow extended raise the arm to the ear, as they can the sound arm, nor move it about as formerly in this direction and that. These, then, are the symptoms of dislocation at the shoulder. (as cited in Hutchins, 1952, pp. 94–95)

The Hippocratic writings with their emphasis on dietetics, exercise, and natural methods were the complete holistic guide for the ancient physician.

### 1.3.3 Galen

Greek medicine provided the foundation for medical practice in the Western world. Galen, a product of the Roman civilization, was the next link in the chain of medicine. He was born in Pergamum, Greece, in the second century AD when Roman civilization controlled much of the Western world. Galen was educated in philosophy, mathematics, and natural science. He learned medicine by traveling to places where the great physicians practiced. After acquiring knowledge steeped in the Hippocratic tradition, he became a doctor to the gladiators who performed in the Roman arenas. Galen became an acclaimed practitioner in Rome and later spent his time writing extensively. He is a model for the medical scientist who engages in clinical practice, teaching, and scholarly publication. Galen's genius was in his ability to integrate prior knowledge with his clinical observations of disease. Unfortunately, his writings on medicine became authoritative dogma from the Middle Ages to the time of the rebirth of scientific inquiry in the Renaissance.

The following excerpt from Galen (ca. AD 192/1971) typifies his skill in teaching anatomy, as well as his careful methods of observation:

> Since therefore, the form of the body is assimilated to the bones, to which the nature of the other parts corresponds, I would have you first gain an exact and practical knowledge of human bones. It is not enough to study them casually or read of them in a book; no, not even in mine, which some call Osteologia, others Skeletons, and yet others simply On Bones, though I am persuaded that it excels all earlier works in accuracy, brevity, and lucidity.
>
> Make it rather your serious endeavor not only to acquire accurate book-knowledge of each bone, but also to examine assiduously with your own eyes the human bones themselves. This is quite easy at Alexandria because the physicians there employ ocular demonstration in teaching osteology to students. For this reason, if for no other, try to visit Alexandria. But if you cannot, it is still possible to see something of human bones. I, at least, have done so often on the breaking open of a grave or tomb. Thus once

a river, inundating a recent hastily made grave, broke it up, washing away the body. The flesh had putrefied, though the bones still held together in their proper relations. It was carried down a stadium (roughly 200 yards), and reaching marshy ground, drifted ashore. This skeleton was as though deliberately prepared for such elementary teaching.

If you have not the luck to see anything of this sort, dissect an ape and having removed the flesh, observe each bone with care. Choose those apes likest man with short jaws and small canines. You will find other parts also resembling man's, for they can walk and run on two feet. Those, on the other hand, like the dog-faced baboons with long snouts and large canines, far from walking or running on their hind-legs, can hardly stand upright. The more human sort have a nearly erect posture; but firstly the head of the femur fits into the socket at the hip-joint rather transversely, and secondly, of the muscles which extend downward to the knee, some go further (than in man). Both these features check and impede erectness of posture, as do the feet themselves, which have comparatively narrow heels and are deeply cleft between the toes.

I therefore maintain that the bones must be learnt either from man, or ape, or better from both, before dissecting the muscles, for those two (namely bones and muscles) form the ground-work of the other parts, the foundations, as it were, of a building. And next, study arteries, veins, and nerves. Familiarity with dissection of these will bring you to the inward parts and so to a knowledge of the viscera, the fat, and the glands, which also you should examine separately, in detail. Such should be the order of your training. (as cited in Wightman, 1971, pp. 32–33)

### 1.3.4 Renaissance Medicine in the Sixteenth and Seventeenth Centuries

The history of medicine parallels, in many ways, the rise of Western civilization. The Middle Ages in Europe was a sterile period for the growth of new ideas and experimentation. Medical practice existed then as dogma, closely linked to practices and beliefs of the Catholic Church. Although Medieval Europe adhered to rigid doctrine, medical practice flourished in the Middle East as represented by the Arab physician, Avicenna (980–1037). With the onset of the Renaissance, scientists carried out experiments on human dissection under great risk of public denouncement and physical punishment. In spite of this, a psychological climate was established in the sixteenth century that allowed medical scholars and scientists to seek the truth by experimentation. Physicians made great strides in integrating laboratory observations with clinical practice.

Renaissance physicians rekindled the torch of medical science that had been stagnant for approximately 1,000 years. The scientists of the Renaissance, scholars familiar with Greek and Roman writings, questioned all knowledge and accepted little dogma. Furthermore, they reexamined the anatomical knowledge of Galen, experimented in chemistry, and sought explanations for the life processes in humans. In short, their work marked the beginning of the science of physiology.

### 1.3.5 Andreas Vesalius and the Refinement of Human Anatomy

The most important medical anatomist of the Renaissance was Andreas Vesalius. He was the first medical specialist in human anatomy. By critically examining the work of Galen, Vesalius realized that Galen's observations of anatomy were not based on human dissection, but were descriptions of the bodily structures of monkeys, pigs, and goats. From 1537 to 1542, Vesalius worked on an anatomical atlas, *De humani corporis fabrica libri septea*, which was published in 1593. The book contained 663 folio pages. Vesalius's research on human anatomy became the basis of medical science and provided the necessary knowledge for the surgeon. The interplay between laboratory observations and clinical practice provided scholars with the data they needed for readjusting theory to practice and practice to theory. The model for obtaining anatomical knowledge in the medical sciences was forged in the sixteenth century.

## 1.3.6 Paracelsus, the Medical Chemist

The next great development in medicine was in the area of physiology. Chemistry and physics are the bases of physiology. The understanding of human physiology awaited great discoveries in these areas. The first physician to apply chemistry to an understanding of biological processes was Paracelsus. He advocated using pharmaceutical agents singly or in combination to treat specific illnesses. He used sulphur, lead, antimony, mercury, iron, and copper as therapeutics. Paracelsus emphasized the relationship between practical clinical experience and scientific experimentation as evidenced in the following quotation from his work *Paragranum* written about 1528 (as cited in Wightman, 1971):

> The doctor must therefore be practiced in Experienz; and medicine is nothing but a wide, certain, Experienz, namely that every procedure is based in Experienz. And that is experientia which is correctly and truly founded. Anyone who has learnt his stuff without Experienz is a doubtful doctor.
>
> Experientia is like a judge; and whether a procedure is undertaken or not depends on its approval; wherefore Experienz ought to keep pace with science, for without science Experienz is nothing. Similar an Experiment grounded in Experienz is well founded and its further use understood. …Experiment divorced from science is but a matter of chance. (pp. 50–51)

## 1.3.7 William Harvey

The culmination of knowledge in physiology during the Renaissance was achieved in the publication by William Harvey in 1628. The publication *Exercitatio* described accurately for the first time the circulation of the blood. Harvey, an English physician, was trained in Padua, Italy, where Vesalius had taught human anatomy. After mastering the physiological theories of his time, Harvey proposed questions, such as: What is the pulse? How does breathing affect the actions of the heart? How does the blood move? These questions directed Harvey's experimental procedures. First, he systematically stated a testable hypothesis on the circulation of the blood, and then he proceeded with rigorous experimental observation. He used precise measurements in recording pulse rate and the volume of blood ejected by the heart over time. He observed the movements of the heart and blood in living animals. He also analyzed the blood circulation of the fetus to support his theory. By using the scientific method, Harvey was able to discover the most vital process in human life. He did this by (a) presenting a researchable question, (b) mastering the published literature on blood flow, (c) using accurate observations, (d) being guided by predictive hypothesis, (e) using rigorous procedures for collecting data, (f) applying measurement to the process of blood flow, and (g) making a deductive analysis and conclusions.

Harvey's achievement in describing the circulation of the blood ranks with Newton's discovery of gravity as one of the greatest scientific accomplishments in the seventeenth century. Harvey's work at first was met with the jealousy and suspicion that many times accompanies an important discovery or change of thinking. In the first chapter from *Exercitatio* entitled "The Author's Motives for Writing" (1628/1952), Harvey explained his reasons for publishing his findings and his desire to bring objective criticism to his work.

> I have not hesitated to expose my views upon these subjects, not only in private to my friends, but also in public, in my anatomical lectures, after the manner of the Academy of old.

These views as usual, pleased some more, others less; some chide and calumniated me, and laid it to me as a crime that I had dared to depart from the precepts and opinions of all anatomists; others desired further explanations of the novelties, which they said were both worthy of consideration, and might perchance be found of single use. At length, yielding to the requests of my friends, that all might be made participators in my labors, and partly moved by the envy of others, who receiving my views with uncandid minds and understanding them indifferently, have essayed to traduce me publicly. I have moved to commit these things to the press, in order that all may be enabled to form an opinion both of me and my labours. (pp. 273–274)

By the end of the seventeenth century, the medical scientist had emerged. At this point in history, medical practice was not at all consistent; yet there was a body of knowledge being created that served as the basis for later discoveries and practices. Medical schools were founded in Europe during the seventeenth century, but it was not until the latter half of the nineteenth century that medical education was rigorously evaluated. These discoveries occurred in a comparatively short period of intense activity from the nineteenth century to the present. The early research describing the human organism served as a foundation of scientific knowledge that was later expanded and incorporated into clinical practice.

## 1.4 Methodological Process—Stage II

### 1.4.1 Development of Medical Technology in the Eighteenth and Nineteenth Centuries

The second stage in medical research was the development of precision instruments and test procedures that enabled the medical scientist to examine and measure the internal processes in the body. Typical among early scientific inventors in medicine was Laennec (1781–1826) who, by watching children playing with hollow cylinders, invented the stethoscope. Methodological research over the centuries has brought about technological advances such as the electroencephalogram, electrocardiogram, X-ray, procedures for urine analysis, positron emission tomography (PET), single photon emission computed tomography (SPECT), computed tomographic X-ray (CT or CAT scan), magnetic resonance imaging (MRI), and other important instruments and procedures that have become basic tools in clinical medicine. Moreover, technology is continually being refined and updated.

Methodological research is unique in its application of industrial technology to the problems of diagnosis and treatment. Initially, the great advances in methodology coincided with the rise of the Industrial Revolution in the eighteenth century. Medical scientists who were able to apply industrial technology to medical practice found a wealth of ideas. These advances are examples of interdisciplinary research where investigators from diverse disciplines have applied their special knowledge to a specific research problem.

Norbert Wiener (1948), who proposed the theory of cybernetics, used interdisciplinary seminars as a means of generating new ideas and stimulating creative thinking. Presently, engineers are working in conjunction with medical scientists to create artificial materials and devices that can replace organs in the body. Biomedical engineering is a direct application of methodological research to medicine. Prosthetics, self-help devices, and orthotics are examples of methodological research applied to the field of rehabilitation. Table 1–2 summarizes the major methodological inventions that have impacted medical care.

### 1.4.2 The Practice of Medicine in the First Half of the Nineteenth Century

The latter half of the nineteenth century was a golden period in the history of medicine. During this time, medical schools were given the legal authority to

**TABLE 1-2**

**Methodological Advances—Stage I**

| Medical Events | Dates | Scientists | Implications |
|---|---|---|---|
| Clinical thermometer | 1614 | Santotio Santorio (1561–1636) | Physical examination in clinical medicine |
| Microscopical anatomy | 1661 | Marcello Malpighi (1628–1694) | Diagnostic studies of the blood |
| Clinical microscope | 1695 | Antony Van Leeuwenhoek (1632–1694) | Refinement of microscope |
| Technique of thoracic percussion | 1761 | Leopold Auenbrugger (1722–1809) | Diagnosis of respiratory disorders |
| Stethoscope | 1819 | Rene Laennec (1781–1826) | Diagnosis of circulatory disorders |
| Hypodermic syringe | 1853 | Alexander Wood (1817–1884) | Blood transfusions |
| Method for testing the quantity of sugar in urine | 1848 | Herman von Fehling (1811–1885) | Diagnosis of diabetes mellitus |
| X-ray | 1895 | Wilhelm Roentgen (1845–1923) | Detection of tuberculosis, fractures, and dislocations |
| Ophthalmoscope | 1851 | Hermann von Helmholtz (1821–1894) | Detection of morbid changes in the eye |
| Cystoscope | 1890 | Max Nitze (1847–1907) | Disease of urinary system |
| Electrocardiograph (EKG) | 1903 | Willem Einthoven (1860–1927) | Coronary functioning |
| Electroencephalograph (EEG) | 1929 | Hans Berger (1873–1941) | Cerebral dysfunction |
| Magnetic resonance phenomena used in magnetic resonance imagery | 1952 | Edward M. Purcell (1905–1983) Felix Bloch (1912–1997) | Diagnostic assistance |
| Computed axial tomography (CAT) | 1972 | Allan Cormack (1924–1998) Sir Godfrey Hounsfield (1919–2004) | Diagnostic assistance |
| Pulsed neuromagnetic resonance (NMR) and magnetic resonance imagery (MRI) | 1975 | Richard Ernst (1933– ) | Diagnostic assistance |
| Positron emission tomography (PET) | 1970s | William H. Sweet (1930–2001) Gordon Brownell (1922–2008) | Diagnostic assistance |
| Single photon emission computed tomography (SPECT) | 1970s | R. Q. Edwards D. E. Kuhl | Diagnostic assistance |

**TABLE 1-3**

**Progress in Surgery, Clinical Medicine, and Public Health up until Pasteur's Formulation of the Germ Theory in 1878**

| Surgery | Diagnosis and Treatment | Public Health |
|---|---|---|
| Use of ether and chloroform as anesthetics | Use of microscope, auscultation, and stethoscope in diagnosis | Construction of municipal sewers |
| Setting of broken bones and reduction of dislocated joints | Dynamic understanding of anatomy and physiology | Recording of vital statistics |
| Removal of superficial diseased tissue and kidney stones | Isolation of patients with contagious diseases | Custodial care of people who are insane, intellectually disabled, poor, or homeless |
| Widespread practice of obstetrics and gynecology | Relief of local pain pharmacologically | Prevention of smallpox through vaccination |

certify physicians. Examinations were required for anyone who practiced medicine in the United States and Europe. In England, for example, a Medical Register was established in 1858. Atwater (1973), in an article documenting the medical profession in Rochester, New York, from 1811–1860, described the current state of medical knowledge available to general practitioners. Table 1–3 contains an abstracted description of the advances in medicine made during the prior three centuries, according to Atwater.

Although medicine had achieved great gains up until this period, most contagious diseases except for smallpox were unbeatable. Surgeons worked at a great disadvantage without antiseptic techniques, and hospitals did not provide the care we associate with excellent nursing. Medical advances would have to wait for Pasteur, Lister, Morton, and Nightingale to provide the revolutionary innovations.

## 1.5 Etiological Advances—Stage III

### 1.5.1 Medical Research in the Latter Half of the Nineteenth Century

The third stage in medical research was the integration of physiology and pathology with the use of a reliable methodology to arrive at a diagnosis. The evolution of the *dynamic understanding of the disease process* is described in Table 1–4. During this stage, an understanding of the etiology of a disease through experimental laboratory research was used to verify cause-effect relationships. This breakthrough in treating disease on a scientific basis started with Pasteur's discovery of the germ theory.

From Pasteur's work, laboratory scientists were able to investigate disease processes by identifying a specific microorganism. The age of chemotherapy was initiated. For every microorganism causing a disease (that was isolated in the laboratory), researchers sought a chemical substance harmless to the body to counteract the germ. From 1850 to 1910, the process of identifying the germ responsible for a disease and the discovery of a chemical to eliminate the germ was the basis for the rapid conquest of many communicable diseases. The elimination of many communicable diseases would not have occurred without the microscope and the laboratory techniques of microbiology and biochemistry. The technology for protecting the individual from infectious diseases was a direct result of the understanding of human physiology and cellular theory. Septic techniques for surgery were later developed by Lister (1827–1912), who was greatly influenced by the work of Pasteur, and by Semmelweis (1818–1865), an obstetrician who recognized the importance of hospital surgeons using prophylactic techniques during childbirth to prevent infection.

TABLE 1-4

**Dynamic Understanding of Disease Processes—Stage III**

| Medical Event | Date | Scientist | Implications |
|---|---|---|---|
| Clinical physiology | 1857 | Claude Bernard (1813–1878) | Treatment of physiologic and metabolic disorders through pharmacology |
| Cell theory | 1858 | Rudolf Ludwig Virchow (1821–1902) | Cellular pathology as the basis of treatment |
| Germ theory | 1878 | Louis Pasteur (1822–1895) | The role of microorganisms in disease established |
| Bacteriology | 1882 | Robert Koch (1843–1910) | Treatment of bacterial infections could be controlled by the physician |
| Role of filterable viruses | 1888 | Pierre Roux (1853–1933) | Identification of viruses resulted in the search for preventative measures |
| Immunization process | 1892 | Elie Metchnikoff (1845–1916) | Understanding of the body's "phagocytosis" defense mechanisms against disease was recognized |
| Chemotherapy | 1899 | Paul Ehrlich (1854–1915) | Specific chemical compounds used to treat communicable diseases |

The knowledge of cellular activity by Virchow (1821–1902) was another line of evidence verifying the germ theory of disease. According to Virchow, the cause of disease was a result of changes at the cellular level. Virchow's cellular theory of disease compelled pathologists to use microscopes in searching for lesions and abnormalities within the cells. Metchnikoff (1845–1916) discovered phagocytosis, recognizing that white blood corpuscles in the body counteract disease. The understanding of the dynamics of disease led to the science of clinical medicine.

Physicians were then able to diagnose disease through laboratory microscope techniques, thus replacing vitalism and metaphysics as explanations for the onset of communicable disease. Probably the most important work on medical research in the nineteenth century was Claude Bernard's *Introduction to the Study of Experimental Medicine* published in 1895. Pasteur acknowledged Bernard as an important influence in his own work. Bernard's major contributions to understanding disease included physiology of digestion, neurophysiology, pharmacology, and organic chemistry. Bernard's work has had a profound influence in medical science. Concepts such as homeostasis and stress introduced by Cannon (1932) and Selye (1956) are based on Bernard's experimental findings on the internal gastrointestinal environment. Bernard, through his experimental methodology, established the future direction of medical research based on rigorous observation, repeated replication, and the acceptance or rejection of a hypothesis. "Scientific generalization must proceed from particular facts or principles" (Bernard, 1865/1957, p. 2). This simple statement is the foundation of twentieth-century medical research.

With a refined scientific methodology and a comprehensive theory of disease, medical researchers from about 1880 to 1910 made dramatic progress in identifying disease agents. This advance is exemplified by Koch's work in tuberculosis in 1890, von Behring's work in diphtheria in 1900, and Ehrlich's persistent search for a chemical to counteract syphilis, culminating in the discovery of the drug Salvarsan (arsphenamine) in 1910, after 606 experimental trials.

## 1.6 Prevention—Stage IV

### 1.6.1 Preventive Medicine in the Twentieth Century

The advances in medical research that have had the most dramatic effect in eliminating diseases can be attributed to primary prevention, including public health techniques and mass vaccinations. Public health measures, such as purification of water, elimination of human waste products, and protection against food spoilage, were used by ancient civilizations such as the Egyptians, Greeks, and Romans. When superstition prevailed over using prophylactic methods, however, as during the Middle Ages in Europe, epidemics and widespread disease occurred. Throughout the world, the potential for epidemics still exists in underdeveloped countries or in war and disaster zones where public health measures have been disregarded. The elimination of typhus, cholera, bubonic plague, polio, and smallpox in areas with access to modern medicine has been accomplished through the combination of medical advances and public health technology. Vaccination as a means of preventing disease has provided the means to control widespread epidemics that dramatically reduced populations in the past.

The first physician to conceive the use of vaccinations to prevent disease was Jenner (1749–1823), who experimented with cowpox infection, a mild disease, as a means of protecting against smallpox, one of the leading causes of death in the eighteenth century. Jenner noted that dairymaids who contracted cowpox by milking infected cows developed a natural immunity to smallpox. This observation led him to believe that if people were deliberately infected with cowpox, they would escape the dreaded smallpox. In 1798, Jenner published his findings, which included 23 case histories of individuals inoculated with cowpox.

Initially, the medical community in England did not accept Jenner's work. He gradually gained recognition after other physicians replicated his work. Jenner's original research on vaccinations remained singularly unique until Pasteur's discovery of the germ theory about 100 years later in 1878. Jenner's method of inoculation to prevent disease was rediscovered by medical researchers who were later able to isolate pathogenic bacteria and viruses. Table 1–5 lists many of the communicable diseases that are now controlled by vaccination.

Presently, the concept of preventive medicine includes the following health procedures:

- Inoculation to prevent communicable diseases
- Environmental health to reduce atmospheric and water pollution
- Prenatal care to prevent birth defects
- Mental health community services to prevent institutionalization
- Family planning and population control
- Supervision of food handling and processing of foods to prevent botulism
- Prevention of industrial accidents through ergonomics
- Sanitary engineering to prevent typhus and cholera

Until the twentieth century, physicians were able to do little for a patient who was severely ill. The introduction of chemotherapy, aseptic surgery, and efficient hospital care changed the course of medical practice.

## 1.7 Chemotherapy, Surgery, and Hospital Care: The Bases of Treatment—Stage V

### 1.7.1 Chemotherapy

As knowledge about anatomy and physiology progressed, technology was developed to improve the diagnoses of illnesses. The foundations, created to produce a body of knowledge underlying therapeutics, resulted in chemotherapy, surgery, and hospital care as the bases of modern-day treatment. Although ancient civilizations, and primitive cultures existing

| TABLE 1-5 | | | |
|---|---|---|---|

**Control of Communicable Diseases through Immunization**

| Disease | Causative Agent | Medical Researcher | Discovery Date |
|---|---|---|---|
| Bubonic plague | Bacterium | Shibasaburō Kitasato Alexandre Yersin | 1893–1894 |
| Cholera | Bacterium | Robert Koch | 1884 |
| Diphtheria | Bacterium | Emil Von Behring | 1890 |
| Measles | Virus | Francesio Cenci | 1901 |
| Poliomyelitis | Virus | Jonas Salk | 1954 |
| Rabies | Virus | Louis Pasteur | 1885 |
| Rocky Mountain spotted fever | Virus | Howard Ricketts | 1909 |
| Smallpox | Virus | Edward Jenner | 1796 |
| Tuberculosis | Bacterium | Albert Calmette Camille Guerin | 1921 |
| Typhoid fever | Bacterium | Almroth Wright | 1906 |
| Typhus | Virus | Charles Nicolle | 1910 |
| Yellow fever | Virus | Max Thieler | 1936 |

today, have used various effective treatments, the causes of diseases and the rationale for understanding the processes were veiled in mystery. For example, rauwolfia serpentine was used in India (AD 100) as the "medicine of sad men" (Thornwald, 1963, p. 205) without the present understanding of the biochemical process of a tranquilizer. Ancient Egyptian doctors used mud and soil in the treatment of eye diseases. This type of "sewerage pharmacology" was not understood until 1948 when Dr. Benjamin M. Dugger, a professor of plant physiology at the University of Wisconsin, discovered the drug aureomycin, a chemical similar to natural substances found near the Nile River. Aureomycin has been highly effective in the treatment of trachoma.

For centuries, practical treatment for many disabilities, diseases, and illnesses has been applied by trial and error without an understanding of the theoretical dynamics of the disease processes. Healers, such as shamans and witch doctors, intersperse treatment with superstition, sometimes attaining positive results. The important difference between applying therapeutics in modern science and in prescientific civilizations is in the explanation of why a specific treatment cures a disease. The search for cures to diseases, beginning with the germ theory of Pasteur and continuing through Alexander Fleming's discovery of penicillin in 1928 and Selman A. Waksman's discovery of streptomycin in 1944, spurred the corporate growth of therapeutic pharmaceutics. Modern medicine is heavily dependent on the availability of various drugs to control abnormal physical conditions, such as hypertension, arteriosclerosis, blood clotting, edema, and emotional illness. Hormone therapy and uses of vitamins and dietetics are other common methods akin to chemical therapy as forms of treatment.

## 1.7.2 Surgery

Surgical interventions in the twenty-first century continue to make traumatic gains in improving health care throughout the world. In a recent report from the U. S. National Center for Health Statistics (Cullen, Hall, & Golosinskiy, 2009), it is estimated that 53.3 million surgical type procedures were performed in the United States in 2006 (latest statistics available). Surgery is increasingly used as an outpatient procedure that has reduced the time in surgery and the time for patient recuperation. There was a 300 percent increase in the rates of visits to free-standing ambulatory surgery centers from 1996–2006. A list of the most frequent surgical procedures performed in the United States is shown in Table 1–6 (Cullen et al.).

Surgery as an advanced medical intervention has a long evolution in the history of humanity. Ancient civilizations such as the Incas of Peru in 200 BC used trepanation (removing parts of a skull) as a method to relieve epileptic fits and intractable headaches (Ellis, 2001). The ancient Romans (ca. 70 BC–200 BC) used up to 200 different surgical instruments in various operations. In addition, ligature of blood

---

| TABLE 1-6 |
|---|

**Most Frequent Surgical Procedures in the United States in 2006**

| Procedure | Number (in thousands) | Rate per 10,000 Population |
|---|---|---|
| Endoscopy of large intestine with or without biopsy | 5,741 | 192.5 |
| Endoscopy of small intestine with or without biopsy | 3,467 | 116.3 |
| Extraction of lens | 3,058 | 102.5 |
| Insertion of prosthetic lens (pseudophakos) | 2,582 | 86.6 |
| Injection of agent into spinal canal | 1,991 | 66.6 |
| Operation on muscle, tendon, fascia, and bursa | 1,465 | 49.1 |
| Injection or infusion of therapeutic or prophylactic substance | 1,462 | 49.0 |
| Endoscopic polypectomy of large intestine | 1,399 | 46.9 |
| Excision or destruction of lesion on tissue of skin and subcutaneous tissue | 1,092 | 36.6 |
| Arteriography and angiocardiography using contrast material | 1,054 | 35.3 |

**Note:** The information contained in this table is based on data from the *Vital and Health Statistics, Ambulatory and Inpatient Procedures in the United States, 2006*, Report #11, by K. A. Cullen, M. J. Hall, and A. Golosinskiy, 2009, U.S. Department of Health and Human Services, Centers for Disease Control and Prevention, National Centers for Health Statistics, pp. 16–19. This publication is available through http://www.cdc.gov/nchs/data/nhsr/nhsr011.pdf

vessels was performed; obstetric surgery, specifically Caesarean section, was known; and even anesthesia was used (Marti-Ibanez, 1962).

Modern surgery as an effective and safe method was the result of two important events: the development of antiseptics by Lister in 1867, who tested the capacity of carbolic acid in preventing infection in general surgery, and the discovery of ether anesthesia as a practical method by William Morton, a dentist, in 1846 (Ellis, 2001; Haeger, 1988).

### 1.7.3 Hospital Care

The third component in the development of modern treatment, parallel to chemotherapy and surgery, was the rise of hospital nursing care. Florence Nightingale's role in developing the nursing profession is legendary. Singlehandedly, she aroused world public opinion about the plight of hospital patients, who were often left to die because of neglect. The story of Florence Nightingale's success is well known. During the Crimean War of 1854, she organized a group of nurses to tend wounded British soldiers. Her experience gave her the insight into the need for clean, efficient hospitals. Reform in hospital care became a national issue in England after the Crimean War, and social legislation was enacted to provide governmental support. Florence Nightingale also started the first school of nursing at St. Thomas' Hospital, London, in 1860. With hospital reform enacted through legislation and a nursing school started, the foundation for progress in the treatment of the hospitalized patient was established.

Below is a short outline of the historical development of hospitals as documented by Rene Sand (1952):

1. *Ancient Greece, Sixth Century, BC:* A large open building was provided for the Greek physician. It comprised a waiting room, consulting room, and theater for operations and dressings.
2. *Ancient Rome, First Century, AD:* Sick bays were attached to the family estates of the wealthy.
3. *Early Medieval Europe, Fourth Century,* AD: Early Christians established "hospitia" for travelers, abandoned children, and the sick who were traveling on their way to pilgrimages. Care

was under the direction of monastic and sisterly orders.
4. *Middle East, Twelfth Century:* Moslems in Baghdad founded the first hospitals where physicians cared for the ill. Special wards for mental illness, blindness, and leprosy were established.
5. *Later Middle Ages, Europe, Fifth to Fourteenth Centuries:* Hostelries under the jurisdiction of the Roman Catholic Church provided care for the sick. Brothers and sisters of the Roman Catholic Church in attached ecclesiastical hospitals provided treatment remedies, performed simple operations, and attended those with serious illnesses.
6. *Renaissance Europe, Fifteenth Century:* For the first time in the Western world, physicians and midwives treated the sick in hospitals. Terminal patients were segregated from the acutely ill.
7. *Europe, Eighteenth Century:* Gradually hospitals began to treat emergency care patients, outpatient departments grew, and hospitals served as training facilities for medical students.
8. *Europe and America, Nineteenth Century:* Nursing care was established in hospitals. Antiseptic surgery, anesthesia, and improvement in general care of the hospitalized patient were initiated.
9. *Worldwide, Twentieth Century:* The growth of specialized hospitals, regional planning, and national health services. A world movement exists in extending health care to underdeveloped countries under the auspices of the United Nations, World Health Organization (WHO).

Current medical treatment is based on the principle of healing—stopping the progression of a disease and promoting natural bodily processes. Chemotherapy, surgery, and nursing care are the three basic methods that have made medical practice effective in treating many communicable diseases and physiological disorders and anatomical defects. The limitations of medical treatment for individuals with severe chronic disabilities, such as schizophrenia, arthritis, cardiovascular disease, and cerebral vascular accident (CVA) are clearly evident. Medical treatment alone is effective only when the disease process can be narrowed down to

| TABLE 1-7 |
| --- |

**Historical Factors Leading to the Rehabilitation Movement in the Twentieth Century**

- Incorporation of scientific methodology into clinical medicine
- Industrialization and its impact on clinical procedures for diagnosis and treatment
- Large population of veterans with disabilities from World War 1
- The availability of financial resources through Social Security and National Health Insurance schemes
- Medical specialties and the development of allied health professions
- Public acceptance that individuals with disabilities can be restored to independence through rehabilitation
- Public acceptance of individuals with disabilities in social and work situations

© Cengage Learning 2013

a specific etiology. Chronic diseases present problems of multiple etiologies and treatment requiring complex solutions and interdisciplinary efforts. The search for solutions to the chronic disabilities led to the rehabilitation movement.

## 1.8 Rehabilitation Movement— Stage VI

The emergence of rehabilitation as a distinct entity in the health care system began in 1916 during World War I. The aftermath of World War I and the devastation it brought saw the beginning of the rehabilitation movement, coinciding with the need for restoring function to those who were permanently disabled. One may ask why the rehabilitation field developed at that time and not in prior periods of recovery from war. The historical factors that led to the rehabilitation movement are outlined in Table 1–7.

Until the eighteenth century, chronic illness and permanent disability in general were not always considered medical problems. For instance, psychiatric illness and epilepsy were considered problems of morality and satanic possession. Treatment of psychiatric illness, if any, was stark, brutal, or radical. Before the rise of large institutions providing custodial care for patients needing psychiatric care, the attitude toward chronic mental illness was at best benign neglect and at worst rejection and punishment. In a related area, birth injuries such as cerebral palsy were misunderstood by ancient cultures. Not until 1862, when W. T. Little, an English orthopedic surgeon, described the relationship between birth injury and neurological disorders, was there any dynamic understanding of this disability. Individuals with other chronic disabilities, such as arthritis, emphysema, stroke, cardiovascular disease, and spinal cord injuries, were left either to the custodial care of the family or were placed into the hands of charlatans who promised miraculous cures.

### 1.8.1 Social Welfare and Rehabilitation

The change from custodial care to therapeutic treatment of the individual with chronic disabilities occurred at a period of time in history when social welfare had become a worldwide concern. Social Security was the forerunner in public health and medicine for the indigent with chronic disabilities. Germany, in 1883, and England, in 1897, were the first countries in Europe to enact legislation providing worker's compensation to cover disability and illness resulting from occupational accidents. The progress toward social and occupational health and safety is described in Figure 1–2. Governmental financial support, resulting from national policies

**Antiquity**
- Manual labor and tradesmen neglected
- Occupational diseases ignored

**Society of Artificers**
- Established apprenticeship system
- Workday regulated 12-13 hours

**Medieval Guilds**
- Voluntary associations formed for mutual aid protection of tradesman
- Assist worker with disabilities
- Assist in funeral expenses

**Protection of Miners** (16th Century)
- Ventilating machines for mines

**Occupational Medicine** (Established 17th Century)
- Relationship between occupation and disease investigated medically
- Prevention measures introduced—rest intervals, positioning, cleanliness, protective clothing

**Compiling of Vital Statistics on Occupational Disease** (18th Century)
- Use of medical inspectors

**Protection of Vulnerable Workers in Dangerous Trades** (19th Century)
- Public health legislation to regulate child labor
- Work day reduced to 10 hours

**Workmen's Compensation** (1890–1910)
- Compensate workers for occupational accidents and diseases

**National Women's Trade Union** (1920)
- Protection of women from dangerous industries

**Worker Health Bureau** (Established 1927)

**Social Security Legislation** (1930s)
- Place safety and health activities within Labor Department

**Occupational Safety and Health Agencies** (OSHA; Established 1970)
- Onsite inspections, regulations, and enforcement of laws relating to dangerous and unhealthy conditions in all industries

**The National Institute for Occupational Safety and Health** (NIOSH; Established 1970)
- Provide information through research, information, education, and training to aid in improving safe and healthful working conditions

**Scientific Investigations of Prevention and Treatment of Occupational Injuries and Diseases** (1980s)
- Application of ergonomics and rehabilitation of principles

**Future Trends in Occupational Medicine**
- Occupational health teams: ergonomist, occupational therapist, physician, industrial hygienist, physical therapist, safety officer, and nurse
- Investigation of physical, chemical, biological, and psychological factors in work environment that may cause or aggravate disease in individuals who are vulnerable
- Investigation of long-term effects of exposure to toxic chemicals, repetitive motion, vibration, excessive noise, extreme temperature, radiation, dust, bacteria
- Prevention of accidents or disease

**FIGURE 1-2**  Progress toward Social Reform in Occupational Health and Safety

on health and welfare, was necessary because of the enormous hospital resources and health personnel required in the rehabilitation of individuals with disabilities. In the United States, Social Security legislation, first enacted in 1935, has been a major impetus for the development of the rehabilitation movement. Change in societies' attitudes toward the individual with chronic disabilities, as evidenced in the social welfare movement, has encouraged the growth of the allied health professions.

### 1.8.2 The Development of Allied Health Professions—Phase I

Three major phases in the history of rehabilitation have affected the growth of the allied health professions. The first phase occurred shortly after World War I. During this period, the medical community recognized the need for physical and social rehabilitation of the individual with disabilities. Casualties from the war included individuals with lower extremity amputation, victims of poisonous gas resulting in neurological disabilities, and soldiers with psychiatric disabilities caused by shell shock. At that time, these veterans of the war needed assistance in readjusting to community living. Reconstruction workers recruited from nursing staffs were the first health personnel in rehabilitation.

Immediately after World War I, the goal of rehabilitation was primarily humane and supportive to the medical treatment. There was no direct effort by the rehabilitation workers to change the course of a disability or to make the individual with disabilities more functional. During the late 1920s, rehabilitation departments were established for the first time in hospitals. The health personnel recruited to work in these departments were, on the whole, dedicated people who applied caring support and activity to facilitate the patient's readjustment to the community.

### 1.8.3 The Education and Professionalization—Phase II

The second phase of rehabilitation, during the 1930s, 1940s, and 1950s, can be identified as the *educational and professionalization* phase. Table 1–8 lists the major landmarks in physical rehabilitation. Dur-

ing this time, programs in colleges and universities were initiated, professional associations grew, and rehabilitation services evolved. The training of allied health specialists who had a unique combination of knowledge in the application of activities and rehabilitation techniques, an understanding of medical treatment, and a background in the social sciences was considered necessary preparation for working in a hospital setting. The concepts underlying rehabilitation at that time were taken from other clinical and applied disciplines such as anatomy, physiology, nutrition, language development, psychology, clinical medicine, and education.

### 1.8.4 Physical Medicine and Rehabilitation

The first rehabilitation medical service in a general hospital was created in 1946, in Bellevue Hospital, New York City (Rusk, 1971). This unit served as a model for the interdisciplinary rehabilitation team. In addition, the physiatry specialty in rehabilitation medicine was started. Conceptually, **rehabilitation** was defined as restoring the individual to the highest level of cognitive, physical, economic, social, and emotional independence. This process, involving a team evaluation of the patient's functions, establishment of treatment goals and priorities, and an interdisciplinary approach to treatment, became the model for rehabilitation. This process is listed in Figure 1–3.

Parallel to the evolution of a medical rehabilitation team was the involvement of the federal and state governments in providing vocational rehabilitation services that resulted from the Vocational Rehabilitation Act of 1954. Sheltered workshops, such as Abilities, Inc. in New York City, Epi-Hab in Phoenix and Los Angeles, Community Workshops in Boston, and Goodwill Industries, provided the vocational training component and the specialized employment placement that helped reemploy individuals with disabilities.

### 1.8.5 Allied Health Treatment Technologies

As the training of allied health professionals developed during the 1940s and 1950s, a treatment

TABLE 1-8

**Early Landmarks in Rehabilitation Movement—Stage VI**

| Rehabilitation Events | Dates | Contributors | Significance |
|---|---|---|---|
| First comprehensive rehabilitation program | 1946 | Howard Rusk | Served as model for physical medicine program in a general hospital rehabilitation team approach |
| Physical therapy methods | 1949 | H. O. Kendall and F. P. Kendall | Basis for physical therapy techniques for muscle testing and patient evaluation |
| Retraining methods of activities of daily living | 1956 | Edith Buchwald Lawton | Provided functional rehabilitation methods for increasing independence |
| Vocational rehabilitation | 1957 | Lloyd H. Lofquist | Established the role of the rehabilitation counselor |
| Aphasia rehabilitation | 1955 | Martha L. Taylor and M. Marks | Provided rehabilitation techniques for speech therapy |
| Prosthetics | 1959 | M. H. Anderson, et al. | Led to cooperative research by physicians, engineers, and prosthetists in the design of artificial limbs |
| Orthotics | 1962 | Muriel Zimmerman | Led to the development of self-help devices for the homemaker and worker with physical disabilities |

© Cengage Learning 2013

technology emerged, especially in physical therapy. Methods for objectively assessing muscle function were established (Daniels, Williams, & Worthingham, 1956; Kendall & Kendall, 1949). Electrodiagnosis of muscle function; measurement of range of motion; and techniques for improving muscle and joint action through heat, ultraviolet rays, electrical stimulation, whirlpool, and cold packs were developed through trial and error and clinical practice. These techniques were a major part of the physical therapist's treatment procedures (Downer, 1970).

Therapists recognized the need for retraining patients in activities of daily living (ADLs) as an important area for intervention. Lawton (1956), working with Howard Rusk at the Institute of Physical Medicine and Rehabilitation, published a manual for therapists describing methods to retrain patients to become functionally independent in their everyday activities. The need to retrain patients with aphasia to regain their use of language as the result of a stroke or brain injury led to the development of sequentially programmed techniques (Taylor & Marks, 1955).

Another important component of rehabilitation was in the area of vocational rehabilitation. Lofquist (1957), McGowan (1960), and Patterson (1958) were some of the early workers who defined the role of the rehabilitation counselor in prevocational evaluation, special placement, and vocational training. Occupational therapy progressed as an integral part of the rehabilitation movement in a more general direction than physical therapy or speech therapy. The use of activities as treatment modalities in work, leisure, and ADLs was applied to a broader spectrum of disabilities. Occupational

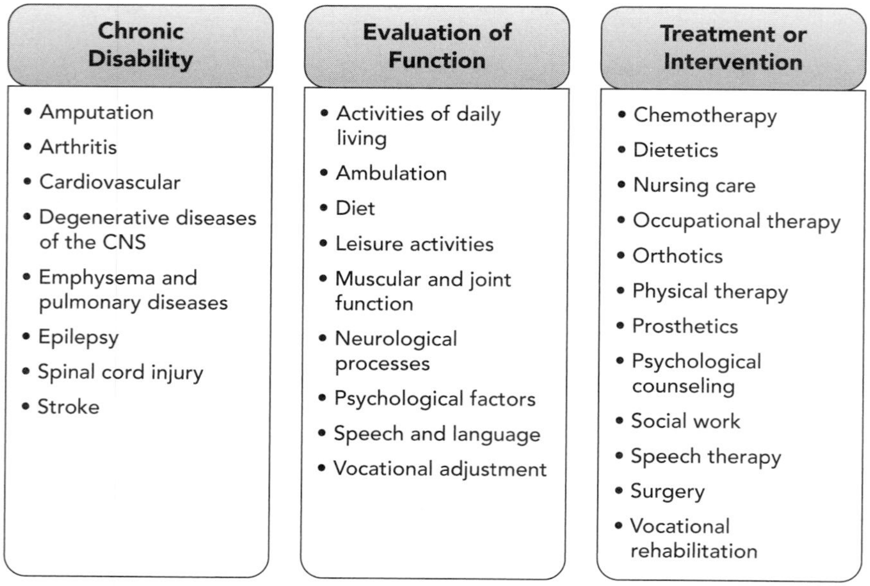

| Chronic Disability | Evaluation of Function | Treatment or Intervention |
|---|---|---|
| • Amputation<br>• Arthritis<br>• Cardiovascular<br>• Degenerative diseases of the CNS<br>• Emphysema and pulmonary diseases<br>• Epilepsy<br>• Spinal cord injury<br>• Stroke | • Activities of daily living<br>• Ambulation<br>• Diet<br>• Leisure activities<br>• Muscular and joint function<br>• Neurological processes<br>• Psychological factors<br>• Speech and language<br>• Vocational adjustment | • Chemotherapy<br>• Dietetics<br>• Nursing care<br>• Occupational therapy<br>• Orthotics<br>• Physical therapy<br>• Prosthetics<br>• Psychological counseling<br>• Social work<br>• Speech therapy<br>• Surgery<br>• Vocational rehabilitation |

© Cengage Learning 2013

**FIGURE 1-3** The Process of Physical Medicine and Rehabilitation: Rehabilitation is the process of restoring function in individuals with severe disabilities. Assessment of the physical, cognitive, psychosocial, and vocational factors are carried out before intervention is planned and implemented.

therapists worked mainly in rehabilitation departments, psychiatric state hospitals, Veteran Administration facilities, and state schools for those with physical and mental disabilities (Willard & Spackman, 1971).

As the rehabilitation movement gained momentum in the 1950s, biomedical research in the replacement of limbs and joints led to the field of prosthetics. The design of component parts, fitting of the prosthesis, and gait training gave rise to another member of the physical rehabilitation team, the prosthetist (Anderson, Bechtol, & Sollars, 1959). Specialization in rehabilitation also occurred at a rapid rate within the fields of nutrition, social work, psychology, and nursing.

## 1.8.6 Psychiatric Rehabilitation

In comparison with physical rehabilitation techniques, psychiatric treatment has lagged behind in developing the technology to treat the individual with mental illness. The initial optimism from 1930 to 1950 that was generated by biological interventions, such as electric convulsive therapy (ECT), insulin therapy, Metrazol treatment, and psychosurgery, has faded. From the 1960s to the 1990s psychiatric treatment remained in a state of disarray. The onset of neuroleptic drugs and the community mental health movement in the 1960s led to the dismantling of large psychiatric hospitals that served as custodial "warehouses" for the patients who were chronically mentally ill.

Since the 1960s, the length of hospitalization for patients with psychiatric disorders has been reduced, but the number of individuals with mental illness living in the community and without treatment has increased. Current enlightened psychiatric treatment emphasizes early return to the community in combination with outpatient vocational rehabilitation. In many state hospitals for those with mental illness, a large percentage of older patients form a residual population from the custodial period. This population is mainly rejected, untreated, and provided mainly with maintenance care. Other individuals with mental illness are in nursing homes, custodial care facilities, and prison facilities, or are left untreated in large cities as members of homeless populations.

Evaluation of psychiatric treatment still remains a fertile area for clinical researchers. Apart from descriptive observations, few comprehensive studies have analyzed treatment techniques in depth. Although many clinicians believe that what they are doing is beneficial, there is little evidence or hard data to support their claims.

Why has psychiatric rehabilitation lagged behind other areas of medical progress? First, there has been wide disagreement in identifying, diagnosing, and treating mental illness in spite of the attempt to classify it as exemplified in the *Diagnostic and Statistical Manual of Mental Disorders—Text Revision* (DSM-IV-TR; American Psychiatric Association [APA], 2000). Theorists have differed widely in their approaches in psychiatry, advocating specific treatment techniques for the broad spectrum of mental illness. Many clinical researchers have failed to recognize the individual needs of patients and the differential effects of treatment.

A second reason for the lag in scientific progress in psychiatric rehabilitation is the lack of comprehensive studies. Psychiatric research has been fixed at the nineteenth-century two-variable research stage model, which assumed a single-factor cause for mental illness. If progress in psychiatric rehabilitation is to occur, multidisciplinary efforts must investigate mental illness on a broad front, using a biopsychosocial model, rather than narrow, one-dimensional research. The promise in psychiatric rehabilitation lies in a holistic approach, the incorporation of a community mental health model relying on halfway houses, vocational programs, and support groups, with an individualized approach to evaluation, education, psychotherapy, counseling, and drug treatment.

## 1.8.7 Third Phase of Allied Health—1960 to Present

This development led to the present period of rehabilitation, which has been characterized by various treatment theories. Unfortunately, these theories have become so specialized that professionals in allied health fields can no longer change from one disability area to another without familiarizing themselves with a vast amount of knowledge and technology. For example, allied health professionals have specialized in diverse areas such as constraint therapy, augmentative communication, computer technology, sensory integration therapy (SI), neurodevelopmental therapy (NDT), robotics, telemetry, cinematography, and biofeedback. These areas of rehabilitation are unique. They are interdisciplinary in nature and incorporate theories and findings from the physical and social sciences. Table 1–9 shows the rapid growth of the allied health professions from 1950 to the present.

The extraordinary growth of the allied health professions since 1950 is apparent if one examines the percentage increase in the number of active practitioners and the number of professional schools. In comparison with the U.S. population increase from 150 million in 1949 to 210 million in 1972, one would have expected the professions to increase about 40 percent. We find, however, that professions such as occupational therapy and physical therapy increased 300 percent during the same period. The number of radiologic technologists increased 685 percent, registered nurses increased 149 percent, and physicians increased 58 percent during this period. On the other hand, the smallest increases were in the numbers of chiropractic, osteopathy, optometry, and pharmacy professionals. The growth of the allied health professions has continued into the 1980s and 1990s with forecasts of continued growth far into the twenty-first century.

Another indication of the rapid expansion of the allied health professions is the emergence of new fields that did not exist 40 years ago. *The Occupational Outlook Handbook* (1951) did not include many allied health professions, which

TABLE 1-9

**The Growth of Health Profession, 1950 to 2008**

| Health Specialty | Postsecondary Training (Years) | Active Practitioners | | | |
|---|---|---|---|---|---|
| | | 1950 | 1972 | 1992 | 2008 |
| Audiologist[1] | 6–8 | — | — | — | 12,800 |
| Chiropractor | 6–8 | 14,000 | 16,000 | 46,000 | 49,100 |
| Dentist | 8 | 75,300 | 105,000 | 183,000 | 141,900 |
| Dietitian and nutritionists | 4–5 | 15,000 | 33,000 | 50,000 | 60,300 |
| Occupational therapist | 5–6 | 2,300 | 7,500 | 40,000 | 104,500 |
| Optometrist | 7–8 | 17,000 | 18,700 | 31,000 | 34,800 |
| Pharmacist | 6–7 | 100,000 | 131,000 | 163,000 | 269,900 |
| Physical therapist | 6–7 | 4,500 | 18,000 | 90,000 | 185,500 |
| Physician and surgeon[2] | 8–16 | 200,000 | 316,500 | 556,000 | 661,400 |
| Physician assistant[3] | 4–6 | — | 303 | 22,305 | 74,800 |
| Podiatrist | 10–12 | 6,400 | 7,300 | 14,700 | 12,200 |
| Psychologist | 9–10 | 10,000 | 57,000 | 144,000 | 170,200 |
| Registered nurse | 3–5 | 300,500 | 750,000 | 1,835,000 | 2,600,000 |
| Speech-language pathologist | 6 | 2,000 | 27,000 | 73,000 | 119,300 |
| Social worker | 4–8 | 100,000 | 185,000 | 484,000 | 642,000 |

[1] Audiologists were included with speech/language pathologists until 2008.
[2] Surgeons were added in 2008.
[3] Physician assistant programs were started in 1967.

**Note:** The information contained in this table is based on data from U.S. Department of Labor, *Occupational Outlook Handbook* (1951, 1974–1975, 1982–1983, 1992–1993, 1994–1995, 1998–1999, 2010–11). Retrieved from http://stats.bls.gov/oco/ and from information obtained from professional societies.

appeared in later editions, starting with 1972. (See Table 1–10).

### 1.8.8 Rehabilitation Research Trends (1950–Current)

Goldberg (1974), in an analysis of rehabilitation research, identified 10 areas that are related to clinical practice:

- **Program Evaluation:** the assessment of the effectiveness of a clinical program in reaching stated objectives or meeting a list of criteria
- **Management:** the study of factors related to health labor, cost effectiveness, and comprehensive planning in providing health care to those in need of services

## TABLE 1-10

**The Growth of Health Professions of Technologists and Assistants, 1972–2008**

| Health Field | 1972 | 1986 | 1996 | 2008 |
|---|---|---|---|---|
| Dental hygienist | 17,000 | 87,000 | 133,000 | 174,100 |
| Electrocardiograph (ECG) technician | 10,000 | 18,000 | 15,000 | 49,500 |
| Electroencephalogram (EEG) technician | 3,500 | 5,900 | 64,000 | 82,000 |
| Medical record technician | 8,000 | 40,000 | 87,000 | 172,500 |
| Nuclear medicine technologist | — | 9,700 | 13,000 | 21,800 |
| Occupational therapy assistant | 6,000 | 9,000 | 16,000 | 34,400 |
| Physical therapy assistant | 10,000 | 12,000 | 84,000 | 109,900 |
| Radiology technologist | 55,000 | 1 15,000 | 174,000 | 214,700 |
| Respiratory therapist | 17,000 | 56,000 | 82,000 | 105,900 |
| Surgical technician | 25,000 | 37,000 | 49,000 | 91,500 |

**Note:** Data in this table are taken from the U.S. Department of Labor, *Occupational Outlook Handbook* (1972–1973, 1988–1989, 1992–1993, 1998–1999, 2010–2011), retrieved from http://stats.bls.gov/oco, and from professional associations.

- **Dissemination:** the process of communicating research findings over a wide area, including to professional and lay persons
- **Involvement of Consumer Groups:** the identification of research problems
- **Chronic Severe Disability:** functional problems as a major focus of research in rehabilitation
- **Social Problems:** alcoholism, adult crime, drug addiction, and juvenile delinquency as areas included under health-related problems instead of correctional problems
- **Functional Assessment Methods:** targeted to the individuals with severe disabilities who are in supported employment and working at home
- **Need for Follow-Up and Follow-Along Research:** evaluation of the continuity of care
- **Rehabilitation Utilization:** incorporation of rehabilitation research in clinical practices
- **Rehabilitation Engineering:** interdisciplinary research in solving practical rehabilitation problems especially in the fields of prosthetics, orthotics, communication, mobility, and independent living

These trends continued to have an impact on rehabilitation research in the 1990s. From the initial emphasis on the physical restoration of the individual, researchers turned to the more complex chronic social problems that are associated with poverty, substandard housing, undernourishment, alienation, and addiction. Evidence was present that severe chronic disabilities, such as polio, tuberculosis, stroke, emphysema, and coronary thrombosis, could be alleviated or reduced through public health immunization programs, balanced nutrition, exercise regimes, and self-monitoring of symptoms. The cost of preventing chronic illnesses was much less than the cost of rehabilitation. Primary, secondary, and tertiary prevention began to make an impact in the work of allied health professionals. Research had an important part in justifying the efficacy of treatment intervention, either in restoring function or preventing chronic disability.

---

**TABLE 1-11**

**Current Trends in Rehabilitation Research (2011)**

- Development of standardized (norm-referenced and criterion-referenced) outcome measures that have acceptable levels of reliability and validity

- Evaluation of treatment techniques using prospective designs

- Operational definitions of treatment methods that can be replicated in clinical practice

- Controlled observation of normal developmental landmarks that serve as reference points for populations with disabilities

- Fundamental investigations of the biopsychosocial nature of disease and underlying dynamics

- Survey of the perceptions of patients with chronic disabilities toward their disability and their evaluation of treatment techniques

- The incorporation of high technology instrumentation in evaluation and treatment, such as microcomputers, cinematography, and psychophysiological measures

- Qualitative and action research methods

- Application of research findings to evidence-based practice

---

Current trends in rehabilitation research are listed in Table 1–11, whereas Table 1–12 gives some examples of current review of rehabilitation and habilitation research.

## 1.9 Habilitation and Special Education—Stage VII

The success of the rehabilitation movement led to the field of habilitation, which goes beyond the medical model. Whereas the medical model traditionally relies on etiology, diagnosis, and treatment, habilitation includes the integration of psychological, sociological, and educational fields of knowledge emphasizing research in developmental theory and educational technology. Rehabilitation is traditionally defined as the restoration of function and the maximization of abilities in individuals with chronic disabilities. In contrast, **habilitation** is defined as the development of functions and capabilities in individuals with disabilities occurring at birth, during childhood, or during a traumatic incident (e.g., traumatic brain injury, posttraumatic

stress). The process of habilitation is presented in Figure 1–4.

The child who is intellectually disabled, the individual who is congenitally blind or deaf, the child born with a missing limb or with cerebral palsy, the child with autism, and the child who is extremely disadvantaged have needs that are different from adults who acquired a physical disability. Helping the child develop independence, coping skills, and physical and mental capabilities to adapt to societal demands requires specialized techniques. The child who is developmentally delayed, unlike the adult with a disability, has not lost a capacity or skill that requires remedial education, sensory retraining, or vocational readjustment. Instead, the child with a disability needs special education, sensorimotor or language training, occupational preparation, and training for activities of daily living basic to the habilitation process. Special education services, available for individuals with special needs, have been developed to provide training and instruction in functional skills necessary for independent living and self-support. What were the early historical precursors to the field of habilitation?

## TABLE 1-12

### Examples of Current Reviews of Research in Rehabilitation and Habilitation from Published Abstracts

| Anxiety And Depression | Ravindran, A. V., Lam, R. W., Filteau, M. J., Lespérance, F., Kennedy, S. H., Parikh, S. V., & Patten, S. B. (with the Canadian Network for Mood and Anxiety Treatments; CANMAT). (2009). Clinical guidelines for the management of major depressive disorder in adults. V. Complementary and alternative medicine treatments. *Journal of Affective Disorders, 117*(Suppl 1), S54–64. |
|---|---|
| | **Abstract:** BACKGROUND: In 2001, the Canadian Psychiatric Association and the Canadian Network for Mood and Anxiety Treatments (CANMAT) partnered to produce evidence-based clinical guidelines for the treatment of depressive disorders. A revision of these guidelines was undertaken by CANMAT in 2008–2009 to reflect advances in the field. There is widespread interest in complementary and alternative medicine (CAM) therapies in the treatment of major depressive disorder (MDD). METHODS: The CANMAT guidelines are based on a question-answer format to enhance accessibility to clinicians. An evidence-based format was used with updated systematic reviews of the literature and recommendations were graded according to Level of Evidence using pre-defined criteria. Lines of Treatment were identified based on criteria that included evidence and expert clinical support. This section on "Complementary and Alternative Medicine Treatments" is one of 5 guideline articles. RESULTS: There is Level 1 evidence to support light therapy in seasonal MDD and St. John's wort in mild to moderate MDD. There is also some evidence for the use of exercise, yoga and sleep deprivation, as well as for omega-3 fatty acids and SAM-e. Support for other natural health products and therapies is still limited. LIMITATIONS: The evidence base remains limited and studies often have methodological problems, including small samples, variability in dose, short duration of treatment, unknown quality of the agent and limited long-term data. Safety data are also sparse with little information about drug interactions. CONCLUSIONS: Some CAM treatments have evidence of benefit in MDD. However, problems with standardization and safety concerns may limit their applicability in clinical practice. |
| Autism | Cotugno, A. J. (2009). Social competence and social skills training and intervention for children with Autism Spectrum Disorders. *Journal of Autism and Developmental Disorders, 39,* 1268–1277. |
| | **Abstract:** This study examined the effectiveness of a 30-week social competence and social skills group intervention program with children, ages 7–11, diagnosed with Autism Spectrum Disorders (ASD). Eighteen children with ASD were assessed with pretreatment and posttreatment measures on the *Walker-McConnell Scale* (WMS) and the *MGH YouthCare Social Competence Development Scale.* Each received the 30-week intervention program. For comparison, a matched sample of ten non-ASD children was also assessed, but received no treatment. The findings indicated that each ASD intervention group demonstrated significant gains on the WMS and significant improvement in the areas of anxiety management, joint attention, and flexibility/transitions. Results suggest that this approach can be effective in improving core social deficits in individuals with ASD. |
| Pediatric Disorders | Parsons, T. D., Rizzo, A. A., Rogers, S., & York, P. (2009). Virtual reality in paediatric rehabilitation: A review. *Developmental Neurorehabilitation, 12,* 224–238. |
| | **Abstract:** OBJECTIVE: To provide a narrative review of studies regarding the outcomes of Virtual Reality (VR)-based treatment and rehabilitation programmes within the paediatric population. METHODS: Studies related to the use of VR across a number of paediatric areas (e.g. cerebral palsy, autism, foetal alcohol syndrome and attention deficits) were identified and summarized. RESULTS: Outcomes from the studies reviewed provide preliminary support for the use of VR. CONCLUSION: VR may be an effective treatment method for specific disorders, although the generalizability of this literature is hindered by several methodological limitations, such as small samples and the absence of appropriate control participants. |

*continues*

**TABLE 1-12**

## Examples of Current Reviews of Research in Rehabilitation and Habilitation from Published Abstracts *continued*

**Schizophrenia**

Taylor, T. L., Killaspy, H., Wright, C., Turton, P., White, S., Kallert, T. W., … King, M. B. (2009). A systematic review of the international published literature relating to quality of institutional care for people with longer term mental health problems. *BMC Psychiatry, 9,* 55. doi:10.1186/1471-244X-9-55.

**Abstract:** BACKGROUND: A proportion of people with mental health problems require longer term care in a psychiatric or social care institution. However, there are no internationally agreed quality standards for institutional care and no method to assess common care standards across countries. We aimed to identify the key components of institutional care for people with longer term mental health problems and the effectiveness of these components. METHODS: We undertook a systematic review of the literature using comprehensive search terms in 11 electronic databases and identified 12,182 titles. We viewed 550 abstracts, reviewed 223 papers and included 110 of these. A "critical interpretative synthesis" of the evidence was used to identify domains of institutional care that are key to service users' recovery. RESULTS: We identified eight domains of institutional care that were key to service users' recovery: living conditions; interventions for schizophrenia; physical health; restraint and seclusion; staff training and support; therapeutic relationship; autonomy and service user involvement; and clinical governance. Evidence was strongest for specific interventions for the treatment of schizophrenia (family psychoeducation, cognitive behavioural therapy (CBT) and vocational rehabilitation). CONCLUSION: Institutions should, ideally, be community based, operate a flexible regime, maintain a low density of residents, and maximise residents' privacy. For service users with a diagnosis of schizophrenia, specific interventions (CBT, family interventions involving psychoeducation, and supported employment) should be provided through integrated programmes. Restraint and seclusion should be avoided wherever possible and staff should have adequate training in de-escalation techniques. Regular staff supervision should be provided and this should support service user involvement in decision making and positive therapeutic relationships between staff and service users. There should be clear lines of clinical governance that ensure adherence to evidence-based guidelines and attention should be paid to service users' physical health through regular screening.

**Spinal Cord Injury**

Cooper, R. A., & Cooper, R. (2010) Quality-of-life technology for people with spinal cord injuries. *Physical Medicine and Rehabilitation Clinics of North America, 21,* 1–13.

**Abstract:** Technology plays a critical role in promoting well-being, activity, and participation for individuals with spinal cord injury (SCI). As technology has improved, so has the realm of possibilities open to people with SCI. School, work, travel, and leisure activities are all facilitated by technology. Advances in materials have made wheelchairs lighter, and developments in design have made wheelchairs that fit individual needs. Software has made computer interfaces adaptive and in some case intelligent, through learning the user's behavior and optimizing its structure. As participatory action design and aware systems take greater hold, transformational change is likely to take place in the technology available to people with SCI.

**Stroke**

Carter, A.R., Connor, L. T., & Dromerick, A. W. (2010). Rehabilitation after stroke: Current state of the science. *Current Neurology and Neuroscience Reports, 10*, 158–166.

**Abstract:** Stroke rehabilitation is evolving into a clinical field based on the neuroscience of recovery and restoration. There has been substantial growth in the number and quality of clinical trials performed. Much effort now is directed toward motor restoration and is being led by trials of constraint-induced movement therapy. Although the results do not necessarily support that constraint-induced movement therapy is superior to other training methods, this treatment has become an important vehicle for developing clinical trial methods and studying the physiology underlying activity-based rehabilitation strategies. Other promising interventions include robotic therapy delivery, magnetic and electrical cortical stimulation, visualization, and constraint-driven aphasia therapies. Amphetamine has not been demonstrated to be effective, and studies of other pharmacologic agents are still preliminary. Future studies will incorporate refinements in clinical trial methods and improved activity- and technology-based interventions.

**Traumatic Brain Injury**

Devine, J. M., & Zafonte, R. D. (2009). Physical exercise and cognitive recovery in acquired brain injury: A review of the literature. *PM & R: The Journal of Injury, Function, and Rehabilitation, 1*, 560–575.

**Abstract:** OBJECTIVE: Physical exercise has been shown to play an ever-broadening role in the maintenance of overall health and has been implicated in the preservation of cognitive function in both healthy elderly and demented populations. Animal and human studies of acquired brain injury (ABI) from trauma or vascular causes also suggest a possible role for physical exercise in enhancing cognitive recovery. DATA SOURCES: A review of the literature was conducted to explore the current understanding of how physical exercise impacts the molecular, functional, and neuroanatomic status of both intact and brain-injured animals and humans. STUDY SELECTION: Searches of the MEDLINE, CINHAL, and PsychInfo databases yielded an extensive collection of animal studies of physical exercise in ABI. Animal studies strongly tie physical exercise to the upregulation of multiple neural growth factor pathways in brain-injured animals, resulting in both hippocampal neurogenesis and functional improvements in memory. DATA EXTRACTION: A search of the same databases for publications involving physical exercise in human subjects with ABI yielded 24 prospective and retrospective studies. DATA SYNTHESIS: Four of these evaluated cognitive outcomes in persons with ABI who were involved in physical exercise. Three studies cited a positive association between exercise and improvements in cognitive function, whereas one observed no effect. Human exercise interventions varied greatly in duration, intensity, and level of subject supervision, and tools for assessing neurocognitive changes were inconsistent. CONCLUSIONS: There is strong evidence in animal ABI models that physical exercise facilitates neurocognitive recovery. Physical exercise interventions are safe in the subacute and rehabilitative phases of recovery for humans with ABI. In light of strong evidence of positive effects in animal studies, more controlled, prospective human interventions are warranted to better explore the neurocognitive effects of physical exercise on persons with ABI.

| Childhood Disabilities Related to Genetic, Embryologic, or Trauma Injury | Evaluation of Function | Educational and Treatment Techniques |
|---|---|---|
| • Attention Deficit/Hyperactivity Disorder<br>• Autism Spectrum Disorders (ASD)<br>• Cerebral palsy<br>• Childhood amputee<br>• Dyslexia<br>• Epilepsy<br>• Fetal Alcohol Spectrum Disorders<br>• Hearing impairment<br>• Intellectual disabilities and developmental delay<br>• Juvenile arthritis<br>• Learning disabilities<br>• Neuromotor impairments<br>• Orthopedic impairments<br>• Sensory integration disorder<br>• Traumatic brain injury<br>• Visual Impairments | • Academic<br>• Activities of daily living (ADL)<br>• Cognitive<br>• Leisure interests<br>• Neuromuscular<br>• Mental health<br>• Memory<br>• Neuropsychological<br>• Prevocational<br>• Psychosocial<br>• Sensory | • Augmentative and alternative communication (AAC)<br>• Braille<br>• Community-based instruction (CBI)<br>• Computer-assisted instruction (CAI)<br>• Explicit or direct instruction<br>• Inclusive education<br>• Individualized learning<br>• Medical treatment<br>• Motor therapy (OT and PT)<br>• Orientation and mobility (O/M)<br>• Psychological counseling<br>• Response to intervention (RtI)<br>• Self-care skills<br>• Sensorimotor training<br>• Sign language<br>• Speech and language therapy (SLP)<br>• Strategic teaching<br>• Vocational development |

© Cengage Learning 2013

**FIGURE 1-4** The Process of Habilitation, or Development of Function: Children with special needs are evaluated and then taught using appropriate educational and treatment techniques.

### 1.9.1 Initial Concern for Those with Disabilities

Although prior to the twentieth century some services were available for individuals with disabilities, these services were minimal, generally no more than custodial care and assistance through the efforts of religious orders and voluntary charities. The earliest report of attempts to treat and educate the blind was the establishment of a hospital in 1260 (Hallahan & Kauffman, 1993; Juul, 1981). Rousseau (1712–1779),

a philosopher and theorist, petitioned in his treatise "Emile" for the study of children directly rather than using what was known about adults and applying that knowledge to children. "Nature intends that children shall be children before they are men.... Treat your pupil as his age demands" (Rousseau, 1762/1883, pp. 52, 54).

During the mid-1800s, Jacob Rodreques Péreire (1715–1780), a Spanish medical doctor living in France, developed an oral method to teach individuals with severe hearing loss to read and speak. At the same time, a Frenchman, Abbé de l'Epée (1712–1789) developed a manual sign language for "deaf-mutes." "The natural language of the Deaf and Dumb is the language of signs; nature and their different wants are their only tutors in it: and they have no other language as long as they have no further instructors" (Epée, 1784/1820, as cited in Lane, 1976, p. 79).

Sicard (1742–1833), a French medical doctor influential in the education of the "deaf-mutes" expanded Epée's methods, producing a way to teach "deaf-mutes" to read and write:

> [Epée] saw that the deaf-mute expressed his physical needs without instruction; that one could, with the same signs, communicate to him the expression of the same needs and could indicate the things that one wanted to designate: these were the first words of a new language which this great man has enriched, to the astonishment of all of Europe. (Sicard, 1795, as cited in Lane, 1976, p. 79)

### 1.9.2 Itard's Influence

The earliest reported case of enlightened intervention with children identified as being intellectually disabled was Jean-Marc Gaspard Itard's (1774–1838) work with Victor, "the wild boy of Aveyron" (Lane, 1976). Victor (ca. 1785–1828), who emerged from the forests of Aveyron between 1797 and 1800, was thought to have been abandoned by his parents as an infant or young child. Itard, a young physician, was assigned the responsibility to teach Victor. Itard applied methods developed earlier by Epée and Sicard. These methods included breaking up each task into small segments and using techniques that had been successful for "deaf-mutes." In this way, Itard believed that he could teach Victor to be social and use language (Lane, 1976; Winnie, 1912). After six years, even though Itard considered his work a failure, Victor had developed some social skills and could read a few words. On the other hand, Itard's work with Victor inspired him to further his methods for teaching "deaf-mutes":

> The child, who was called the wild boy of Aveyron, did not receive from my intensive care all the advantages that I had hoped. But the many observations that I could make and the techniques of instruction inspired by the inflexibility of his organs were not entirely fruitless, and I later found a more suitable application for them with some of our children whose mutism is the result of obstacles that are more easily overcome. (Itard, 1825, as cited in Lane, 1976, p. 185)

Several authors in education (Forness & Kavale, 1984; Hunt & Marshall, 1994; McDermott, 1994; Smith & Tyler, 2010) have recognized the significant contribution of Itard's work with Victor to present-day methods used in special education classes. In his effort to teach Victor, Itard developed methods that encompassed multiple senses (auditory, visual, kinesthetic) and demonstrated that individual instruction could be successful. Eduardo Séquin (1812–1880), a student of Itard, advanced these methods. He opened the first school for the "intellectually deficient" in 1837 and demonstrated that they could be systematically trained and educated. Finally, as a physician involved in the education and treatment of individuals with disabilities, Itard played a significant part in the development of educational and treatment services for individuals with disabilities (Forness & Kavale, 1984). Initially, the emphasis of special education relied on a medical model using etiology, symptomology, differential diagnosis, and specialized treatment. This resulted in an educational system based on classification and segregation, rather than a system based on community participation and mainstreaming in general education. It is notable that Itard's work using a single case study has led to the development of general methods for teaching children with disabilities (Kirk & Gallagher, 1989).

### 1.9.3 Montessori's Contribution to Special Education

The following quote is from Marie Montessori who, as a physician and teacher, established the basis for special education in Italy at the end of the nineteenth century. "In this method the lesson corresponds to an experiment, the more fully the teacher is acquainted with the methods of experimental psychology, the better will she understand how to give the lesson" (Montessori, 1912, p. 107).

Montessori advocated that the special education teacher of individuals with intellectual disabilities should use observation and experimentation in sequencing pedagogical activities. Montessori, who acknowledges the influence of Itard and Séquin, was a forerunner in the movement to provide special education methods through perceptual-motor training to the child with disabilities. These materials and methods were based on concrete, three-dimensional manipulatives (hands-on activities) that allowed exploration and learning through discovery. Today these methods are used with populations of typical children and children with special needs (Shea & Bauer, 1994).

Theoretically, Montessori's method changed the direction of treatment from a medical model to a model based on education, psychology, and child development. This approach was not limited to the child with intellectual disabilities. For example, Louis Braille, who was blind, developed a system of reading for the blind over a period from 1825 to 1852 (Illingworth, 1910). This method of teaching was the basis of special education for the blind in the early 1900s. Analogous to Braille as a method for teaching the blind was sign language for the deaf, devised by Abbé de l'Epée around 1755 (Winnie, 1912). The oral method was later practiced in Germany by Heinicke and Hill, who felt that speech development in the deaf child should parallel normal speech development (Winnie, 1912). Because of the complexity in educating blind and deaf children, special schools that segregated them from the public schools were founded. The significance of the Montessori method for those with intellectual disability, of the Braille system for the blind, and of sign language for the deaf is that these methods compensate for the child's inability to learn in a typical classroom. They are specific, technological advances designed to help the child to learn. These methods have allowed special education to be effective for children who are blind, deaf, or intellectually disabled.

## 1.9.4 Early Services in the United States

Séquin's contribution to the education of individuals with disabilities extended to the United States. Through the efforts of Samuel Gridley Howe, Séquin immigrated to the United States in 1848 where he shared his knowledge of educational methods for teaching individuals with mental retardation. He was later instrumental in founding the American Association on Intellectual and Developmental Disabilities (AAIDD), formerly known as the American Association on Mental Deficiency (AAMD). This association "promotes progressive policies, sound research, effective practices and universal human rights for people with intellectual and developmental disabilities" (AAIDD, 2010, para 1).

In the United States, Reverend Thomas Gallaudet, Horace Mann, and Samuel Gridley Howe were pioneers in the early development of special schools for children with disabilities. In 1817, in Hartford Connecticut, Gallaudet, assisted by Clerc, a "deaf-mute" trained by Sicard, founded the first residential school for the deaf (Lane, 1976). This outstanding school still exists. Gallaudet University, located in Washington, DC, is the only liberal arts college established for students with hearing impairments. The university was founded by Gallaudet's grandson in 1864 (Lane, 1976). In 1829, Howe opened the Perkins Institute at Watertown, Massachusetts, a residential school for students with visual impairments. This school is well known because Anne Sullivan, teacher of Helen Keller, was trained there. Fernald State School, the first institution for individuals with intellectual disabilities, was opened in 1848, with the Commonwealth of Massachusetts assuming full financial responsibility (Sigmon, 1987). In addition to Séquin and his work in intellectual disability, individuals such as Louis Braille and Alexander Graham Bell, who was instrumental in the amplification of sound for the hearing impaired, greatly influenced the teaching methods used in these early institutions (Kirk & Gallagher, 1989).

A major change in educational practices in the United States occurred when individual states mandated compulsory education between 1852 and 1918. Although some students with disabilities were taught in the general education program, the degree of severity in these individuals resulted in the creation of residential institutions, segregated day schools, and special classes. The first special education day school in the United States, the Horace Mann School, was opened in 1868 in Roxbury, Massachusetts. New Jersey, in 1911, was the first state to mandate programs for students with disabilities (Sigmon, 1987). Individuals confined to wheelchairs or with severe disabilities continued to be excluded from public schools until the 1960s and 1970s. The right for children with disabilities to be educated in a public school was mandated by court decisions such as *Pennsylvania Association of Retarded Citizens (PARC) v. Pennsylvania* (1971) and *Mills v. Board of Education, Washington, DC* (1971). Decisions from these judicial cases supported the position that individuals with disabilities were entitled to a free and appropriate public education (FAPE), regardless of the degree of severity or educational need (Turnbull, 1998).

### 1.9.5 Special Education Assessment and Programming

In 1905, the French government commissioned Alfred Binet (1857–1911), a French psychologist, to provide a useful assessment tool that would identify those children who needed special techniques to learn. Binet began working to develop methods of assessing intelligence in 1886. His first book, published at that time, was entitled *Psychologie du Raissonnement (The Psychology of Reasoning; 1899/1912)*. This was the beginning of intelligence testing as we know it today. (More information regarding Binet and the development of intelligence tests can be found in Chapter 9 in the discussion on intelligence testing.)

In the United States, Lewis Terman (1877–1956) and Henry Herbert Goddard (1866–1957), strongly influenced by Binet, continued the development of intelligence tests. Both believed that intelligence was inherited, stable, and did not change over time. A student's failure in the general education curriculum was explained by his or her inadequate intellectual level, not by methods of teaching or environmental factors. As a result, in the first half of the twentieth century, institutionalization and segregation of those individuals with severe intellectual deficits and physical disabilities became the norm. It was not until the 1960s when there was a major push toward normalization (Wolfensberger, 1972) and deinstitutionalization that individuals with intellectual disabilities and physical impairments were returned to the community and local school programs.

Historically, the habilitation of those with mild intellectual disability, blindness, and deafness has been more successful than the habilitation of individuals with brain damage, learning disabilities, autism, or social deprivation. One reason for these differences has been in the specialized educational curricula that have been developed to compensate for the child's disability. Methods for educating students with brain damage, learning disabilities, autism, or social deprivation were slower to develop.

During the latter half of the nineteenth century and the beginnings of the twentieth century, physicians such as James Hinshelwood (1917) and Samuel T. Orton (1879–1948) used adult models to understand reasons for learning difficulties in children who were not deaf, blind, or intellectually disabled. Both clinicians developed a multisensory method for teaching reading. Later, their ideas were expanded by special educators. The methods developed are still used today in many classrooms (Mercer, Mercer, & Pullen, 2011).

The aftermath of World War I was another turning point in the development of educational programs for individuals with brain injuries. Kurt Goldstein (1878–1965), in his experimental work with soldiers who had sustained head injuries during battle, contributed much to the understanding of the consequences of brain damage. His work inspired Alfred Strauss and Heinz Werner (Strauss & Werner, 1943) to study children with brain damage during the 1930s and 1940s at Wayne County Training School in Michigan. Their findings led to the identification of a group of children with brain damage. Although these children appeared to be intellectually disabled, the cause of the disability was not genetic. Moreover, their behavioral characteristics were similar to the symptoms displayed by soldiers with brain injuries, such as perseveration, distractibility, inattention, and memory problems (Mercer, 1983). In their classic book, *Psychopathology and Education of the Brain-Injured Child,* Strauss and Lehtinen (1947) described symptoms and behaviors of the child with brain injury and justified special education methods for teaching this group of children. Prior to the published works by Strauss and collaborators (Strauss & Kephart, 1940; Strauss & Lehtinen, 1947; Strauss & Werner, 1941), treatment for the child with brain damage was undifferentiated. Strauss and Lehtinen (1947) described the problem as follows: "The response of the brain-injured child to the school situation is frequently inadequate, conspicuously disturbing, and persistently troublesome" (p. 127).

A. R. Luria (1961) and L. Vygotsky (1934/1961), Russian neuropsychologists, were influential in the understanding of brain functioning and language development. Luria believed that the brain was made up of three functional units: the brainstem, involved with arousal and attention; the posterior portion, involved with taking in and processing of sensory information; and the anterior portion, implicated in planning, monitoring, and verifying one's performance. Luria and Vygotsky postulated that the development of language played an important part in one's ability to organize tasks involving planning, self-monitoring, and self-regulating. Individuals with brain damage who no longer use language for organization manifest extreme difficulties in self-regulatory and self-monitoring activities. Likewise, children who do not use language for organization do not develop self-regulation or planning skills. These ideas of Luria and Vygotsky have influenced the way we teach all students in developmentally appropriate early childhood classes.

Until recently, children with autism faced an even more uncertain future because of the lack of effective methods to compensate for their disability. For example, Bettelheim (1967) described the initial reaction to the orthogenic school and the problems of communication in an 11-year-old girl with autism:

At first what little speech she had consisted of very rare, simple, highly selective and only whispered echolalia. For example, when we asked her if she wanted some candy she would merely echo "candy." She would say "no" but never "yes"....It was not our language she used, but a private one of her own. (p. 162)

Currently, programs such as TEACCH (Treatment and Education of Autistic Children and Communication Handicapped Children) at the University of North Carolina in Chapel Hill provide expertise and technical assistance in diagnosis and treatment to teachers and parents of students with autism (Edwards & Bristol, 1991).

As with the child with brain damage or autism, the child who is socially disadvantaged has been an enigma in the classroom. Gordon (1968) characterized the child who is socially disadvantaged as unprepared for a normal educational experience. He wrote: "As a consequence, these children show in school disproportionately high rates of social maladjustment, behavioral disturbance, physical disability, academic retardation and mental subnormality" (p. 6). Many of the children formerly characterized as socially disadvantaged are now diagnosed with Attention Deficit/Hyperactivity Disorder (ADHD).

In 1963, at the first national meeting of what later became the Association for Children with Learning Disabilities (now named the Learning Disabilities Association of America), the term *learning disabilities* was identified by Samuel A. Kirk (1963):

Recently I have used the term "learning disabilities" to describe a group of children who have disorders in development, in language, speech, reading, and associated communication skills needed for social interaction. In this group I do not include children who have sensory handicaps such as blindness or deafness, because we have methods of managing and training the deaf and the blind. I also exclude from this group children who have generalized mental retardation. (p. 3)

Another impetus for the development of appropriate educational programs for individuals with disabilities was the formation of various organizations, such as the March of Dimes, National Easter Seal Society, and United Cerebral Palsy, designed to provide community-based services. Although these organizations originally provided resources for equipment and medical care for children with disabilities, parents of these children became politically proactive in obtaining rehabilitation hospitals and clinics, special education programs, community services, and barrier-free environments. These organizations have been instrumental in the development of support groups for families and in the publication and distribution of educational materials on prevention and treatment of disabilities.

Compared with children who have disabilities that cause severe problems in communication and learning; children with physical impairment who have normal language and sensory functions present different problems in habilitation. Physical barriers present problems in architectural design. Emotional and social adjustment is affected by the self-concept of children with disabilities, as well as by their feelings of competence. Other chronic disabilities of childhood such as juvenile arthritis, ulcerative colitis, childhood diabetes, heart defects, and epilepsy profoundly affect the child's development and require adaptive or specialized treatment methods.

### 1.9.6 Services for Individuals with Disabilities

Since the passing of Section 504 of the Rehabilitation Act in 1973, the Education for the Handicapped Act (EHA; Public Law 94–142) in 1974, the reauthorization and amendment of EHA as Public Law 99–457, the passing of the Americans with Disabilities Act (1990), the reauthorization and amendment of EHA as Public Law 101–456, also known as Individuals with Disabilities Education Act (IDEA) in 1990, the Individuals with Disabilities Education Act Amendments of 1997 (IDEA; PL. 105–17), No Child Left Behind in 2002 (NCLB, PL 107 – 110) and the reauthorization of IDEA through the Individuals

with Disabilities Education Improvement (IDEIA; PL 108–446) in December, 2004, programs for students with special needs have grown by leaps and bounds. For example, in 1976–1977, approximately 3.5 million students, ages 6 to 18, were served in special education. By 1987–1988, this number had risen to 4.1 million; and by 1996–1997, there were 5.3 million students, ages 6 to 21, or approximately 8.5 percent of the population (U.S. Department of Education, 1998). The latest figures, from 2004 show approximately 6 million students, ages 6 to 21, or approximately 9.2 percent of the population served in special education. This increase is a result of the increased number of students identified as autistic and ADHD since 1995. Additionally, the number of students ages 3 to 5 served in special education during the period 1995–2004 had grown 28 percent (U.S. Department of Education, Office of Special Education and Rehabilitative Services, Office of Special Education Programs, 2009).

Approximately 13.1 thousand occupational therapists were employed in educational and school settings during the 2007–2008 school year (Bureau of Labor Statistics, U.S. Department of Labor, 2010). Treatment and educational services are provided by public schools for any student from birth to age 21 who is at risk or is disabled. In addition, a continuum of services are available that range from consulting with the general education teacher about a student's needs, to providing an intense, restrictive residential setting for a student. Augmentative communication, life-skills training, and assistive technology are provided to the student when needed (Meyen & Skrtic, 1988; Smith & Tyler, 2010).

During the 1950s, 1960s, and 1970s, services for students with special needs were available primarily in residential institutions, special day schools, or special classes that were often physically isolated and segregated from the mainstreamed students. The concept of Least Restrictive Environment (LRE), delineated in EHA (PL. 94–142), states that each student will be educated in the program that allows him or her to be educated with his or her own peers to the maximum extent possible. Efficacy studies examining the effectiveness of special classes show mixed results. Earlier studies (Dunn, 1968;

Epps & Tindall, 1987; Haynes & Jenkins, 1986) found special education to be ineffective; however, more recent studies have suggested that students with learning disabilities and behavior disorders often show greater improvement in the special education classroom (Fuchs, Fuchs, & Fernstrom, 1993; Marston, 1987–1988). Madeline Will (1986), the Assistant Secretary of Education, strongly recommended that students with mild disabilities be returned to general education. She argued that general educators should take more responsibility for teaching these students. This position, originally called the Regular Education Initiative (REI), is now known as the General Education Initiative. Although some individuals, such as Sailor (1991) and Stainback and Stainback (1992) proposed total inclusion, that is, placement of all students, regardless of their educational needs, into their home schools and into the regular classroom, others (Vergason & Anderegg, 1992) encouraged a range of inclusiveness, with each student's placement based on individual needs and related to specific long-term goals. This latter stance appears to be more in accord with the concept of Least Restrictive Environment (LRE) as stated in IDEA and IDEIA.

Two factors have influenced changes in how services are provided to students in special education. First, NCLB mandated that students with special needs have access to the general education curriculum. Second, following the passage of IDEIA (2004), the Office of Special Education and Rehabilitation mandated the "implementation of a process known as response to intervention (RTI)" (Reynolds, 2008, p. 15) be used with students with learning disabilities. As a result, more than half of the students in special education are taught in the general education classroom with supports provided as needed (U.S. Department of Education, Office of Special Education and Rehabilitative Services, Office of Special Education Programs, 2009). With the increase in inclusive classes, additional training in collaborative techniques has been provided for general educators, special educators, occupational therapists, physical therapists, speech-language pathologists, school psychologists, and audiologists. Students with severe disabilities may continue to receive educational services in special class placements, especially when the educational needs include self-care skills and independent living skills.

Although much has been achieved in the development of programs and services for those individuals with special needs, there is much more to accomplish. There continue to be a greater percentage of students from minority groups placed in special education than those from the majority population. We are only beginning to understand how to remediate and improve cognitive and processing deficits. Augmentative communication, assistive technology (AT), and the use of computer-assisted instruction in education and training are still in the infancy stage of development. Although increased medical technology has made it possible to keep infants and patients with severe disabilities alive, we have only just begun to develop educational and training needs for these individuals.

Habilitation is the latest frontier in health research. Much research remains to develop the knowledge and technology that will facilitate growth and learning in the child with disabilities. The progress that has been made is the result of the persistent efforts of investigators devoting a lifetime of work to specific problems.

## 1.10 Research and the Future of Health Care

What are the future directions and goals of health care? The physician, an individual educated in the arts and science of healing, historically has been the primary health practitioner. At first, education of the physician was "at the foot of a master"; later, formal training permitted one to legally practice medicine. It is only in the last 130 years that medicine has become a science with reliable and valid methods. The science of modern medicine began with Claude Bernard and Louis Pasteur, who provided the research methods and theory of disease that underlie clinical practice. Progress has been dramatic since the late 1800s, culminating with the elimination of many major diseases through vaccination, chemotherapy, surgery, and effective hospital care. Preventive medicine is now the cornerstone of health maintenance. At the beginning of the twenty-first century, researchers are mobilizing their efforts to discover means to prevent premature deaths from heart disease, stroke, cancer, arthritis, emphysema, and AIDS. Ironically, chronic disabilities continue to persist as people live longer. As new diseases emerge (e.g., ebola virus), they present new challenges for medical researchers.

A second trend in medical progress is toward self-regulation of health care through education and monitoring of bodily symptoms. The individual's understanding of one's own anatomical, physiological, and psychological makeup through public health education continues to play an increasingly important role. Present trends have included Wellness as part of the curriculum. Educating the public toward an understanding of the relationship between mind and body is an example of the Wellness movement. The trend toward self-regulation in health will lead to more responsibility for one's own well-being in preventing illness through activities such as exercise, stress management, diet, and complementary medicines. Scientific research will explore the effectiveness of these methods.

Another trend in health care is the growth of specialized health professions. Up until 1920, the doctor and the nurse were the main health care providers. More than 100 health-related professions now exist. These new positions, such as cardiovascular technologist, respiratory therapist, nuclear medicine technologist, sanitarian, and public health educator, are the result of progress made in medical technology and the advancement of public health methods. New professions will continue to emerge from advanced technology. As research refines the diagnosis and treatment of illness, there will be a parallel growth in specialized health professions.

The medical practice of the future may well be dominated by machines that monitor physiological changes; control the heart rate; stimulate nerves, muscle, and skin; replace bodily organs; and, in general, receive and transmit information to and from the body (Longmore, 1970). These medical machines will be designed to adapt to the internal organism of the body. Computers connected to the machines will be programmed to interpret accurately the information received. This relationship is shown in Table 1–13.

Another trend in rehabilitation medicine is the merging of technology in assisting individuals with disabilities. For many years, professionals in rehabilitation have recognized the need to develop devices and apparati to help individuals with disabilities maximize their independence and functional activities. The growth of the fields of orthotics (braces and splints), self-help devices, prosthetics (design of artificial limbs), and assistive technology is a direct result of this vision. Methodological research in health care is an example of interdisciplinary cooperation

## TABLE 1-13

**Computer Application in Diagnosis and Treatment**

| Bodily Processes | Machine Monitoring | Computer Diagnosis |
| --- | --- | --- |
| • Circulatory | • Electrocardiogram | • Aids health professionals in diagnosis and prescription of treatment |
| • Gastrointestinal | • Electroencephalogram | |
| • Neurophysiological | • Respirator | |
| • Genitourinary | • Magnetic resonance imagery (MRI) | |
| • Skeletal-muscular | • Computerized axial tomography (CT-Scan) | |
| • Respiration | | |

between scientists. Biomedical engineering, which emerged as a complex multidisciplinary field incorporating medicine, engineering, psychology, economics, computer technology, law, sociology, and the environmental sciences, has grown rapidly in the last 60 years. Rushmer (1972), a researcher at the Center for Bioengineering, University of Washington, Seattle, was one of the first to describe the interaction of these multidisciplines. Table 1–14 is adapted from his description.

The Defense Advanced Research Projects Agency (DARPA) launched an initiative to develop technologically sophisticated upper extremity prosthetic devices. Titled *Revolutionizing Prosthetics 2007* and *Revolutionizing Prosthetics 2009*, the goals were to develop a prosthetic device that could mimic the functioning of a normal healthy upper extremity, including having five dexterous fingers, an articulating wrist with "normal" motion including flexion, extension, abduction, adduction, supination, and pronation. The limb is required to have an elbow strong enough to lift weight and a shoulder with range of motion to allow flexion above the head and internal rotation to reach behind the back. Additionally, the device is required to have a power source to last an entire day, be waterproof, have "normal" looking skin and weigh no more than 8 pounds (Beard, 2008).)

The merging of medicine with the social sciences to find solutions to the complex problems of mental illness, alcoholism, drug addiction, and criminology is inevitable. Interdisciplinary approaches to prevention and rehabilitation will result in the merging of the physical and social sciences. The study of the relationship between psychology and physiology and the immune system has led to the field of psychoneuroimmuniology. The relationship of poverty, alienation, malaise, and hopelessness (which are social variables) to the onset of disease, self-destruction, and social aggression have attracted the attention of health researchers who work closely with social scientists.

The controversy in the United States during the 1990s regarding the creation of a national health care system was influenced by the health consumer's concern about being denied the right to choose a health plan. The rise of health maintenance organizations (HMOs) and managed care in the 1990s brought attention to the issue of quality health care.

The Health Care Reform Bill of 2010 was signed into law by President Obama March 23, 2010 (Meckler & Hitt, 2010). This bill provides many substantial changes to the health care system in the United States. Some of these changes will begin to take place in a graded fashion for several years after being signed into law:

- In 2010, subsidies were made available to small businesses to help offset the cost of providing health insurance coverage for their employees. A notable change during 2010 was that insurance companies were barred from denying health insurance coverage for children with preexisting illnesses. Additionally, children were allowed to stay on their parent's health insurance until the age of 26 years.

- During 2011, a long-term care program initiative will begin where people who pay premiums into the long-term care program will become eligible for long-term care support payments if they require assistance in daily living.

- In 2014, "exchanges" will be created where individuals without employer health-care insurance, as well as small businesses, can shop for health-care coverage. Another significant change for 2014 is that insurance companies are barred from denying health insurance coverage to anyone with preexisting conditions. Additionally, 2014 is the year where most people are required to have health insurance. People at or below 133 percent of the federal poverty level will be required to pay a maximum of 3 percent of their income for coverage; people at 400 percent of the poverty level will be required to pay up to 9.5 percent of their income for coverage (the poverty level in 2010 for a family of 4 was $22,000). 2014 also marks the year when Medicaid expands to all Americans with income up to 133 percent of the federal poverty level. Additionally, subsidies will be available for small businesses to provide health insurance coverage.

## TABLE 1-14

### Examples of Biomedical Engineering to Health Care and Ecology

| Developments in Technology | | | |
| --- | --- | --- | --- |
| **Research Tools in Diagnosis** | **Clinical Interventions in Organ Systems** | **Diagnostic Procedures** | **Computer Applications** |
| Physical Measure (e.g., bone density) | Auditory (Hearing) | Chemical analysis | Data processing, such as in epidemiological studies |
| Chemical Composition (e.g., DNA) | Cardiovascular | Clinical microbiology | Analysis of large data sets to make clinical decisions |
| Microscopy (e.g., studying articular cartilage) | Gastrointestinal | Multiphasic screening (e.g., screening for multiple illnesses) | Retrieval of research findings for meta-analysis |
| Radiological (e.g., CAT-scan, MRI, fMRI, PET-scan) | Genitourinary | Pathology | |
| | Musculoskeletal | Robotic instruments | |
| | Neurological | | |
| | Respiratory | | |

| Therapeutic Techniques | | | |
| --- | --- | --- | --- |
| **Applied Therapies and Services** | **Inpatient Monitoring** | **Artificial and Replacement Organs** | **Transplants** |
| Assistive technology | Emergency care | Sensory aids | Liver |
| Occupational therapy | Intensive care | Heart-lung machine | Heart |
| Pharmaceutics | Nursing care | Artificial kidneys | Blood vessels |
| Physical therapy | Ward supervision | Artificial extremities: (e.g., myoelectric prostheses and mechanical arms and legs) | Kidneys |
| Radiation therapy | | | |
| Respiratory treatments | | | |
| Special education | | | |
| Speech-language therapy | | | |
| Surgical interventions | | | |

| Health Care System | | | |
| --- | --- | --- | --- |
| **Components** | **Methods and Improvements** | **Operations Research** | **Cost Benefit Analysis** |
| Organization of state health care systems (e.g., Medicaid) | Support functions (e.g., patient care) | Optimization of laboratories | Cost accounting |
| Medical economics (e.g., cost of Medicare) | Service functions | Personnel selection and retention | Evaluation of results |
| Long-range planning (e.g., single payment and its implication for quality care) | • Nursing | Processing and scheduling of patients in hospitals and clinics | Continuous quality improvement |
| Facilities design (e.g., hospital and clinical buildings) | • Medical care | | |
| | • Community care | | |
| | • Independent living | | |

| Environmental Engineering | |
| --- | --- |
| **Pollution Control** | **Aerospace** |
| Air | Environment control (e.g., in creating living habitation in alien environments) |
| Water | Closed ecological systems (e.g., in space travel) |
| Noise | Physiological adaptation to extreme environments (e.g., on the moon) |
| Solid waste | Heat conservation (e.g., NASA space suits) |
| Food | Communication (e.g., in telemedicine) |

The plan to finance these changes involves a combination of cost-saving Medicare policies, increased Medicare wage taxes, a new tax on unearned income, annual fees for pharmaceutical and insurance companies (in the billions of dollars), other taxes, and fines/penalties for those who don't carry health-care coverage. In summary, the Health Care Reform Bill of 2010 promises that more people will have health insurance coverage, regardless of preexisting illnesses. Although there is some controversy over this bill (e.g., the magnitude of changes and its associated costs), it does increase accessibility of health care insurance to many individuals who otherwise would and have gone without such health care insurance (Meckler & Hitt, 2010).

Currently, health care is dominated by a biomedical model in which prescriptive drugs have dominated treatment. The overprescribing of drugs such as Prozac®, Ritalin®, Tagamet®, and the overuse of drugs such as Ibuprofen® by the general public have led many health care consumers to alternative medicines. It is hoped that research will resolve the conflict between the biomedical model and alternative medicine, promoting a holistic approach to health care.

A delicate balance between governmental intervention and the respect for the sanctity and privacy of the individual must be maintained. The right of every individual to the very best health care should be among the most important priorities for every nation. In evaluating and treating clients, occupational therapy and special education should be guided by the application of sound research. In the following chapters, the methods and procedures intrinsic to scientific research applied to occupational therapy and special education are presented.

In 1998, the World Health Organization examined the international health trends. This report can be obtained at http://www.who.int/whr/1998/media_centre/50facts/en/index.html and is reproduced in the following chart.

---

**50 Facts: Global Health Situation and Trends 1955–2025**

*(Source: Reproduced with permission from the World Health Organization, http://www.who.int/whr/1998/media_centre/50facts/en/index.html)*

Population

1. The global population was 2.8 billion in 1955 and is 5.8 billion now. It will increase by nearly 80 million people a year to reach about 8 billion by the year 2025.

2. In 1955, 68% of the global population lived in rural areas and 32% in urban areas. In 1995 the ratio was 55% rural and 45% urban; by 2025 it will be 41% rural and 59% urban.

3. Every day in 1997, about 365,000 babies were born, and about 140,000 people died, giving a natural increase of about 220,000 people a day.

4. Today's population is made up of 6 million children under 5; 1.7 billion children and adolescents aged 5–19; 3.1 billion adults aged 20–64; and 390 million over 65.

5. The proportion of older people requiring support from adults of working age will increase from 10.5% in 1955 and 12.3% in 1995 to 17.2% in 2025.

6. In 1955, there were 12 people aged over 65 for every 100 aged under 20. By 1995, the old/young ratio was 16/100; by 2025 it will be 31/100.

7. The proportion of young people under 20 years will fall from 40% now to 32% of the total population by 2025, despite reaching 2.6 billion—an actual increase of 252 million.

8. The number of people aged over 65 will rise from 390 million now to 800 million by 2025—reaching 10% of the total population.

9. By 2025, increases of up to 300% of the older population are expected in many developing countries, especially in Latin America and Asia.

10. Globally, the population of children under 5 will grow by just 0.25% annually between 1995–2025, while the population over 65 years will grow by 2.6%.

11. The average number of babies per woman of child-bearing age was 5.0 in 1955, falling to 2.9 in 1995 and reaching 2.3 in 2025. While only 3 countries were below the population replacement level of 2.1 babies in 1955, there will be 102 such countries by 2025.

Life expectancy

12. Average life expectancy at birth in 1955 was just 48 years; in 1995 it was 65 years; in 2025 it will reach 73 years.

13. By the year 2025, it is expected that no country will have a life expectancy of less than 50 years.

14. More than 50 million people live today in countries with a life expectancy of less than 45 years.

15. Over 5 billion people in 120 countries today have life expectancy of more than 60 years.

16. About 300 million people live in 16 countries where life expectancy actually decreased between 1975–1995.

17. Many thousands of people born this year will live through the 21st century and see the advent of the 22nd century. For example, while there were only 200 centenarians in France in 1950, by the year 2050, the number is projected to reach 150,000—a 750-fold increase in 100 years.

Age structure of deaths

18. In 1955, 40% of all deaths were among children under 5 years, 10% were in the 5–19 year-olds, 28% were among adults aged 20–64, and 21% were among the over-65s.

19. In 1995, only 21% of all deaths were among the under-5s, 7% among those 5–19, 29% among those 20–64, and 43% among the over-65s.

20. By 2025, 8% of all deaths will be in the under-5s, 3% among 5–19 year-olds, 27% among 20–64 year-olds and 63% among the over-65s.

Leading causes of global deaths

21. In 1997, of a global total of 52.2 million deaths, 17.3 million were due to infectious and parasitic diseases; 15.3 million were due to circulatory diseases; 6.2 million were due to cancer; 2.9 million were due to respiratory diseases, mainly chronic obstructive pulmonary disease; and 3.6 million were due to perinatal conditions.

22. Leading causes of death from infectious diseases were acute lower respiratory infections (3.7 million), tuberculosis (2.9 million), diarrhea (2.5 million), HIV/AIDS (2.3 million) and malaria (1.5–2.7 million).

23. Most deaths from circulatory diseases were coronary heart disease (7.2 million), cerebrovascular disease (4.6 million), other heart diseases (3 million).

24. Leading causes of death from cancers were those of the lung (1.1 million), stomach (765,000), colon and rectum (525,000), liver, (505,000), and breast (385,000).

Health of infants and small children

25. Spectacular progress in reducing under-5 mortality achieved in the last few decades is projected to continue. There were about 10 million such deaths in 1997 compared to 21 million in 1955.

26. The infant mortality rate per 1,000 live births was 148 in 1955; 59 in 1995; and is projected to be 29 in 2025. The under-5 mortality rates per 1,000 live births for the same years are 210, 78, and 37 respectively.

*continues*

**50 Facts: Global Health Situation and Trends 1955–2025** *continued*

27. By 2025 there will still be 5 million deaths among children under five—97% of them in the developing world, and most of them due to infectious diseases such as pneumonia and diarrhea, combined with malnutrition.

28. There are still 24 million low-birth weight babies born every year. They are more likely to die early, and those who survive may suffer illness, stunted growth or even problems into adult life.

29. In 1995, 27% (168 million) of all children under 5 were underweight. Mortality rates are 5 times higher among severely underweight children than those of normal weight.

30. About 50% of deaths among children under 5 are associated with malnutrition.

31. At least two million a year of the under-5 deaths could be prevented by existing vaccines. Most of the rest are preventable by other means.

Health of older children and adolescents

32. One of the biggest 21st century hazards to children will be the continuing spread of HIV/AIDS. In 1997, 590,000 children age under 15 became infected with HIV. The disease could reverse some of the major gains in child health in the last 50 years.

33. The transition from childhood to adulthood will be marked for many in the coming years by such potentially deadly "rites of passage" as violence, delinquency, drugs, alcohol, motor accidents and sexual hazards such as HIV and other sexually transmitted diseases. Those growing up in poor urban areas are more likely to be most at risk.

34. The number of young women aged 15–19 will increase from 251 million in 1995 to 307 million in 2025.

35. In 1995, young women aged 15–19 gave birth to 17 million babies. Because of population increase, that number is expected to drop only to 16 million in 2025. Pregnancy and childbirth in adolescence pose higher risks for both mother and child.

Health of adults

36. Infectious diseases will still dominate in developing countries. As the economies of these countries grow, non-communicable diseases will become more prevalent. This will be due largely to the adoption of "western" lifestyles and their accompanying risk factors—smoking, high-fat diet, obesity and lack of exercise.

37. In developed countries, non-communicable diseases will remain dominant. Heart disease and stroke have declined as causes of death in recent decades, while death rates from some cancers have risen.

38. About 1.8 million adults died of AIDS in 1997 and the annual death toll is likely to continue to rise for some years.

39. Diabetes cases in adults will more than double globally from 143 million in 1997 to 300 million by 2025 largely because of dietary and other lifestyle factors.

40. Cancer will remain one of the leading causes of death worldwide. Only one-third of all cancers can be cured by earlier detection combined with effective treatment.

41. By 2025 the risk of cancer will continue to increase in developing countries, with stable if not declining rates in industrialized countries.

42. Cases and deaths of lung cancer and colon or rectal cancer will increase, largely due to smoking and unhealthy diet, respectively. Lung cancer deaths among women will rise in virtually all industrialized countries, but stomach cancer will become less common generally, mainly because of improved food conservation, dietary changes and declining related infection.

43. Cervical cancer is expected to decrease further in industrialized countries due to screening. The incidence is almost four times greater in the developing world. The possible advent of a vaccine would greatly benefit both the developed and developing countries.

44. Liver cancer will decrease because of the results of current and future immunization against the hepatitis B virus in many countries.

45. In general, more than 15 million adults aged 20–64 are dying every year. Most of these deaths are premature and preventable.

46. Among the premature deaths are those of 585,000 young women who die each year in pregnancy or childbirth. Most of these deaths are preventable. Where women have many pregnancies the risk of related death over the course of a lifetime is compounded. While the risk in Europe is just one in 1,400, in Asia it is one in 65, and in Africa, one in 16.

Health of older people

47. Cancer and heart disease are more related to the 70–75 age group than any other; people over 75 become more prone to impairments of hearing, vision, mobility and mental function.

48. Over 80% of circulatory disease deaths occur in people over 65. Worldwide, circulatory disease is the leading cause of death and disability in people over 65 years.

49. Data from France and the United States show breast cancer on average deprives women of at least 10 years of life expectancy, while prostate cancer reduces male average life expectancy by only one year.

50. The risk of developing dementia rises steeply with age in people over 60 years. Women are more likely to suffer than men because of their greater longevity.

# CHAPTER 2

# The Scientific Method and Research Models

*Scientific research is a systematic, controlled, empirical, and critical investigation of hypothetical propositions about presumed relations among natural phenomena.*

—F. N. Kerlinger, 1973,
*Foundations of Behavioral Research* (2nd ed.), p. 11

## Operational Learning Objectives

By the end of this chapter, the learner will:
- Define the following terms:
  - *research*
  - *theory*
  - *scientific method*
  - *independent and dependent variable*
  - *associational or statistical relationship*
  - *hypothesis*
- Give examples of common fallacies in scientific thinking.

- Outline and analyze the components of a research article.
- Identify overall objectives of the researcher.
- Contrast the nomothetic and idiographic methods of scientific inquiry.
- Compare and contrast research models.
- Compare and contrast quantitative, qualitative, and action research.

## 2.1 Science, Research, and Theory

The concept of the scientific method was first introduced by the Greeks, who proposed that knowledge is enacted by a hypothesis that leads to observation and logical reasoning (Northrop, 1931). The scientific method ensures an empirical view of the world. In general, the scientific method can be summarized in four steps:

1. A hypothesis that is testable is proposed.
2. Objective observations are collected.
3. Results are analyzed in an unbiased manner.
4. Conclusions proposed are based on the results of the study and previous knowledge.

The dictionary definition of **research** is "the diligent and systematic inquiry, or investigation into a subject in order to discuss facts or principles" (Barnhard, 1948). *Science* is defined as the "systematic, objective study of empirical phenomena and the resultant bodies of knowledge" (Gould & Kolb, 1964). Research and science are almost identical in definition; both imply systematic objective inquiry resulting in knowledge. Scientific **theory**, on the other hand, is a comprehensive explanation of empirical data. Theory predicts what will be observed through research. A theory represents a *deductive* system of understanding the world. It predicts laws in nature that form consistent cause-effect relationships. Theories are developed by considering the underlying processes, linking an observed cause with an effect.

For example, when medical scientists investigated the relationship between a specific bacteria and the cause of a disease, a theory was proposed to explain this relationship. The theory served as the *underlying explanation*, that is, the link between the **independent variable** (presumed cause) and **dependent variable** (presumed effect). This relationship is schematically diagramed in Figure 2–1 (Gould & Kolb, 1964).

### 2.1.1 Theory Building

Theory building is a key part of research. Many assumed cause-effect relationships instead may be in actuality *associational* or *statistical relationships* where a direct one-to-one ratio between cause and effect does not exist. Instances of associational relationships are those phenomena in nature that may occur together, such as precipitation in India and an increased birth rate or solar activity and wars. By proposing a theory, a researcher seeks to explain the direct relationship between observed causes and effects. Theory building is a way of distinguishing those relationships that are interdependent. Theories may also be developed by scientists who have systematically collected data. Generally, scientific theories generate research and predict relationships between variables.

### 2.1.2 Characteristics of a Theory

A *theory* is defined "as a set of interrelated constructs (concepts), definitions and propositions

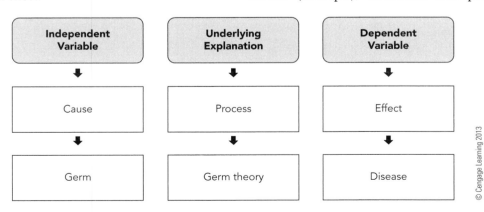

**FIGURE 2-1**   The Relationship Between the Independent and Dependent Variable

that present a systematic view of phenomena by specifying relations among variables, with the purpose of explaining and predicting phenomena" (Kerlinger, 1986, p. 9). In general, scientific theories are characterized by certain assumptions:

- **Technical vocabulary, language, or terms are generated by a theory.** For example, Piaget, in developing a theory of cognitive development, introduced the terms *assimilation, accommodation,* and *differentiation.* Theorists now use these terms in child development to explain how a child thinks. Freud, in introducing the theory of psychoanalysis, gave new meaning to familiar terms such as *ego, id, super ego, unconscious, libido,* and *catharsis.* These terms lose their ordinary connotations and take on the precise meanings of the theorist.

- **Natural phenomena or behavior can be explained by a theory.** For example, Darwin's theory of evolution was shaped by his observations of animal behavior and the examination of fossils. He formulated a theory from years of painstaking field observation. The pieces of evidence he amassed on animal and plant evolution were mosaics that he put together like a picture puzzle to form a theory. His research expeditions were guided by questions that sought to explain the wide variations in animal behavior that he observed in his travel expeditions to South America.

- **A theory is a tentative set of beliefs that can be verified by scientific research.** Pasteur, in 1863, proposed the germ theory after proving that microorganisms caused the processes of putrefaction and fermentation. In 1880, Koch built on the work of Pasteur by completing scientific laboratory investigation of tuberculosis and cholera, thus demonstrating the validity of the germ theory. Koch's (1878/1880) postulates were an example of deterministic causality. To prove that an organism causes a disease, he required that (a) the organism must be isolated in every case of the disease (i.e., be necessary); (b) the organism must be grown in pure culture; (c) the organism must always cause the disease when inoculated into an experimental animal (i.e., be sufficient) and (d) the organism must then be recovered from the experimental animal and identified.

- **A theory predicts events that can be simulated in the laboratory or observed under controlled conditions.** The theory of genetic determinacy predicts that a child born with a chromosomal deficit such as Down syndrome will be intellectually disabled. An infant is diagnosed with Down syndrome when an extra chromosome 21 is detected through genetic screening.

- **A theory allows a researcher to interpret results and form conclusions.** Konrad Lorenz (1937/1957), an ethnologist who received the Nobel Prize in Medicine, studied instinctive behavior patterns and proposed a theory of aggression. This theory seeks to explain the presence of conflicts and wars throughout human history.

- **A theory generates knowledge and leads to the development of further theories.** Gesell's (1928) theory of development predicted that normal human growth is based on sequential, hierarchical stages that unfold at critical ages. Other theorists, such as Erikson (1950; eight stages of psychosocial development), Kohlberg (1981; theory of moral reasoning), and Brofenbrenner (1979; theory of ecological systems), were greatly influenced by Gesell's works in the 1920s.

- **A theory can be completely or partially true or completely or partially false.** When Freud proposed the psychoanalytic theory at the turn of the nineteenth century, many of his colleagues completely rejected his work as unsubstantiated and based on clinical speculation. Psychoanalysis was later incorporated into psychiatric treatment programs, especially in the United States, from the beginning of the twentieth century until about 1960 when criticism started to appear in the professional journals. Many parts of Freud's theory, such as the terms he defined, are widely used in many studies of psychotherapy. Is psychoanalysis a valid theory of behavior? This question is still unresolved.

For clinical research, theories are a critical component in a study. To paraphrase Kurt Lewin (1939), nothing is as practical as a good theory. A scientific theory implies that phenomena or events in the world can be explained in a logical or rational way. Theories are the engines for scientific research that encompass an inductive system of knowledge. Data, which are collections of facts or information, result from research and, in turn, can eventually generate scientific laws. The systematic collection of data entails procedures for the review of previous results, the selection of research subjects, and the use of measuring instruments.

The relationship between theories and laws are diagramed in Figure 2–2. In all scientific research, the objectivity of the investigator is the most crucial variable. How a clinician or practitioner gains knowledge is often through the process of constructivism. Proponents of this paradigm of learning (constructivism) believe that a person gains knowledge through relating a personal experience to what he or she already knows. Constructivism is learner-driven, rather than teacher-initiated (Dewey, 1964; Piaget, 1977; Steffe & Gale 1995; Vygotsky, 1986). A person can construct his or her knowledge base in a number of ways. Figure 2–3 describes major factors that promote constructivism.

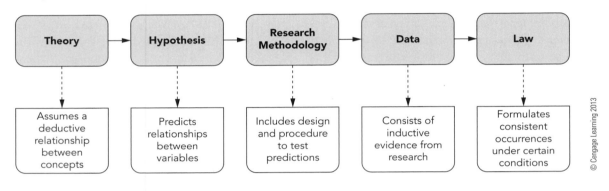

© Cengage Learning 2013

**FIGURE 2-2** Relationship between theory and law: A theory can become a law only through accurate and systematic research.

### CONSTRUCTING A KNOWLEDGE BASE

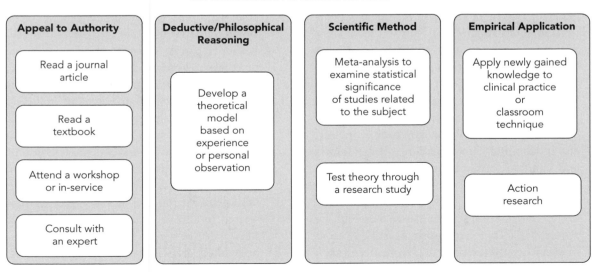

© Cengage Learning 2013

**FIGURE 2-3** Factors that promote constructivism or the construction of one's knowledge base

## 2.2 Fallacies Related to Research

Before the development of scientific research at the turn of the century, our knowledge of medicine rested on a combination of trial and error methodology and deductive reasoning based on a priori assumption. Fallacies growing out of the acceptance of invalid methods of treatment were common during times of superstition, such as in the Dark Ages in Europe and in primitive societies. These fallacies are incorrect arguments that are psychologically persuasive and, in some societies, continue to influence health practices. For example, contemporary practitioners who treat patients with methods that have no theoretical foundation act as if there were data supporting their methods. Some clinicians advocate a particular treatment method or drug based on the fallacious premise that a disease is highly prevalent, and therefore, any treatment is better than no treatment. Also, explanations by "authorities in the field" are used to support therapeutic applications. In the past, experimentation with radical procedures, such as the use of psychosurgery with psychiatric patients, was rationalized as relevant to treatment merely because the patients were severely psychotic and considered hopeless.

Or, to cite another fallacy, people refuse to accept data linking smoking to lung cancer and heart disease because they assume it cannot happen to them, but only to other persons. A knowledge of the more common fallacies is helpful to analyze objectively the validity of published studies. Copi (1953) proposed common fallacies that can occur in scientific research. These fallacies and others applied to health research and clinical practice are listed here.

### 2.2.1 Irrelevant Conclusion

This fallacy is evident when investigators intend to establish a particular conclusion by shifting their argument to another conclusion. For example, a clinician seeks support for a treatment method for patients with arthritis by arguing that arthritis is a crippling disease affecting millions of individuals. The fallacy in this argument is that the clinician proposes the acceptance of a treatment method based on the irrelevant fact that a specific disease is widespread. In this case, the specific treatment method that is introduced requires objective data to support its use, irrespective of the pressing need to help patients with arthritis. Another example of this fallacy in research is the use of unreliable or invalid tests because no other tests for measuring a specific variable exist. For example, a test written in English is given to a speaker whose first language is Navajo because there are no tests written in Navajo. Results obtained are questionable and probably invalid. If a test is invalid or unreliable, it should not be used to measure function.

### 2.2.2 Appeal to Authority

It is fallacious for a researcher to accept the opinions of respected scientists on the sole basis of their reputation but without any supporting data. For example, in recognizing an authority's knowledge of nutrition, investigators may use their opinions to support a position that megavitamins are an effective treatment for patients with schizophrenia. The authority on nutrition may not have any research data to support or negate this position. A respected authority's personal opinion is not valid scientific evidence. Researchers who appeal to authorities as supporting evidence fail to separate the scientists' previous reputations from their current opinions. In an age of specialization, scientists are no longer encyclopedists who are knowledgeable in all areas. The intensive study required for excellence in one area makes it almost impossible to have expertise even in related areas. When researchers use greatly respected scientists' opinions as supporting evidence, especially outside their area of competence, they are committing the fallacy of appeal to authority.

### 2.2.3 False Cause

This fallacy is common in societies where superstition and ignorance of cause and effect exist. Curing diseases through special amulets, magical words, or patent medicines are examples of the use of false cause. It is also common in nonexperimental research where correlational relationships are observed. For example, it may be noted that a full moon is associated with an increase in admissions to psychiatric hospitals. The relationship between the full moon and insanity (Raison, Klein, & Steckler, 1999) is then fallaciously transposed to the conclusion that a full moon causes insanity. A cause-and-effect relationship is not established by correlational data.

In the absence of valid causes of a disease, simple and reductive explanations often are accepted. For example, a researcher investigating a complex variable, such as a learning disability, may accept *prima facie evidence* that the learning disability is caused by hyperactivity. The researcher bases this conclusion on correlational evidence that children with a learning disability are also hyperactive. The fallaciousness of the argument is illustrated in Figure 2–4.

In this hypothetical example, not all individuals with ADHD have a learning disability, although a large number of individuals with a learning disability do have ADHD. Nonetheless, there is no evidence to support the conclusion that ADHD causes a learning disability or that a learning disability causes ADHD. The very nature of a complex variable presupposes multiple causes and interactional effects among variables.

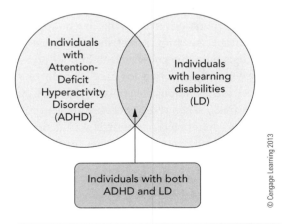

© Cengage Learning 2013

**FIGURE 2-4** The diagram depicts the fallacy of the argument that all individuals with Attention-Deficit/Hyperactivity Disorder (ADHD) are learning disabled. In fact, there are two populations: individuals with ADHD and those with learning disabilities. A few individuals have both conditions.

Another example of false cause in clinical practice is observing the effectiveness of a treatment method without adequately explaining the direct effect of treatment on improvement. Even though a treatment method is associated sequentially with improvement, it does not logically follow that it alone changed the patient's condition. There may be other factors in a patient's experience or in the research conditions that could have contributed to a patient's or subject's improvement. These potential factors, which could affect the result of an experiment, must be controlled before a researcher can conclude that a specific treatment affects improvement. For example, the **placebo effect** (or "dummy treatment") is widely recognized in drug research as a change in a condition brought about seemingly by a drug, but in reality by the power of suggestion that is attached to a drug. The **Hawthorne effect** is another example of a camouflaged relationship between cause and effect. In the Hawthorne effect, the change in behavior is produced by the attention of the researcher or clinician to the subjects or patients, rather than solely by the specific treatment method applied. False cause is a fallacy based on traditional thinking or superstition and without supporting research evidence.

### 2.2.4 Ambiguity

The lack of rigor in operationally defining terms and variables used in research produces the fallacy of ambiguity. When researchers compare outcome studies of wellness, perception, functional capacity, or weight loss, false conclusions may result if their comparisons fail to acknowledge the differences in defining and measuring these variables. Wellness can be defined in multiple ways and is measured by various tests and outcome measures. How the researcher defines and measures wellness will affect the conclusions and comparisons made. When a researcher states that there is a direct relationship between healthy living and wellness, one must denote how these variables were operationally defined. Otherwise, one may be operating on a simplistic and false basis that fails to take into consideration the various ways of operationally defining wellness.

For the purpose of explanation, let us examine a hypothetical example of ambiguity as shown in Table 2–1. In this example, if the researcher did not state how these two variables—healthy living and wellness—are operationally defined, then there is no basis for comparing the results. In actuality, there are many different studies measuring the relationship between these two abstract variables. For example, in one study, the researcher could examine the effects of nutrition on the four outcome measures; in another study, exercise could be substituted for nutrition. Each of these presumed causes and effects will need to be elaborated on further so that another researcher can replicate the study.

Researchers must operationally define complex abstract variables that they investigate; that is, the measuring instrument or procedure must be clearly identified before studies can be compared and conclusions proposed. Ambiguity is an example of comparing "apples with oranges." For example, an investigator decides to use diet therapy as an *independent variable* (presumed cause) and weight reduction as the *dependent variable* (presumed effect); however, the specific method employed in diet therapy and the method used in measuring weight reduction are the variables that are, in fact, being investigated, not diet therapy or weight reduction per se. Clearly, operationally defining variables is important in eliminating the fallacy of ambiguity.

## 2.2.5 Generalization

Much scientific research involves collecting group data from a representative sample of a target population. Group data represent the average of all individual scores. Also, the data imply a range of scores from high to low on specific measured variables. The fallacy of generalization occurs when a researcher applies group data to a specific individual subject. For example, a researcher collects evidence of a statistically significant relationship between the absence of epilepsy and the occurrence of schizophrenia. The researcher concludes this from a study of seizures in which there were fewer individuals with epilepsy among patients with schizophrenia compared to the general population.

The statistics are based on probability factors, not on a one-to-one relationship, however. The investigator can conclude only that there are fewer individuals with epilepsy in a population of individuals also exhibiting schizophrenia than in the general population, but not that every individual with epilepsy will not become schizophrenic, nor that every individual with schizophrenia will not be epileptic. Nor can one conclude that if epilepsy is produced through electric shock, schizophrenia can be prevented or treated. This is a fallacy where group data describing a population is generalized to every individual in the population.

### TABLE 2-1

**Operationally Defining Ambiguous Terms**

| Presumed Cause: Healthy Living | Presumed Effect (outcome measures): Wellness |
| --- | --- |
| 1. Balanced diet | 1. Trips to a physician |
| 2. Adequate exercise | 2. Self-report |
| 3. Reduction of stress | 3. Findings from a physical examination |
| 4. Positive interpersonal relationship | 4. Standardized test of wellness |

Group data cannot be applied to individuals whenever probability statistics do not approach 100 percent. The error variance in probability makes it impossible to make predictions about the specific individual from group data. One can only describe the general characteristics of groups, not the individual subjects that comprise the group. From probability statistics, we can describe groups of patients, students, hospitals, or schools, but we are unable to predict the individual case with any complete certainty. For example, Alberg and Samet (2003), in reviewing the literature, reported that 90 percent of people who get lung cancer are smokers; however, we cannot predict which of those individuals who smoke will actually develop lung cancer.

Another example of generalization fallacy is in the selection of students based on entry examinations, such as the Scholastic Aptitude Test or Graduate Record Examination (GRE). For example, a researcher interested in predicting academic success in an occupational therapy program may find a positive correlation of $r = .73$ between aptitude test scores and grade point averages. This is not a perfect correlation however; it indicates only that many students with high aptitude test scores will attain relatively high grade point averages. If a program director has to predict a specific individual's success or failure, the data cannot support complete accuracy. In fact, the chance of error in predicting a specific individual's grade point average is high, although there may be accuracy in predicting a group's success in a program.

An example of the fallacy of generalization applied to clinical treatment is the **"Procrustean bed."** In this case, clinicians who advocate a specific treatment method apply this method as a panacea to all patients, regardless of individual differences. The clinician falsely applies the treatment method as a cure-all. For example, in the fifteenth and sixteenth centuries, tobacco was thought to have several therapeutic purposes and was considered to be a panacea for health. In the mid-twentieth century, the harmful effect of tobacco was established (Fraga, 2010). Good treatment implies fitting the best available treatment method to the individual based on his or her needs, rather than fitting the patient to a panacea.

In spite of the strong arguments used to convince researchers and clinicians to accept the findings of a study or the efficacy of a treatment method, consumers of research must recognize the fallacies of irrelevant conclusion, appeal to authority, false cause, ambiguity, and generalization as totally unacceptable means of advancing knowledge. The following discussion includes positive guidelines for analyzing the research process and the qualities of the researcher.

## 2.3 Critical Analysis of the Research Process

How is a research study judged to be either adequate or valid? How does one analyze the components of research and detect the biases of the investigator, the limitations of the design, and the deficiencies of the sampling procedure? The consumer of research must critically evaluate the methodology of a study before fully accepting the results and conclusions. Many times, the results of a study are reported in the media without evaluating the methodology. The results of research can play a prominent role in supporting or negating a particular theory or social action.

Governmental policies affecting funding patterns and priorities of social programs are influenced by the results of research studies. For example, continued funding of the children's television program *Sesame Street* is dependent on data that support the position that the program has educational value. Early childhood programs such as Head Start, manpower retraining, state mental health systems, and graduate training programs in occupational therapy professions are examples where evaluation research is used to justify federal grant support. The unfortunate policy of "benign neglect" toward minority groups during the latter half of the 1960s and the 1970s was a result of government-sponsored research that supported the discontinuance of many antipoverty programs. When research is used as evidence to initiate or discontinue social programs, there is an obvious need to evaluate methodology before accepting or rejecting the conclusions. Research is not acceptable merely on the basis of social appeal, no matter how noble the conclusions. Political considerations are one of the abuses of research that confront investigators of controversial social issues, such as community health programs or family planning.

In spite of the diversity in content and the differences in application to treatment, all research has a common methodological format. When a researcher poses a question, the process of research is initiated. The question generates a search of the literature, predictions of results, and a controlled objective procedure for collecting data. An investigator generates background questions to help lead into specific research questions. This is a way of helping students to discover research topics of interest to them and to narrow a research study to feasible dimensions.

Raising background questions is a "brainstorming" tactic to lead one into a review of the literature. The student or clinical investigator is encouraged to list as many basic questions as possible to initiate a study. For example, if the goal of a clinical research is to determine the most effective treatment methods for children with traumatic brain injury (TBI), the background questions related to TBI would include:

- How is TBI operationally defined?
- What are the diagnostic tests to identify TBI?
- What are the prevalence and incidence rates of TBI?
- What are the most common treatment methods for children with TBI?
- What are the research data supporting treatment interventions for TBI?
- What outcome measures are used to measure treatment effectiveness?
- What is the typical course of the disability?
- What is the prognosis of TBI?
- How can vocational rehabilitation be used to treat individuals with TBI?
- How are functional capacity evaluations applied?

The investigator uses a literature review to answer some of these background questions. This process enables the investigator to become familiar with the research literature and to begin narrowing the study. In general, research is a process of systematically accumulating knowledge. What has been done previously is incorporated into current research. Background questions generate the research process and set in motion the beginning stages of completing a research study. Figure 2–5 describes this process.

The following outline of a research study is based on the scientific method. It is a systematic and objective way to investigate a topic.

I. A *Title* includes variables investigated, populations studied, and the setting to which the results can be generalized to such as a hospital or outpatient clinic.

II. An *Abstract* is usually between 150 and 300 words, contains one or two sentences from each section of the research study, and summarizes the findings, limitations of the methods, and recommendations for further research.

III. The *Problem* includes the research questions examined and the stated need and significance of the study.

IV. A *Literature Review* contains the findings of related studies obtained through a systematic search.

V. *Stated Hypotheses* include the operationally defined variables and research predictions.

VI. A *Method* section includes procedures for selecting subjects, screening criteria, measuring instruments, and collecting data, as well as a plan for statistical analysis and obtaining human ethics approval.

VII. *Results* include objective findings that are statistically analyzed and organized into tables, charts, and graphs.

VIII. *Discussion, Conclusions, Limitations, and Recommendations* include the significance of the findings related to previous research and the implications for further investigations.

Each of the subsections can be analyzed by posing specific questions relating to the objectivity of

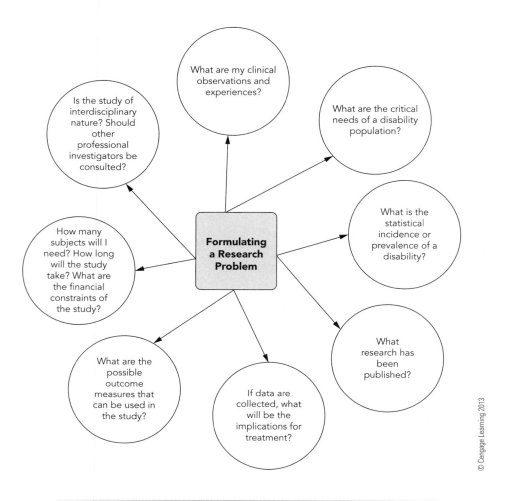

© Cengage Learning 2013

**FIGURE 2-5**  Raising basic questions, such as those in this figure, lead to a review of the literature as the beginning of a research study.

the investigator and the validity of the methods. For example:

**I.** Title

    **a.** Does the title of the study clearly define what the investigator actually did, or does it refer only to a segment of the study?

    **b.** Can the results of the study be generalized to the population identified by the title?

    **c.** Are the variables stated in the title identifiable and unambiguous?

**II.** Abstract

    **a.** Are the number of words between 150 and 300?

    **b.** Does the abstract include the highlights from each section of the study?

    **c.** Does the abstract summarize the findings or results of the study?

    **d.** Are implications or recommendations for further research summarized?

**III.** The Problem or Research Question

    **a.** Are the purposes or objectives of the study stated clearly?

    **b.** Are the research questions clearly identified?

    **c.** Is the study justified in relation to social need, significance, or potential contribution to occupational therapy?

**d.** Are statistics used to support the incidence and prevalence of a disability or to justify the investigation?

**e.** What is the relationship of the study to occupational therapy?

**f.** Does the study have a potential significant contribution to evaluation methods, treatment techniques, student training, or program administration?

**g.** Are the projected results of the study practical so they can be implemented into practice?

**h.** Is the researcher being objective in selecting a specific problem for investigation, or is there evidence that personal biases will affect the results?

**IV.** Literature Review

**a.** What information retrieval systems and primary sources of data did the investigator use in systematically reviewing the literature?

**b.** Are there theoretical assumptions that are unstated but are tacitly accepted?

**c.** What major areas were reviewed?

**d.** Was the literature search exhaustive in regard to the research problem?

**e.** Did the investigator use primary or secondary sources of information?

**f.** Was the investigator objective in listing results from studies that refute the stated hypotheses, as well as those studies that support the hypotheses?

**g.** How were previous studies reported? Did the investigator describe the number and characteristics of subjects and tests used when reporting the results of studies?

**h.** Are references up to date?

**i.** Did the researcher review a wide range of computer databases and journals related to the research topic?

**V.** Stated Hypotheses

**a.** Are independent and dependent variables identifiable?

**b.** Are variables operationally defined?

**c.** Did the investigator present guiding questions?

**d.** Were hypotheses generated from a review of the literature, and did the investigator cite previous findings?

**e.** Were the hypotheses stated in null form or directionally?

**VI.** Research Methods

**a.** How were the subjects selected for the study: randomly, convenience sample, or volunteers?

**b.** Were screening criteria used in selecting a representative sample?

**c.** Were subjects a representative sample for a specified target population?

**d.** How were the measuring instruments selected?

**e.** Did the investigator state the reliability and validity of measuring instruments?

**f.** Do the measuring instruments have a test manual including standardized procedures for data collection and scoring?

**g.** How did the researcher inform subjects of the risks and benefits of the study?

**h.** Can the research study be replicated?

**i.** Did the investigator carefully outline the procedure for data collection?

**VII.** Results

**a.** What statistical techniques were used in analyzing the data?

**b.** How were the results reported?

**c.** At what level of statistical significance were results accepted?

**d.** Were limitations of the study presented?

**VIII.** Discussion, Conclusions, and Recommendations

**a.** Were the findings incorporated with previous literature?

**b.** Were conclusions justified from reported results?

**c.** Is researcher bias evident in interpreting results or "rationalizing away" results?

**d.** Were there unforeseen events that influenced results?

**e.** Are results omitted that contradict the hypothesis?

**f.** Is further research indicated?

## 2.4 Qualities of a Researcher

What are the qualities of a researcher? Scholars analyzing the process of research consider that the researcher's attitudes and integrity are sometimes more important than the rigor of the methodology and the veneer of scientism. The following has been enlarged from Gee's (1950) discussion of a researcher's qualities.

### 2.4.1 Dissonance

The researcher feels uncomfortable with an aspect of the world and the problem serves as the motivation for carrying out the research. Research is perceived as problem oriented. For example, Semmelweis's concern over the large number of maternal deaths after pregnancy in the nineteenth century spurred him to initiate research into the causes of puerperal fever. Salk's experimenting with a vaccine to prevent polio was concerned with the alarming incidence of polio worldwide. These are two examples of medical researchers who were motivated by dissonance. Investigators starting with a problem such as delinquency, malnutrition, AIDS, cancer, or homelessness are energized and moved to action by the amount of pain, anxiety, and degradation that a problem produces in society and arouses public empathy.

### 2.4.2 Objectivity

This quality enables an investigator to follow the data where it takes one, instead of arriving at a conclusion first and then collecting data to support personal biases. Objectivity many times leads to accidental discoveries made through serendipity and happenstance. The researcher is open to accepting whatever the data reveal. Accidental discoveries of major significance are numerous in the history of science and technology: Bell's discovery of the telephone (1875); Edison's stumbling upon the phonograph (1877); Goodyear's accidentally inventing a process to vulcanize rubber (1839); Roentgen's noticing chemical changes on paper, which led to the invention of the X-ray (1895); and Fleming's discovery of penicillin (1928).

### 2.4.3 Perseverance

The scientist's persistence and dedication to an area of research are prominent in medicine. The history of medical research is filled with researchers such as the Curies, who devoted their entire professional lives to uncovering the properties of radium. Perseverance and persistence are necessary qualities if a researcher wants to uncover ample evidence before publishing findings. The pressure on the contemporary researcher to rush to publish results discourages persistent and painstaking efforts to accumulate overwhelming evidence. The tendency to release findings prematurely, such as in pharmaceutics, has led to medical calamities such as the effects of the drug Thalidomide on fetal development. The need still remains for the researcher to persevere in the face of the pressure to publish.

### 2.4.4 Intellectual Curiosity

The scientist pursues a topic not only for the practical benefits that may result from the study, but because of the desire to know. Basic research is ordinarily carried out because of the investigator's intellectual curiosity. The basic research that produced the breakthrough in understanding the anatomy and physiology of humans came about because of Renaissance scientists' need to know. How does the body function? What are the basic processes in cell division? What is the basic chemistry of living protoplasm? Questions regarding the essential nature of the universe and matter can be answered only by research conducted by individuals with intellectual curiosity. The researcher who earnestly seeks knowledge is likely to be diligent and persevere in attaining some significant goal.

### 2.4.5 Self-Criticism

The investigator pursuing an area of interest needs to evaluate work critically by redesigning problems, reworking hypotheses, and initiating new methods for collecting data. The ability to examine one's work critically is important in preventing stagnation. Research involves a continual process of questioning, of obtaining evidence, and of requestioning.

The data from research serve as feedback for the reformulation of hypotheses only if the researcher is able to criticize oneself objectively.

## 2.4.6 Creativity

Being creative does not necessarily mean being novel or different. The creative researcher juxtaposes different ideas and integrates previous knowledge with contemporary issues. The qualities of risk, innovation, and independence are aspects of creativity. At odds with creativity are conformity and the need to please others while denying one's own ideas. Creativity may be a necessary quality in the researcher who desires more than fulfilling the needs of a corporate body or serving as a data collector for someone else's mission. Formulating and planning a research design is a creative act. The process of identifying a research problem and designing an objective method to test a hypothesis demands a creative quality.

## 2.4.7 Integrity

The researcher represents an attitude of mind. In applied health and educational fields, the researcher must be guided by ethical principles that involve a respect for the rights of participants and the honesty to bide by one's own research design and report data as found. The researcher who is engaging in human research is ethically bound not to abuse participants. The demand by social action groups and consumer advocates for formalized regulations in regard to the use of human subjects—especially in institutional environments such as prisons, psychiatric centers, chronic disease hospitals, and state schools for individuals with intellectual disabilities—reflects the past abuses in human research. An informed consent contract between researcher and subject must be included in every research design. The contract shall include the following considerations:

1. The exact procedure to be carried out must be explained in language that is understandable to the participants. Jargon and technical terms should be avoided.
2. The possible physical and psychological side effects in the study and the steps taken by the researcher to prevent harm to the participants should be stated.
3. The participant's time commitment in the study, procedures involved, and place of study should be clearly stated.
4. If the participants are mentally or physically incompetent or under age, then legal guardians or parents should be asked to provide written consent for the participants' inclusion in a study.
5. If the researcher requires that the purposes of the study not be revealed to the participants, then the researcher should explain this openly to the participants.
6. The researcher should not use coercion through any means that imply social disapproval or penalize the participants for not participating in the study.
7. If participants are paid for participation in an experiment, it should be based on work and time considerations, not as a camouflaged attempt to disguise the risks involved in being a participant or as an inducement to vulnerable individuals.
8. The findings of the research are to be treated as confidential: an individual participant's data should not be identified. Ongoing research data should be stored in a locked cabinet or password protected computer located in a secure area.

No research is so important that it disregards the rights of participants. The practices during World War II by the Nazis who engaged in human research without any regard for human rights (Lipton, 2000) is an extreme example of the abuse of research done with fanaticism and conformity to political goals. A researcher's integrity should be within the confines of an ethical code that must go beyond the mere search for data. Research with human subjects is not a pure or amoral theoretical activity.

Integrity in research also involves honesty in abiding by a research design and in reporting data accurately. Many times overzealous researchers are eager to present a theory of treatment or technological advance without having conclusive evidence. The pressure to present significant or dramatic findings sometimes is a result of the researcher's ego.

Unfortunately, it may become more important for the researcher to gain personal distinction than to report one's data honestly. The scientific community frequently has witnessed personality struggles in which rival researchers engaged competitively while striving for national recognition (Watson, 1968). The research in heart transplants, cancer, and DNA has been marked by personality conflicts.

### 2.4.8 Replication

Scientific research does not exist in a vacuum, nor is it usually the product of a single individual. When researchers investigate something, they typically build on the work of others. Even the giants of science, such as Newton, Einstein, Pasteur, and Edison, were vitally aware of previous research findings in the literature. Replication means that the researcher is able to repeat an experiment that was reported previously. The researcher who initially carries through an experiment must be able to describe the methodology in sufficient detail to allow other researchers to repeat the experiment. Research is not a mysterious activity carefully guarded and left to mystics. It is an open activity in which a scientific community of scholars engages. Without replication, knowledge would be stagnant, as in the Dark Ages when researchers carefully hid their methods of alchemy and magic. In clinical research, it is vital that investigators share their findings with the clinical community and also receive feedback from clinicians who undertake pilot studies of new practices and treatments.

## 2.5 Nomothetic Versus Idiographic Methods

One of the most important goals in scientific research is prediction. Whether it is the prediction that a drug will cause certain beneficial effects in the body or that a surgical operation will improve the functioning of a bodily organ, the scientific investigator seeks to discover relationships that may be universally true. The search for general laws in nature is defined as a **nomothetic approach** to science. However, the individual is affected by numerous idiosyncratic factors, such as physiological, emotional, and social influences, that are complex, unique, and sometimes unpredictable. The **idiographic approach** to science pertains to the intensive study of individuals within their own particular genetic milieu and environment. The nomothetic approach tends to be quantitative research, whereas qualitative research is generally used with idiographic approaches.

### 2.5.1 Nomothetic Approach to Science

In nomothetic research, large groups are studied in order to find general laws and principles that apply to a specific population (Babbie, 2010). Therefore, a certain level of probability is assumed in that any given individual's behavior or response to an independent variable can be predicted with a certain level of confidence. Behavior modification and operant conditioning assume that individuals are operating under general laws of nature, especially defined as *reward* and *punishment* (Skinner, 1953). The precursors of behaviorism were the logical positivists who theorized that all meaningful scientific propositions are derived from experience and can be expressed in quantifiable physicalistic language (Spence, 1948). This concept of physicalism has tried to incorporate empirical methods of collecting data into the social sciences. The technology of the logical positivists in social science is based on empirical methods of experimental control and objective observation.

The major limitation of a nomothetic approach to social science is in the inability to operationally define and measure social variables such as motivation, interests, attitudes, emotions, and thinking. Another limitation of the nomothetic approach is that the naming of the disability or disease (e.g., autism or depression) can appear to the patient as a cure. For example, the naming of the disease or disability does not necessarily lead to successful treatment such as when a patient is diagnosed with bipolar depression. This patient may feel that the problem has been solved by naming the disease (Babbie, 2010).

Behaviorism and scientific empiricism apply a psychophysiological model; historically, the major contributions of behaviorism to social science has been by pioneers such as Pavlov (1927) in classical conditioning, Wolpe(1969) in desensitization experiments, and Miller (1969) in biofeedback and conditioning experiments of the autonomic nervous systems of the body.

### 2.5.2 Idiographic Approach to Science

Psychoanalysis (Tyson, 2009), phenomenology (Van Boven, Kane, McGraw, & Dale, 1998), Gestalt psychology (Ventegodt, Clausen, & Merrick, 2006), and the humanistic movement (Videler, van Royen, & van Alphen, 2010) in the social sciences are examples of idiographic approaches. The subjective nature of experience and the uniqueness of the individual are, in these approaches, the vantage points for investigations. Social scientists use the case study approach in trying to understand the dynamic forces that influence an individual's behavior. The individual is perceived as an active agent interacting with the world continuously and always in the process of change. Gestalt investigations are concerned with the perceptual processes and individual differences among people and within a humanistic framework (Perls, 1969). These idiographic approaches to scientific knowledge assume that prediction in human beings is limited to the single individual, as no two individuals share the same genetic background, physiological makeup, or psychological experiences.

How does an understanding of these two approaches, nomothetic and idiographic, affect our understanding of research in occupational therapy? In the nomothetic approach, we assume that general laws control human behavior and physiological responses. For example, in medicine, when an individual is treated with a drug for a specific illness, the physician assumes this patient will react as other individuals do to the same drug. Treatment is presented in relation to the illness, not in relation to the specific individual. Researchers investigating cause-and-effect relationships frequently assume a nomothetic approach. By contrast, with the idiographic approach, the clinician evaluates the patient by considering individual differences and idiosyncratic traits and treats by prescribing a specific regimen.

Case studies, single-subject design, and naturalistic observations are the methods used in idiographic approaches. The history of medicine, occupational therapy, rehabilitation, and special education contains many examples of both approaches. In analyzing a research study or designing an experiment, either a nomothetic (quantitative) or idiographic (qualitative) approach may be appropriate.

## 2.6 Types of Inquiry

There are two categories of scientific inquiry: retrospective and prospective. Each has its own advantages and disadvantages (Hill, 1971).

**Retrospective research** examines data or events from an historical viewpoint. For example, the investigator may be interested in the causes of multiple sclerosis or the evolution of multisensory teaching. In both cases, the investigation includes the analysis of sequential events leading to the current understanding of disease, events, or methodology. In correlational research, the investigator examines the relationship between two variables or two groups. For example, one might examine the relationship between perceptual abilities and intelligence. In retrospective designs, the investigator does not establish a cause-effect relationship.

**Prospective research**, on the other hand, predicts the effect of the independent variable on the dependent variable, thereby establishing a cause-effect relationship. In experimental prospective designs, the research manipulates the independent variable and observes its effect on the dependent variable. For example, in a study examining the effects of aquatic therapy on the reduction of symptoms in individuals with multiple sclerosis, the researcher provides aquatic therapy to an experimental group and compares it to a control group in which no aquatic therapy is provided.

The prospective design is also used in longitudinal research where a researcher examines the effects of a variable over time. For example, longitudinal research would be used in studies examining the effects of prenatal exposure to cocaine on academic success (Delaney-Black et al., 1998; Richardson, 1998).

The following are specific advantages and disadvantages (Hill, 1971):

- In a prospective method, the sample is more easily defined and may be more representative of a target population than in the retrospective design.
- Extraneous variables are more easily controlled in an experimental prospective design.
- In a longitudinal prospective design, such as in the Framingham Heart Study (Dawber & Kannel, 1958), individuals can be followed up over a long period of time to determine the impact of risk factors.
- In a retrospective design, the subjects can be identified as a convenient sample, and events or variables contributing to the condition can be studied in depth.
- One disadvantage of a retrospective design is that cause-effect cannot be determined by the results of the research; rather, a statistical or correlational relationship can be established and used as the basis for a prospective experimental design.

## 2.7 Models of Research

*Research* is defined as objective systematic investigation. The process of designing a research study is one of the most creative acts in science. In this process, the researcher can generate new knowledge, synthesize findings from different studies, and develop new theories by being innovative. The research design is an outline of the systematic plan for collecting data. From this outline, the investigator develops a plan of action. Table 2–2 describes the steps involved in designing a research study, and Figure 2–6 gives an example.

The diversity of research designs in occupational therapy is characterized by **problem-based research**. These studies might include the following: (a) evaluating the efficacy of a treatment method in occupational therapy, (b) surveying the attitudes of a population of individuals with spinal cord injury, (c) carrying out an organizational case study of a sheltered workshop for adults, (d) constructing a rating scale to evaluate student teachers or interns,

### TABLE 2-2

**Steps in Formulating a Feasible Question in Qualitative, Quantitative, and Action Research**

| Step | Tasks | Rationale | Example |
|------|-------|-----------|---------|
| 1 | List numerous questions about topics in which the clinician, teacher, or student is interested. | Allows the investigator to select areas of interest and locate relevant studies. | What are the most effective treatment methods for treating spasticity? |
| 2 | Locate a secondary source, such as a text or review article. | Enables the researcher to have an overview of the topic and provides a means for locating research articles. | A recent (within the last five years) textbook or review article on cerebral palsy. |
| 3 | Do a mini-literature review using primary sources (e.g., research articles). | Investigator becomes familiar with the current research in the area of interest. | A current (within the last three years) research article on treatment of spasticity. |
| 4 | Identify an expert in the field. | This expert can serve as an informal consultant for locating resources, identifying additional aspects, and narrowing the research. | A clinician or special educator who has worked with children with cerebral palsy. |

| Step | Tasks | Rationale | Example |
|------|-------|-----------|---------|
| 5 | Narrow the research topic. | When a research topic is too broad, the researcher has difficulty operationally defining the variables or generalizing the results. | Is Neurodevelopmental Treatment (NDT) more effective than Sensory-Integration (SI) therapy in reducing spasticity in children with cerebral palsy? |
| 6 | Determine the feasibility of the research question. | The ability to do the research is dependent on several factors, such as the availability of participants, time elements, costs of the study, or the ability to control extraneous variables. | NDT and SI are used with children with cerebral palsy in a children's care facility. |

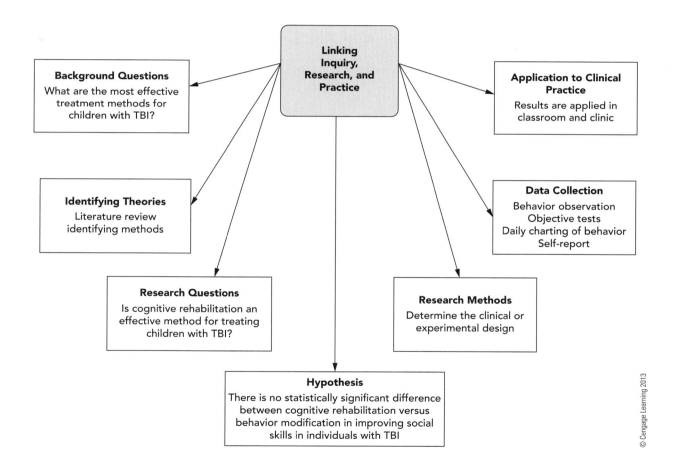

**FIGURE 2-6** Relationship among Scientific Inquiry, Theory, Research, and Clinical Practice: This relationship is pictured using an example of research in traumatic brain injury (TBI).

or (e) correlating a relationship between perceptual skills and academic ability. In each of these research examples, a method of data collection serves as the "skeleton" for the study. The research approach chosen is a decision based on the purposes of the study and the data collection methods available to the investigator. Approaches to research may include qualitative or quantitative analysis, action research, or a combination of any of these. Table 2–3 describes these approaches.

Research models appropriate to problems in occupational therapy, rehabilitation, and habilitation

## TABLE 2-3

### Comparison of Quantitative and Qualitative Research Methods

| | Quantitative | Qualitative |
|---|---|---|
| **Definition** | • Empirical method that is based on hypothesis testing and control and measurement of variables within a value-free framework | • Study of people and events in a natural setting to make sense of and obtain meaning from the phenomena observed and experienced, emphasizing a value-laden nature of inquiry (Denzin & Lincoln, 1994a) |
| **Underlying assumptions** | • Reality is based on natural laws that predict outcome (nomothetic). | • Reality is based on the subjective interpretation of the study (idiographic approach). |
| | • Variables are operationalized and the relationships between the variables can be measured. | • Variables are difficult to measure because of the complexity and interconnectedness. |
| | • The hypothesis is stated before data collection occurs. | • Analysis of data collection is heuristic and ends with grounded theory. |
| | • In experimental design, the investigator manipulates the independent variable(s) and measures the dependent variable(s). | • Variables emerge as the researcher collects and analyzes subjective data. |
| | • Standardized tests or procedures are used to collect data. | • Researcher as an interviewer serves as the instrument for collecting data. |
| | • The researcher assumes an objective, unbiased attitude toward participants. | • The researcher interacts on a personal, subjective level with the participants. |
| | • Representative samples of a target population are obtained through random sampling. | • A "snowballing effect" is used to obtain a convenience sample of the target population. |
| **Models for conducting research** | • Experimental | • Case study (retrospective or prospective) |
| | • Correlational | • Phenomenology |
| | • Methodological | • Biographical or historiography |
| | • Evaluation | • Ethnography |

| | Quantitative | Qualitative |
|---|---|---|
| | • Heuristic | • Grounded theory or heuristic |
| | • Case study (prospective) | • Survey (interview) |
| | • Survey (assessment) | |
| Techniques of data collection | • Structured forced-choice questionnaire and surveys | • Structured and unstructured interviews |
| | • Standardized tests or procedures (performance or paper and pencil) | • Case studies |
| | • Frequency count or interval recording | • Observation |
| | • Rate of response | • Diaries, journals, and personal experiences |
| | • Triangulation | • Introspection |
| | | • Interactional and visual texts |
| | | • Archival records |
| | | • Field notes |
| | | • Triangulation |
| Analysis of data | • Application of descriptive and inferential statistics to test hypothesis or guiding question | • Content analysis to develop naturalistic generalizations (e.g., themes, meanings, theories) |

**Note:** Adapted from "Introduction: Entering the Field of Qualitative Research," by N. K. Denzin and Y. S. Lincoln, 1994. In N. K. Denzin & Y. S. Lincoln (Eds.), *Handbook of Qualitative Research* (pp. 1–17). Thousand Oaks, CA: Sage. Copyright 1994 by Sage. *Becoming Qualitative Researchers: An Introduction*, by C. Glesne and A. Peshkin, 1992, New York: Longman. Copyright 1992 by Longman. *Nursing and Health Care Research; A Skills-Based Introduction* (2nd ed.), by C. Clifford, 1990, London: Prentice-Hall. Copyright 1990 by Prentice-Hall. *Qualitative Inquiry and Research Design: Choosing Among Five Traditions*, by J. W. Creswell, 1998, Thousand Oaks, CA: Sage. Copyright 1998 by Sage.

are summarized in Table 2–4 and described in Chapters 3 and 4. These models were identified by analyzing the methods used in the important landmark studies in the biological and social sciences and in the Allied Health and Rehabilitation literature.

Research is not limited to one method. Investigators who carry out an unbiased research plan and collect objective data are engaging in research whether they wear a white coat in a laboratory or do historical research in a library. In practice, some investigators combine both qualitative and quantitative research models. For example, the same study may involve constructing an instrument for measuring clinical effectiveness and then carrying out an experimental design. Another frequently used research method is to survey two populations (survey research models) and then compare differences between the two samples (correlational research model).

The diversity of research models available for the multiple problems of a disability is illustrated by the varied approaches in investigating the aging process. For example, amyloid has been identified hypothetically as a protein that, when accumulating in the body, may be a factor in accelerating the general process of aging. The relationship between amyloid and aging can be analyzed from many perspectives by using more than one research model.

TABLE 2-4

**Research Models**

| Quantitative Models | | |
| --- | --- | --- |
| **Research Models** | **Tasks of Researcher** | **Significance** |
| Experimental (group or case study) | Direct manipulation of independent variables and examination of effects in highly controlled settings | Determine empirically the effectiveness of treatment or classroom procedures |
| Methodological | Construction of a measuring instrument, curriculum, or therapeutic procedure/approach | Develop innovative methods or procedures, including technology |
| Correlational (retrospective design) | Test of the relationships between nonmanipulated variables | Identify factors that are presumed to have an associational relationship |
| **Qualitative Models** | | |
| **Research Models** | **Tasks of Researcher** | **Significance** |
| Observation (child development, ethnography, descriptive case study) | In-depth study of individuals, groups, or systems | Identify underlying dynamics in individuals or groups or organizational models of practice to affect change |
| Historical | Investigation of past events through primary sources (e.g., interviews, documents) | Reconstruct past events to understand contemporary problems |
| **Either Quantitative or Qualitative Models** | | |
| **Research Models** | **Tasks of Researcher** | **Significance** |
| Evaluation | Critical analysis of health care delivery systems and educational programs | Objective and/or qualitative assessment of the effectiveness of systems and treatment programs |
| Heuristic and Operations | Discovery of possible causative factors in chronic disabilities, analysis of time, space, and cost factors | Generate further research by identifying significant variables |
| Longitudinal (prospective studies) | Follow-up studies to determine the effectiveness of a treatment technique or the effects of variable on maturation | Determine long-term effects of variables (e.g., genetic, environment, and intervention) |
| Survey | Study of the characteristics of homogeneous populations | Describe general factors that characterize a group |

© Cengage Learning 2013

For instance, an experimental design using animal research is one possibility (Flood & Morley, 1998). Here, the investigator can form two animal groups, one receiving amyloid injections and the other as a control. The results of this hypothetical design could yield empirical data regarding the direct relationship between amyloid and aging in mammals.

Another design applying a correlational model could be created by testing retrospectively the relationship between explicit memory with Alzheimer's disease as compared to control subjects without impairment (Fleischman & Gabriele, 1998). A methodologist may be interested in devising an instrument for detecting the presence of amyloid in the bloodstream (Ronald and Nancy Reagan Research Institute of the Alzheimer's Association and the National Institute on Aging Working Group, 1998). A retrospective clinical case study of Alzheimer's and the examination of neurological changes is another research possibility (Fukutani et al., 1997). An examination of the relationship between diet and the precursors to amyloid would add another dimension to data collection (Howland et al., 1998).

The research models employed by investigators imply certain hypotheses in generating data collection procedures. Research investigations into specific problems can take place from many perspectives. Knowledge of specific research models enables the investigator to attack problems from more than one dimension. Table 2–5 demonstrates how several research models can be applied to a multifaceted investigation of the aging process.

## 2.7.1 Action Research

Another application to the scientific method is action research. Action research developed out of Dewey's (1933) concept of learning by doing through creative problem solving. Lewin's (1939) field theory in which he examined the forces in the environment that impacted on the individual is the theoretical foundation for action research. **Action research** is defined as a problem-oriented investigation that is applied in site-specific environments such as an industry, school, classroom, hospital, clinic, or home setting. In action research, the teacher or clinician, as the researcher, applies quantitative and qualitative research methods to specific problems originating out of a curriculum, treatment program, or ergonomic situation.

## TABLE 2-5

### Relationship between Research Models: Aging Example

| | |
|---|---|
| **Experimental or Prospective:** | Use laboratory animals (induce aging or retard aging) and study physiological variables (Okuma & Nomura, 1998). |
| **Methodological:** | Construct tests and instruments to measure neuropsychological aspects of aging (Schinka et al., 2010). |
| **Evaluation:** | Evaluate the effectiveness of an independent living facility for individuals who are older to increase quality of life (Wang, Kane, Eberly, Virnig, & Chang, 2009). |
| **Heuristic:** | Discover the underlying factors related to premature aging, such as in progeria (Domínguez-Gerpe & Araújo-Vilar, 2008). |
| **Correlational or retrospective:** | Compare individuals who have retired and who are active in the community with comparable individuals who are inactive (Remsburg, Bennett, Inez Wendel, & Durso, 2002). |
| **Qualitative case study:** | Use a case study analysis of an individual who is older expressing feelings of hopelessness (Markowitz, 2007). |
| **Survey:** | Identify the attitudes of young people regarding Alzheimer's disease (Lundquist, & Ready, 2008). |
| **Historical:** | Document through a study of federal legislation a society's changing attitudes toward individuals who have Alzheimer's disease (Ahmed, 2001). |

### Where Can Action Research Be Applied?

Action research can be applied in the following ways:

- Within the school setting, when there is concern about overall achievement, teachers or occupational therapists may use action research to develop ways of changing or modifying the curriculum to allow all students to benefit from instruction.
- When occupational therapists and special education teachers work collaboratively to develop methods for students with developmental disabilities to become more functionally independent in self-care tasks, they may use action research. For example, they examine the effectiveness of teaching work adjustment skills to a student who has a goal of local employment. The success of the student may possibly enable this method to be applied to another student in the same school or may lead to a revision of the method.
- An occupational therapist fabricates a splint in a hand therapy clinic for patients who have had carpel tunnel release surgery. Using action research, the occupational therapist seeks to devise a splint that keeps the wrist in a neutral position and facilities the healing process.
- In a psychosocial setting, the occupational therapist designs strategies to help patients with a diagnosis of depression to be self-motivated and to self-regulate their symptoms. Action research is used to enable the therapist to select the most effective strategies.
- Within the home, an occupational therapist uses action research to modify the home environment so that an individual with a stroke is able to be independent. The occupational therapist considers accessibility, kitchen adaptations, placement for furniture and electronic equipment to enable an individual to be functional.

### Characteristics of Action Research

- Action research occurs in a local, naturalistic setting, sometimes referred to as *site-based*.
- Research may be applied to a setting (e.g., school, organization, hospital, or home), to a classroom or clinic, or to a single individual (e.g., single-subject design).
- The results of the research are usually not generalized outside of the specific setting.
- Quantitative and qualitative research methods can be applied to the investigation. For example, use of standardized tests, observational methods, and statistical analysis may be used to examine the effectiveness of the program.
- Occupational therapists and teachers act as the participant-observer by planning the research, collecting data, and analyzing and interpreting the results. The research is designed and conducted in the teachers' or therapists' own setting as a means of improving one's teaching, therapy, or ergonomic adaptations.
- Problem-solving methods are used to generate possible solutions. For example, a therapist working in a long-term care facility may be looking for ways to increase the morale among staff, or a teacher may be looking for better ways to teach students with ADHD.

### Possible Outcomes of Action Research for Occupational Therapists

- Students in special education who are receiving services either in a pull-out program (i.e., where students leave the general education classroom to go into a special classroom) or in the general education program will benefit as changes are made in their individualized program because of the outcome of the action research.
- Occupational therapists and special educators work together to modify the program for a student who is having difficulty with handwriting. The special educator and the therapist will look at building up the size of the pencil to make it easier to grasp, use of a neutral position and pincer grip for handwriting, perceptual motor activities to increase performance, methods for improving posture, or changes of furniture to improve ergonomic adaptations.
- Students with intellectual disabilities will be taught how to be more independent in activities of daily living (ADLs) within the community.

- Within occupational therapy, results of action research will enable individuals with spinal cord injuries to become employable in a local community.
- The occupational therapist will devise methods to decrease carpel tunnel syndrome in individuals working in a meatpacking plant.
- Occupational therapists working with an individual with depression will develop strategies for sleep hygiene to enable the individual to sleep better.

## 2.7.2 Scholarly Models Not Based on the Scientific Method

These research models are not the only methods of organizing knowledge. A theoretical paper in which a scientist integrates and synthesizes knowledge by creating a conceptual model and a position paper in which a health practitioner advocates a governmental policy such as National Health Insurance are both examples of nonresearch that are scholarly and original. The important difference between research and a scholarly essay or exposition is that in research the investigator formulates a problem first and then objectively collects data related to the problem. In a nonresearch scholarly article, the investigator presents a position or theory and then cites evidence in its support. Another scholarly model is a case study in which a clinician describes a disease process or a treatment technique with a specific individual. Because this model is case-specific, the author does not usually attempt to control variables or generalize the information to another situation. A review paper can also be a model of scholarly work. In this paper, the author integrates studies to generate a body of knowledge. A summary of scholarly manuscripts is described in Table 2–6.

For the last 100 years, the scientific method has generated many research models. Although for many years research generally was limited to those who did not teach or conduct therapy, there is a need for clinicians and teachers to apply evidence-based practice in their everyday work. Qualitative and quantitative methods can be applied within one's own setting through action research, whereas scholarly papers can be written through a review of articles in the literature. It is incumbent on those of us in the clinical and teaching fields to use an evidence-based practice model to establish the efficacy of our practices.

## TABLE 2-6

### Examples of Types of Scholarly Manuscripts

| Scholarly Manuscripts | Tasks of Writer | Significance |
|---|---|---|
| Position paper | Advocate reforms of health care or educational systems, legislation, ethics of research, standards of practice | Presentation of policy statements and editorials |
| Theoretical exposition | Explain relationships between variables and predict outcomes | Logical explanation in natural or social science using deductive reasoning |
| Case study presentation* | Present chronological history of an individual, such as one's course of illness, or treatment effectiveness | Sequential description of disease process or treatment in an individual |
| Review Paper | Integrate and synthesize published research | Exploration of current state of knowledge in specified field |

*A case study can be used as a research model in both qualitative and quantitative research.

## CHAPTER 3

# Quantitative Research Models

*The clinical trial is a carefully, and ethically, designed experiment with the aim of answering some precisely framed question. In its most rigorous form it demands equivalent groups of patients concurrently treated in different ways.*

—Sir A. B. Hill, 1971, *Principles of Medical Statistics*, p. 273

## Operational Learning Objectives

By the end of this chapter, the learner will:
- Define *quantitative research*.
- Define key terms in quantitative research methods.

- Critically analyze examples of research from the occupational therapy and special education literature.
- Identify types of quantitative research.

**Quantitative research** involves the systematic use of empirical methods to test relationships between variables. Quantitative research is often employed to investigate whether there are statistically significant differences among dependent variables based on an independent variable. The research hypothesis usually describes the research question and establishes the anticipated relationships between the dependent and independent variables.

**Empiricism** is defined as gaining observable, objective, and verifiable data through the senses. An example of empirical data is measuring hand strength with a dynometer. Another example is mea-suring the rate of words per minute that a student reads. Empirical data must be operationally defined so that another investigator can reproduce them. In quantitative research, the investigator begins with a hypothesis that predicts the results of the investigation. Although this chapter focuses specifically on quantitative research models, the concepts of research design and methodology (Chapter 7) are closely related to many of the concepts introduced in this chapter. Indeed, successful research amalgamates the concepts from this chapter with many of the concepts found in Chapter 7. Some key terms used in quantitative research are described in Table 3–1.

---

## TABLE 3-1

### Key Definitions in Quantitative Research

| | |
|---|---|
| Control group: | A group selected to compare with the experimental group. This group may be a nonintervention group with no treatment, or it may receive a different treatment method. For example, the researcher may wish to determine the effects of splinting on reducing carpal tunnel syndrome and may introduce exercise in the control group. |
| Dependent variable: | In clinical research, the treatment effect or outcome resulting from the intervention of the independent variable. For example, the dependent variable in a study of sensory integration therapy could be a reduction of tactile defensiveness in children. |
| Empirical data: | Data based on controlled observation that can be observed, measured, verified, and replicated. |
| Evidence-based practice (EBP): | The most common definition of EBP is taken from Dr. David Sackett, a pioneer in evidence-based practice. EBP is "the conscientious, explicit and judicious use of current best evidence in making decisions about the care of the individual patient. It means integrating individual clinical expertise with the best available external clinical evidence from systematic research" (Sackett et al., 1996). |
| Experimental group: | A group that the researcher manipulates. For example, the experimental group could receive heart-rate biofeedback or relaxation therapy or handwriting instruction. The treatment represents the independent variable in experimental research. |
| External validity: | The degree to which results can be generalized to a target population. External validity depends on the representativeness of a sample and the rigor of the experiment. Replication of a study producing consistent results increases the external validity. |
| Extraneous variable: | A variable that the researcher does not manipulate but one that can potentially affect the results of a study. Extraneous variables can include such factors as gender, intelligence, severity of disability, or socioeconomic status. These variables, if they are uncontrolled, can threaten the internal validity of a study. |

| | |
|---|---|
| **Hypothesis–Directional:** | A statement that predicts results and is testable by a systematic methodology. A hypothesis can be either null or directional. An example of a stated hypothesis is: *There is a statistically significant difference in reducing spasticity in children with cerebral palsy when using neurodevelopmental treatment as compared to splinting.* |
| **Hypothesis–Null:** | A researcher's statement that predicts no statistically significant difference or relationship between variables. For example, a clinical researcher may state, "There is no statistically significant difference between a prescriptive aerobic exercise and Prozac® in reducing clinical depression." |
| **Independent variable:** | A variable that the researcher manipulates. In clinical research, it represents the treatment method, such as aquatic therapy, progressive relaxation, or phonemic awareness. |
| **Internal validity:** | The degree of rigor in an experiment in controlling for extraneous variables and error variance. Potential threats to internal validity have been identified as extraneous historical factors, maturation, instrumentation, and lack of random sampling. Internal validity is an indication of the trustworthiness of the results. Well-designed studies with good control of variables that can potentially distort the results have high internal validity. The quality of a research study is increased by eliminating the threats to internal validity. |
| **Intervention protocol:** | The operational definition of the independent variable or intervention method. The intervention protocol should have enough detail so that it can be replicated. One purpose of designing a treatment protocol is to evaluate its effectiveness. |
| **Operational definition of a variable:** | Specific measure, observation, or a criterion that defines a variable. For example, activities of daily living (ADL) skills may be defined as the score obtained on the Barthel Index. An operational definition is important in replicating a study or in evaluating a group of studies using meta-analysis. |
| **Pre-post group design with control group:** | Classical experimental design where the investigator compares the results obtained by both groups. |
| **Random sampling:** | An unbiased portion of a target population selected by chance, such as through random numbers. |
| **Reliability:** | A measure of the consistency/stability of a test instrument. For example, on a test with high reliability, one would expect approximately the same results on two different administrations when there is no change in subject. |
| **Replicability:** | The ability to repeat an experiment or scientific procedure. The purpose is to strengthen generalizability of the findings and to ensure external validity. |
| **Validity:** | As pertaining to measurement, the degree to which a test or measuring instrument actually measures what it purports to measure. |

## 3.1  Factors in Quantitative Research Models

The following factors are the sine qua non (i.e., the essential ingredients) of quantitative research models.

- **A justification and rationale for the research:** This includes a justification for the research based on the significance of the research. For example, a researcher justifies the need for research in spinal cord injury by describing the number of individuals who incur such an injury and by the cost of the injury. In special education, a teacher may justify the examination of different ways to work with students with autism based on the increasing incidence of this population.

- **An extensive review of literature:** The researcher identifies and analyzes previous research related to the topic of study. For example, a researcher examining animal-assisted therapy would search the databases for previous studies.
- **Operational definitions of research variables:** The researcher must operationally define each of the variables being examined. These variables include the intervention, the outcome measures, the participants, and the setting where the experiment takes place.
- **Identification of extraneous variables that could confound the results:** The investigator tries to control the static variables, such as gender, age, socioeconomic status, ethnicity, and handedness.
- **Statement of hypothesis or guiding question:** Prior to collecting data, the researcher predicts or hypothesizes the results of the study.
- **An objective, unbiased method for collecting data:** The investigator develops a research design that can be reproduced.
- **Separate sections for results and discussion:** After the data are collected, the investigator designs tables, figures, and graphs to depict the results in an objective manner. A discussion of the results is more subjective and allows the investigator to speculate on the implications of the study.
- **Limitations of the study and recommendations for further research:** The researcher acknowledges limitations in the methodology or uncontrolled variables that could affect the results and makes recommendations that could improve future studies. For example, one limitation might be the limited number of subjects or an unreliable outcome measure.

## 3.2 Experimental Research

### 3.2.1 Purposes of Experimental Research

The researcher uses experimental methods to collect empirical data by manipulating independent variables and observing their effects, seeking maximum control of the data collection procedure and environmental conditions. Experimenters achieve **internal validity** when they are able to control extraneous variables that could affect the results (see Table 3–2). The degree of experimental rigor depends on these controls.

Figure 3–1 shows the relationship between experimental research and clinical practice. Working together, their purposes are to:

- Compare the effectiveness of clinical intervention methods;
- Observe cause-effect relationships established in a laboratory; and
- Examine biopsychosocial factors underlying human responses.

### 3.2.2 Comparison of Intervention Methods

Is intervention method "A" more effective than intervention method "B"? This question is a clinical problem affecting every individual an occupational therapist treats in a hospital, home, or school setting. Nonetheless, the impact of clinical research remains limited. Many occupational therapists continue to cling to traditional methods of intervention without searching the literature to determine whether their effectiveness has been established experimentally. The classical research design employed in testing the relative effectiveness of clinical intervention methods is the paradigm:

**CLASSIC CLINICAL TREATMENT PARADIGM**

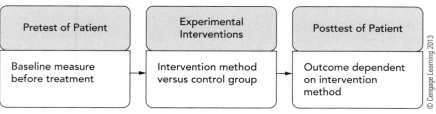

© Cengage Learning 2013

TABLE 3-2

### Control of Extraneous Variables

| Possible Confounding Extraneous Variables | Methods to Control Extraneous Variables |
| --- | --- |
| Demographic variables | Establish screening criteria that includes range of ages, gender, SES, ethnic groups, home language, and/or hand dominance. |
| Cognitive and academic variables (e.g., intelligence, academic achievement, processing abilities) | Administer a screening test to ensure equivalent groups. |
| Test anxiety | Establish rapport, answer questions, and set the participant at ease prior to any data collection. |
| Low motivation | Screen out individuals who show reluctance to participate in the study. |
| Hawthorne effect | Establish a control group and ensure that each group within the study has equal attention. |
| Test conditions | Ensure that environmental conditions (e.g., lighting, noise, temperature, presence of other people, distractions) do not interfere with data collection. |
| Reliability and validity of procedure | Use a double-blind control in which the data collector is not aware of the participant's group. |
| Experimental bias | Ensure that all individuals collecting data have been trained and that interrater reliability is high. |
| Data collection methods | Do a pilot study to examine the reliability and validity of the procedure, or use tests and procedures that have established high validity and reliability. |
| Test Administration | Ensure administrator has read or reviewed test manual and procedures, and follows standardization procedures without deviation. |

© Cengage Learning 2013

In this example, the experimental intervention represents the independent or manipulated variable, whereas the degree of improvement represents the dependent variable. The experimenter directly observes a cause-effect relationship.

Traditionally, the control group has been a non-intervention group or a comparative intervention group. In a nonintervention group, there is a possibility of a Hawthorne effect in which each group does not get equal attention, and the results may be attributable to the attention of the experimental group rather than to the intervention effect. Campbell and Stanley (1963), in their classical work on experimental design, used the term "quasiexperimental" to indicate experimental designs in which there is no comparative control group. For example,

in a pilot study, a researcher may want to examine the effects of a stress management program on the reduction of depression by using an experimental group without a control group (Stein & Smith, 1989). This would be considered a quasiexperimental design.

An example of a clinical research design using a control group is a study by Callinan and Mathiowetz (1996). In this study, the researchers compared soft and hard resting hand splints on pain and hand function for 39 persons with rheumatoid arthritis. "A repeated measures research design was used to compare the two experimental conditions, wearing a soft splint versus a hard splint on the dominant hand for 28 days at night only, and an unsplinted control period of 28 days" (p. 347).

PURPOSES OF EXPERIMENTAL RESEARCH

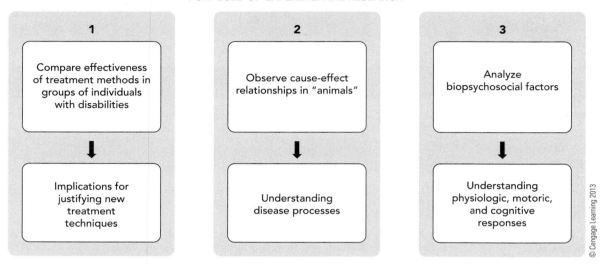

**FIGURE 3-1** Purposes of Experimental Research: Note that there are three purposes for research, all of which lead to implications for treatment or intervention.

Table 3–3 compares the features of two studies: Stein and Smith (1989) and Callinan and Mathiowetz (1996). Although the basic design is similar, the former study has no control group and uses a smaller sample.

### 3.2.3 Clinical Research

The clinician's major concern is the effectiveness of a specific intervention method for a specific client. The clinician evaluates the client, establishes intervention goals using RUMBA (i.e., **R**elevant, **U**nderstandable, **M**easurable, **B**ehavioral, and **A**chievable), applies appropriate intervention methods, reevaluates the client's improvement made prior to discharge, and concludes that if the client improved, then the treatment intervention was effective. If the intervention method is effective, can the clinician assume that it could be applied to similar clients (**external validity**)? Before one can generalize the results, further data must be obtained to validate the results.

Using an evidence-based intervention is one way clinicians may validate intervention (Brown & Rodger, 1999). Clinicians may also postulate that the selected intervention method is better than other comparable methods. Again, this must be confirmed by comparing the effectiveness of various intervention methods. Another assumption is that the evaluation of intervention outcome is objective. The technique of measuring the effectiveness of an intervention method can make the difference between labeling it successful or ineffective. The test for an adequate outcome measure or evaluation of intervention effectiveness is its reproducibility by other clinicians. General application to other clients, relative effectiveness compared with other methods of intervention, and objective measurement of improvement are factors that clinicians must examine if their results are to be considered valid and generalizable.

Experimental research enables clinicians to compare the relative effectiveness of intervention

TABLE 3-3

**Comparison of Quasiexperimental and Experimental Designs**

|  | Quasiexperimental | Experimental with Control |
|---|---|---|
| **Citation** | Stein, F., & Smith, J. (1989). Short-term stress management programme with acutely depressed in-patients. *Canadian Journal of Occupational Therapy, 56,* 185-192. | Callinan, N. J., & Mathiowetz, V. (1996). Soft versus hard resting hand splints in rheumatoid arthritis: Pain relief, preference, and compliance. *American Journal of Occupational Therapy, 50,* 347-353. |
| **Subjects** | 7 hospitalized patients with acute depression | 39 clients with rheumatoid arthritis |
| **Experimental group** | 7 hospitalized patients with acute depression | 39 clients with rheumatoid arthritis using the soft and hard splints |
| **Control group** | None | Patients served as their own control when no splint was used. |
| **Design** | Pre- and post-design with no control group | Repeated measures design |
| **Treatment program** | Six sessions using various relaxation therapy techniques, including Benson relaxation response, progressive relaxation, visual imagery, back massage, biofeedback, behavioral rehearsal, deep breathing, and paradoxical intention | "Experimental treatment periods (28 nights each) included treatment with the soft splint, treatment with the hard splint, and unsplinted (control). The order of assignment to treatment periods was randomized" (p. 349). |
| **Assessment of outcome** | *Stress Management Questionnaire*; (Stein, 1987), *State-Trait Anxiety Inventory* (STAI; Spielberger, 1983), and self-evaluation | *Arthritis Impact Measurement Scales* (AIMS; Meenan, Gertman, & Mason, 1980), self-evaluation of pain localization, grip strength, diary, and a splint rating form |
| **Results and conclusions** | "Results showed that there was a significant reduction in anxiety… and patients indicated that the sessions had a positive effect in increasing their ability to relax and in learning to recognize individual stress reactions" (p. 185). | "The findings indicate that resting hand splints are effective for pain relief and that persons with rheumatoid arthritis are more likely to prefer and comply with soft splint use for this purpose" (p. 347). |

© Cengage Learning 2013

methods. In clinical research, the occupational therapist carefully documents the effects of intervention over time. The therapist can carry out the research in a group experiment or single-subject design. (See Boxes 3–1 and 3–2 for examples of research studies using experimental design with single subject or groups.) In a group experiment, the researcher compares intervention methods with groups of clients. Intervention groups are set up ahead of time, and clients are randomly assigned to each group. Analysis of results is by group statistics. In a single-subject design, the therapist may alternate different intervention methods with the same client (alternating interventions) who may act as his or her own control.

BOX 3-1

## Example of an Experimental Case Study (Prospective Design)

### 1. Bibliographical Notation

Flinn, N., Smith, J., Tripp, C., & White, M. (2009). Effects of robotic-aided rehabilitation on recovery of upper extremity function in chronic stroke: A single case study. *Occupational Therapy International, 16,* 232–243.

### 2. Abstract

The objective of the study was to examine the results of robotic therapy in a single client. A 48-year-old female client 15 months post-stroke, with right hemiparesis, received robotic therapy as an outpatient in a large Midwestern rehabilitation hospital. Robotic therapy was provided three times a week for 6 weeks. Robotic therapy consisted of goal-directed, robotic-aided reaching tasks to exercise the hemiparetic shoulder and elbow. No other therapeutic intervention for the affected upper extremity (UE) was provided during the study or 3 months follow-up period. The outcome measures included the *Fugl-Meyer, Graded Wolf Motor Function Test* (GWMFT), *Motor Activity Log* (MAL), active range of motion and *Canadian Occupational Performance Measure* (COPM). The participant made gains in active movement; performance; and satisfaction of functional tasks, GWMFT and functional use. Limitations involved in this study relate to the generalizability of the sample size, effect of medications, expense of robotic technologies and the impact of aphasia. Future research should incorporate functional use training along with robotic therapy.

### 3. Justification and Need for Study

The authors list several popular therapeutic strategies used in occupational therapy to treat persons with stroke while at the same time discussing associated limitations with these approaches. The authors also discuss some of the successes from using robotics for upper extremity (UE) rehabilitation with the stroke population. The study's first purpose was to elucidate robotics as an additional treatment option for persons with stroke whose recovery plateaued from the more traditional therapy strategies. The second purpose was to study the effectiveness of using robotics to enhance the motor abilities of the affected UE.

### 4. Literature Review

Twenty-three references from a wide variety of sources were used. Cited journals included, but were not limited to: *Archives of Physical Medicine and Rehabilitation, Clinical Rehabilitation, Journal of Rehabilitation Research and Development, NeuroRehabilitation, Scandinavian Journal of Rehabilitation Medicine, Stroke,* and *Topics in Stroke Rehabilitation.* The years of cited publications ranged from 1975 through 2008.

### 5. Research Hypothesis or Guiding Questions

The guiding question for this research was to investigate "the relationship of robotic-aided treatment on return of spontaneous, functional use of the UE" (p. 233).

### 6. Methods

The participant was a female aged 48 years who suffered an ischemic stroke. She was initially hospitalized 1 week then received 4 weeks of inpatient therapy. She was enrolled in this study 15 months after her discharge from her in-patient rehabilitation stay. At the initiation of the study, she presented with "dense right hemiplegia, an inferior and anterior shoulder sublux-ation with mild shoulder hand syndrome. Her shoulder hand syndrome symptoms included pain with movement, especially active or passive shoulder range beyond 40 degrees of shoulder flexion" (p. 234). The intervention involved the use of an InMotion2 robot by Interactive Motion Technologies. This device provided the ability "to practice reaching motions in a gravity-reduced horizontal plane. The motions required shoulder flexion and extension, internal and external rotation, and elbow flexion and extension" (p. 235). The intervention included 18 one-hour sessions dispersed across 6 weeks with 3 sessions per week. The outcome measures included AROM measurements, the *Fugl-Meyer*, the GWMFT, the MAL, and the COPM. This study used a pretest/posttest/follow-up single experimental case design that employed descriptive statistics to compare performances across time. The timeline involved 6 weeks between the pre- and posttests and 3 months between the posttest and the follow-up.

### 7. Results

Improvements on the GWMFT and the *Fugl-Meyer* were the most dramatic between the pre- and posttests; additionally, performance on these two measures showed little decline at the follow-up time period. The variation in performance on the MAL varied very little between the three testing periods. The same was largely true for the COPM measures of satisfaction and performance. AROM improvements were seen in "shoulder abduction, external rotation, elbow extension and wrist flexion and extension. Of these, some of the shoulder external rotation and elbow extension AROM gains were not maintained at the time of the follow-up testing. The participant also reported decreases in pain, and stiffness over the course of the study" (p. 239).

### 8. Conclusions

Flinn et al. concluded that:

1. "Robotic therapy was successful in gaining active movement in the involved UE...." (p. 242).
2. "The participant also made small gains in functional use" (p. 242).
3. "Improvement in motor function does not necessarily translate to functional use" (p. 242).

### 9. Limitations of the Study

Because this is a single-case clinical experimental study, generalization of these results is very limiting. Future research is needed using a larger population to increase the external validity of this line of research.

*continues*

BOX 3-1

## Example of an Experimental Case Study
### (Prospective Design) *continued*

### 10. Major References Cited in the Study

Fasoli, S. E., Krebs, H. I., Stein, J., Frontera, W. R., & Hogan, N. (2003). Effects of robotic therapy on motor impairments and recovery in chronic stroke. *Archives of Physical Medicine and Rehabilitation, 84,* 477–482.

Fugl-Meyer, A. R., Jaasko, L., Leyman, I. Olsson, S., & Steglind, S. (1975). The post-stroke hemiplegic patient: A method for evaluation of physical performance. *Scandinavian Journal of Rehabilitation Medicine, 7,* 13–31.

Law, M., Baptiste, S., Carswell, A., McColl, M. A., Polatajko, H., & Pollock, N. (1998). *The Canadian Occupational Performance Measure* (3rd ed.). Ottawa, Ontario, Canada: Canadian Association of Occupational Therapists Publications, Ace.

Taub, E., Uswatte, G., & Pidikiti, R. (1999). Constraint-induced movement therapy: A new family of techniques with broad application to physical rehabilitation—A clinical review. *Journal of Rehabilitation Research and Development, 36,* 1–17.

BOX 3-2

## Example of Experimental Research Group Study

### 1. Bibliographical Notation

Maitra, K., Philips, K., & Rice, M. (2010). Grasping naturally versus grasping with a reacher in people without disability: Motor control and muscle activation differences. *American Journal of Occupational Therapy, 64,* 95–104.

### 2. Abstract

We investigated motor control and muscle activation when reaching for and grasping objects with a reacher compared with the unaided hand. In a repeated-measures counterbalanced design, 41 healthy participants with no previous experience using a reacher were randomly assigned to a sequence of four conditions. Movements of the wrist and fingers were recorded using a three-dimensional Qualisys camera system for assessing reach and grasp. Muscle activations from finger and arm flexors and extensors were recorded by surface electromyography. Participants exhibited a smaller grasp aperture, longer reaching time, and more muscle activity when they used a reacher. Efficient motor control, which requires both time and practice, is needed to successfully use a reacher. Clients presented with reachers without sufficient time to develop motor skills unique to reacher use may be more likely to abandon this assistive device and fail to benefit from its function.

### 3. Justification and Need for Study

Occupational therapists frequently recommend a client to utilize assistive devices to enhance functional independence in daily life activities. A reacher is a device that is commonly recommended for clients with decreased grip strength and range of motion. There is currently a dearth of research examining the extent to which function is impaired by utilizing a reacher. The purpose of this study is to systematically investigate the movement characteristics and muscle activation patterns of the upper extremity when reaching or grasping different objects with a reacher and with the unaided hand.

### 4. Literature Review

Twenty-one references from a variety of sources were identified. Cited journals included, but were not limited to: *Quarterly Journal of Experimental Psychology*, *American Journal of Occupational Therapy*, *Journal of Psychiatric Research*, *Journal of Neuroscience*, *Psychological Review*, *Physical and Occupational Therapy in Geriatrics*, and *Experimental Brain Research*. The years of publications cited in this article ranged from 1971 through 2006.

### 5. Research Hypothesis or Guiding Questions

The study consisted of two hypotheses. The first hypothesis was that the use of a reacher, compared with use of the hand, would yield significant mean differences in kinematic parameters when participants reach for and grasp four objects of different shapes and sizes. The second hypothesis stated that the use of a reacher, compared with use of the hand, would yield significant mean differences in muscle activation patterns, as measured by net and relative muscle excitation, when participants reach for and grasp four objects of different shapes and sizes.

### 6. Methods

For the study, participants included 41 healthy adults ages 19 to 55 from the Toledo, Ohio, area. To be included in the study participants had to have an absence of any physical or cognitive impairment, needed to be right-hand dominant, and have normal vision with or without corrective lenses. Prescreening was conducted, which consisted of testing of the upper extremity for normal range of motion and hand strength testing with a cutoff at 40 lb; the *Mini-Mental State Exam* with a required score range of 26 to 30; and the *Edinburgh Handedness Inventory*. Participants were blinded to the experimental hypotheses and could not have any previous experience using a reacher. A 2 x 2 x 2 repeated-measures analysis of variance (ANOVA) design was employed to analyze the differences

*continues*

BOX 3-2

## Example of Experimental
## Research Group Study *continued*

among reacher grasp and hand grasp. The grasping apparatus had two levels: the hand and the reacher. The object characteristics were defined by shape (round and square), and size (small and large). This created four types of object characteristics: small round (golf ball), large round (baseball), small square (small Rubik's Cube), and large square (large Rubik's Cube). Using a repeated-measures counter balance design, participants were randomly assigned to a sequence of four conditions: Condition A: reaching-grasping a golf ball; Condition B: reaching-grasping a baseball; Condition C: reaching-grasping a small Rubik's Cube; and Condition D: reaching-grasping a large Rubik's Cube. Participants sat in a chair facing a table with hips and knees at 90 degrees and trunk in midline. The starting position for natural grasp consisted of having the participant's right hand with index thumb in a pinch position on a red disk switch at the edge of the table. The participants were instructed to reach and grasp the object 15 cm in front of them without bending the trunk and place the object 20 cm to the left. The reacher condition setup was the same, except the object was moved farther forward so the object was 15 cm away from the end of the reacher. Each trial consisted of picking up each of the four objects in a randomly assigned sequence. The study included 12 trials each using the reacher and the natural grasp (three trials for each object). A three-dimensional movement recording system was used to record arm, hand, and finger movements. For noninvasive surface electromyography, a Bagnoli EMG system was used, which analyzed muscle activation patterns. The dependent variables for the reach task included peak velocity of reach, reach time, and percentage of time to reach peak velocity.

## 7. Results

- The mean maximal grasp aperture was significantly larger when reaching naturally than when reaching with a reacher.
- The mean maximal grasp aperture was significantly larger when reaching for a larger object than a smaller object.
- A significant interaction was yielded between the main factor of grasp size.
- Main effects of shape and other interactions were not significant.
- Peak velocity of finger aperture was significantly increased when reaching naturally than reaching with the reacher.
- The time it took to reach peak velocity of maximal finger aperture was significantly longer when reaching naturally opposed to reaching with the reacher.
- Time to reach peak velocity of finger aperture was significantly shorter when reaching for a round object than reaching for a square object.
- Reach time was significantly shorter when using a natural reach compared to using a reacher.

- The peak velocity of reach was increased significantly when using the hand compared to the reacher.
- Acceleration time was significantly different when reaching naturally compared to using a reacher.
- The global electromyographic activity was significantly less when using a natural reach compared to using a reacher.
- The global electromyographic activity was significantly more when reaching for larger objects compared to smaller objects.
- The contribution of the biceps was relatively higher when reaching for smaller objects than reaching for larger objects.
- The relative excitation of the triceps was significantly higher when reaching for smaller objects than reaching for the larger objects.
- There were no significant differences in grasping when reaching naturally compared to using a reacher.
- The excitation of the wrist flexors was significantly higher when reaching for larger objects than smaller objects.
- The wrist extensors were significantly lower when reaching naturally than when reaching with the reacher.
- The wrist extensors were significantly higher when reaching for larger objects compared to smaller objects.
- The contribution from the pollicis was significantly larger when reaching naturally compared to using a reacher.

## 8. Conclusions

Maitra et al. concluded that:

1. "Motor control characteristics are different in a reacher grasp than in a natural grasp" (p. 102).
2. Characteristics of a natural grasp include faster reach and larger grasp aperture with higher peak velocity. Characteristics of a reacher grasp include smaller grasp aperture and shorter acceleration profile.
3. "Muscular activations were less in a natural grasp than in a reacher grasp; combined muscular activations were also sensitive to size…" (p.102).
4. "With practice, the brain may begin to think of the reacher as a useful alternative to hand grasp" (p. 103).
5. "Some level of motor planning is needed to accomplish tasks using a reacher in non clinical populations" (p. 103).
6. "A sufficient amount of training and practice is needed before patients will develop motor learning and control needed to master reacher use…" (p. 103).

## 9. Limitations of the Study

The sample size appears to be adequate, but may have been a limiting factor. Many variables were involved; a larger sample may have given more generalizable results. Participants

*continues*

BOX 3-2

## Example of Experimental Research Group Study *continued*

were all from the same area, which may decrease generalizability of the results. Finally, the study was conducted in a nonnaturalistic lab environment.

### 10. Major References Cited in the Study

Gentilucci, M. (2002). Object motor representation and reaching grasping control. *Neuropsychologia, 40*, 1139–1153.

Gentilucci, M., Roy, A. C., & Stefanini, S. (2004). Grasping an object naturally or with a tool: Are these tasks guided by a common motor representation? *Experimental Brain Research, 157*, 383–387.

Jeannerod, M. (1988). *The neural and behavioral organization of goal-directed movements.* Oxford, England: Oxford University Press.

Maruishi, M., Tanaka, Y., Muranaka, H., Tsuji, T., Ozawa, Y., Imaizumi, S., Miyatani, M., & Kawahara, J. (2004). Brain activation during manipulation of the myoelectric prosthetic hand: A functional magnetic resonance imaging study. *NeuroImage, 21*, 1604–1611.

For example, in a group design, clients with arthritis are referred to occupational therapy for intervention. The clinician can employ physical agent modalities, exercise, purposeful activity, and hydrotherapy methods randomly. Functional skills, range of motion, and self-evaluation in the shoulder joint can be used as measures of improvement. Each intervention group is charted, and statistical analysis can be used to compare the relative effectiveness of each intervention method. On the other hand, with a single-subject design, the effect of using an upper extremity inhibitive casting to reduce spasticity is used for a single child with cerebral palsy (Tona & Schneck, 1993). In this case, the investigators measured pre-post performance using the *Modified Ashworth Scale*, a clinical measure of spasticity. Results could not be generalized without further replication. Figure 3–2 illustrates how a clinical researcher could chart progress by using a graph.

Other variables that can potentially affect the results should be recorded for each client. In this way, systematic patterns can be noted. A data collection sheet containing information can be statistically analyzed later to compare the relative effectiveness of intervention methods and the systematic influence of extraneous variables. An example of a data collection sheet is illustrated in Figure 3–3.

### 3.2.4 Designing Experimental Groups

The advantage of using clinical research is that the experimenter does not need large numbers of subjects to initiate research. The major disadvantage is the experimenter's lack of control in matching the groups on specific variables. For example, there will always be demographic and biopsychosocial differences between two intervention groups. Experimental research with matched groups increases the internal validity or rigor of the experiment.

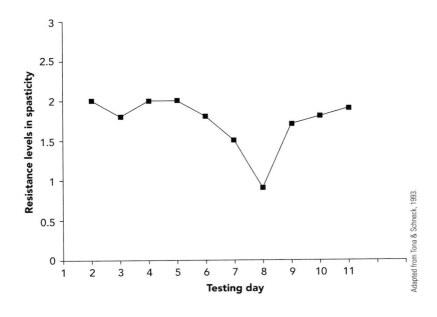

Adapted from Tona & Schneck, 1993.

**FIGURE 3-2** Example of Progress Chart: On the horizontal axis (X) are the testing days, and on the vertical axis (Y) is the passive resistance to spasticity for each day.

| Data Collection Sheet | | |
|---|---|---|
| **Background Data** | | |
| 1    Patient code number (based on intervention group) | | |
| 2    Gender | 3    Date of Birth | 4    Handedness |
| 5    Diagnosis | | |
| 6    Date of onset of illness | | |
| 7    Occupation | | |
| 8    Years of formal education | | |
| 9    Date of data collection | | |
| **Test Data** | | |
| 10    Pretest Scores on dependent variable | | |
| 11    Posttest scores<br>    a    1 week _____<br>    b    2 weeks _____<br>    c    3 weeks _____ | d    4 weeks _____<br>e    3 months _____ | |
| 12    Intervention | | |
| 13    Other test data, including psychological tests, physiological measures, and self-report | | |

© Cengage Learning 2013

**FIGURE 3-3** Example of a Data Collection Sheet: The information contained on the sheet will change according to the researcher's needs.

CLINICAL GROUP RESEARCH PARADIGM

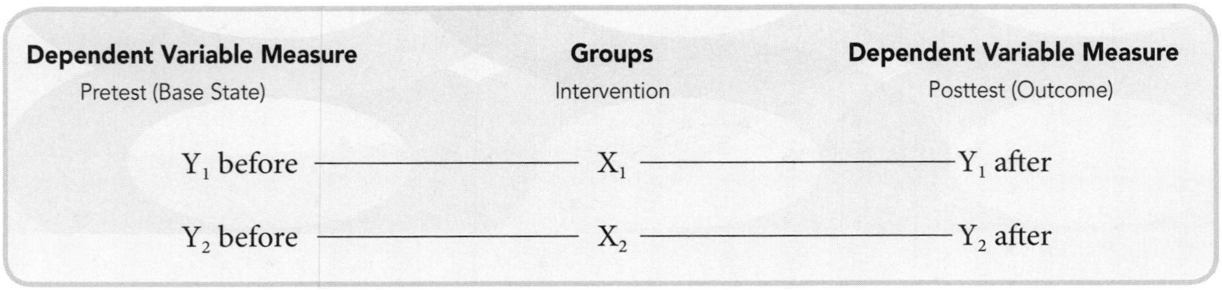

| Dependent Variable Measure | Groups | Dependent Variable Measure |
|---|---|---|
| Pretest (Base State) | Intervention | Posttest (Outcome) |

$$Y_1 \text{ before} \longrightarrow X_1 \longrightarrow Y_1 \text{ after}$$

$$Y_2 \text{ before} \longrightarrow X_2 \longrightarrow Y_2 \text{ after}$$

© Cengage Learning 2013

**FIGURE 3-4**  Pre-Post Experimental Design

In clinical research with groups, the investigator compares the effects of two or more independent variables in a patient population. If clinical researchers want to compare intervention method $X_1$ with intervention method $X_2$, they must create relatively equal groups and employ reliable and valid measures to test outcome. The design is illustrated in Figure 3–4.

Experimental research with two or more groups can potentially eliminate the Hawthorne effect. Each group is given equal time and attention to control the effect. The procedure for guarding against the Hawthorne effect is described in Figure 3–5.

The foregoing sequential analysis illustrates the many controls necessary in isolating the experimental or intervention effect and in controlling for extraneous variables. In designing experimental research with a control group, it is important for the researcher to match the groups on variables that could potentially affect the results of the study, such as age, gender, socioeconomic status, intelligence, and education. For example, how can an investigator design an experiment applying biofeedback techniques in reducing hypertension in patients with post-cardiac disease?

The first step in this hypothetical design is to select a population of clients with cardiovascular disease by establishing screening criteria for inclusion based on age, gender, diagnosis, length of hospitalization, and vital capacities. Statistical and practical considerations determine the number of subjects to be included in the study. (See Chapter 7 for a discussion of these considerations.) Participants are then randomly assigned to an experimental group (e.g.,

biofeedback) and a control group (e.g., medication). The investigator should review the participants' backgrounds to determine if the groups are evenly matched on the relevant variables being considered.

After two matched groups have been established, diastolic and systolic blood pressure is taken in various conditions (e.g., at rest and at several stages of exertion) to establish a baseline. Then the investigator checks to determine if both groups have approximately equal mean blood pressure scores. If not, the groups are reformed until the researcher is satisfied that the two groups are comparable. The two groups then undergo the experiment within a specified time period (e.g., two 2-hour sessions per week over a 3-month period). To avoid researcher bias, the test administrator would not know whether a subject was in the biofeedback group or medication group. Research assistants, who would not be told the purpose of the study, would be responsible for implementing the design. This method, called **double-blind control** eliminates experimenter bias. In a double-blind study, neither the investigator nor the subject participant is made aware of the subject's experimental condition assignment.

Subject motivation, fatigue, anxiety, and distractibility or lack of cooperation are major factors that increase the error variance in experimental research and should be carefully monitored because these variables could affect the results. After the 3-month period, a posttest of blood pressures would be obtained from both groups. It would be expected that a training or Hawthorne effect would lower blood pressure in both groups; however, a null hypothesis would be proposed stating that there would be no

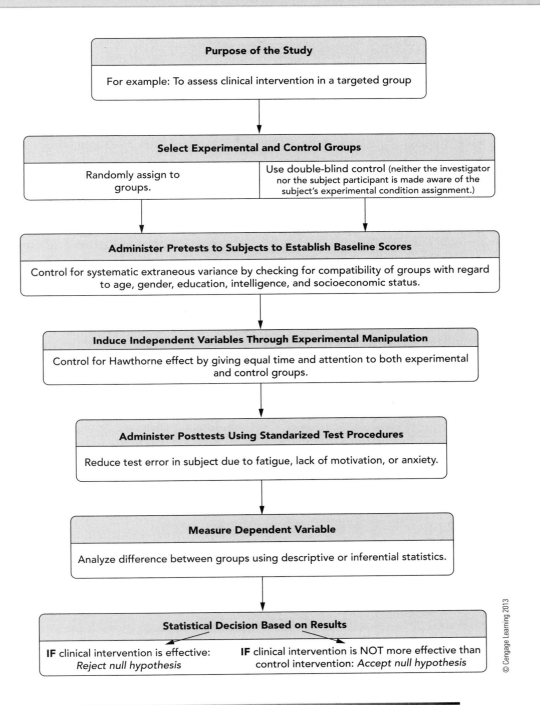

**FIGURE 3-5**  Sequential Analysis of Control Factors in Experimental Research: Controlling for each of these factors helps prevent possible error as a result of the Hawthorne effect.

© Cengage Learning 2013

statistically significant difference between the experimental and control groups. Statistical analysis would be performed to determine whether there is, in fact, a significant difference. The researcher could then propose a conclusion based on statistical analysis of the data. Additionally, the researcher would examine the literature for similar studies to determine if the current results corroborate or contradict these findings.

There are many variations of experimental research. One example of a factorial design is the interactional effect between medication and relaxation therapy in children with Attention-Deficit Hyperactivity Disorder (ADHD).

Before undertaking experimental research with human subjects, ethical and human rights factors must also be considered. Every subject should be informed of the experimental procedures and potential risks involved. (Further discussion regarding this topic is found in Chapter 7.)

### 3.2.5 Experimental Research Methods and the Effects of Clinical Intervention

Researchers and clinicians have various definitions of improvement. For researchers, improvement is operationally defined and measurable, and the variables that caused the improvement are clearly identified. Clinicians, who work with clients every day, use individual goals and, many times, subjective criteria for evaluating a patient's progress. In addition, clinicians present individual cases from their clinical practice to support or to negate a method of intervention. Table 3–4 summarizes the differences between researchers and clinicians in evaluating intervention outcome.

The problem of investigating the effectiveness of an intervention method is a complex issue. What criteria are used in evaluating improvement? How can other variables in a patient's life space, such as family, friends, diet, activities, and work, be separated from the intervention procedure in the evaluation of improvement? How can the therapeutic relationship be separated from the intervention method in determining its effect on intervention outcome? The interactional effects between the therapist and client, intervention method and client, and external environment and client make it difficult for the experimenter to isolate the specific variables causing specific results. These interrelationships are schematically shown in Figure 3–6.

Before it is possible to determine if one intervention method is more effective than another, the clinical researcher must identify and control possible

### TABLE 3-4

**Researcher-Clinician Comparison for Evaluating Intervention Outcome**

| Variable | Research Methods (Nomothetic Approach) | Clinician Methods (Idiographic Approach) |
|---|---|---|
| Intervention method | Experimental variable that is manipulated, mutually exclusive, and can be replicated in other studies | Clinical method that is modifiable, dependent on the observed needs of patient and the experiences of clinician |
| Other factors affecting intervention | Systematic, extraneous variables that must be controlled (e.g., by matching, random assignment, or narrowing the scope of the study) | Individual factors in the patient that account for some patients improving, whereas other patients remain the same or regress |
| Assessing improvement | Operational definition of measurement instruments for improvement and control for the Hawthorne effect | Clinical impression of patient's progress based on the clinician's initial evaluation and subsequent observed changes at discharge |

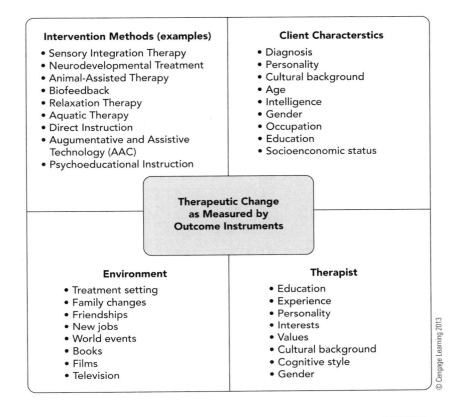

**Intervention Methods (examples)**
- Sensory Integration Therapy
- Neurodevelopmental Treatment
- Animal-Assisted Therapy
- Biofeedback
- Relaxation Therapy
- Aquatic Therapy
- Direct Instruction
- Augumentative and Assistive Technology (AAC)
- Psychoeducational Instruction

**Client Characterstics**
- Diagnosis
- Personality
- Cultural background
- Age
- Intelligence
- Gender
- Occupation
- Education
- Socioenconomic status

**Therapeutic Change as Measured by Outcome Instruments**

**Environment**
- Treatment setting
- Family changes
- Friendships
- New jobs
- World events
- Books
- Films
- Television

**Therapist**
- Education
- Experience
- Personality
- Interests
- Values
- Cultural background
- Cognitive style
- Gender

© Cengage Learning 2013

**FIGURE 3-6**   Potential Factors Affecting Change in a Patient: Each of these factors (i.e., intervention method, patient, intervention setting, and therapist) is multifaceted.

extraneous variables that could influence the results. Four areas of influence, as shown in Figure 3–6, include variables within the client, therapist, and environment, as well as within the intervention method. All of these factors potentially can affect outcome. Knowing this, the researcher must ask: What specific *intervention* method by what specific *therapist* for what specific *patient* in what specific *environment* is effective as measured by what specific *outcome instruments*? The interactional effects of these variables are shown in Figure 3–7.

### 3.2.6 Control of Factors Affecting Patient Improvement

When controlling for factors that may account for patient improvement, the researcher considers the following questions within each of the variables listed.

#### Therapist Variables

- Is the therapist's age or gender significant in affecting outcome?
- Is cognitive style (the characteristic way that the individual perceives the world) a factor?
- How does the therapist's personality affect change?
- Is the therapist's level of education or expertise a factor in improvement?
- What part does the therapist's experience play in client improvement?
- Does the therapist have cultural or ethnic factors that facilitate or retard client progress?
- What other qualities of the therapist can potentially affect patient improvement?

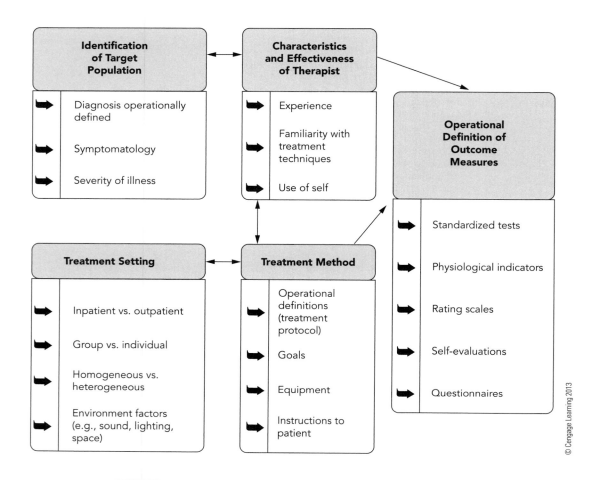

**FIGURE 3-7** Interactional Effects of Intervention, Therapist, Patient, and Intervention Setting: Although the operational definition remains the same, the results obtained on the outcome measures are dependent on the interactional effects of method, therapist, patient, and setting.

## Client Variables

- Do specific demographic factors (e.g., age, gender, or marital status) affect intervention outcome?
- What are the effects of diagnosis and severity of illness on intervention?
- How do the client's intelligence, education, occupation, and social class affect the intervention process?
- Does the congruence or conflict between the personality of the patient and therapist affect outcome?
- Is the patient's environment a factor?

## Intervention Method Variables

- Does the therapist need special training to apply the intervention method?
- Is the intervention method reliable, that is, does it allow the therapist to apply a standard operational procedure or protocol to clients?
- Is there an underlying theoretical explanation for treatment intervention effect on patient improvement?

## Environmental Variables

- Does the setting where intervention takes place affect outcome? (Examples include hospital, clinic, patient's home, classroom, special school, transitional housing, or supported employment.)

- How does the timing (the length of individual intervention sessions and frequency of interventions during a week) affect outcome?
- Does group versus individual intervention affect outcome?
- What are the effects of interactions of co-therapists who are simultaneously treating the same patients?
- Do physical variables in the intervention setting (e.g., lighting, background, sound, color, temperature, atmospheric pressure, and visual distractions) affect intervention outcome?

In addition to these four variables (therapist, patient, intervention method, and environment), the researcher must pose the following questions regarding the measurement of outcome.

### Measurement of Intervention

What criteria are used for measuring outcome? These criteria include the following:

- Change in physical capacity, such as grip strength, spasticity, fine motor dexterity, heart rate, upper extremity strength, gross motor abilities
- Increase in psychosocial functioning, such as the ability to work, improved self-esteem, improved interpersonal relationships (e.g., with family, peers, authority figures), and the ability to cope with stress
- Cognitive functioning, such as alertness, attention span, memory or information processing, problem solving, organization
- Improved behavioral performance with regard to insomnia, eating disorders, smoking, substance abuse, or sexual dysfunction
- Increase in health-related knowledge, such as nutrition, stress management techniques, the use of activity or exercise, family relationships, and use of and compliance with pharmaceutical drugs

### Interactional Effects on Intervention Outcome

The researcher must also account for interactional effects among variables. For example, a therapist with a penchant for order may be more effective using a behavioral modification intervention method than a therapist who has a personality characterized by a strong need for nurturing others. An intervention method that is effectively employed with one therapist may not be as effective with another therapist. The therapist's personality, values, and characteristics impact his ability to work with specific clients and may affect the outcome. The therapist's preferences for working with specific patients are usually indicative of personality variables, although the self-selecting process of the therapist's preference for a specific intervention method in a specific intervention setting with a designated diagnostic group, may be limited by the therapist's education and experience. As a therapist gains insight into his own skills and perceived effectiveness in working with patients, he will develop specific preferences. For the researcher evaluating the effectiveness of an intervention procedure, sensitivity to and awareness of the interactional effects of variables on intervention outcome is a necessity.

An example of a hypothetical research study examining the interaction between intervention methods in occupational therapy and a therapist's characteristics is shown in Figure 3–8. In this example, four methods for treating ADHD in children are compared: behavior therapy, stress management, group psychodynamic, and psychoeducational. The therapist's characteristics in working with clients are typified as:

1. *Laissez-faire*: The therapist is permissive in approaching clients.
2. *Authoritarian*: The therapist is directive in working with clients.
3. *Democratic*: The therapist allows the clients' input into developing interventions.

The hypothetical results may show that behavior therapy is most effective with therapists who are authoritarian and that a group psychodynamic approach may be most effective with a therapist who is laissez-faire. The stress management or psychoeducational approaches may be most effective with therapists who use a democratic approach.

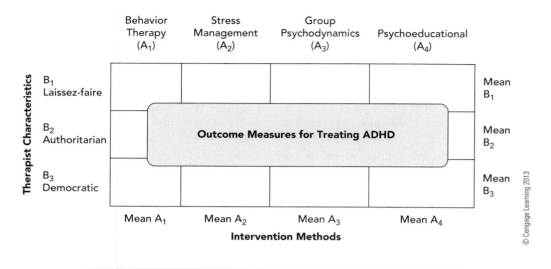

**FIGURE 3-8** Interaction between Intervention Methods and Therapist Characteristics in Treating Clients with ADHD

### 3.2.7 Analysis of Human Processes in Typical Subjects

Experimental research models have been used to investigate physiological, psychological, and sociological responses to various stimuli with typical ("normal") human subjects. In general, experimental research with typical subjects tends to be *nomothetic* in that the researcher seeks general laws of nature that govern kinesthetic, physiological, neurological, sociological, or psychological processes. The researcher might investigate the most effective means to encourage typical child development, for example. Such a study could involve selection of toys, specific teaching methods, nutrition, sensory motor stimulation, or physical activity. In all of these examples, the investigator can use experimental research to compare the different methods.

Potential relationships that can be studied with experimental research are the following:

- Exercise and mood in typical subjects
- Cooperative learning groups and achievement
- Cognitive style and choice of leisure activities
- Body alignment and mechanical stress on joints
- Dichotic listening and organization of auditory stimuli into meaningful patterns
- Movement patterns and sport skills
- Verbal reinforcement and learning
- Language stimulation and reading achievement
- Activity and normal aging

### 3.2.8 Operational Definitions of Normality

When defining normality and selecting typical subjects, the investigator should be guided by an a priori screening criterion setting forth attributes in the continuous range of typical functioning. Each screening criterion (e.g., intelligence, muscle strength, range of motion, blood pressure, heart rate, reading achievement) must be operationally defined and the range of scores determined to be typical or normal before the study begins. If this guideline is followed, the researcher can generalize the results from the data to all typical human subjects within the age ranges represented.

In some experiments, **normality** is defined as an ideal state of health without the presence of a disability or disease. In other cases, *normality* refers to a statistical average of a population where disease and disability are evenly distributed. The following example illustrates the fallacy of rigid criteria for defining "normality": A physician evaluating an older individual's blood pressure would take into consideration the individual's age in concluding that the blood pressure is within the normal range. A pregnant woman would be expected to have a higher blood pressure than a non-pregnant woman. An individual with obesity would be expected to have a higher blood pressure than a person without obesity, and so forth. The concept of "normal blood pressure" is dependent on age, gender, and weight as is indicated.

Relative normality needs to be considered when a researcher reports data for typical subjects. Many researchers assume that normality exists as an absolute and that the healthiest age is young adulthood. Concluding that young adults are usually healthy, the researcher many times is tempted to select young college students as representative samples of normally healthy individuals. The data derived from such a study would be representative only of a young adult population of college students, however. Whatever group is selected, the researcher must also demonstrate that the subjects had no physiological abnormalities that could influence results. In sort, a research subject is considered *typical* only when compared to a priori screening criteria.

## 3.3 Methodological Research

### 3.3.1 Purposes of Methodological Research

**Methodological research** involves the objective and systematic investigation for designing instruments, tests, procedures, curriculum, software programs, and intervention programs. Figure 3–9 outlines specific areas of applying methodological research to rehabilitation, occupational therapy, and habilitation.

As seen in Chapter 1, significant advances in medicine and rehabilitation occurred because of technological advances via microscopes, X-ray machines, electrocardiograms, alternative and augmentative communication, computer software, CT scans, and the numerous diagnostic scopes, all of which are results of methodological research. The introduction of psychophysiological measures and functional capacity evaluations are examples of the ongoing importance of methodological research and its relationship to clinical practice.

### 3.3.2 Strategies

In devising an assessment tool, intervention protocol, or assistive device, the researcher poses the question: What are the relevant factors that must be considered in devising a test instrument, intervention method, or self-care device? Factors to consider include developmental age, cognitive functioning, sensory-motor abilities, and educational level. The content and format of the instrument or test should be determined after a systematic review of related literature.

An example of a methodological research study involves developing a feasible method of independent feeding for a population of individuals with severe disabilities. The researcher needs to consider several aspects of feeding, including positioning, utensils, eye-hand coordination, motivational factors, instructional methods, and attention level of the clients. Another example is a researcher interested in devising therapeutic toys for children with cerebral palsy. In this case, factors relating to sensorimotor, cognition, psychosocial aspects, and language should be considered. The sequential analysis shown in Figure 3–10 describes the steps involved in designing a therapeutic toy for children with cerebral palsy.

### 3.3.3 Designing Intervention Protocol

The **intervention protocol** is an operational definition of an intervention method. It includes all the details in the prescription, preparation, initiation, implementation, documentation, and evaluation. The number of interventions per day or week and the length of the sessions are also included. The intervention protocol should be modified or adjusted to meet the individual needs of the client.

What if an occupational therapist is interested in designing a new intervention protocol for cognitive retraining in adult patients who have sustained a traumatic brain injury (TBI)? How can the clinical researcher assist the occupational therapist in this investigation?

| ASSISTIVE TECHNOLOGY | ASSESSMENT INSTRUMENTS | PHYSICAL EVALUATION |
|---|---|---|
| • Augmentative and Alternative Communication (ACC)<br>• Computer hardware and software<br>• Mobility (e.g., wheelchairs, environmental controls)<br>• Prosthetics and orthotics<br>• Self-help devices<br>• Sensory aids (visual, tactile)<br>• Switches and controls<br>• Vocational adaptations | • ADL scales<br>• Developmental inventories<br>• Functional capacity evaluations<br>• Interview schedules<br>• Outcome measures<br>• Perceptual-motor scales<br>• Questionnaires and attitude scales<br>• Rating scales | • Abnormal reflexes<br>• Biofeedback<br>• Grip strength<br>• Gross and fine motor<br>• Manual-muscle testing<br>• Pain sensitivity<br>• Range of motion<br>• Sensory (visual, auditory, tactile) |

| TREATMENT ENVIRONMENTS | CURRICULUM DEVELOPMENT | TREATMENT PROTOCOLS |
|---|---|---|
| • Adult day care programs<br>• Areas for animal-assisted therapy<br>• Community-based settings<br>• General and special education classrooms<br>• Halfway houses<br>• Skilled nursing facilities<br>• Social milieus<br>• Supported employment<br>• Therapy clinics | • Distance learning<br>• Field work (e.g., preceptor, mentoring, internships<br>• Instructional aids (e.g., audiovisual tapes, CD and DVD, anatomical models)<br>• Module development<br>• Problem-based learning<br>• Software programs | • Academic instruction<br>• ADL/IADL programs<br>• Animal-assisted therapy<br>• Aquatic therapy<br>• Cognitive retraining<br>• Functional academics<br>• Neurodevelopmental therapy<br>• Relaxation therapy<br>• Sensory-integration therapy<br>• Speech-language therapy |

© Cengage Learning 2013

**FIGURE 3-9** Methodological Research—Purposes and Content: This figure illustrates the application of methodological research to occupational therapy, rehabilitation, and habilitation.

The overall design of the research is organized into five phases:

- *Phase I* is an examination of the need for developing a new cognitive retraining protocol that takes into consideration the incidence of TBI in the population, as well as the family, social, and economic costs of TBI. The significance of the study is documented.
- *Phase II* includes a search of the literature reviewing the etiology, incidence and prevalence rates, and current intervention methods for cognitive retraining. As part of the literature review, the researcher would ideally complete a descriptive meta-analysis that evaluates and compares the research on cognitive retraining methods.
- *Phase III* considers the variables that enter into the design of a specific intervention protocol. The variables considered in devising the protocol are described in Table 3–5. In this phase, the clinical researcher's goal is to design the intervention method so that it can

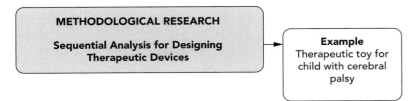

METHODOLOGICAL RESEARCH

**Sequential Analysis for Designing Therapeutic Devices**

→ **Example**
Therapeutic toy for child with cerebral palsy

| **Step 1. Purpose** | **Step 2. Areas for literature review** | **Step 3. Select subjects** | **Step 4. Analyze materials and construction** |
|---|---|---|---|
| Devise toy to stimulate development in child with cerebral palsy | • Theory of play<br>• Cerebral palsy<br>• Child development<br>• Toy construction | Screening criteria for cerebral palsy | Set up laboratory to design the toy |

| **Step 5. Operationalize therapeutic goals for:** | **Step 6. Construct therapeutic toy, considering:** | **Step 7. Observe effects of toy with typical population** |
|---|---|---|
| • Cognitive development<br>• Interpersonal growth<br>• Motor coordination<br>• Language development<br>• Intrapersonal development | • Chronological age<br>• Developmental age<br>• Interests<br>• Materials<br>• Applicability<br>• Goals | • Therapist or teacher completes observational scale<br>• Child completes self-report questionnaire<br>• Examine effectiveness of toy, interest in toy, and developmental areas stimulated |

| **Step 8. Redesign toy based on feedback from typical children** | **Step 9. Use the toy with representative group of children with cerebral palsy** | **Step 10. Use feedback from consumers to modify toy** | **Step 11. Apply use of the toy in therapeutic treatment and evaluate its effectiveness** |
|---|---|---|---|

© Cengage Learning 2013

**FIGURE 3-10** Methodological Research–Construction of a Therapeutic Toy: Note that the construction includes a literature review, operationalized goals, pilot testing on students with and without disabilities, and evaluation of effectiveness.

be used by trained occupational therapists to work with individuals with TBI.

- *Phase IV* includes the pilot testing of the intervention protocol. During this phase, the researcher is concerned with the refinement of the procedure and initial evaluation

by occupational therapists working with TBI. The researcher develops and the clinicians complete a rating scale for assessing the clarity and relevancy of the intervention method. The actual testing of the effectiveness of the intervention protocol cannot be accomplished until

© Cengage Learning 2013

| TABLE 3-5 | | |
|---|---|---|
| **Variables in Devising an Intervention Protocol** | | |
| **Patient** | **Therapist** | **Method** |
| • Diagnosis | • Educational level | • Operationalized intervention goals |
| • Severity of illness | • Experience | • Time factors |
| • Gender | • Specific training | • Manual of directions |
| • Intelligence | • Cognitive style | • Individual versus group factors |
| • Education | | |
| • Socioeconomic status | | |

the protocol has been operationally defined and then tested for its feasibility. The following issues must also be considered:

1. Are the instructions presented clearly to the client?
2. Are all theoretical assumptions considered when developing the method? For example, when developing a cognitive retraining protocol, the researcher must consider the encoding, storage, and retrieval aspects of information processing.
3. Should the intervention be shortened or lengthened in time?
4. Are there limitations to the intervention procedure? For example, clients with limited cognitive abilities may not benefit from a cognitive retraining protocol.

• *Phase V* includes the evaluation of the intervention protocol, its applicability to individuals with TBI, and the level of skill necessary to administer the intervention. The potential effectiveness of the intervention method compared with other procedures as identified in the literature review should also be considered.

### 3.3.4 Assessment Instruments

The design of assessment instruments is a traditional role for psychologists who are trained in measurement theory and test construction. Recently, clinicians of diverse disciplines in rehabilitation and special education have also become involved in developing new assessment measures that are directly related to clinical evaluation.

For example, interest among occupational therapists in perceptual-motor functions and child development has led to the construction of new tests designed for specific intervention populations (Miller, 1988). Application and use of standardized tests is becoming an increasingly important task of the clinician who routinely evaluates the level of patient function. The construction of reliable and valid instruments for measuring human capacities is a relatively fertile area of methodological research in the allied health professions. A more in-depth discussion of testing and measurement is in Chapter 9. Figure 3–11 analyzes the steps involved in test construction.

### 3.3.5 Questionnaires and Interviews

The need to gather information regarding the characteristics and attitudes of populations has led to the wide abuse of interviews and questionnaires, especially in marketing research. Individuals are deluged by interviews and questionnaires asking whether they use a certain brand of toothpaste or deodorant, ad infinitum. Despite abuses, surveys can be useful tools in obtaining information about a target population.

**SEQUENCE OF METHODOLOGICAL TEST CONSTRUCTION**

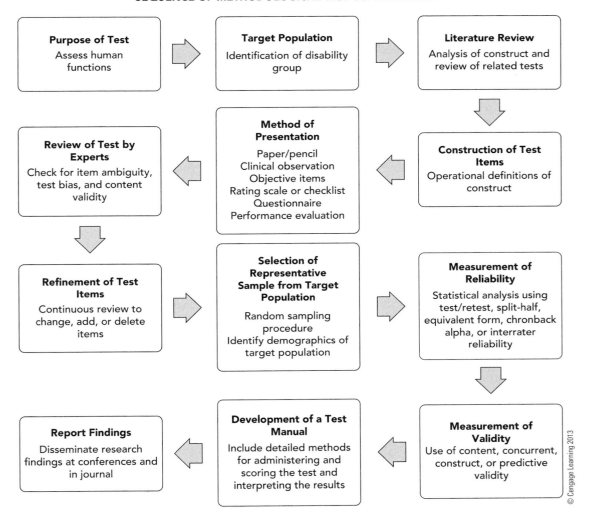

**FIGURE 3-11** Methodological Research–Test Construction, including Rating Scales and Questionnaires: Note that there is a sequential order to the construction, with many validity checks as the task is being completed.

In constructing interviews or questionnaires, the researcher must resolve the following questions:

- Was there an overall theoretical framework or rationale for selecting the items?
- Do the items measure accurately what the researcher purports to measure? (Validity)
- Are the items clear, unambiguous, and consistent? (Reliability)
- Was a representative pilot sample selected for testing reliability?

For a further discussion of interviews and questionnaires see Chapter 9.

### Rating Scales

**Rating scales** are a type of questionnaire that can be used to quantify information. Rating scales are employed most frequently in evaluating the performance of students, clients, and staff. Typically, the evaluator checks off the description most indicative of performance from a list of adjective phrases.

Rating scales are usually of three types: numerical, dichotomous, and descriptive. In a numerical scale, often called a **Likert scale**, ratings are distributed along a continuum, such as in the following example:

Rate each of the following items by circling the number that corresponds to your opinion. (Likert Scale)

| | |
|---|---|
| Strongly agree | 1 |
| Agree | 2 |
| Neutral | 3 |
| Disagree | 4 |
| Strongly disagree | 5 |

a. The United States should adopt a universal health plan for all residents.

   1     2     3     4     5

b. Medicare and Medicaid should be combined into one health care system.

   1     2     3     4     5

In a dichotomous scale, the extremes are identified, and the rater chooses the extreme that indicates the client's performance. For example:

Circle *yes* or *no*.

The patient's ability to assemble small parts is adequate.

              Yes     No

In a descriptive scale, the rater chooses a phrase from a presented list. For example:

Circle the descriptive phrase that is most accurate.
1. On a specific task (e.g., addressing envelopes) the worker in a supported employment needs supervision:

- all of the time
- some of the time
- once in a while
- rarely
- none of the time

## 3.3.6 Treatment Facilities

How can a clinical researcher contribute to the design of an effective intervention environment for clients with disabilities? The tasks of designing sheltered workshops, adult day care, outpatient clinics, and halfway houses are a joint effort by architects, administrators, therapists, and other rehabilitation personnel. The researcher applying methodological research to the construction of an intervention environment should first pose the question: What factors must be considered in designing a therapeutic environment for clients? Using answers to this question, the researcher can generate a plan that considers several variables. A tentative outline for research follows.

## 3.3.7 Methodological Review: Treatment Facilities

1. Formulating the purposes for the treatment facility:

   a. Disabilities serviced (e.g., individuals with mental illness, retardation, or physical impairments)
   b. Intervention or treatment goals (e.g., cognitive and physical development, functional skills, independent living)
   c. Demographic considerations for screening clients (e.g., age, gender, level of care)
   d. Location of treatment facility (e.g., urban, suburban, or rural area) and impact on neighborhood

2. Surveying need for intervention facility by documenting:

   a. Number of potential clients to be serviced
   b. Number of other intervention facilities in service area
   c. Attitudes toward facility's location by potential clients, community residents, and health care providers

3. Reviewing literature describing similar programs:

   a. Identifying model programs
   b. Architectural descriptions of physical layouts

c. Analysis of staff functions and patient ratios

d. Policies regarding patient admissions, discharges, and follow-up

e. Evaluation research of intervention effectiveness

f. Administrative considerations (e.g., budgeting, departmental responsibilities)

4. Stating guiding assumptions and rationale for:

   a. Setting screening criteria for client admission and discharges

   b. Designing physical layout and geographical location

   c. Proposing staff positions

   d. Setting criteria for evaluating effectiveness

5. Surveying resources of community for:

   a. Potential source of staff

   b. Transportation facilities

   c. Consultative services

   d. Community support

6. Survey cost-effectiveness factors:

   a. Construction cost

   b. Cost of providing patient care and intervention

   c. Cost of providing supportive and maintenance services

   d. Sources of potential income:
      i. private pay
      ii. insurance and any third-party payments
      iii. government entitlements (Medicaid and Medicare)
      iv. state and federal grants
      v. private foundations

## 3.3.8 Designing Education Curricula

The training of occupational therapists, dietitians, rehabilitation counselors, speech-language pathologists, audiologists, physical therapists, special educators, school psychologists, and other related professional groups involves interdisciplinary approaches. What knowledge in the areas of physiology, anatomy, psychology, and sociology are necessary? What interpersonal skills in working with clients with disabilities must be developed? What evaluation and intervention procedures should be taught?

These questions regarding the content of educational curricula are continually reevaluated in light of the rapid growth of the occupational therapy profession. Parallel to the growth of the curricula content areas is the interest in designing methods for effectively communicating knowledge to occupational therapy students. How do students learn most effectively? What should be the role of problem-based learning, computer-assisted instruction, distance learning, technology, preceptor and intern supervision, and lecture in the educational curricula? These questions lend themselves to methodological research. The researcher objectively designs a curriculum after identifying the relevant factors from an extensive review of the literature.

## 3.3.9 Physical Evaluation Techniques and Intervention Hardware

Another area of methodological research that is appropriate to the allied health professions pertains to the use of machines and hardware for evaluating a patient's functional capacity Electromyography (EMG), electrodiagnostic recording, perceptual-motor tests, visual, auditory and kinesthesis testing, and manual muscle testing are examples of the broad areas for potential research.

Occupational therapists may use physical agent modalities (PAMs). PAMs include ultrasound, diathermy, infrared light, ultraviolet rays, hydrotherapy, electrical stimulation, hot packs, acupuncture, TENS, biofeedback, and paraffin. New methods of intervention, especially in muscle retraining, are now relying on electrophysiological methods involving oscilloscopes, telemetry, and computers. The growth in the area of prosthetics has been the result of the combined talents of researchers coming from backgrounds in engineering, neurophysiology, and occupational therapy. Orthotics, the development of splints and braces for individuals with physical disabilities, is another area for research development in occupational therapy.

In Box 3–3, the investigators examine the *Useful Field of View* (UFOV), and the *Stroke Drivers' Screening Assessment* (SDSA) to determine which is the more useful to guide clinical practitioners in evaluating the skill of driving after a stroke.

---

### BOX 3-3

## Example of Methodological Research

### 1. Bibliographical Notation

George, S., & Crotty, M. (2010). Establishing criterion validity of the useful field of view assessment and stroke drivers' screening assessment: Comparison to the result of on-road assessment. *American Journal of Occupational Therapy, 64,* 114–122. doi:10.5014/ajot.64.1.114

### 2. Abstract

We sought to determine the criterion validity of the *Useful Field of View* (UFOV; Ball & Roenker, 1998) assessment and *Stroke Drivers' Screening Assessment* (SDSA; Nouri & Lincoln, 1993) through comparison to the results of on-road assessment. This was a prospective study with people with stroke. Outcome measures used were UFOV, SDSA, and the results of on-road assessment. Both the results on UFOV (Divided Attention subtest, $p < .01$; Selective Attention subtest, $p < .05$) and SDSA ($p < .05$) were significantly related to the recommendation from on-road assessment. The Divided Attention subtest of the UFOV had the highest sensitivity value (88.9 %). UFOV and SDSA are valid assessments of driving ability for stroke. The Divided Attention subtest of the UFOV can guide decision making of occupational therapists in stroke driver rehabilitation and in determining those who require further assessment on road because they pose a safety risk. Screening assists people with stroke to decide whether they are ready to have an on-road assessment.

### 3. Justification and Need for Study

Only a small number of research studies investigating the validity of pre-driving assessment tools in stroke have reported sensitivity. In this study, both the UFOV and the SDSA are investigated to determine which is the most useful to guide clinical practice in driving after stroke. The purpose of this study was to determine the criterion validity, including the sensitivity, specificity, and positive and negative predictive values of the UFOV and SDSA, using a comparison with the result of on-road assessment.

### 4. Literature Review

Thirty-six references from a wide variety of sources were cited. The cited journals included, but were not limited to: *Neurorehabiliation and Neural Repair, Archives of Physical Medicine and Rehabilitation, American Journal of Occupational Therapy* (AJOT), *Clinical Rehabilitation, Scandinavian Journal of Psychology, Journal of Mental Health, British Medical Journal, Journal of Clinical Epidemiology,* and *Australian Occupational Therapy Journal.* The years of the cited publications ranged from 1985 to 2008.

### 5. Research Hypothesis or Guiding Questions

The perspective of the study was to determine the criterion validity, including the sensitivity, specificity, and positive and negative predictive values, of the UFOV and SDSA, using a comparison with the result of on-road assessment. No hypotheses were made.

### 6. Methods

This study was a prospective correlation study of a group of drivers with stroke. The participants of the study included the diagnoses of 24 right-hemisphere stroke, 37 left-hemisphere stroke, and five other strokes. All the participants had a stroke, drove before onset, were older than age 18, and were assessed as having adequate cognition to follow instructions to complete the assessments. After informed consent was obtained, the following assessments were performed by the researcher: UFOV, SDSA, and a standardized on-road driving assessment performed within six weeks of completion of the UFOV and SDSA. After the completion of the assessments, the driving assessors, a driving instructor, and a driver-trained occupational therapist determined recommendation, and participants were classified as either a pass or a fail. The on-road driver assessors were blinded to the results of the UFOV and SDSA. Data was analyzed using the Statistical Package for Social Sciences Version 12.0. Relationships between categorical variables for the stroke participants were tested using the Chi-square test for categorical variables and used independent samples $t$-test and Mann-Whitney $U$ test for continuous variables. Pass or fail on the UFOV and the SDSA were compared to the pass or fail recommendations that were given or the on-road assessment. Specificity, sensitivity, positive and negative predictive values, and confidence intervals were calculated for the screening tests that were found to be statistically significantly associated with the outcome of the on-road assessment.

### 7. Results

The SDSA results recommendations were significantly associated with the evaluation of on-road ability, indicating it is a valid assessment of driving ability when using the original discriminant equation. However, when using an alternate discriminant equation there was not a significant association with the outcome of the on-road assessment. The UFOV and outcome of the on-road assessment indicated that divided attention and selective attention were significantly associated with the evaluation of on-road ability. Overall the results indicate that the UFOV and the SDSA are valid tests of driving ability for stroke.

### 8. Conclusions

George and Crotty concluded that:

1. "SDSA and UFOV are valid tests of driving ability after stroke" (p. 121).
2. The divided attention subtest of the UFOV showed high sensitivity, and "indicates the inclusion of the UFOV in an occupational therapist's predriving assessment to determine drivers requiring an on-road assessment" (p. 121).
3. "Predriving assessment assists people with stroke to determine whether they are ready to undergo the on-road assessment" (p.120).

*continues*

---

**BOX 3-3**

**Example of Methodological Research** *continued*

---

### 9. Limitations of the Study

One limitation is the small sample size. Another limitation is the delay between the performance of prescreening assessments and the on-road assessment. Further research needs to be conducted to determine whether performing the UFOV subtests in isolation yields the same findings as the results in this study.

### 10. Major References Cited in the Study

Bouillon, L., Mazer, B., & Gelinas, I. (2006). Validity of the Cognitive Behavioural Driver's Inventory in predicting driving outcome. *American Journal of Occupational Therapy, 60,* 420–427.

Lincoln, N. B., Radford, K. A., & Nouri, F. M. (2004). *Stroke Drivers Screening Assessment: Revised Manual.* Nottingham, England: University of Nottingham.

Mazer, B., Sofer, S., Korner-Bitensky, N., Gelinas, I., Hanley, J., & Wood-Dauphinee, S. (2003). Effectiveness of a visual attention retraining program on driving performance of clients with stroke. *Archives of Physical Medicine and Rehabilitation, 84,* 541–550.

Novack, T. A., Baños, J. H., Alderson, A. L., Schneider, J. J., Weed, W., Blankenship, J., & Salisbury, D. (2006). UFOV performance and driving ability following traumatic brain injury. *Brain Injury, 20,* 455–461.

Visual Awareness, Inc. (2002). UFOV user's guide. Birmingham, AL: Author. Retrieved from http://crag.uab.edu/VAI/PDF%20Pubs/UFOV_Manual_V6.0.6.pdf

---

Figure 3–12 illustrates the steps involved with developing a test for manual dexterity using methodological research.

## 3.4 Evaluation Research

### 3.4.1 Purposes of Evaluation Research

Evaluation research examines the effectiveness of programs that provide direct health care, prepare health personnel, and administer services for private and governmental agencies. When engaged in evaluation research, the investigator considers a total corporate unit and the components that comprise it. Program effectiveness, quality of service, productivity, organizational communication, cost-effectiveness, stated objectives, and personnel practices are areas considered in evaluation research. Evaluation research is commonly applied in the following programs, services, and agencies:

- Certification of hospitals (e.g., The Joint Commission)
- Accreditation of college or educational program (e.g., National College Accreditation of Teacher Education [NCATE] or Accreditation Commission of Occupational Therapy Education [ACOTE])

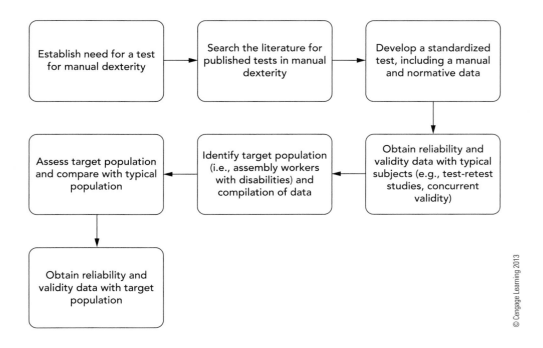

**FIGURE 3-12**  This is an example of a methodological research showing the steps in developing a test for manual dexterity. This process is used in the development of all tests.

- Rehabilitation agency evaluation (e.g., The Rehabilitation Accreditation Commission [CARF])
- Analysis of cost-per-patient intervention (e.g., Medicare guidelines, Diagnostic Related Groups [DRGs])
- Outcome studies of patients or clients
- Needs assessment (e.g., community's health needs, available resources)
- Evaluation of program effectiveness using **a priori** criteria

A historical example of the impact of evaluation research on changing an institution was Abraham Flexner's (1910) report *Medical Education in the United States and Canada*, which was made to the Carnegie Foundation for the Advancement of Training. Flexner personally toured the 155 medical schools that existed at that time in the United States and Canada. Although he did not use

a standardized questionnaire or test instrument for evaluation, Flexner did apply specific criteria in evaluating the quality and effectiveness of medical schools in preparing physicians. These criteria were the following:

1. The entrance requirements for gaining admission to the medical school (e.g., minimal standards, high school graduation or equivalent, or college education)
2. The number of students in full-time or part-time attendance
3. The size of the faculty, including number of full-time professors and part-time instructors
4. The financial resources available to the college from endowments, student tuition, and clinical fees
5. The quality and adequacy of the physical plant, including laboratory classrooms, lecture halls, medical and laboratory equipment, refrigerator

plants, amphitheater for observation of surgery and clinical interviews, and medical library

6. Professional supervision available to the students in the laboratories
7. The opportunities for student practice in clinics and availability of hospital patients

On the basis of these criteria, Flexner found a wide discrepancy in standards of medical education in the schools he visited. He concluded, based on his observations, that many medical schools were doing a disservice to the public by preparing poorly educated physicians. He recommended that there be fewer medical schools.

Flexner's evaluations of the 155 medical schools led to dramatic changes in medical education that occurred between 1910 and 1925. He recommended that (a) medical schools and hospitals enter into teaching relationships, (b) state boards reject applicants for medical degrees who graduate from medical schools that were inadequate, and (c) examinations for state licensure be rigorous. He hoped that "Perhaps the entire country may some day be covered by a health organization engaged in protecting the public health against the formidable combination made by ignorance, incompetency, commercialism, and disease" (p. 173). All of these recommendations were eventually implemented and led to the founding of the American Medical Association (AMA). Evaluation research as used by Flexner was directed toward the improvement of an institution, specifically the medical profession.

When properly used, evaluation research can be useful (Weiss, 1972) in deciding whether to:

- Continue or discontinue a program
- Improve an agency's practices and procedures
- Add or drop specific program strategies and techniques
- Use a program as a model for new agencies
- Utilize more fully the services of a program on a geographical basis
- Accept or reject theoretical approaches underlining an agency's program

These purposes are achieved only after the investigator has collected objective and valid data.

The research steps include (a) the stated need for evaluation research; (b) a review of the literature, comprising a description of programs and criteria used; (c) an objective research design for collecting data through interviews, questionnaires, attitude scales, and clinical observation; (d) statistical analysis of records and examination of the physical plant; (e) comparisons of program with objective criteria; (f) separate sections on results and discussion of findings; and (g) the evaluation team's recommendation for reaccreditation, probation, or closing of the program. Figure 3–13 identifies examples of potential areas for evaluation research in occupational therapy, rehabilitation, and habilitation.

### 3.4.2 Strategies of Evaluation Research

The issue of researcher bias is of prime consideration in evaluation research. The underlying purpose of evaluation research is to apply objective assessment to a facility, an agency, or an intervention program. How does a researcher objectively evaluate an organization? How are criteria established for measuring the effectiveness of a program? Are criteria established by the evaluation research team based on ideal theoretical considerations or by the intervention agency that is being evaluated? What expertise in research is needed in evaluating the competence and abilities of health professionals? What controls should be established in the research methods to reduce investigator bias?

The following hypothetical example explores the process of evaluation research as applied to a residential school for adolescents who have diagnosed emotional disturbance:

1. Stated purposes of evaluation are set forth, such as:

   a. Continued school certification or accreditation
   b. Evaluation of intervention effectiveness
   c. Direct and indirect costs per student intervention
   d. Widening of services to include more diverse client groups

**Treatment Program Located in:**

- General hospitals
- Psychiatric facilities
- Rehabilitation centers
- Home-health services
- Halfway houses
- Residential treatment centers (RTC)
- Independent living complexes
- Special schools
- Sheltered workshops
- Clinics
- Therapy departments

**Preparatory and Advanced Educational Programs for Occupational Therapists**

- Certified occupational therapy assistants
- Basic professional (bachelor's or master's degree) training program
- Advanced professional degree program (master's or doctorate)

**Voluntary and Primary Agencies Related to:**

- AIDS
- Alzheimer's disease
- Arthritis
- ADHD/ADD
- Autism
- Cancer
- Cerebral palsy
- Heart disease
- Learning disabilities
- Mental retardation
- Multiple sclerosis
- Muscular dystrophy
- Psychosocial disorders
- Spinal cord injury
- Stroke
- Traumatic brain injury

**Governmental and Nongovernmental Agencies**

- Division of Vocational Rehabilitation
- Department of Health and Human Services
- Department of Corrections
- Health maintenance organizations (HMOs)
- Social Security Administration
- National Institute of Mental Health
- State Departments of Education
- United States Department of Education
- United States Department of Veteran Affairs

© Cengage Learning 2013

**FIGURE 3-13**    Potential Areas for Evaluation Research in Occupational Therapy, Rehabilitation, and Habilitation

e. Change in delivery of services to reduce residential population and to include more day care or community-based intervention

f. The overall decision to cease operation before evaluation research is undertaken. There must be a mutual understanding of the purpose between the evaluators and those being evaluated. If the purposes are unclear or if there is a hidden agenda, then the research objectivity could become undermined, and the evaluation could serve more as a political maneuver than as a means to collect objective data. For example, if the evaluators seek to close a program by collecting negative or damaging information and by omitting any positive attributes, then the evaluation is worthless as scientific research.

2. The formation of a research team of evaluators is dependent on the stated purposes of

the evaluation and the specific areas considered. Expertise and experience in program administration, budgeting, intervention techniques, special education, vocational rehabilitation, research methodology, interviewing techniques, and familiarity with educational requirements and job descriptions of professional and nonprofessional staff members are necessary to provide appropriate expertise and knowledge levels for the members of an evaluation research team. Evaluation research demands a sophisticated level of expertise that is essential in the research process. The responsibility of judging the effectiveness of the program is delegated to the research team. As the level of effectiveness is a relative judgment, it is important that each member of the evaluation team understand and accept the criteria being used as the "measuring yardsticks." Experience of the members of the team in working in other intervention agencies and familiarity with the evaluation process, either as a supervisor in a clinic or in an educational environment, are necessary requisites for doing evaluation research. The size of the research team, responsibility based on the areas of expertise and experience represented, and the availability of consultants are considered in forming an effective evaluation research team.

3.  The descriptive data will include:
    a.  History of the organization, including why it was established and names and backgrounds of founders
    b.  Flowchart of administration, including lines of responsibility, and departmental components
    c.  Description of the physical plant, including a detailed layout of the facilities
    d.  Staff resumés, including education and experience of administrators, intervention staff, and supporting personnel
    e.  Job descriptions of work responsibilities
    f.  Rehabilitation and intervention services offered, including but not limited to medical, psychological, educational, child care, and prevocational

    g.  Formal and informal meetings, conferences, and patient staffings
    h.  Intake policies, orientation, and discharge procedures
    i.  Follow-up care and evaluation of discharges
    j.  Relationships with community and outside agencies
    k.  Numerical data regarding maximum client capacity of facility, present number of clients, average length of residence, number of referrals, and discharges over time.

4.  Criteria of effectiveness are established by the research team. The criteria are based on a priori standards or objectives furnished by the administrator of the program. Areas for criteria include:

    a.  *Intervention effect:* percentage of clients who have made successful and unsuccessful adjustments after discharge (definition of successful and unsuccessful outcome should be operationally defined)
    b.  *Physical plant:* safety, health, and accessibility for those individuals with mobility impairment meeting the requirements for Americans with Disability Act (ADA, 1990); fire requirements
    c.  *Professional staff:* percentage of staff having professional educational backgrounds (resumés, number of years at facility, reasons for leaving previous position)
    d.  *Staff ratio:* number of clients per intervention staff
    e.  *Staff salaries:* average salaries as compared with national average or salaries in comparable agencies
    f.  *Continuing education:* opportunities for staff to attend conferences, workshops, or in-services
    g.  *Discharges:* number over time and reasons for client discharge

5.  Criteria can also be established by selecting characteristic patterns from programs considered to be successful models, although flexibility in employing these models is necessary when applying criteria. The severity of the

disability in clients serviced and the financial resources available to an agency are factors that must be considered when analyzing outside criteria.

6. Interviews with staff and residents are necessary to transform the highly subjective process of "getting insights into a systematic method for the collection of social data" (Festinger & Katz, 1953, p. 327). The researcher should recognize the limitations of the interview process. The very nature of communicating feelings and attitudes is limited by the natural suspiciousness of the interviewee and his or her reliance on memory to provide information. It is not the authors' intent to discuss interviewing techniques in detail, but it shall be sufficient to note that researchers utilizing interview information must be certain that the interviewers have had training. Leading questions, long and complicated questions, and rambling and unrelated items, which untrained interviewers often use, provide data that subsequently bias the results. (See Festinger & Katz, 1953, for further information.)

7. The next process in evaluation research is the synthesis of objective descriptive data and objective interview material. The Results section of the report should be separated from the Discussion and Conclusions. Results are raw data that are objective findings. Results should not be "flavored" by subjective analysis or "undone" by interpretations. The results should remain separate from critical analysis. Table 3–6 lists hypothetical data that would be included in a Results section.

8. The interpretative summary consists of a qualitative discussion of the results apart from the quantitative results. Qualitative or naturalistic information could include, for example, staff opportunities to innovate new programs, the informality of the communication process, the accessibility of administrators, the feelings of hope and optimism generated by the staff, the willingness of the agency to change the consumer with disabilities' involvement in intervention planning, the use of community resources, the integration of new technology with present methods, and the facilitation of professional growth through supervision.

9. The conclusions and recommendations of evaluation research are a vital part of the report. How does the research team decide that an intervention program is effective and should

---

### TABLE 3-6

**Hypothetical Results of a Residential Treatment Program**

| Variable | Number | Percent |
| --- | --- | --- |
| Capacity of program | 55 | 100 |
| Average daily attendance of residents during last six months | 50 | 90 |
| Average length of residence for each individual discharged in last six months | 3 months | N/A |
| Number of individuals in residence for over one year | 15 | 30 |
| Number of direct care workers (treatment personnel) | 10 | N/A |
| Number of full-time professional staff, excluding administrators | 6 | N/A |
| Number of part-time consultants | 3 | N/A |
| Number of full-time teachers | 5 | N/A |

have continued support by the community, or that an intervention program is ineffective, not responsive to the needs of a community, and should be terminated?

During the last 50 years, we have seen the decline and closing of large, isolated institutions that served individuals with physical and psychiatric disabilities who mainly came from poor backgrounds. These institutions were closed because they became custodial "warehouses" without providing for the needs of the individuals. Nevertheless, when the institutions were supported by governmental agencies in the United States in the 1920s up until the 1960s, there were few alternatives for community-based intervention. Did evaluation research play a role in the closing of institutions during the 1960s and 1970s?

The criteria identified in evaluative research must be consistent with the needs of the target population. These needs relate to values in human society, such as economic independence, social relationships, educational development, self-esteem, and whatever else the research team or agency sets forth as the goals and objectives. It should be clear that if an agency is not meeting "stated needs" of those individuals who are treated, educated, or serviced and if alternative agencies or facilities are available, then the community should not continue to support an institution's existence.

The following research models are *ex post facto* in nature: heuristic, correlational, clinical observation, survey, and historical. Clinical observation is unique in that it can be either ex post facto (retrospective) or prospective. The data collection procedure in ex post facto research is retrospective because the presumed independent variable has already occurred. Kerlinger (1986) differentiated experimental research and ex post facto research on the basis of the lack of direct control by the researcher in **ex post facto designs**. For example, in experimental research, the investigator hypothesizes "if $X$ then $Y$" and manipulates the $X$. In ex post facto research, the investigator observes $Y$ (the dependent variable) and hypothesizes $X$ (the independent variable). The researcher in ex post facto designs can only presume a past cause-effect relationship. In many ex post facto designs, the investigator seeks historically to reconstruct cause-effect relationships.

Suchman (1967) identified several areas of potential abuse as follows:

- "Eyewash" is an attempt to justify an ineffective program by deliberately selecting only those aspects that appear successful and overlooking important parts of the program.
- "Whitewash" is an effort whereby the evaluators try to cover up program failure and inadequacies by avoiding these areas when evaluating the program. The evaluators may solicit "testimonials" to divert attention from the general failure of the program.
- "Submarine" or "torpedo" is a device to destroy a program regardless of its worth or usefulness in delivering health services. This often occurs in administrative power struggles when opponents and their programs are attacked.
- "Posture" is used by evaluators when they want to appear scientific and objective when, in fact, they carry out a superficial and incomplete evaluation.
- "Postponement" is a tactic of using evaluation research, for example, to answer public reaction to scandalous conditions in an institution. The real purpose of this ploy is to defuse public outrage by substituting research for action.
- "Substitution" is an attempt to hide an essential part of a program that is an obvious failure and to shift emphasis to areas that are controversial.

From the foregoing examples, it is evident that evaluation research can serve not only to provide objective data, but also as a tactic to keep an inadequate program operative or to discredit an effective program.

An example of evaluation research in occupational therapy is found in Box 3–4. The authors of this research study evaluated the effectiveness of an occupational therapy program with older adults who were living in independent housing.

BOX 3-4

## Example of Evaluation Research

### 1. Bibliographical Citation

Clark F., Azen, S. P., Zemke R., Jackson, J., Carlson, M., Mandel, D., Hay, J., Josephson, K., Cherry, B., Hessel, C., Palmer, J., and Lipson, L. (1997). Occupational therapy for independent-living older adults. A randomized controlled trial. *The Journal of American Medical Association, 278,*1321–1326.

### 2. Abstract

**CONTEXT:** Preventive health programs may mitigate against the health risks of older adulthood. **OBJECTIVE:** To evaluate the effectiveness of preventive occupational therapy (OT) services specifically tailored for multiethnic, independent-living older adults. **DESIGN:** A randomized controlled trial. **SETTING:** Two government subsidized apartment complexes for independent-living older adults. **SUBJECTS:** A total of 361 culturally diverse volunteers aged 60 years or older. **INTERVENTION:** An OT group, a social activity control group, and a non-treatment control group. The period of treatment was nine months. **MAIN OUTCOME MEASURES:** A battery of self-administered questionnaires designed to measure physical and social function, self-rated health, life satisfaction, and depressive symptoms. **RESULTS:** Benefit attributable to OT treatment was found for the quality of interaction scale on the *Functional Status Questionnaire* ($p = .03$), *Life Satisfaction Index-Z* ($p = .03$), *Medical Outcomes Study Health Perception Survey* ($p = .05$), and for 7 of 8 scales on the *RAND 36-Item Health Status Survey, Short Form*: bodily pain ($p = .03$), physical functioning ($p = .008$), role limitations attributable to health problems ($p = .02$), vitality ($p = .004$), social functioning ($p = .05$), role limitations attributable to emotional problems ($p = .05$), and general mental health ($p = .02$). **CONCLUSIONS:** Significant benefits for the OT preventive treatment group were found across various health, function, and quality-of-life domains. Because the control groups tended to decline over the study interval, our results suggest that preventive health programs based on OT may mitigate against the health risks of older adulthood (Clark et al., 1997, p. 1321).

### 3. Justification and Need for Study

Findings from the literature suggest that effective activity-based interventions are capable of enhancing the lives of older individuals. "In response to this need, we conducted between 1994 and 1996 a randomized controlled trial, the Well Elderly Study, to evaluate the effectiveness of preventative OT specifically targeted for urban, multiethnic, independent-living older adults" (p. 1321).

### 4. Literature Review

The authors examined the literature on normative aging, activity-theory and aging, quality-of-life issues in aging, and the role of occupational therapy with the older adults. Forty-three references were used, selected from the following journals: *Social Indicators Research,*

*continues*

BOX 3-4

### **Example of Evaluation Research** *continued*

*Social Science in Medicine, American Journal of Occupational Therapy* (AJOT), *International Journal of Aging and Human Development, Journal of Gerontology and Psychological Science, Journal of Gerontology, Journal of Clinical Psychology, Journal of the American Medical Association,* and *Research in Nursing Health.*

### 5. Research Hypothesis or Guiding Questions

"We hypothesized that mere participation in a social activity program does not affect the physical health, daily functioning, or psychosocial well-being of well elderly individuals; and compared with participation in a social activity program or an absence of any treatment, preventative OT positively affects the physical health, daily function, and psychosocial well-being of well elderly individuals (1-sided alternative)" (p. 1322).

### 6. Methods

Three hundred sixty-one older adults, ages 60 and above, were assigned randomly to three groups: an occupational therapy group, a social activity group, and a no treatment group. Participants came from government subsidized housing for independent living, private homes, and other facilities in the community. In the occupational therapy group, participants were exposed to didactic teaching of community living and use of adapted equipment, and performed activities emphasizing grooming, nutrition, exercising, and shopping. Those in the social activities group were involved in "community outings, craft projects, films, played games, and attended dances" (p. 1322). Five questionnaires were used to measure outcome.

### 7. Operational Definition of Variables

Functional status, life-satisfaction, depression, perceptions of health, and physical and mental health status were evaluated through self-report.

### 8. Conclusions

The occupational therapy program in general was more effective than the other two groups. "The OT program enabled subjects to construct daily routines that were health promoting and meaningful given the context of their lives" (p. 1325).

### 9. Limitations of the Study

"The results may not generalize to older adults in different living situations (e.g., single-family dwellers, nursing home residents) or of different socioeconomic status" (p. 1326).

### 10. Major References in Study

Carlson, M., Fanchiang, S-R, Zemke, R., & Clark, F. (1996). A meta-analysis of the effectiveness of occupational therapy for older persons. *The American Journal of Occupational Therapy, 50,* 89–98.

Fisher, B. J. (1995). Successful aging, life satisfaction and generativity in later life. *International Journal of Aging and Human Development, 41,* 230–250.

Larson, K. O., Stevens-Ratchford, R. G., Pedretti, L. W., Crabtree, J. L. (1996). *ROTE: The role of occupational therapy with the elderly.* Bethesda, MD: American Occupational Therapy Association.

Levine, R. E., & Gitlan, L. N. (1992). A model to promote activity competence in elders. *The American Journal of Occupational Therapy, 47,*147–153.

## 3.5    Heuristic Research

### 3.5.1 Purposes of Heuristic Research

Kerlinger (1986) described a heuristic view of science as that which "emphasizes theory and interconnected conceptual schemata that are fruitful for further research" (p. 8). The main purpose of **heuristic research** is to discover relationships between variables as a means of generating further investigations. In heuristic research, the researcher "fishes" for correlational relationships as a means to build a theory and design further research.

The researcher engaged in heuristic research seeks to discover significant relationships by correlating variables with a specific disease or factors affecting intervention. Research in cardiovascular diseases, learning disorders, mental illness, arthritis, multiple sclerosis, cancer, and AIDS are appropriate areas for heuristic research, as well as investigations of space, time, and cost factors in the intervention environment.

### 3.5.2 Application of Pilot Studies in Heuristic Research

**Pilot studies** are innovative studies that examine a problem or question to determine if the research is viable. These studies often have a small number of participants. The investigator does not control all of the extraneous variables. Limitations of the research methodology are identified. Although pilot studies are carried out in other research designs, pilot studies in heuristic research require both an exploration of a theoretical basis and recommendations for further research.

The following list gives examples of pilot studies from occupational therapy, medicine, and special education that are heuristic:

- Allen, S., & Donald, M. (1995). The effect of occupational therapy on the motor proficiency of children with motor/ learning difficulties: A pilot study. *British Journal of Occupational Therapy, 58,* 385–391.
- Bone, C., Cheung, G., & Wade, B. (2010). Evaluating person centred care and dementia care mapping in a psychogeriatric hospital in New Zealand: A pilot study. *New Zealand Journal of Occupational Therapy, 57,* 35–40.
- Cutler, S. K. (1992). *Executive functioning in middle school students who have learning disabilities.* Unpublished doctoral dissertation. University of New Mexico, Albuquerque.
- Dunn, W. (1990). A comparison of service provision models in school-based occupational therapy services: A pilot study. *Occupational Therapy Journal of Research, 10,* 300–320.
- Gagné, D. E. (2003). The effects of collaborative goal-focused occupational therapy on self-care skills: A pilot study. *American Journal of Occupational Therapy, 57,* 215–219.
- Hammer, A. M. (2009). Effects of forced use on arm function in the subacute phase after stroke: A randomized, clinical pilot study... including commentary by J. H. Cauraugh, J. J. Summers, and J. Charles with authors' response. *Physical Therapy, 89,* 526–545.

Hoppes, S. (1997). Can play increase standing tolerance? A pilot-study. *Physical and Occupational Therapy in Geriatrics, 15,* 65–73.

Lloyd, C. (2007). The association between leisure motivation and recovery: A pilot study. *Australian Occupational Therapy Journal, 54,* 33–41.

Lo, J., & Zemke, R. (1997). The relationship between affective experiences during daily occupations and subjective well-being measures: A pilot study. *Occupational Therapy in Mental Health, 13,* 1–21.

May-Benson, T. A. (2007). Identifying gravitational insecurity in children: A pilot study. *American Journal of Occupational Therapy, 61,* 142–147.

Miller, L. J. (2007). Lessons learned: A pilot study on occupational therapy effectiveness for children with sensory modulation disorder. *American Journal of Occupational Therapy, 61,* 161–169.

Prince, F., Winter, D. A., Sjonnensen, G., Powell, C., Wheeldon, R. K. (1998). Mechanical efficiency during gait of adults with transtibial amputation: A pilot study comparing the SACH, Seattle, and Golden-Ankle. *Journal of Rehabilitation Research and Development, 35,* 177–185.

Rabadi, M. H. (2008). A pilot study of activity-based therapy in the arm motor recovery post stroke: A randomized controlled trial. *Clinical Rehabilitation, 22,* 1071–1082.

Reid, D. T., & Jutai, J. (1997). A pilot study of perceived clinical usefulness of a new computer-based tool for assessment of visual perception in occupational therapy practice. *Occupational Therapy International, 4,* 81–98.

Seidman, L. J., Biederman, J., Faraone, S. V., Weber, W., Mennin, D., & Jones, J. (1997). A pilot study of neuropsychological function in girls with ADHD. *Journal of the American Academic of Child and Adolescent Psychiatry, 36,* 366–373.

Stefanyshyn, D. J., Engsberg, J. R., Tedford, K. G., & Harder, J. A. (1994). A pilot study to test the influence of specific prosthetic features in preventing transtibial amputees from walking like able-bodied subjects. *Prosthetics and Orthotics International, 18,* 180–190.

Wille, D. (2009). Virtual reality-based paediatric interactive therapy system (PITS) for improvement of arm and hand function in children with motor impairment—A pilot study. *Developmental NeuroRehabilitation, 12,* 44–52.

Zinzi, P. (2007). Effects of an intensive rehabilitation programme on patients with Huntington's disease: A pilot study. *Clinical Rehabilitation, 21,* 603–613.

### 3.5.3 Assumptions Underlying Heuristic Research

In engaging in heuristic research, the investigator:

- Seeks to discover statistically significant relationships between variables
- Seeks data for theory building; the result of research provides the basis for theoretical formulations
- Uses deductive methods to analyze a research problem
- Analyzes a research problem retrospectively; that is, the researcher starts with the presumed effect (dependent variable) and works back to the presumed causative factors (independent variables)
- Understands that results derived from heuristic research are not conclusive, implying that further investigation using prospective research is needed to substantiate cause-effect relationships

### 3.5.4 Method of Heuristic Research

The use of factor analytic studies with computer technology enables an investigator to correlate many variables and to systematically analyze interactional patterns. This method is especially appropriate in analyzing psychophysiological illnesses where there is a combination of presumed causative factors rather than a single etiological factor. Warren Weaver (1947) characterized research in the seventeenth, eighteenth, and nineteenth centuries as typifying the era of the two-variable problems in simplicity. In medicine during the early part of the twentieth century, a single etiological factor was correlated with the effects of disease (two-variable research).

Today, however, both modern medical research and social sciences research are engaged in investigating complex health problems that involve multiple causes. For example, drug addiction, mental retardation, arteriosclerosis, Alzheimer's disease, and dyslexia have multiple causes. An application of a two-variable model, where the investigator searches for the single cause of the disease, is inadequate in biopsychosocial research. On the other hand, heuristic research lends itself to the study of multiple factors that are interactive in nature. The Framingham Study of heart disease (Dawber, Meaders, & Moore, 1951) is an example of heuristic research. The strategy involved in these studies was to identify numerous risk factors that are significantly more frequent in patients with heart disease than in the normal population. The purposes of heuristic research are diagramed in Figure 3–14.

### 3.5.5 Identification of Correlating Factors

In heuristic research, the investigator seeks to derive the major factors that correlate significantly to assess their relative importance. Descriptive and inferential statistics, as well as multiple regression, factor analysis, and path analysis, are appropriate for analyzing the relative significance of factors that are important in generating further research.

A major problem in this research model is in the selection of a diagnostic group. It is critical that screening criteria be used in selecting a research sample. The researcher cannot assume that a patient's diagnosis is accurate. There is much controversy in

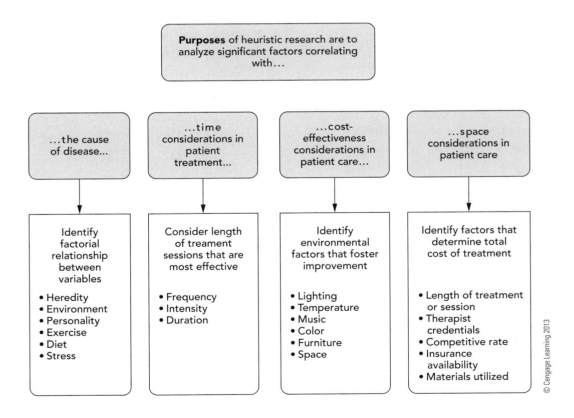

**FIGURE 3-14**  Four Examples of the Application of Heuristic Research

the diagnosis of chronic illnesses such as asthma, schizophrenia, arthritis, fetal alcohol syndrome (FAS), and failure to thrive that requires the investigator to use rigorous methods for operationalizing diagnostic categories. After the investigator has developed and refined the screening criteria for subject selection, the next problem is to select a population of subjects that will be the source for a representative sample.

Parallel to the process of subject selection is the compiling of investigative variables. These variables are derived by analyzing the following areas:

- *Demographic:* age, gender, occupation, educational level, marital status, income
- *Psychosocial:* personality, intelligence, attitude, lifestyle
- *Biochemical:* physiological, somatotype, nutritional, genetic

### 3.5.6 Interactional Effects in Heuristic Research

Heuristic research requires the investigator to make an exhaustive search for variables that can potentially contribute to the onset of a disease. It is necessary for the investigator to take a holistic view of the problem of etiology so as to avoid the trap of two-variable research that lacks an analysis of interactional effects. As an example, let us

suppose hypothetically that schizophrenia is a result of the interactional effects of genetics, child development, and lack of competence in educational, vocational, or social areas. In studying the exclusive relationship between genetics and schizophrenia, a researcher will have mixed results because other major factors have not been taken into account. Results cannot be generalized to all patients with schizophrenia. Figure 3–15 illustrates hypothetically the interaction between the three independent variables (genetics, child development, and competence) and the dependent variable (diagnosis of schizophrenia).

The diagram shows that those individuals who have effective parenting and educational and vocational competence are the least likely to develop schizophrenia, even if they have a genetic vulnerability factor. Schizophrenia results only through the interaction of three variables: genetic, parental, and educational-vocational competence.

This hypothetical example shows the complexity of factorial designs that test the interactional effects of multiple causes. It is highly probable that many chronic illnesses result from this type of interactional pattern. Nonetheless, only through rigorous, painstaking research will it be possible to identify interactional effects. Heuristic research provides the framework to investigate multiple factors in the development of a disease process.

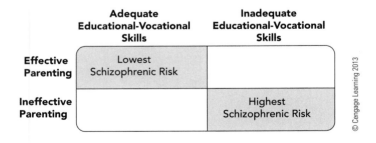

**FIGURE 3-15** Interaction between Independent and Dependent Variables in the Risk of Developing Schizophrenia: An explanation of the development of schizophrenia must take into account all major variables, not just a single variable.

### 3.5.7 Analysis of Time Factors in Client Intervention

What are the determining factors in planning intervention time for patients? Why is 1 hour a week sufficient for some clients, whereas 2 hours a week are prescribed for others? What proportion of intervention time is a function of pragmatic issues, such as the availability of a therapist? What consideration for time is given to the client's physical and emotional needs? How is intervention time planned for client groups? All of these questions are suitable for research analysis. In general, only a few studies have analyzed time factors in patient care (Atalay, 2009; Granger, et al., 2010). Yet, time is one of the most basic factors in clinical intervention. An analysis of the factors considered in determining the length of time for interventions should consider both the ideal factors and pragmatic issues (see Table 3–7).

### 3.5.8 Analysis of Cost-Effectiveness Factors in Intervention

What are the real economic costs for intervention? What does it cost to treat a patient in a hospital compared with the intervention in an outpatient clinic? What are the costs for direct patient care by professionals as compared with nonprofessional health technicians trained for specific health purposes? What is the cost of a massive public health prevention program compared with existing costs for treating a specific disability group? What fac-

tors are considered in determining fees for health services? How are salaries for health workers determined? What is the economic worth of a health professional?

These questions are typical of the pressing economic problems facing industrialized and developing countries where the demand for health care far outreaches the resources that countries can allocate for prevention and intervention. If a society is to determine rationally how its economic resources can be used most effectively for implementation, then it must examine objectively the underlying factors affecting the costs of health care (Blumstein, 1997; Timpka, Leijon, Karlsson, Svensson, & Bjurulf, 1997).

### 3.5.9 Analysis of Space Factors in Patient Care

As with time and cost, space has received little attention from clinical researchers. Ethnologists and social anthropologists (e.g., Hall, 1966; Hemsworth, 1986; Jensen, 1998) analyzed the effect of space in animal behavior and health. There are a few studies that suggest a direct relationship between life space and psychological reactions (Barnes, 2007; Crump, 1997; Hewitt, 1997).

In psychiatry, it has been evident that space affects a client's emotions and behavioral patterns. Goffman (1961), in a classical study, described the syndrome of passivity and depersonalization as being the result of institutionalization. A contemporary definition of space is not limited to

| TABLE 3-7 | |
|---|---|
| **Analysis of Time Factors in Intervention** | |
| **Ideal** | **Pragmatic** |
| 1. Time needed for application of intervention method: dependent on the client's treatment goals | 1. Number of patients under care in proportion to the number of hours allocated for intervention (client load) |
| 2. Time needed to meet short-term objectives or goals | 2. Traditional practices (therapy schedules) |
| 3. Time needed for preparation and progress notes | 3. Third-party reimbursement for service (insurance) |

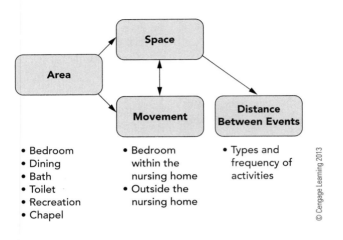

© Cengage Learning 2013

**FIGURE 3-16**  Analysis of Space Factors in a Nursing Home

the traditional nineteenth-century view that space represents *area*. Since Einstein's theory of relativity, space has taken on new meaning, implying in conceptual terms that space is the distance between two events. Space involves events, occurrences, or movement. An individual's space represents the potential area for movement. In this concept of space, factors related to increasing or diminishing space are appropriate.

Hospitalization, imprisonment, and institutionalization are situations in which the patient, prisoner, or inmate are deprived of space and consequently has fewer movements and events. In treating a patient, what considerations are given to space? Are wards or private rooms considered on any other basis than economic? Do groups occupying space limit the number of events or increase the movement of patients? Questions involving space are invariably linked to issues of group versus individual intervention. What is the relationship between the number of clients in a group, the area of movement, and the events taking place in a group? Issues related to the size of client groups in occupational therapy clinics involve space factors.

A researcher employing a heuristic research model seeks to discover underlying factors affecting space. For example, how would a researcher analyze the problem of determining the space needs of

geriatric clients in a nursing home? Figure 3–16 illustrates this example.

The first step is to define operationally the space of geriatric clients. The next step is to discover the physical, psychological, and social needs of geriatric clients. A review of the literature and a survey of existing programs would provide the data. Maslow's (1954) theory of a hierarchy of needs and Havighurst's (1952) activity theory could be applied to an analysis of psychological and emotional needs. Theories of aging and health could provide the framework for setting physical and health goals. The third step in the research process is to integrate the data derived from analyzing space factors in a nursing home with biopsychosocial needs. This is illustrated in Figure 3–17.

The goals of heuristic research in this example are to:

- Discover the factors comprising space in a nursing home
- Analyze the effects of these factors in psychological adjustment, social relationships, and physical health maintenance
- Identify in the literature the needs of the aged
- Integrate space factors with need theory

The reader may be puzzled with the example in Figure 3–17. How, the reader may ask, does the

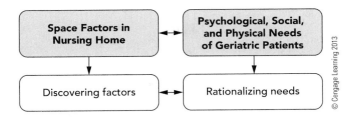

© Cengage Learning 2013

**FIGURE 3-17** Integration of Data with Need Theory: In this example, the data obtained from analyzing space factors in the nursing home with the needs of elderly patients (obtained through a literature review) is integrated.

heuristic researcher know that all factors related to space and all needs of geriatric patients have been identified? The answer is that researchers cannot conclude that the data collection is complete. Heuristic research is a method of discovery, and research in general is an ongoing process that functions as a feedback loop. As more information is gathered, analyzed, and integrated with previous data, the researcher comes closer to solving questions. Box 3–5 gives an example of heuristic research.

---

**BOX 3-5**

## Example of Heuristic Research

### 1. Bibliographical Notation

Rabadi, M., Galgano, M., Lynch, D., Akerman, M., Lesser, M., & Volpe, B. (2008). A pilot study of activity-based therapy in the arm motor recovery post stroke: A randomized controlled trial. *Clinical Rehabilitation, 22,* 1071–1082.

### 2. Abstract

**OBJECTIVE:** To determine the efficacy of activity-based therapies using arm ergometer or robotic or group occupational therapy for motor recovery of the paretic arm in patients with an acute stroke (< or = 4 weeks) admitted to an inpatient rehabilitation facility, and to obtain information to plan a large randomized controlled trial. **DESIGN:** Prospective, randomized controlled study. **SETTING:** Stroke unit in a rehabilitation hospital. **SUBJECTS:** Thirty patients with an acute stroke (< or = 4 weeks) who had arm weakness (Medical Research Council grade 2 or less at the shoulder joint). **INTERVENTION:** Occupational therapy (OT) group (control) (n = 10), arm ergometer (n = 10) or robotic (n = 10) therapy group. All patients received standard, inpatient, post-stroke rehabilitation training for three hours a day, plus 12 additional 40-minute sessions of the activity-based therapy. **MAIN MEASURES:** The primary outcome measures were discharge scores in the *Fugl-Meyer Assessment Scale* for upper limb impairment, *Motor Status Scale*, total *Functional Independence Measure*

*continues*

BOX 3-5

## **Example of Heuristic Research** *continued*

(FIM) and FIM-motor and FIM-cognition subscores. The three groups (OT group versus arm ergometer versus robotic) were comparable on clinical demographic measures except the robotic group was significantly older and there were more haemorrhagic stroke patients in the arm ergometer group. After adjusting for age, stroke type and outcome measures at baseline, a similar degree of improvement in the discharge scores was found in all of the primary outcome measures. **CONCLUSION:** This study suggests that activity-based therapies using an arm ergometer or robot when used over shortened training periods have the same effect as OT group therapy in decreasing impairment and improving disability in the paretic arm of severely affected stroke patients in the subacute phase (p.1071).

### 3. Justification and Need for Study

This study lists multiple novel rehabilitation techniques such as constraint-induced therapy, robotic training and other intensive activity tasks, (e.g., bilateral arm training with rhythmic cueing to increase functional motor recovery). Recently the amount of time of hospitalization in the inpatient rehabilitation has been reduced as a cost-containment measure which has motivated the evaluation of techniques that complement conventional therapies to enhance potential post-stroke motor recovery. The researchers in this study decided to investigate whether an activity-based program (of bilateral arm training using the ergometer or unilateral arm training with a robot) would be more effective than occupational group therapy for the same amount of intensity and duration of treatment in decreasing arm motor impairment and improving disability in patients with moderately severe stroke during their acute rehabilitation hospital stay. This study also hopes to use the findings to design a larger randomized controlled trial study.

### 4. Literature Review

This study had 51 references from a wide variety of sources. Cited journals included but were not limited to: *Archives of Physical Medical Rehabilitation, Neurology, Stroke, Neurorehabilitation and Neural Repair, Behavior Brain Science, Scandinavian Journal of Rehabilitation Medicine, Physical Therapy,* and *American Journal of Physical Medicine Rehabilitation.* The years of cited publications ranged from 1951 to 2008.

### 5. Research Hypothesis or Guiding Questions

No hypotheses or questions were stated in the article.

### 6. Methods

Thirty-three participants were recruited with an acute stroke (less than or at four weeks) who had arm weakness (Medical Research Council grade two or less at the shoulder joint). Each patient received standard occupational and physical therapy by their assigned therapist for three hours per day. Each participant also received 12 additional sessions of 40 minutes/day,

5 days/week, consisting of arm ergometer, robot, or occupational therapy alone based on randomization.

The Monark arm ergometer is a bidirectional hand cycle that is used for upper body aerobic exercise. It uses all muscle groups of the upper limb. The intensity to which the paretic arm was subjected was a count of the number of movements completed at one minute and over the 40-minute session. Each participant exercised for 20 minutes of continuous cycling at zero resistance, had a 5-minute break, and then again cycled for 20 minutes. The unaffected arm helped move the paretic arm

The robot-aided therapy consists of goal-directed, robot-assisted arm movement, and a customized interactive computer-generated video programme provides visual feedback to the participant about the accuracy and speed of reaching a given target. The participants paralyzed arm initially receives passive movement, but as the voluntary movement returns, the robot assists the participant to initiate, guide, and complete the motor activity required for point-to-point movements. Each participant completed two, 20-minute programmes with a 5-minute break between each session. The intensity of this treatment is displayed electronically by the robot.

The control occupational therapy group received 40 minutes of group therapy led by a certified occupational therapist assigned to that specific stroke unit who is competent in the group therapy protocol. Therapy focused on self-range of motion exercises focusing on patient-directed movements at the affected shoulder, elbow and hand when able. Each participant was encouraged to use his or her unaffected arm in actively assisting the paretic arm movement. The participants in this group had moved his or her arm an average of 16 to 18 times/minute either by the participant supporting or assisting the paretic arm, or helped by the therapist. The primary outcomes measured arm motor weakness by a variety of tests that are commonly implemented in rehabilitation settings and whose change scores have been correlated with functional motor improvement. The assessments used include the discharge scores in *the Fugl-Meyer Assessment Scale* for upper limb motor impairments, the *Functional Independence Measure* (FIM), the FIM-motor, and the FIM-cognition subscores for disability. The secondary outcome measures were discharge scores on the following assessments: *Motor Power Scale* for muscle strength, *Action Research Arm Test* for arm-hand function, *Modified Ashworth Scale* for muscle tone, and the *Fugl-Meyer Assessment Scale* for arm pain and range of motion.

## 7. Results

All three of the groups demonstrated improvements in both motor impairment and functional scores. Among the three groups there were no differences in the discharge *Fugl-Meyer Assessment Scale* upper extremity impairment score, the *Motor Status Scale*, FIM-total, FIM-motor subscore, and FIM-cognition subscore. The ergometer group performed better than the occupational therapy group on the *Fugl-Meyer Assessment Scale* wrist-hand score, and the robot group performed better on the *Motor Status Scale* shoulder-elbow score than the occupational therapy group. The robot group performed better on the *Motor Power Scale*, *Modified Ashworth Scale*, and the pain score than the occupational therapy group. The ergometer group performed better on the *Modified Ashworth Scale* and the

*continues*

BOX 3-5

**Example of Heuristic Research** *continued*

pain score than the occupational therapy group did. The degree in these impairment and functional scores overall favored the occupational therapy group compared to the robot group or the arm ergometer group.

### 8. Conclusions

Rabadi et al. concluded that the activity-based therapies, which include the arm ergometer and robot, were no more effective in improving disability and decreasing impairment than occupational therapy during the subacute phase of stroke.

### 9. Limitations of the Study

The first limitation is that this study was a single-center study. Secondly there was a small sample size. Thirdly, the treatment plan is debatable whether the 12 sessions of 40 minutes a day 5 days a week is sufficient to induce cerebral reorganization to supplement a change. Finally, these techniques do require supervision.

### 10. Major References Cited in the Study

Broeks, J. G., Lankhorst, G. J., Rumping, K., & Prevo, A. J. (1999). The long-term outcome of arm function after stroke: Results of a follow-up study. *Disability Rehabilitation, 21,* 357–364.

Kunkel, A., Kopp, B., Muller, G. Villringer, K., Villringer, A., Taub, E., & Flor, H. (1999). Constraint-induced movement therapy for motor recovery in chronic stroke patients. *Archives of Physical and Medicine and Rehabilitation, 80,* 624–628.

Nakayama, H., Jorgensen, H. S., Raaschou, H. O., & Olsen, T. S. (1994). Recovery of upper extremity function in stroke patients: The Copenhagen Stroke Study. *Archives of Physical and Medicine and Rehabilitation, 75,* 394–398.

Taub, E., Miller, N. E., Novack, T. A., Cook, E. W., Fleming, W. C., Nepomuceno, C. S., … Crago, J. E. (1993). Technique to improve chronic motor deficit after stroke. *Archives of Physical and Medicine and Rehabilitation, 74,* 347–354.

Taub, E., Unswatte, G., & Pidikiti, R. (1999). Constraint induced movement therapy: A new family of techniques with broad application to physical rehabilitation—A clinical review. *Journal of Rehabilitation Research and Development, 36,* 237–251.

## 3.6  Correlational Research

### 3.6.1 Purposes of Correlational Research

Many studies published in occupational therapy are primarily correlational and retrospective. This research is analogous to experimental research in that the investigator tests a hypothesis. Unlike the experimental researcher, however, the investigator does not manipulate independent variables, nor is a cause-effect relationship simulated. In **correlational research**, the investigator compares the relationships between variables by measuring differences. It is applied frequently to areas in the social sciences because the very nature of the problem limits the experimenter from inducing causal effects. If, for example, a researcher's purpose is to correlate characteristics in the individual who is alcoholic with causative factors, then the researcher is limited to an ex post facto design where it is not possible to induce experimentally the onset of alcoholism. The researcher in this example is limited to a retrospective analysis of the assumed causes of alcoholism. Kerlinger (1986), in discussing the value of nonexperimental research, concluded that "social, scientific, and educational problems do not lend themselves to experimentation, although many of them do lend themselves to controlled inquiry of the nonexperimental kind" (p. 359).

A sequential analysis of correlational research is diagramed in Figure 3–18. These steps are reviewed in the section below.

### 3.6.2 Identification of Research Variables

As clinicians in the health fields, we are all concerned with the question of etiology. Why did this patient develop symptoms of schizophrenia when he was 16 years old? Why did this individual develop learning problems? What factors led to arthritis? What environmental factors contributed to juvenile delinquency? These questions regarding etiology and relationships between variables are feasible for correlational research.

The first step in correlational research is to identify the variables in a target population to be studied. These variables are presumed causative factors and may be genetic, neurophysiological, psychosocial, or cultural. The variables are identified from clinical observations, by examining previous studies or theoretical papers, or through deductive reasoning. The presumed independent variables and presumed dependent variables are identified. Because the researcher does not actively induce the independent variables, an associational or statistical relationship can only be assumed.

### 3.6.3 Formulating Hypotheses in Correlational Research

The researcher formulates a hypothesis after reviewing the related literature. The hypothesis can be a **directional hypothesis**, that is, predicting a significant positive or negative relationship between two variables. For example, the researcher predicts that there is an increase of abnormal reflexes in children with cerebral palsy compared with typical children. A hypothesis stated in a null form predicts no significant relationship. For example, the **null hypothesis** may be stated as, "There is no statistically significant difference between the presence of abnormal reflexes in children with cerebral palsy compared with typical children." The decision whether to formulate a directional hypothesis or null hypothesis is based on direct or implied evidence from previous research. If previous studies indicate directionality, then the researcher should state a directional hypothesis. On the other hand, if the researcher finds no evidence for a directional hypothesis in a review of the literature, then a null hypothesis should be stated. The form in which the hypothesis is stated has implications when analyzing the data statistically. For those readers without statistical background, it will suffice to say that when a researcher is comparing statistically significant differences between two variables with a *t*-test, a null hypothesis usually indicates a two-tail test of significance, and a directional hypothesis usually indicates a one-tail test of significance.

Other examples of directional hypotheses in correlational research are as follows:

- Individuals who are blind have a significantly greater kinesthetic ability than individuals with normal vision.
- Individuals with intellectual disabilities educated in an inclusive setting will show higher self-concept than those educated in a self-contained program.
- Carpal tunnel syndrome occurs more frequently among individuals using a computer for six or more hours daily when compared with individuals using a computer for fewer than four hours daily.
- Children from dysfunctional, low-income families have better visual perceptual abilities than auditory processing abilities.
- There is a higher percentage of cancer among asbestos workers than in the population at large.

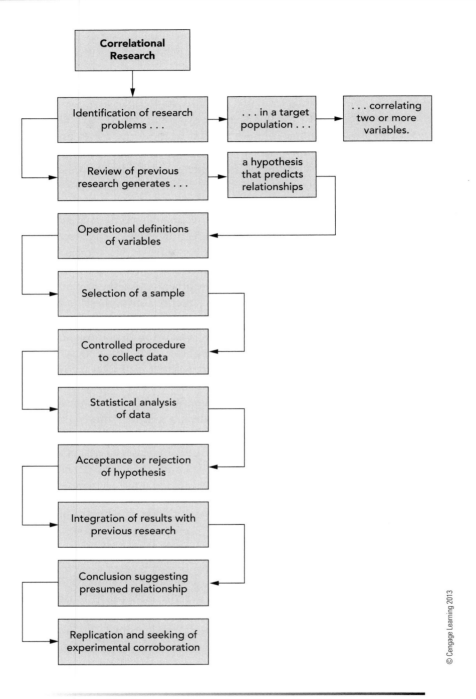

**FIGURE 3-18** The Sequential Analysis of Correlational Research

In all of the foregoing examples of directional hypotheses, the variables are associated with a target population. Analyzing the hypotheses one by one, we find the relationships shown in Table 3–8.

In the foregoing hypotheses, variables and populations are compared. Hypotheses can test the effects of multiple variables in one population or, conversely, the differences among multiple populations on one variable. A researcher cannot test multiple variables in multiple populations in one hypothesis. For example, it is fallacious to offer a hypothesis such as the following: "High cholesterol level and hypertension are more prevalent among cardiac patients than among a normal population." Each variable, high cholesterol level and hypertension, should be stated in a separate hypothesis.

### 3.6.4 Operational Definitions of Variables

Before a hypothesis can be tested, the investigator must operationally define the **variables** stated in the hypothesis. The operational definition includes the specific test or procedure used in measuring a variable. If an investigator is measuring mild cognitive deficits, then the procedure given by Geslani (2005) (e.g., "Mild Cognitive Impairment: An Operational Definition and Its Conversion Rate to Alzheimer's Disease") might be indicated as the operational measure.

### 3.6.5 Selection of Sample

Screening criteria is necessary when selecting a sample. It is not sufficient simply to state that patients with diabetes or epilepsy will be compared with a typical population. The investigator must indicate how the patients have been diagnosed, the severity of the illness considered, and other demographics identifying the population such as age, gender, occupation, socioeconomic status, education, and geographical area. The screening criteria devised by the investigator serve as a reference point in generalizing the results to a population. Universality and external validity depend on the screening criteria devised for subject selection.

### 3.6.6 Data Collection Procedure

Can the test procedure be replicated? Has the investigator tried to reduce factors such as subject fatigue, anxiety, extraneous distractions, lack of cooperation,

TABLE 3-8

**Associational Relationships between Variables**

| Variables | Populations Compared |
| --- | --- |
| Kinesthetic ability | Blind<br>Normal vision |
| Self-concept | Children with intellectual disabilities in inclusive settings<br>Children with intellectual disabilities in self-contained settings |
| Carpal tunnel syndrome | Computer operators using the computer 6 or more hours a day<br>Computer operators using the computer fewer than 4 hours a day |
| Visual-motor perception | Children from dysfunctional families<br>Children with mental health disorders |
| Auditory processing | Individuals with autism<br>Individuals with learning disabilities |
| Cancer | Asbestos workers<br>Typical individuals |

and any other factors that threaten the internal validity of the investigation? The investigator should describe in detail the test procedure, including the time of day when the subjects are tested, the number in the group, the environmental conditions, the length of time for testing each subject, and the sequence in presenting the operational measures.

### 3.6.7 Interpretation of Results

In general, research has a cumulative effect. Usually, the results of one study are not sufficient to be conclusive. Many factors affect the results in correlational research that are not directly controlled by the investigator. These limitations affecting internal validity do not negate correlational research. The advantages of correlational research are that investigations can be easily replicated and subjects can be easily tested. Before proposing a conclusion based on the results of one study, the investigator must integrate the results with previous research. If the results are contradictory, then perhaps further research is indicated. If the results are consistent with previous literature, then it may be valid to suggest that conclusive evidence has been found. There is a need in research to be conservative rather than premature.

An example of correlational research is found in Box 3–6.

---

### BOX 3-6

## Example of Correlational Research

### 1. Bibliographical Notation

Goldberg B., Brintnell, E. S., & Goldberg, J. (2002). The relationship between engagement in meaningful activities and quality of life in persons disabled by mental illness. *Occupational Therapy in Mental Health*, *18*, 17–44.

### 2. Abstract

A hypothesized relationship between engagement in meaningful activities and quality of life was tested for 32 individuals attending a community mental health agency's programs. They completed the *Lehman Quality of Life Interview* (QOLI; Lehman, 1988), the *Derogatis Symptom Checklist-90-Revised* (SCL-90-R), and the *Engagement in Meaningful Activities Survey* (EMAS; Goldberg, Brintnell, & Goldberg, 2002), constructed for this study. It measures 12 facets of the meaningfulness of activities and includes some open-ended questions. Its test-retest reliability and Cronbach Alpha were .69 and .84, respectively. Participants were involved in a wide range of activities that were most lacking in providing appropriate challenge and a sense of control. Engagement in meaningful activities was significantly correlated with satisfaction with life as a whole ($p < .05$), but depression accounted for most of the variance. Some support is provided for the theorized value of meaningful activity engagement and recommends strategies to increase the meaningfulness of activities. Findings alert clinicians to the importance of treating depression (p. 17).

### 3. Justification and Need for Study

A basic theory of occupational therapy is that "engagement in meaningful activities/occupations leads not only to enhanced occupational performance, but also to life satisfaction" (p.18). Two developments have developed this study. The first is the demonstration that the quality of life construct can be used as an index of life satisfaction. The second is that occupational therapy literature suggests criteria to measure meaningfulness of occupations, but there have not been any studies that have measured meaningfulness of occupations in previous research. The current study tests the hypothesis that life satisfaction, as it is measured by quality of life, of a person with severe and persistent mental illness is correlated to his or her engagement in activities that are meaningful.

### 4. Literature Review

This study had 82 references from a variety of sources. Cited journals included but were not limited to: *Psychosocial Rehabilitation Journal, Journal of Affective Disorders, Occupational Therapy in Mental Health, Social Psychiatry and Psychiatric Epidemiology, Community Mental Health in New Zealand, Journal of Chronic Disease, Archives of General Psychiatry, Journal of Nervous and Mental Disease, Journal of Health and Social Behavior, Journal of Social Psychiatry, International Journal of Social Psychiatry, American Journal of Occupational Therapy* (AJOT), and *Canada's Mental Health*. The years of cited publications ranged from 1962 through 2000.

### 5. Research Hypothesis or Guiding Questions

The hypotheses include:

- That there is a positive relationship between the degree of engagement in meaningful activities and subjective quality of life in people living in the community with disabilities related to mental illness.
- There are positive relationships between the degree of engagement in meaningful activities and subjective satisfaction with eight domains of life: living situation; daily activities and functioning; family; social relations; finances; work and school; legal and safety issues; and health of people living in the community with disabilities related to mental illness.
- There is a negative relationship between the degree of psychopathology and subjective quality of life in people living in the community with disabilities related to mental illness.

### 6. Methods

The study consisted of 32 participants. The participants for this cross-sectional correlation study consisted of those who have a mental illness living in the community and attend programs at a private, non-profit mental health agency. At the first session the EMAS, the QOLI, and the SCL-90-R were administered. The interviews lasted around 79 minutes. Following a 2- to 10-week interval, 15 of the participants repeated the EMAS in order to receive data on its test-retest reliability. Those who did relate relevant changes were asked to repeat the SCL-90-R.

### 7. Results

The engagement in occupations and meaningful activities was significantly correlated with satisfaction with the participant's life as a whole, but depression accounted for most of the

*continues*

BOX 3-6

**Example of Correlational Research** *continued*

variance. It is very likely that an individual who cannot engage successfully in meaningful activities or that his or her occupations will not be perceived as meaningful as long as he or she is having symptoms of depression. The study also found that there were significant negative correlations between depression and anxiety, and satisfaction with life as a whole.

### 8. Conclusions

Goldberg et al. concluded that:

1. "There is a relationship between the extent of engagement in meaningful activities and QOL, but depression and anxiety confound this relationship" (p.38).
2. "Quality of life can best be enhanced when both psychosocial and medical interventions are used simultaneously for this purpose, and occupational therapists in community practice have a paramount role in identifying symptoms, addressing them within the scope of practice, and advocating for additional treatment as necessary" (p. 37).
3. "Depression and anxiety need to be actively treated" (p.37).

### 9. Limitations of the Study

This study had a small sample size. Further research needs to be conducted on the activities and social participation of this population and other subsets of people with first-episode psychosis.

### 10. Major References Cited in the Study

Dickerson, D. B., Ringel, N. B., & Parente, F. (1998). Subjective quality of life in out-patients with schizophrenia: Clinical and utilization correlates. *Acta Psychiatrica Scandinavica, 98,* 124–127.

Koivumaa-Honkanen, H. T., Honkanen, R., Antikainen, R., Hinitkka, J., & Viinamaki, H. (1999). Self-reported life satisfaction and treatment factors in patients with schizophrenia, major depression and anxiety disorder. *Acta Psychiatrica Scandinavica, 99,* 377–384.

Packer, S., Husted, J., Cohen, S., & Tomlinson, G. (1997). Psychopathology and quality of life. *Journal of Psychiatry & Neuroscience, 22,* 231–234.

Tollefson, G. D., & Anderson, S. W. (1999). Should we consider mood disturbance in schizophrenia as an important determinant of quality of life? *Journal of Clinical Psychiatry, 60,* 23–29.

## 3.7 Survey Research

### 3.7.1 Definition of Survey Research

**Survey research**, as defined in this text, is the descriptive study of populations. The main purpose of survey research is to obtain accurate objective descriptions about a specific universe of people or entities, such as a group of individuals with disabilities or the curriculum requirements in occupational therapy. The major task of the survey researcher is to obtain reliable and valid data from a representative sample of a population. In some cases, the researcher will be able to survey the total population or universe without relying on a representative sample.

### 3.7.2 Purposes of Survey Research

Health, social, and educational planners use descriptive survey research as the basis for needs assessment for developing health strategies, programs, and physical plants. The changing needs of populations as derived from surveys can contribute to the planning of health centers, inclusion practices for individuals with disabilities, allied health training programs, community mental health centers, and adult day care centers. Survey research should play an essential part in assessing the needs of a population where the planning of services is involved.

Along with community planning, survey research is an important tool for learning about the general attitudes of people. Governmental agencies and legislators sponsor many studies to solicit general opinion on topics such as national health insurance, malpractice in health, legalization of abortion, ethics in research, inclusion of individuals with disabilities in educational and community settings, and other controversial issues where majority opinion is used to formulate national policy and to guide the enactment of laws.

Survey research need not be limited to questioning individuals. Methodologies in survey research assessing the physical characteristics of groups are also applicable. Recently, governmental grants in health research have funded studies that screen a population for the presence of a disability. School populations are screened for deficits in hearing and vision acuity. Diabetes tests, chest X-rays to detect tuberculosis and lung cancer, cardiovascular screening utilizing blood cholesterol counts, blood pressure measurements, and testing for HIV are some of the examples of survey research utilizing physical measurements to screen for health defects in large populations. Public health agencies use survey research as a means of identifying trends in the incidence of diseases and health problems. The information comprising the survey data is obtained from physicians, hospitals, clinics, and other health agencies that compile disease statistics. Table 3–9 from the *Morbidity and Mortality Weekly Report* is an example of epidemiological statistics, that is, data showing cases of specified notifiable diseases in the United States.

### TABLE 3-9

**Provisional Cases of Infrequently Reported Notifiable Diseases (<1,000 cases reported during the preceding year) in the United States for the Week Ending July 3, 2010**

| Disease | Cumulative Number (through 7/3/2010) |
| --- | --- |
| Botulism, total | 35 |
|    foodborne | 4 |
|    infant | 23 |
|    other (wound & unspecified) | 8 |
| Brucellosis | 53 |
| Chancroid | 27 |
| Cholera | 2 |
| Cyclosporiasis | 54 |

*continues*

## TABLE 3-9

**Provisional Cases of Infrequently Reported Notifiable Diseases (<1,000 cases reported during the preceding year) in the United States for the Week Ending July 3, 2010** *continued*

| Disease | Cumulative Number (through 7/3/2010) |
| --- | --- |
| Hansen disease | 18 |
| Hanta virus pulmonary syndrome | 4 |
| Hemolytic uremic syndrome, post-diarrheal | 70 |
| Influenza-associated pediatric mortality | 54 |
| Listeriosis | 283 |
| Measles | 28 |
| A, C, Y, and W-135 | 132 |
| serogroup b | 62 |
| other serogroup | 6 |
| unknown serogroup | 206 |
| Mumps | 2,064 |
| Novel influenza A infection virus | 1 |
| Psittacosis | 4 |
| Q fever total | 47 |
| acute | 36 |
| chronic | 11 |
| Rabies, human | 1 |
| Rubella | 4 |
| Streptococcal toxic-shock syndrome | 91 |
| Syphilis, congenital (age < 1yr) | 80 |
| Tetanus | 1 |
| Toxic-shock syndrome (staphylococcal) | 45 |
| Trichinellosis | 1 |
| Tularemia | 22 |
| Typhoid fever | 164 |
| Vancomycin-intermediate *Staphylococcus aureus* | 50 |
| Vancomycin-resistant *Staphylococcus aureus* | 1 |
| Vibriosis (non-cholera *Vibrio* species infections) | 162 |
| Viral hemorrhagic fever | 1 |

**Note:** Table adapted from TABLE I of the *Morbidity and Mortality Weekly Report, 59* (26), pp. 820-833 by the Centers for Disease Control and Prevention, National Center for Health Statistics, 7/9/2010. Data are cumulative through the week ending 7/3/2010. Retrieved from http://wonder.cdc.gov/mmwr/mmwr_reps.asp?mmwr_year=2010&mmwr_week=26&mmwr_table=1

### 3.7.3 Statement of Problem in Survey Research

The first step in survey research is to state the problem in question form. The problem should be researchable, requiring measurable data that can be collected and analyzed. In stating a problem in survey research, the investigator must operationally define the population to be surveyed in terms of geographical area and demographic characteristics, such as age, gender, socioeconomic level, education, and marital status. The identified population must be rigorously defined, otherwise there can be confusion in the external validity or in generalizing the results from the representative sample to the larger population. This, of course, is not a problem when the total population is surveyed. The following are hypothetical questions related to survey research:

- What is the present occupational status of clients who have been discharged from a supported employment program where they had been for a least one year?
- What are the minimal competencies required in different programs for teacher preparation in special education?
- What rehabilitation services do individuals with spinal cord injuries perceive as the most important?
- What are the socioeconomic characteristics of individuals using community mental health centers?
- What are the cholesterol levels of sedentary office workers?
- How do occupational therapists use service dogs as adjunctive therapy?
- What are the specific intervention techniques that occupational therapists use in working with clients with AIDS?
- What methods are used for teaching reading in resource rooms?

### 3.7.4 Survey Research Methodology

After identifying a researchable problem, the target population, and the variables to be measured in the sample, the investigator formulates the procedure for collecting data and the measuring instruments. Sampling procedures (discussed in more detail in Chapter 7) should be objective and unbiased and provide a true description of the population. **Random sampling**, where the investigator selects a **sample** out of the total population, is the best method to achieve an unbiased, representative sample. The external validity of the results is, of course, increased as the percentage of the population sampled increases. For example, a random sample of 50 percent of the population will be more accurate than a random sample of 30 percent of the population. Use of stratified samples also increases the external validity. In a stratified sample, the sample is divided into strata, such as gender, age, diagnostic, or SES groups. Of course, the determination of how large a sample to include in a survey is often times based on practical considerations, such as the cost of the survey and the time allocated to the research project.

The principle methods for collecting data in survey research are the personal interview, mail (regular or e-mail), and telephone. Table 3–10 lists the relative merits of these three procedures.

### 3.7.5 Selection of Questionnaire

In selecting a measuring instrument for data collection, the survey researcher often is found in the position of devising a self-made questionnaire. Whether the questionnaire is custom designed for a study or has already been published, the researcher must account for the reliability and validity of the instrument. Before the investigator devises the instrument, a thorough search of published questionnaires should be undertaken. The latest edition of the *Buros Mental Measurements Yearbook* (BMMI; Spies, Carlson, & Geisinger, 2010; http://www.unl.edu/buros/bimm/html/catalog.html#mmy), other compendiums of tests and questionnaires, and abstracting journals are excellent sources for locating specific instruments for a study.

Surveys involving the measurement of physical variables in human research are also dependent on the reliability and validity of the instruments used. Procedures are employed for increasing the validity

## TABLE 3-10

### Relative Merits of the Principle Survey Methods

| Advantages | | | |
|---|---|---|---|
| **Personal Interview** | **Mail** | **Telephone** | **E-mail/Internet-based** |
| Most flexible means of obtaining data because questions can be elaborated upon or revised during the interview | Wider and more representative distribution of sample possible | Cost per response relatively low | Wide and large representative distribution of sample possible |
| Open-ended questions are possible | No field staff | Control over interviewer bias easier; supervisor can be present at interview | Cost per response is low or minimal |
| Accountability of the respondent is increased | Cost per questionnaire relatively low | Quick way of obtaining data | Quick way of obtaining data |
| Nonverbal cues can be observed | People may be more frank on certain issues (e.g., sex) | Flexibility possible by elaborating or revising questions | E-mail addresses readily available |
| Lack of response generally very low | No interviewer bias; answers in respondent's own words | Current lists of telephone numbers easily obtained | Respondent can answer at leisure |
| Equalize the types of subjects (e.g., men vs. women) | Respondent can answer at leisure; has time to "think things over" | | Certain segments of population more easily approachable |
| Establishment of rapport may increase validity and reliability of the response | Certain segments of population more easily approachable | | Enhanced ability to automate and tabulate responses |
| **Disadvantages** | | | |
| **Personal Interview** | **Mail** | **Telephone** | **E-mail/Internet-based** |
| Likely to be the most expensive of all methods | Bias as a result of poor response rate (e.g., <30%) | Shortened interviews because of time | Bias as a result of poor response rate (e.g., <30%) |
| Training the interviewer is required | Control over who answers the questionnaire may be lost | Questions must be short and to the point | Control over who answers the questionnaire may be lost |
| Dangers of interviewer bias that may result in skewed results (Halo or devil effect) | Interpretation of omissions to questions may be difficult | Open-ended questions usually avoided because of possibility of misinterpretation | Interpretation of omissions to questions may be difficult |
| Scheduling | Cost per return may be high if the response rate is poor | Certain types of questions cannot be used (e.g., visual material) | Certain segments of population are not available (e.g., those without e-mail) |
| Time required for obtaining data | Open-ended questions may result in poorer response rate or difficulty interpreting | Certain segments of population are not available (e.g., those without telephones) | Open-ended questions may result in poorer response rate or difficulty interpreting |

| Disadvantages | | | |
| --- | --- | --- | --- |
| Personal Interview | Mail | Telephone | E-mail/Internet-based |
| | Only those interested in subject may reply | | Only those interested in subject may reply |
| | Likely to be slowest response time of all | | Ambiguities in questions |
| | | | Technology may hinder responses |

© Cengage Learning 2013

of a subject's response, such as taking three blood pressure readings or two different grip strength readings. Usually, the instruments used in collecting data are reliable and valid, such as the X-ray, electrocardiogram, and blood typing; but sometimes, because of subject anxiety or variability caused by external circumstances, one test result can be inaccurate. Figure 3–19 describes the sequential steps in undertaking survey research.

### 3.7.6 Constructing a Questionnaire in Survey Research

The questionnaire is the most commonly used and most frequently self-devised measuring instrument. Simply defined, a **questionnaire** is a standardized list of objective questions or personal opinions. The purpose of a questionnaire is to obtain information directly from a sample. Ultimately, the goal may be

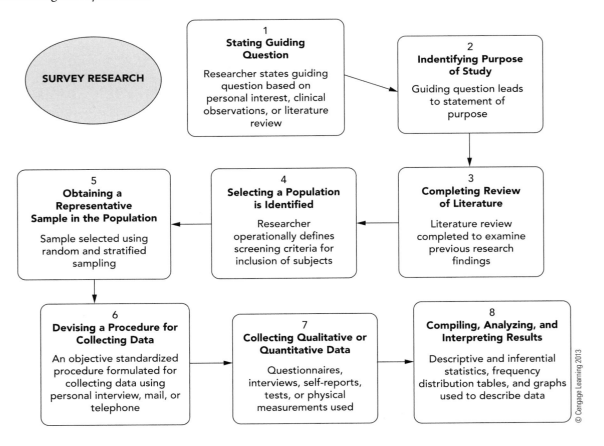

**FIGURE 3-19** The Sequential Steps in Survey Research

to make generalizations to a larger population. The format of a questionnaire considers the following:

- Content: (e.g., demographic variables, personality characteristics, behavioral patterns, health history)
- Form of question: (e.g., forced-choice or open-ended)
- Level of data collected: (e.g., objective or attitudinal)

The steps in devising a questionnaire are listed in Table 3–11.

### 3.7.7 Item Construction

In constructing items, the researcher should be aware of the following:

- The choices available to the subjects should be exhaustive. On some items, a place for "other; please specify" should be provided.
- The choices should be mutually exclusive.
- The items presented should be unambiguous and precise. A pilot study testing the reliability of items is essential.

---

**TABLE 3-11**

#### An Example of the Steps in Creating a Mail Questionnaire

| | |
|---|---|
| **State research question:** | What are the role functions of a public school occupational therapist? |
| **Carry out literature review:** | Locate studies on public school occupational therapists |
| **Identify key areas for items in the questionnaire:** | Description of school environment, faculty, and staff |
| | Description of occupational therapists |
| | Occupational therapy facilities and space |
| | Student demographics |
| | Classification of students treated by occupational therapist |
| | Treatment techniques employed by occupational therapists |
| | Occupational therapy treatment goals for diagnostic groups |
| | Treatment modalities used by occupational therapists |
| | Outcome measures for diagnostic groups |
| | Quality assurance through progress monitoring of individual students |
| **Devise survey format:** | Forced-choice check off |
| | Rank priorities |
| | Avoid open-ended questions |
| | Allow opportunity for comment |
| **Expert evaluation:** | Send questionnaire to three public school occupational therapists asking them to evaluate each item using a specified form and make suggestions for improvement. |
| | Send questionnaire to research design expert. |
| **Revise questionnaire:** | Make revisions based on expert recommendations. |
| | Limit time for completion to 10–15 minutes. |
| **Final draft:** | Have local public school occupational therapist complete questionnaire before mailing to participants |
| | Work out final "bugs" and consider aesthetics of format |

- Items should ask only one question. Avoid double-barreled questions.
- The respondent should have enough information to answer the item.
- The researcher should have a rationale for each item asked. The questionnaire should not be padded with irrelevant items.
- Negative questions should be avoided.
- Leading questions that force a response should be omitted. The respondents should not be in a position to give expected answers or opinions.

Examples of questionnaire items using various formats are described below:

- *Likert-type scales* rate subjects by their agreement or disagreement with a statement on a scale usually of 1 to 5 or 1 to 7. For example, if an investigator is interested in surveying the attitudes of the general public with respect to research on children, an item such as shown in Figure 3–20 could be considered for inclusion in the study.
- *Multiple-choice questions* can be used to elicit opinions or attitudes. Suppose a researcher is interested in surveying a group of patients with postmyocardial infarction on their attitudes toward the disability. The multiple-choice question in Figure 3–21 is one example.
- *Rank-order items* are used by researchers as a way of determining priorities. For example, a survey soliciting perceptions of intervention from former patients with psychiatric problems could include the item shown in Figure 3–22.
- *Incomplete sentences* are used in questionnaires to measure informational level, personality traits, and attitudes. (Figure 3–23)

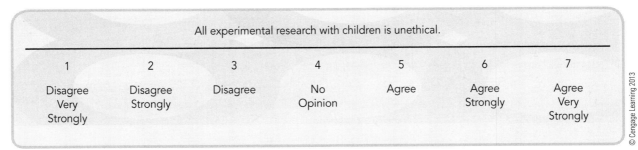

All experimental research with children is unethical.

| 1 | 2 | 3 | 4 | 5 | 6 | 7 |
|---|---|---|---|---|---|---|
| Disagree Very Strongly | Disagree Strongly | Disagree | No Opinion | Agree | Agree Strongly | Agree Very Strongly |

© Cengage Learning 2013

**FIGURE 3-20**   Example of Likert-type Scale

If I had a severe pain in my chest, I would first do the following:

1. Call my private physician.
2. Call an ambulance.
3. Call the emergency rescue unit of the police.
4. Lie down and rest.
5. Other; please specify.

© Cengage Learning 2013

**FIGURE 3-21**   Example of Multiple Choice Question

From the list below of mental health workers, rank in order the most important persons who helped you improve in the hospital. Start numbering with 1 as the person who helped you most; 2, the second most helpful person, and so on:

**Mental Health Worker Rank**

Attendant ＿＿＿

Nurse ＿＿＿

Occupational Therapist ＿＿＿

Psychiatrist ＿＿＿

Psychologist ＿＿＿

Social Worker ＿＿＿

Other: Please specify occupation: ＿＿＿＿＿＿

© Cengage Learning 2013

**FIGURE 3-22**   Example of Rank Order Item

- *Multiple adjective checklists* (Figure 3–24) can be used to elicit effective perception.
- *Open-ended questions* are used in the interviews when the researcher wants the subject to discuss a particular issue in detail. Examples of open-ended questions are shown in Figure 3–25.

> Children with intellectual disabilities are different from typical children in . . .

© Cengage Learning 2013

**FIGURE 3-23** Example of Sentence Completion Item

> *Circle the appropriate adjectives.*
>
> In general, older patients in nursing homes are:
>
> | | |
> |---|---|
> | independent | dependent |
> | happy | sad |
> | well-nourished | poorly fed |
> | active | passive |
> | neglected | supervised |
> | healthy | sick |

© Cengage Learning 2013

**FIGURE 3-24** Example of Multiple Adjective Checklist

Depending on the researcher's ingenuity and creativeness, other types of questionnaire items can be constructed, such as true-false questions, analogies, and rating scales. As with constructing any test instrument, it is critical that the investigator check the reliability and validity of the questionnaire before collecting data.

### 3.7.8 Evaluation of Survey

Once the survey has been developed, it will be important to have experts in the field evaluate it. This will improve reliability and validity and eliminate ambiguous questions. An example of an evaluation form is found in Figure 3–26. This form can be adapted as necessary.

> 1. What is your opinion of including students with disabilities in the general education program?
> 2. What do you think the purpose(s) of prisons are?
> 3. Do you think the United States should adopt a national health insurance program?

© Cengage Learning 2013

**FIGURE 3-25** Example of Open-Ended Question

**Please read the survey.**
1. For each question on the survey, indicate whether the question is stated clearly or if it should be restated or eliminated.
2. Add additional questions that you feel would improve the validity of the questionnaire.

**Answer the following questions.**
3. Do you feel the survey is too lengthy? _____ Yes _____ No
   If you feel the questionnaire is too long, please place a line through the questions that you would omit.
4. Do you find the questionnaire interesting? _____ Yes _____ No
   If you answered no, please tell us what you found uninteresting or irrelevant.
   _____
   _____
5. Were the questions arranged in a logical sequence? _____ Yes _____ No
   If you answered no, please indicate how you would rearrange the questions.
   _____
   _____
6. List further comments and include suggestions for decreasing research bias when administering questionnaires.
   _____
   _____

Thank you for your time. Any feedback you can give us will greatly enhance our study.

© Cengage Learning 2013

**FIGURE 3-26** Evaluation Form for Survey Questionnaires

### 3.7.9 Application of Survey Research to Occupational Therapy

In recent years, occupational therapists have expanded their role functions to include health planning and research. The future role of occupational therapists in planning community health services and health programs in schools is related to needs assessment research (Soderback & Paulsson, 1997). Figure 3–27 gives examples of the application of survey research and needs assessment.

#### Distribution of Health Care

One of the essential purposes of survey research is to guide the direction and planning of health services in a community. Health planners need hard data before they can recommend the construction of a health facility or hospital or the allocation of additional financial resources to a community health agency. Community health planning, therefore, is vitally linked to survey research. Legislators and developers who are persuaded by community pressures for new facilities need data to justify their positions.

Survey research has taken on new importance in the current debate on whether the federal government should be responsible for the total health needs of the population. The data provided by survey research, such as the distribution of health personnel, the proportion of hospital beds for a designated population, and the number of various services provided in defined health catchment areas, can enable legislators to decide whether the present system of delivering health services is adequate for the country or whether a national system for health care would meet the needs of the population more equitably. Survey research can be combined with evaluation research in examining the effectiveness of a health delivery system.

#### Planning Therapeutic Services

Community organization of health services is a good example of the applicability of survey research

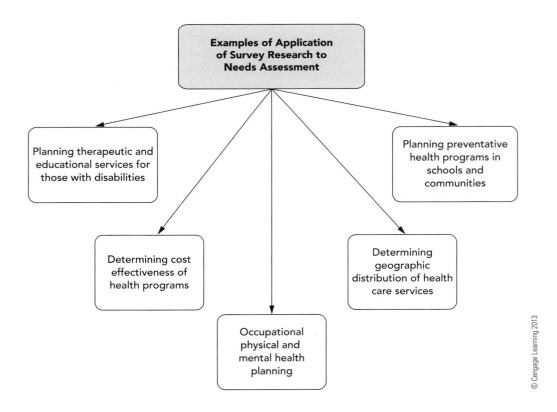

FIGURE 3-27 Application of Survey Research to Allied Health and Education

to the needs of a population. Questions such as "What are the health needs of a community?" and "What are the health resources available?" are areas that occupational therapy researchers can directly examine through survey research. Survey research in health is comparable to market research in advertising. In market research, the individuals in a business collect data regarding the need for a product in the community and the community's attitude toward the introduction of new merchandise. Health planners have sometimes failed miserably in surveying a community before introducing a halfway house, a clinic for treating individuals with addictions, or a child health center. The failure usually has been the result of unexpected resistance from the community to the apparent visibility of individuals with social or physical disabilities in a neighborhood. Survey research can be used to anticipate a community's negative attitudes or even to expose the unrealistic fears that are attached to individuals with disabilities.

### Educational Planning

Deans and presidents of colleges often ask educational planners and administrators to determine if there is a need for a specific allied health training program (e.g., occupational therapy). Are there positions in schools, hospitals, or community agencies for occupational therapists when they graduate from a new program? Do vacancies in occupational therapy exist in hospitals and community clinics at present? Will there be an increased demand for occupational therapists in the future? In what geographic areas are the needs most pressing? These questions are directly accessible through survey research. Questions regarding level of training (i.e., associate, bachelor's, graduate, postgraduate, and continuing education) can be answered through a survey methodology.

Other important concerns that health educators should consider in designing curriculums are course content, clinical reasoning, and skill knowledge. What theoretical content and level of training should the occupational therapy program provide? In designing curriculums, health educators must be aware of the expectations of administrators. Have graduates of an occupational therapy program been adequately prepared to provide services needed by

individuals with disabilities? On what basis does the educator determine the content of a training program? The need for continual feedback and interaction between educators and health administrators is necessary to create meaningful development of the occupational therapy profession. The occupational therapy educator must decide whether the education provided is directly or indirectly related to the needs of the individual with disabilities. If the education of the occupational therapists is directed toward clinical practice and specialization, then occupational therapist educators must be responsive to the community's needs. Survey research can provide the data gathered from the community to answer many questions in educational planning in occupational therapy.

### Occupational Health Planning

There is an increasing need to investigate the prevention of occupational injuries through ergonomics. Other areas include the relationship between mental health and job satisfaction and the study of environmental conditions such as noise, ventilation, chemical contamination, and radiation. The distribution of accidents and the statistical relationship between occupation and disease are related to the application of survey research to occupational health. Occupational therapists in consultation with industrial researchers can provide information about workers' occupation patterns, nutritional needs, and protective equipment. Occupational health planning should not be done in a vacuum. There are obvious needs for descriptive data regarding frequency of diseases or accidents and the attitudes of workers toward using ergonomic methods before preventive programs can be implemented.

Research in occupational health must also consider psychosocial factors, such as the relationship between personality and accident-proneness; the effects of boredom, low morale, and poor motivation on job satisfaction and mental health; and the effects of job modification on productivity and injury prevention.

### Preventive Programs in Schools and Communities

For the child from a low-income or socially disadvantaged family, school represents the greatest potential escape from a life of deprivation and misery. The school is one of the few institutions that can help the child overcome parental neglect or other disadvantages. It was not by happenstance, but through careful research, that during the 1960s social reformers saw the need to incorporate Head Start programs, work-study curriculums, nutritional programs, and vocational education into schools located in inner-city slums and poor rural regions. Survey research has been used in the past as a means to justify the existence of new programs in the schools, but there has been a backlash to the abuse of survey research in areas where data have been gathered and the needs of a community identified without any program implementation. Community leaders are now suspicious of researchers who come into a neighborhood or community for the purpose of determining the need for services and promising to start new programs, only to leave without any follow-up.

Occupational therapists, in conjunction with allied health professionals and educators, have much to contribute in the areas of nutrition, health education, career planning, recreation, and developmental screening in schools and community centers. Survey research can provide the data for planning these services. Nonetheless, community support and follow-up are necessary if survey research is to have any impact on planning preventive programs. Box 3–7 gives an example of survey research.

---

### BOX 3-7

### Example of Survey Research

#### 1. Bibliographical Notation

Freeman, A. R., MacKinnon, J. R., & Miller, L. T. (2004). Assistive technology and handwriting problems: What do occupational therapists recommend? *Canadian Journal of Occupational Therapy. Revue Canadienne D'ergothérapie, 71*, 150–160.

#### 2. Abstract

Handwriting difficulties for students are a common reason for referral to occupational therapy. Little research evidence is available concerning the factors guiding technology recommendations for these children. The objective of this survey research was to describe the technology-related recommendations and factors involved in the decisions made by Canadian occupational therapists for these students. More therapists recommended the use of keyboard-based strategies (93%) than dictation-based strategies (72%). Experienced therapists were more likely to prescribe technology tools. Dictation to a scribe (93%) and desktop computers (89%) were the strategies most frequently recommended. Equipment cost and availability of funding, and the availability of support in the school for the student were the most influential factors, respectively, on the keyboard and dictation strategy type prescribed. The results confirmed that occupational therapists prescribe a range of technology solutions. Factors influencing these recommendations differ depending on the nature of the technology, the person, environment, or occupation. Knowing the factors guiding occupational therapist technology recommendations will help provide valuable information about the practical implications of the available technologies (p. 150).

*continues*

**BOX 3-7**

**Example of Survey Research** *continued*

### 3. Justification and Need for Study

The authors state that there is little known about the nature of different technology strategies that are being recommended by occupational therapists for students who have handwriting problems. Having more information could help determine the extent to which occupational therapy practice in this area is appropriate. The objective of the current study is to collect data on the nature of the technology-related recommendations made by occupational therapists for school-aged children who have handwriting problems, and the factors influencing these recommendations.

### 4. Literature Review

This study had 79 references from a variety of sources. Cited journals included but were not limited to: *American Journal of Occupational Therapy, Review of Educational Research, Journal of School Psychology, Journal of Educational Measurement, International Journal of Special Education, Learning Disability Quarterly, Journal of Educational Psychology, Canadian Journal of Occupational Therapy, Physical and Occupational Therapy in Pediatrics, British Journal of Educational Technology, Computers and Composition, Topics in Language Disorders, School Psychology Review, Occupational Therapy in Pediatrics,* and *Journal of Computing in Childhood Education.* The years of cited publications ranged from 1978 through 2004.

### 5. Research Hypothesis or Guiding Questions

No hypotheses or guiding questions were stated.

### 6. Methods

Survey research was conducted and distributed to 1,468 occupational therapists who had indicated both working with school-aged children and agreement to receive such surveys. The therapists were required to have provided services to the target population within six months prior to receiving the survey due to rapid changes in technology. Eight hundred and thirty-five surveys were returned (57%). Of these, 382 respondents indicated not providing services to the target population. Additionally, two respondents indicated having little experience in the area and four were excluded because they had not provided services within the six-month exclusion criterion. Also, three were excluded due to working in the United States and one was excluded because it was completed by two respondents. So, in total there were 443 useable surveys, response rate was calculated as 41.95%. The survey questions used were formulated based on clinical experience and a review of literature on occupational therapy and technology. The survey had summated rating scale questions, therapists were asked to identify how influential (1 = not at all influential; 5 = highly influential) were 10 different factors on their recommendations of keyboard strategies, dictation strategies, and keyboard or dictation strategies.

## 7. Results

The majority of the therapists who participated (57%) had worked for more than five years, and only 6% worked less than one year. The greatest proportion of therapists (88–91%) supplied services to children from kindergarten through grade three, with a steady decrease from grade four and above. The results show that 93% of the therapists recommended that students with handwriting problems complete all or part of their work using keyboard strategies. Of the therapists surveyed, 72% used dictation-based strategies. More experienced therapists were more likely to recommend technology tools. The strategies more frequently recommended included dictation to a scribe (93%) and desktop computers (89%). The most influential factors on the keyboard and dictation strategy type prescribed were equipment cost and availability of funding and the availability of support in the school for the student.

## 8. Conclusions

Freeman et al. concluded that:

1. "Ensure that any technological strategies recommended are clearly related to student's education goals" (p.158).
2. "Developing user-friendly training guidelines, which can be readily supported by parents as well as school personnel, will be essential in successfully implementing technology" (p. 158).
3. "As technology becomes increasingly integrated into education practice, occupational therapists will need to be involved in the ongoing debate regarding the importance of handwriting in the school curriculum and collect evidence to support this position (p. 158).

## 9. Limitations of the Study

In the survey, 5% of the therapists who had reported recommending the use of keyboard strategies promoted the use of assistive software, which may have been an under-representation of the number of therapists who recommended the use of software. Also on the surveys, there were missing responses on some questions. Finally, some survey respondents reported being frustrated about completing the summated rating scales in the survey, reporting that they felt obliged to be somewhat prescriptive in their responses regarding the critical thinking process that was implemented in their work with students. Further evidence is needed regarding the development of keyboarding competency by students experiencing handwriting difficulties.

## 10. Major References Cited in the Study

Gardner, M. (2002, October 14). Using speech dictation software as an occupational therapy medium. *OT Practice, 7*(18), 20–21.

Penso, D. E. (1990). *Keyboard, graphic and handwriting skills: Helping people with motor disabilities.* London: Chapman & Hall.

Priest, N., & May, E. (2001). Laptop computers and children with disabilities: Factors influencing success. *Australian Occupational Therapy Journal, 48*, 11–23.

Reed, B. G., & Kanny, E. M. (1993). The use of computers in school system practice by occupational therapists. *Physical and Occupational Therapy in Pediatrics, 13*, 37–55.

## 3.8 Summary

Quantitative research offers occupational therapy clinicians the means to demonstrate the effectiveness of their intervention protocols. The importance of evidence-based practice is established primarily through the results of quantitative research. The various quantitative research models described in this chapter can assist clinicians in developing new ways to evaluate outcome, design intervention methods, and implement a needs assessment. Action research provides the occupational therapist with data to solve clinical problems at the local level. Qualitative research, as described in the next chapter, can be integrated with quantitative research to investigate research problems more thoroughly.

## CHAPTER 4

# Qualitative Research Models

*It is undesirable to believe a proposition when there is no ground whatever for supposing it is true.*

—Bertrand Russell, 1928, *Sceptical Essays*, p. 1

*What do researchers seek when they carry out qualitative research? They seek understandings and insights. And subjectivity is what qualitative researchers seek to understand—the meanings of human phenomena, the nature of human experiences, and the dynamics of the processual elements of living.*

—Betty R. Hasselkus, 2003,
*The Voices of Qualitative Researchers:
Sharing the Conversation*, p.7

## Operational Learning Objectives

By the end of this chapter, the learner will:

- Identify the characteristics of qualitative research.
- Explain the qualitative research process.
- Recognize the difference between quantitative and qualitative research designs.
- Identify qualitative data collection methods.
- Identify the principles of qualitative data analysis.
- Critically analyze examples of qualitative research from the health literature.

## 4.1 Defining Qualitative Research

**Qualitative research** can be defined as the study of people and events in their natural setting.

> Qualitative research is multi–method in focus, involving an interpretive natural-istic approach to its subject matter. This means that qualitative researchers study things in their natural settings, attempting to make sense of or interpret phenomena in terms of the meanings people bring to them. Qualitative research involves the studied use and collection of a variety of empirical materials—case study, personal experience, introspective, life story, interview, observational, historical, inter-active, and visual texts—that describe routine and problematic moments and meaning in individuals' lives. (Denzin & Lincoln, 1994b, p. 2)

In this method, researchers use multiple and interconnected methods, seeking to explore percep-tions and experiences to understand phenomena in terms of the meanings that people bring to them. These phenomena are examined in context and from the individual's point of view. In rehabilita-tion settings, the phenomena investigated include the experience of disability or of a chronic medical condition. The people involved may be clients, their family members, or health personnel.

One example of the application of qualitative research to the understanding of disability has been the growing interest in exploring the views of clients and their families (Ferguson, Ferguson, & Taylor, 1992; Llewellyn, 1995; Morse, 1994; Westby & Back-man, 2010). This interest is being shaped by two forces. The first is the disability movement. Con-sumers of health and related services are actively campaigning for a less medical approach to dis-ability and a more positive acceptance of people with disabilities' place in society (French, 1994). The second is the coming together of researchers in medical and social science disciplines. This has led to the demise of the traditional illness–based view of disability. In its place, disability is regarded as a social construct. This view takes into account the ways in which particular societies regard impair-ments and the influence of situational factors such as poor socioeconomic conditions on the incidence of disability (Oliver, 1991). Another trend in patient physician relationships is the sharing of medical records with patients. Fisher, Bhavani, and Winfield (2009), in a study in the United Kingdom, described how patients' electronic access to medical records helped patients to make more informed decisions and reinforced trust and confidence in their doctors.

Exploring the viewpoint of individuals requires different research designs from those usually employed in the medical and health sciences. Health researchers are turning to sociology (the study of groups) and to anthropology (the study of cultures) for more appropriate research models. Investigators in these disciplines have been "unraveling" the com-plex interactions between individuals since the turn of the century (Parsons, 1964).

Qualitative research models differ from those in the positivist quantitative tradition in three fun-damental ways. First, qualitative researchers are interested in "participatory and holistic knowing" (Reason, 1988, p. 12). This contrasts with the dis-tance and objectivity found particularly in experi-mental research designs. Second, there is a focus on critical subjectivity in qualitative research. This involves researchers acknowledging their primary subjective experience. Researchers become their own "research instrument." This is in direct con-trast to the notion of the objective researcher in experimental research designs. Third, researchers working in the qualitative tradition hold the view "that knowledge is formed in and for action" (Rea-son, p. 12). Action, as it naturally occurs, is viewed as the appropriate context for the development of knowledge. It is also important for the qualitative researcher to investigate how things work.

For example, Stake (2010) discussed how Gali-leo rejected Aristotle's view of gravity by deduction and subjective intuition. Of course, Galileo also used quantitative experimentation to test gravity's influ-ence on planetary movements. Qualitative research does not always work in isolation; it often works hand in hand with experimental methods to explore complex questions. In health care, we may be able to discover a cause-effect relationship for many diseases, but there are qualitative factors that may affect the course of a disease and may be unknown or puzzling to the clinician. For example, many individuals who have a diagnosis of cancer live for many years even though the original prognosis could have predicted death within a short period of time. Qualitative research may help us to answer these questions on how things work when an individual survives a deadly prognosis.

The final issue at the end of a qualitative study is transferability or how the results can be used pragmatically such as in applying the findings to a treatment setting in occupational therapy. This is also a question of generalizing the results within the context of intervention. For example, say, a qualitative researcher in occupational therapy found in a study of children with autism that the mother's manner in helping the child to learn how to dress oneself is sometimes facilitated by modeling behavior. Can this strategy also work in the clinic? It is important in transferability that the researcher describes in detail the methods in the study and the specific reactions of the mother and child. This will help in specific settings to transfer the results found from the study to similar contexts. The occupational therapist, using results from a qualitative study, is functioning in an experimental mode and uses clinical judgment in applying the results to practice.

## 4.2 Characteristics of Qualitative Research

There are four fundamental characteristics of qualitative research:

1. **Phenomena are investigated and interpreted in their natural settings, taking into account the socio–cultural–historical context.** Qualitative research takes place in the field. Qualitative researchers get involved in the natural setting to understand the meanings that participants hold about the phenomena under investigation. From this involvement and understanding, qualitative researchers develop knowledge. This knowledge may be in the form of patterns or themes or a fully developed theory about the phenomena studied. Whatever the case, the resulting knowledge is grounded in direct field research experience rather than imposed a priori through hypotheses or deductive propositions (Glaser & Strauss, 1967).

2. **Multiple methods are used to understand and offer interpretations of the meanings that participants hold about the phenomena under investigation.** Qualitative researchers use an array of methods to collect information about, describe, and interpret events and meanings in individuals' lives. The basic methods used for gathering data are interviews, observation, and documentary analysis. The strategies most commonly used to analyze data include content or theme analysis, grounded theory procedures, and story analysis. These strategies are employed in the search for regularities in the meanings that participants hold about the phenomena under investigation. For some researchers, these regularities are viewed as a form of conceptual order; for others, their interest lies in the repetition of patterns across the data.

3. **The researcher occupies a central place in the qualitative research process.** In qualitative research, the researcher is acknowledged as an individual located within a historical context and within a research tradition or traditions. Researchers bring to the research process particular sets of beliefs about the world that guide their actions. In contrast to experimentally based research designs, however, qualitative researchers do not impose preexisting expectations on the phenomena or setting under study. Rather, the researchers' set of beliefs functions as an interpretive framework (Guba, 1990). This interpretive framework guides the research purpose and also shapes the research questions and the methods employed to address these questions. In addition to an interpretive framework, qualitative researchers become familiar with the literature and develop a guiding question to focus the purpose of the research.

4. **An inductive process is used to develop general principles from the study of specific instances.** In qualitative research, the analysis begins with specific instances of data and builds toward general principles. This contrasts with the deductive process employed in the quantitative tradition in which hypotheses are constructed prior to data collection and then tested. In qualitative research, preparing the research text is the final stage of the inductive analysis process. The **research text** is a construction that integrates and interprets data and researcher understanding of the area of study. The completed product is the public text, which may be delivered either as a research report, journal article, book, or seminar paper.

## 4.3 Types of Qualitative Research

*Qualitative research* is a term widely used to indicate methods that subscribe to the characteristics described above. Tesch (1990), for example, listed 46 different research approaches under the rubric of qualitative research. Some research methods more closely fit the characteristics described; others are less closely associated. Several qualitative methods have become standard in the medical literature and in the related health professional literature (Morse, 1994). These include case study, field study, focus group research, ethnography, and oral history (Table 4–1). Other methods, such as ethnoscience, discourse analysis, transformative research, and hermeneutics are not as familiar.

Discourse analysis and ethnoscience are concerned with the study of the characteristics of language as a communication tool and as culture, respectively. **Transformational research** involves the research subjects as active participants in developing and implementing the research project to overcome the usually passive nature of the research process by turning this into a "transforming" activity. Researchers employing hermeneutics take as their central theme the understanding of events in relation to the context of which these are part, with special reference to the historical context.

Tesch (1990) proposed that working with words is a basic requirement of qualitative research. She developed a continuum of qualitative research types based on the degree of focus on language. At one end of this continuum is research primarily concerned with the characteristics of language. At the other end is research with an interest solely in reflection. In between, some types of research focus on the discovery of regularities in text; others focus on the comprehension of the meaning of text or action. Those approaches that focus on language are more structured and employ more codified methods of data collection and analysis. In contrast, the approaches that rely mainly on reflection employ more holistic procedures that "build on intuition and on insight that are achieved through deep immersion in and dwelling with the data" (Tesch, 1990, p. 60).

Another way of classifying the different approaches used in qualitative research is by the research purpose. Some approaches are ideal for identifying regularities, patterns, or themes. Others are better suited to generating and refining tentative theoretical propositions. Still others are more useful for intense, intimate study of a particular phenomenon using personal reflection. There is ongoing debate in the qualitative research literature about this diversity of approaches and associated methodological issues (Denzin & Lincoln, 1994a; Higgs, 1997). Each approach has adherents in the core disciplines of psychology, psychiatry, sociology, and anthropology.

It is not by chance that many important contributions in the history of the social sciences have emerged from clinical observation methods (Dukes, 1965). Sigmund Freud in his search for an understanding of the psychodynamics of mental illness, Arnold Gesell's (1928) rigorous observation of child development, Jean Piaget's (1926) conceptualization of cognitive development through detailed analysis of clinical responses, and Jules Henry's (1971) naturalistic observation of families of children with emotional disturbance have all made a significant impact through qualitative research. Clinical observation as a research method has the potential to contribute greatly to occupational therapy. Table 4–2 lists some of the landmark studies in the social sciences based on clinical observation research methods.

## TABLE 4-1

### Five Approaches to Qualitative Research

| | Case Study (Retrospective or Prospective) | Grounded Theory or Heuristic Study | Phenomenological | Ethnography or Field Study | Biographical |
|---|---|---|---|---|---|
| **Definition** | Exploration of an individual, organization, program, or event through an in-depth data collection using multiple sources of information (Creswell, 1998) | General method for generating or discovering theory during the data collection (Strauss & Corbin, 1994) | "From the individual descriptions, general or universal meanings are derived, in other words, the essences of structures of the experience" (Moustakas, 1994, p. 13). | Examination of a cultural or social group through extended participant observations to determine the meanings of behavior, language and interactions of the group (Creswell, 1998; Vidich & Lyman, 1994) | Study of an individual. This study may be through "portrayals, portraits, profiles, memoirs, life stories, life histories, case studies, autobiographies, journals, diaries, and on and on—each suggesting a slightly different perspective under consideration" (Smith, 1994, p. 278). |
| **Example of Study** | Emerson, H., Cook, J., Polatajko, H., & Segal, R. (1998). Enjoyment experiences as described by persons with schizophrenia: A qualitative study. *Canadian Journal of Occupational Therapy, 65*, 183–192. | Creighton, C., Dijkers, M., Bennett, N., & Brown, K. (1995). Reasoning and the art of therapy for spinal cord injury. *American Journal of Occupational Therapy, 49*, 311–317. | Hasselkus, B. R., & Dickie, V. A. (1993). Doing occupational therapy: Dimensions of satisfaction and dissatisfaction. *American Journal of Occupational Therapy, 48*, 145–154. | Frank, G., et al. (1997). Jewish spirituality through actions in time: Daily occupations of young Orthodox Jewish couples in Los Angeles. *American Journal of Occupational Therapy, 51*, 199–206. | Frank, G. (1996). Life histories in occupational therapy clinical practice. *American Journal of Occupational Therapy, 50*, 251–264. |
| **Methods of Data Reporting** | • Interviews<br>• Naturalistic observational techniques | • Mute evidence<br>• Personal experience | | | |

## TABLE 4-2

### Major Contributions from Clinical Observation Methodologies in the Social Sciences

| Social Scientist | Major Works | Methods | Publication Dates | Fields of Investigation |
|---|---|---|---|---|
| Sigmund Freud and Josef Breuer | Studies in Hysteria | Case study | 1895/1955 | Psychiatry |
| Margaret Mead | Coming of Age in Samoa | Field observation | 1928 | Cultural anthropology |
| Arnold Gesell | Infancy and Human Growth | Developmental observation | 1929 | Child development |
| Jean Piaget | The Psychology of Intelligence | Developmental observation | 1947/1950 | Cognitive development |
| Alfred Stanton and Morris S. Schwartz | The Mental Hospital: A Study of Institutional Participation in Psychiatric Illness and Treatment | Operations research | 1954 | Psychiatry |
| Robert White | Lives in Progress | Case study | 1952 | Personality |
| Jules Henry | Pathways to Madness | Field observation | 1965 | Family casework |
| Rene A. Spitz | The First Year of Life: A Psychoanalytic Study of Normal and Deviant Development of Object Relations | Developmental observation | 1965 | Child psychiatry |
| Joseph Church | Three Babies: Biographies of Cognitive Development | Case study | 1966 | Cognition |
| Oscar Lewis | La Vida | Field observation | 1966 | Cultural anthropology |
| Bruno Bettelheim | The Empty Fortress | Case study | 1967 | Child psychiatry |
| Robert Coles | Children of Crisis | Field observation | 1967 | Social psychiatry |
| Eric Bermann | Scapegoat: The Impact of Death-Fear on an American Family | Field observation | 1973 | Family casework |
| Mary Ainsworth et al. | Patterns of Attachment: A Psychological Study of the Strange Situation | Clinical observation | 1978 | Social psychology |

| Social Scientist | Major Works | Methods | Publication Dates | Fields of Investigation |
|---|---|---|---|---|
| Jack Fadely and Virginia Hosler | Case Studies in Left and Right Hemispheric Functioning | Case study | 1983 | Perception |
| Stephen Marks | Three Corners: Exploring Marriage and the Self | Case study | 1986 | Family relationships |
| Sylvia Kenig (Ed.) | Who Plays? Who Pays? Who Cares? A Case Study in Applied Sociology, Political Economy and the Community Mental Health Centers Movement | Case Study | 1992 | Community mental health |
| Kelley Johnson | Deinstitutionalizing Women: An Ethnographic Study of Institutional Closure | Case Study | 1998 | Deinstitutionalization |
| Steven Pinker | The Blank Slate: The Modern Denial of Human Nature | Clinical observation | 2002 | Psychology |
| Jonathan Kozol | The Shame of the Nation: The Restoration of Apartheid Schooling in America | Field observation | 2005 | Educational philosophy |
| Oliver Sacks | Musicophilia: Tales of Music and the Brain | Case study | 2007 | Neuropsychology |
| Temple Grandin | The Way I See It: A Personal Look at Autism and Asperger's | Case study | 2008 | Autism |

Clinical observation research employs four methods: individual case study, child development studies, field observation (ethnography), and operations research. The definition, purposes, procedure, and application to occupational therapy and special education are listed in Table 4–3.

## 4.3.1 Case Study

There is much criticism by experimentalists of the case study approach as a model for research, primarily directed toward the researcher's subjectivity and the inability to generalize to a population on the basis of one subject. The most important purpose of the **case study** is in the intensive investigation about one individual. Through a thorough study, the researcher can examine factors that ordinarily would be difficult either in an experimental study involving a group of subjects, or in a correlational study.

To illustrate, let us suppose an investigator is interested in learning why individuals who are older and living in a nursing home develop feelings of hopelessness and disengage from the mainstream of society. The researcher poses the question: What factors in an older person's life contribute to feelings of hopelessness and disengagement? In this study, the investigator is limited to an ex post facto research model. It would be possible to answer this

### TABLE 4-3

**Application of Clinical Observation Methods**

| Methods | Purposes | Procedures for Collecting Data | Application to Fields |
|---|---|---|---|
| Individual case study | Understanding of underlying dynamics of illness | • interviewing<br>• testing<br>• examining personal documents<br>• conducting case research | Investigation of health problems, chronic diseases, and individual factors |
| Child development studies | Description of the sequential and hierarchical processes in human development | • objective observation in a controlled setting<br>• mechanical audiovisual recordings | Examination of normal and abnormal patterns in development |
| Field observations (ethnography) | Examination of the interaction between members of a social group, educational group, or family | • naturalistic observation<br>• processing of recordings of interactions<br>• unobtrusive measurement | Description of group interaction in:<br>• dysfunctional families<br>• halfway houses<br>• residential treatment programs<br>• education classrooms<br>• socioeconomic units |
| Operations research | Analysis of administrative problems in organization systems | • flowcharts of organizational structure<br>• job descriptions<br>• communication patterns<br>• decision-making process | Examination of interrelationships among systems:<br>• political<br>• economic<br>• health care<br>• educational |

question by comparing a group of older individuals who display feelings of hopelessness with another group of older individuals who are actively engaged in independent activities. In this hypothetical study, the researcher could test whether individuals who have personalities characterized by an external locus of control feel more hopeless than a similar geriatric sample who characteristically have more internal locus of control and feel less hopeless.

The reader will recognize this research model as correlational. In a correlational model, the researcher is restricted by the test instruments used in measuring the variables of locus of control and hopelessness and by the limitations in controlling for the individual differences among participants. On the other hand, a case study approach would allow the investigator the freedom to search for individual factors that could easily be overlooked in a correlational study, but on closer investigation prove to be a critical variable in generating dependency and hopelessness. The flexibility of a case study and the creativity afforded to the researcher compensate for the apparent lack of external validity or the ability to generalize to a representative population.

The general outline of case study research is similar to all aspects of research in that the researcher justifies the need for investigation, reviews previous literature, states guiding questions for data collection, and obtains data through observation. In contrast to experimental and correlational research, in the case study the researcher does not initially state a statistical hypothesis or collect group data from a representative sample of a population. Rather, the researcher draws inferences from an analysis and review of data collected from and about the individual during the study. The general format of a case study follows.

### Need for the Study

The need for the study comes from a broad societal context and from contemporary psychosocial problems such as aggression and hopelessness in disadvantaged youth, obesity as related to diabetes, or underachievement in gifted students. In this section of the study, the investigator explores the multiple effects of a problem on family, educational

and health institutions, and society in general. The investigator examines the prevalence and epidemiology of the problem and its relationship to occupational therapy. The investigator should also discuss the appropriateness of using a qualitative case study model in contrast to an experimental or correlational design.

If a case study is used as a pilot study or preliminary study, such as to collect data about a problem before undertaking a larger study, then it should also be stated. A case study should not be used in place of an experimental or correlational study. For example, a case study is more appropriate than experimental or correlational methods in an in-depth study of a complex chronic disability such as osteoarthritis. The investigator should also consider the indirect effects of a problem, such as economic loss to society as a result of the inability of the individual with a disability to work and the emotional and family turmoil that accompany chronic disability. The number and percentage of a population affected by a health problem should be documented.

What statistics are available regarding mortality rates, hospitalization admissions, physician visits, and costs of special education, and related services? What evaluation tests and treatment methods do health or educational professionals provide at present, and what is the potential of generating therapeutic techniques and interventions? These questions are pertinent in demonstrating the need for a study. The investigator should also discuss in this section what the possible implications of the results from a case study could provide such as changes in treatment. Investigations into the dynamic factors affecting the onset of multiple sclerosis, schizophrenia, delinquency, anorexia, dementia, reading or math disability, and ADHD are particularly appropriate for case study research.

### Review of Literature

The investigator should do an extensive review of the literature on the question and critically examine the variables in the case study. Research related to etiology and treatment is particularly important in a case study. The literature review should provide the investigator with a general overview of the current state of knowledge. Research journals, textbooks, and conference proceedings, electronic databases, and other sources of information should be reviewed. An outline should guide the investigator in deciding what aspects of the research problem to include, the extensiveness of the review, and the sources used to obtain information. (For a more detailed discussion on reviewing literature, see Chapter 6.)

The literature review also should include an examination of case study methods for collecting data, such as interviewing, reliability of case records, medical history recording, and psychological testing. These areas are especially important to the investigator who is unfamiliar with the case study methods.

### Research Methods

In this section, critical variables are operationally defined, screening criteria for subject selection are delineated, a procedure for interviewing and testing the subject is stated, test instruments are identified, and reliability and validity data are reported. Screening criteria should be based on a rationale considering representative statistical data

for a target population. For example, if investigators are interested in doing a case study of a youth who is delinquent, they would consider gender, age when most delinquency occurs, socioeconomic group factors, school status, cognitive level, family, and delinquent acts committed. The variables identified should be obtained from a review of the literature, statistical abstracts, and clinical observations. From these sources, researchers operationalize the screening criteria as outlined in Table 4–4.

The investigator should also consider **exclusion criteria**, that is, factors that should not be present in the subject. These could include brain damage, mental illness, language difficulty, or language difference. After the researcher has determined inclusion and exclusion criteria, the next task is to plan a procedure for selecting a subject or subjects if the project involves several case studies (Llewellyn, Sullivan, & Minichiello, 1999). This entails contacting a juvenile facility, a court, or an agency working with delinquent youth. The agency's cooperation is crucial to the research. The participant and the parent or guardian must be told of the purposes of the study through informed consent. The plan for collecting data is another important part of the

---

### TABLE 4-4

#### Example of Screening Criteria (Youth Who are Delinquent)

| | |
|---|---|
| Age: | 16 years old |
| Gender: | Male |
| Socioeconomic factor: | Working-class family |
| Intelligence: | Average nonverbal IQ |
| Family: | Dysfunctional, non-intact as a result of divorce, separation, or parent desertion |
| School status: | Special education setting |
| Geographic area: | Urban |
| Behavior: | Delinquent, with vandalism, truancy, and deviant behavior resulting in adjudication, probation, or referral to residential treatment setting |

research methodology. This includes the following questions:

- At what setting will the study take place?
- What psychological tests, evaluation instruments, questionnaires, and interview schedules will be employed?
- During what period of time will the study take place (e.g., hours of day, school time or evening, time of year)?
- What are the costs of the study?

### Results

The data gathered for a case study include the subject's history, informal and formal assessments, collateral information from case records, interviews with the individual and family members, and clinical reports. Difficulties can arise in a case study that threatens the researcher's objectivity. Robert White (1952), in his classic study *Lives in Progress* felt, "It is impossible to study another person without making evaluations, and it is hard to keep the evaluations from being seriously distorted by one's personal reactions to the subject" (p. 99). How does the investigator control some of the limitations of a case study? One way to do this is to have more than one interviewer obtain an independent history on the same individual. In this way, the investigator bias and personal views can be isolated. Another method is to make the investigators aware of their own rigidities, assumptions, and prejudices "through increased familiarity with their own personalities" (p. 100). Most important, however, is the need to acknowledge that there will always be investigator influence in the conduct and reporting of any study, particularly in intensive works such as a case study.

The preferred way to demonstrate that the reported results accurately reflect the case study individual or individuals, and the investigator's perceptions, is to ensure that the investigator states up front (a) his or her perspectives, assumptions, and biases and (b) the interpretative theoretical framework used to examine the case material. Most investigators, in reporting a case study, use a chronological outline starting from the subject's early childhood and continuing through his or her

current age. A topical biography is another way to organize data. For example, in a case study of a subject with arthritis, the investigator may want to report data under subject headings, such as possible etiological factors (joint injuries, allergies, emotional disturbances, endocrine disorders) or treatment intervention (occupational therapy, physical therapy, chemotherapy, and psychological counseling). An interpretive summary and a recommendation for further research follow the reporting of results.

In short, case study research is a viable method for obtaining credible data pertaining to the life of an individual with disabilities. It is an idiographic approach to research that considers individual differences in etiology of disease and specific adaptations in coping with a disability. Box 4–1 gives an example of a qualitative case study.

### 4.3.2 Operations Research

Ackoff and Rivett (1963) described the three essential characteristics of **operations research**: "(1) systems orientation, (2) the use of interdisciplinary teams, and (3) the adaptation of scientific method" (p. 10). Operations research was developed in Great Britain during World War II mainly for the purpose of using radar effectively to combat German air attacks (Crowther & Whiddington, 1948). Subsequently, during the 1950s, large corporations employed operations research teams to analyze production methods as a way of increasing efficiency. Norbert Wiener's (1948) contribution in cybernetics and the application of the feedback principle expanded systems theory to biological, sociological, and psychological dimensions. Using the technology of cybernetics, the methodology of operations research, and systems theory, researchers have examined the physiology of respiration (Pribram, 1958), equipment design and human engineering (Schrader, 2006; United States Department of Defense, Joint Services Steering Committee, 1963), political life (Easton, 1961), the city as a system (Blumberg, 1972), clinical rotation (Reid, Seavor, & Taylor, 1991), higher education (Cheng, 1993), family planning (Huezo, 1997), obstetric

BOX 4-1

## Example of Qualitative Case Study

### 1. Bibliographical Notation

Chan, A. S., Tsang, H. W., & Li, S. M. (2009). Case report of integrated supported employment for a person with severe mental illness. *American Journal of Occupational Therapy, 63*, 238–244.

### 2. Abstract

**OBJECTIVE:** We illustrate the implementation of an integrated supported employment (ISE) program that augments the individual placement and support model with social skills training in helping people with severe mental illness (SMI) achieve and maintain employment. **METHOD:** A case illustration demonstrates how ISE helped a 41-year-old woman with SMI to get and keep a job with support from an employment specialist. An independent, blinded assessor conducted data collection of employment information, including self-efficacy and quality of life, at pretreatment and at 3–month, 7–month, 11–month, and 15–month follow-up assessments. **RESULTS:** The participant eventually stayed in a job for 8 months and reported improved self-efficacy and quality of life. **CONCLUSION:** The case report suggests that ISE could improve the employment outcomes of people with SMI. Moreover, changes in the participant's self-efficacy and quality of life were shown to be driven by the successful employment experience.

### 3. Justification and Need for Study

The authors document the need for individuals with severe mental illness to obtain and maintain competitive employment since only 15 to 30 percent are employed. A protocol for the integrated supported employment program was tested and evaluated with one individual diagnosed with depression.

### 4. Literature Review

Twenty-nine references were cited in the study. Primary sources came from *Community Mental Health Journal, American Journal of Occupational Therapy, Psychiatric Rehabilitation Journal, American Journal of Psychiatry, Schizophrenia Bulletin, British Journal of Medical Psychology, Psychiatric Services, Psychiatric Quarterly, Archives of General Psychiatry, Social Indicators Research, Psychiatry: Interpersonal and Biological Processes, Social Psychiatry and Psychiatric Epidemiology, Journal of Nervous and Mental Disease, Journal of Behavior Therapy and Experimental Psychiatry, International Journal of Psychosocial Rehabilitation, Psychologia,* and the *American Journal of Rehabilitation.*

### 5. Research Hypothesis or Guiding Questions

The authors assessed how integrated supported employment can improve the employment outcome of an adult individual with chronic depression.

### 6. Methods

The integrated supported employment program was operationally defined applying vocational assessment, individual employment plan, social skills training, vocational placement and follow-along support. The program was in place for 7 months.

### 7. Results

The individual stayed in her job for 8 months. She expressed that she was satisfied in her job and was able to maintain a good relationship with her supervisor and co-workers.

### 8. Conclusions

The authors felt that the program supported the application of an integrated supported employment program and were developing an e-learning package for clinicians.

### 9. Limitations of the Study

Because this was a qualitative study without a control group, more research is needed to validate the conclusions. The protocol developed in the study needs to be replicated to assess its applicability in a wide range of vocational rehabilitation programs.

### 10. Major References Cited in the Study

Bond, G. R. (2004). Supported employment: Evidence for an evidence-based practice. *Psychiatric Rehabilitation Journal, 27*, 345–359.

Drake, R. E., McHugo, G. J., Bebout, R. R., Becker, D. R., Harris, M., Bond, G. R., & Quimby, E. (1999). A randomized clinical trial of supported employment for inner-city patients with severe mental illness. *Archives of General Psychiatry, 56*, 627–633.

McGurk, S. R, Mueser, K. T., & Pascaris, A. (2005). Cognitive training and supported employment of persons with severe mental illness: One year results from a randomized controlled trial. *Schizophrenia Bulletin, 31*, 898–909.

care (Sibley & Armbruster, 1997), and rehabilitation (Doarn, McVeigh, & Poropatich, 2010).

Efficiency in industrial production has been one of the areas in which operations research has been widely applied. Feigin, An, Connors, and Crawford (1996) applied operations research to restructure IBM's manufacturing strategy. The goal of the efficiency expert in a factory is to minimize expenditures and maximize production. By analyzing the industrial system of production, the operations researcher can determine where costs can be reduced and production increased. Factors such as competitive costs of raw materials and plant machinery, redeployment of labor, employee morale, and distribution of goods are all considered in operations research. Essentially,

operations research analyzes a system by identifying all those factors that affect input or raw materials and output or finished product. Operations research is subjective in that the researcher selects various processes to analyze. For example, if trying to determine the factors that lead to job satisfaction in a company, then the researcher will identify these factors through previous research, on-site observation, or intuition. The research per se can also generate findings and change the researcher's assumptions.

The feedback in this system represents the critical analysis of input and output and the resultant changes in the total system of production. In the input, the investigator identifies the factors that determine job satisfaction. The process is the feedback from the workers' survey or interviews. The output can change, depending upon the results of the study. Operations research in general is a dynamic process where feedback is continuous in building a product. This simple feedback model is illustrated in the following diagram:

**Simple Feedback Model**

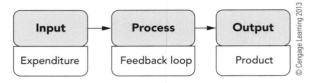

© Cengage Learning 2013

The concept of operations research and systems theory can also be applied to research problems in health care (Dickinson et al., 2010; Jacob & Shapiro, 2010; Uomoto & Wiliams, 2009). For example, hospital management provides an excellent area for operations research. For hospital administrators, the problems of expanding costs and depersonalized care for health consumers have become increasingly more aggravated during the last two decades. Although society seeks improved expanded health care for larger portions of the population, hospitals have to find more efficient methods to service more clients and to provide them with sophisticated diagnostic methods for detecting and treating illnesses with the most advanced technology. Specifically, these problems include (a) architectural design; (b) medical equipment; (c) hospital staffing, including availability of consultants; (d) cost sharing for using expensive machinery; and (e) issues such as managed care. Operations research as applied to the fields of health and rehabilitation uses observational data and systems analysis to identify critical issues and solve problems. Health problems appropriate for operations research include the following:

- The lack of health care workers in rural areas (Rosenblatt, 1991)
- Depersonalization of clients in long–term care (Kliebsch, Sturmer, Siebert, & Brenner, 1998)
- Inadequate funding for long-term care (Xakellis, Frantz, Lewis, & Harvey, 1998)
- Recurrence of chronic disease among vulnerable populations (Woods et al., 1997)

- Lack of rehabilitation services in forensic psychiatry (Lloyd, 1995)
- Inefficient emergency care in urban hospitals (Ernst, Houry, & Weiss, 1997)
- Day care for elderly or adults with severe disabilities (Macdonald, Epstein, & Vastano, 1986)
- Quality of life for patients with post-polio (Jacob & Shapira, 2010)
- Integrated care for returning veterans (Uomoto & Williams, 2009)
- Computer-based cognitive remediation for schizophrenia (Dickinson et al., 2010)
- Learning difficulties in children with ADHD (Bennett et al., 2009)
- Characteristics of TBI assessed in the workplace (Bootes & Chapparo, 2002)
- Waiting time for total hip replacement (Hajat et al., 2002)
- Computerized contingency management in a drug addiction treatment program (Vahabzadeh, Lin, Mezghanni, Epstein, & Preston, 2009)
- Roles of nonmedical health care workers (Mitchell, 2009)
- Challenges in occupational therapy (Gewurtz, Stergiou–Kita, Shaw, Kirsh, & Rappolt, 2008)

In all the foregoing problems, the underlying assumption is that a system, a unified interconnected whole, exists. The systems researcher analyzes the specific components of the system and their interrelationships. In these examples, the systems are identified as rural health, long-term care, legislation process, general hospitals, chronic illness, emergency care, and adult day care. Box 4–2 provides an example of an operational research study.

### 4.3.3 Developmental Observations

"Experimental observation, with conditions so clearly defined that they can be duplicated and so delimited that only a single variable remains for study is scientifically a goal to work toward" (Gesell, 1928, p. 23). This description stated over three-quarters of a century ago remains the benchmark for research on child development. **Developmental observation research** is concerned with the rigorous investigations into the process, stages, and hierarchical steps

BOX 4-2

## Example of Operations Research

### 1. Bibliographical Notation

Bennett, A. E., Power, T. J., Eiraldi, R. B., Leff, S.S., & Blum, N. J. (2009). Identifying learning problems in children evaluated for ADHD: The Academic Performance Questionnaire. *Pediatrics, 124*, e633–e639. doi: 10.1542/peds.2009–0143

### 2. Abstract

**OBJECTIVE:** The objective of this study was to assess the usefulness of the *Academic Performance Questionnaire* (APQ) to identify low reading and math achievement in children who are being evaluated for attention-deficit/hyperactivity disorder (ADHD). **METHODS:** Charts of 997 patients who were seen in a multidisciplinary ADHD evaluation program were reviewed. Pupils who were in first- through sixth-grade and had completed *Academic Performance Questionnaire* (APQ) and *Wechsler Individual Achievement Test II* (WIAT–II) Basic Reading and Numerical Operations subtests were enrolled in this study. The 271 eligible pupils were randomly assigned to a score-development group ($n = 215$) and a validation group ($n = 56$). By using data from the score-development sample, APQ questions that predicted low academic achievement were identified, and the scores for these questions were entered into a logistic regression to identify the APQ questions that independently predicted low achievement. **RESULTS:** Only two APQ questions, one about reading and one about math, independently predicted low achievement. By using these two questions, the area under the receiver operating characteristic curve was 0.834, and the optimal combination of sensitivity and specificity occurred when the total score for the two items was >4. This cutoff had a sensitivity of 0.86 and a specificity of 0.63 in the score-development group and a sensitivity of 1.0 and a specificity of 0.53 in the validation sample. **CONCLUSIONS:** The APQ may be a useful screening tool to identify children being evaluated for ADHD who need additional testing for learning problems. Although the predictive value of a negative screen on the APQ is good, the predictive value of a positive test is relatively low.

**Keywords:** attention-deficit/hyperactivity disorder; learning disorder; screening; developmental-behavioral pediatrics; school-aged children (p. 633)

### 3. Justification and Need for Study

The authors stated that learning disorders co-occur with ADHD in 20 to 30 percent of children and are typically identified by a psychoeducational assessment. Primary care physicians who evaluate children for ADHD often find it difficult to identify which children they should refer for additional assessment of academic skills. The purposes of this study were to (a) examine the test-retest reliability of the APQ and (b) evaluate the validity of the APQ with regard to predicting low achievement in reading and/or math.

*continues*

BOX 4-2

**Example of Operations Research** *continued*

### 4. Literature Review

The authors cited 17 references. The primary sources came from the journals, *Pediatrics*, *Journal of Pediatric Psychology, Journal of Learning Disabilities, School Psychology Review,* and the *Journal of Developmental Behavior Pediatrics.*

### 5. Research Hypothesis or Guiding Question

Is the APQ helpful in identifying those students with ADHD who will have difficulty in reading and math achievement?

### 6. Methods

The charts of 997 students who were seen in a multidisciplinary ADHD evaluation program were reviewed. Students who were in first- through sixth-grade and had completed APQ and WIAT–II Basic Reading and Numerical Operations subtests were enrolled in this study. The 271 eligible students were randomly assigned to a score-development group ($n = 215$) and a validation group ($n = 56$). By using data from the score-development sample, APQ questions that predicted low academic achievement were identified, and the scores for these questions were entered into a logistic regression to identify the APQ questions that independently predicted low achievement.

### 7. Results

Results of this study demonstrate that using only two questions from the APQ, one about math and one about reading, as a screen produces a test with acceptable test-retest reliability and sensitivity.

### 8. Conclusion

The APQ may be a useful initial screening tool for assessing learning problems among children who present with symptoms of ADHD or other school problems. Before the APQ can be implemented as a primary care screening tool, additional research is needed to confirm its predictive validity in a primary care setting assessing children with a diverse range of demographic characteristics.

### 9. Limitations of the Study

This study was a retrospective chart analysis of children with ADHD who attended a multidisciplinary center. The results of this study should be considered in the context of the following limitation. The children in this study did not have a full psychoeducational assessment. For clinical efficiency, only the two subtests of the WIAT–II that best correlate with overall reading and math scores were selected. A more complete academic assessment may have changed the classification of some children who scored near the cutoff. In addition, we did not assess other important skills, such as writing, spelling, and phonics. Thus, the ability of the APQ questions to detect children with low achievement in these areas could not be assessed.

## 10. Major References Cited In The Study

Glascoe, F. P. (2001). Can teachers' global ratings identify children with academic problems? *Journal of Developmental and Behavioral Pediatrics, 22*, 163–168.

Gresham, F. M., & MacMillan, D. L. (1997). Teachers as "tests": Differential validity of teacher judgments in identifying students at-risk for learning difficulties. *School Psychology Review, 26*, 47–60.

Leslie, L. K., Weckerly, J., Plemmons, D., Landsverk, J., & Eastman, S. (2004). Implementing the American Academy of Pediatrics attention-deficit/hyperactivity disorder diagnostic guidelines in primary care settings. *Pediatrics, 114*, 129–140.

Polaha, J., Cooper, S., Meadows, T., & Kratochvil, C. J. (2005). The assessment of attention-deficit/hyperactivity disorder in rural primary care: The portability of the American Academy of Pediatrics guidelines to the "real world". *Pediatrics, 115*, e120–126.

in human development. How does speech develop? What are the sequential stages in the areas of language, ambulation, psychosocial development, and cognition? These and other questions are examples of research problems that lend themselves best to developmental observation methods. The investigator seeks to identify the processes involved in development, the approximate ages when landmarks are reached, and the biopsychosocial factors that shape development.

A key assumption in developmental research is that human behavior unfolds at critical stages. In Table 4–5, some examples of approximate ages are given for achieving a developmental landmark. The typical child is expected to pass a test item related to a chronological age. The child's rate of development is

## TABLE 4-5

### Denver Developmental Screening Test–II

| Developmental Skills | Hierarchical Sequential Activities from Birth to 6 Years |
| --- | --- |
| Gross motor | Lifts head at 2 months to walks backward (heel to toe) at 6 years |
| Fine motor | Visually tracks objects to midline at 2 months to draws a man with six distinct parts at 6 years |
| Language | Responds to bell at 2 months to defines six words at 6 years |
| Personal-social | Regards face at 2 months to dresses without supervision at 5 years |

**Note:** From normative data, age levels were established as to when children develop individual skills. Normal limits (upper and lower) were validated for each hierarchical activity. Adapted from *The Denver Developmental Screening Test–II* (DDST–II) by W. R. Frankenburg, J. B. Dodds, P. Archer, H. Shapiro, and B. Bresnick, 1990, Denver, CO: Denver Developmental Materials. Copyright 1990 by Denver Developmental Materials. The DDST is also available as an online tool at http://www.denverii.com/

relative to the norm response for specific chronological age groups. The basic assumption in the *Denver Developmental Screening Test*, DDST–II (Frankenburg, Dodds, Archer, Shapiro, & Bresnick, 1990) is that human development progresses in a linear direction originating from genetic forces and shaped by environmental factors. In this model, the typical child is biologically ready at a specific age to learn to roll over, stand, walk, play games cooperatively with other children, write, speak, or perform any number of other developmental tasks. Environmental experiences provide the opportunities for development to unfold during critical stages in the child's life.

### Stating the Guiding Question

The researcher's first task is to state a research question that generates data. Piaget (1926), in the first sentence of his book *The Language and Thought of the Child* stated: "The question which we shall attempt to answer in this book may be stated as follows: What are the needs which a child tends to satisfy when he talks?" (p. 1). Gesell and Thompson (1923), in their research on infant behavior, also began with a guiding question: "When does this orthogenetic patterning of the human individual begin?" (p. 9).

The potential areas for research using developmental observation are considerable. An outline of the broad areas of development and specific research questions, listed in Table 4–6, demonstrates the wide perspective in doing developmental research.

The research questions listed in Table 4–6 represent only a fraction of the potential areas appropriate for developmental observation. The area of development selected by a researcher and the research questions generated provide the engine for the study. The justification and need for the study are many times based on contemporary and controversial issues such as the causes of and effective interventions in autism. For example, how can we use developmental observation to diagnose autism? In observing children with autism, what are effective interventions such as sensory intervention? Spitzer (2003) described how participant observation can be used with young children with autism who do not have language skills. The researcher can use toys or other occupations with the child in trying to understand the child's individual way of communicating.

### Need for Study in Developmental Observation

For the occupational therapist, developmental research provides the data for evaluating the progress of children as they mature. Is this individual functioning within normal limits? To answer this

---

### TABLE 4-6

**Suggested Areas for Research Questions**

| Areas of Development | Examples of Research Questions |
|---|---|
| Social | What are the sequential stages that lead to cooperative play in children? |
| Emotional | What are the origins of anxiety? |
| Cognitive | What types of logic do 3-year-old children use? |
| Language | What is the most favorable age for learning a second language? |
| Academic | What cognitive processes are related to reading? |
| Moral | What factors facilitate moral learning in 8-year-old children? |
| Motor | What are the sequential stages of development in eye-hand coordination? |
| Feeding | What is the relationship between obesity in infancy and obesity in adolescence? |

question, data regarding typical development are needed. Developmental studies therefore provide benchmarks for (a) interpreting the developmental level and (b) constructing sequential treatment programs. For children with developmental disabilities, such as cerebral palsy, intellectual disabilities, autism, or severe social deprivation, occupational therapists use data from developmental observations to monitor the progress within the treatment or intervention.

The rationale behind this approach is that development progresses in a sequential and hierarchal manner in the typical child, but is delayed, incomplete, or impaired in the child with a developmental disability. Using evidence-based practice, the pediatric occupational therapist tries to reconstruct the sequential stages in an area of development and intervenes with the child by facilitating progress through each stage. Steps along a linear developmental progression are programmed for the individual child starting at the child's base level of performance. Research is essential in identifying the critical stages in development for evidence-based practice in pediatrics.

The results of developmental observation research have a direct effect on evaluating and treating children with developmental disabilities. After delineating the need for the study, the researcher designs an observational method for collecting data.

## Observational Methods for Collecting Data

"The technique of observing infant behavior in a controlled environment" (Gesell, 1928, p. 23), as first demonstrated by Gesell, demands objective and painstaking research. Children are unique and it is difficult to establish norms in development without replication in various settings and cultures. What is the best way to observe children's behavior in pediatric occupational therapy during sensory integration sessions? "Observation methods must vary considerably with the age of the infant and, of course, with the objectives in view" (p. 23).

The observational method that the developmental researcher selects should provide objective descriptive data that are representative of the child's repertoire of behavior. This is accomplished by providing the child with a stimulus that will elicit the desired behavior, schematically represented in Figure 4–1.

The researcher selects the stimulus after operationally defining the area of development in terms of the behavioral response. Tests for assessing a child's

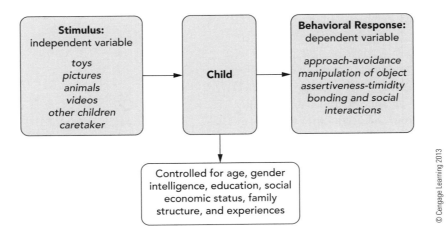

© Cengage Learning 2013

**FIGURE 4-1**  Schematic Representation of Observational Research: Notice that the child is provided with stimuli so as to elicit a response. The data collected, using video cameras and computers, are the behaviors elicited by the stimuli.

level of development such as the *Bayley Scales of Infant Development-2* (BSID–2; Bayley, 1993), the *Mullen Scales of Early Learning* (MSEL; Mullen, 1995), and the *Miller Assessment for Preschoolers* (MAP; Miller, 1988) are examples of this method. In the BSID–2, cognitive abilities are operationally defined by the following tasks:

| Developmental Factors | Operational Definition |
|---|---|
| Object Permanence | An object is wrapped in a sheet of paper while the child is watching. The child is asked to find the object. |
| Manual Dexterity | Child puts pegs into a peg board in a timed or untimed condition. The time taken to complete the task is age-specific. |

© Cengage Learning 2013

Questions arise in this context. How does the researcher know that all aspects of a developmental factor are being considered and that the operational definition of a developmental factor is valid? These questions are pertinent in developmental research, and they demand a rationale from the investigator.

In reporting developmental data, the researcher should describe factors in the child that affect the results. These factors include age, gender, intelligence, education, socioeconomic status, family structure, and experiences. The selection and control of these factors by inclusion in the research eliminates ambiguity in interpreting the results.

As well as operationally defining the developmental factors and identifying variables within the child, the researcher must also construct an objective environment for collecting valid data. Examples of experimental environment in developmental research are shown in Figure 4–2 and Figure 4–3. Arrangements for observation are part of a standard procedure. Adaptations in this method include

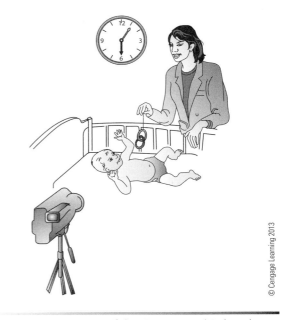

© Cengage Learning 2013

**FIGURE 4-2**  Position of the Camera and Baby when Taking Observational Data

the use of a photographic dome as developed by Gesell (1928) or the use of experimental rooms with one-way mirrors, where the subject cannot see the observer. Box 4–3 gives an example of a study using developmental research.

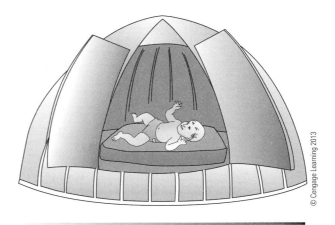

© Cengage Learning 2013

**FIGURE 4-3**  Illustration of a Photographic Dome Used by Gesell (1928) in Observational Research

BOX 4-3

## Example of Developmental Observation

### 1. Bibliographic Notation

Kawaguchi, H., Murakami, B., & Kawai, M. (2010). Behavioral characteristics of children with high functioning pervasive developmental disorders during a game. *Journal of Epidemiology, 20* (Suppl. 2), S490–S497.

### 2. Abstract

**BACKGROUND:** To evaluate children's sociability through their behavior, we compared the motion features of children with high functioning pervasive developmental disorders (HFPDD) and typical development (TD) during a game. We selected "Jenga" as the game because this is an interactive game played by two people. **METHODS:** We observed the behavior of seven children with HFPDD and 10 children with TD. An optical motion capture system was used to follow the movement of three-dimensional position markers attached to caps worn by the players. **RESULTS:** The range of head motion of the children with HFPDD was narrower than that of the control group, especially in the X-axis direction (perpendicular to the line connecting the two players). In each game, we calculated the range of motion in the X-axis of each child and divided that figure by the matched adult player's range. The average ratios of children with HFPDD and TD were 0.64 and 0.89 (number of games are 61 and 18), and the difference of these two ratios is significant ($P < 0.001$). **CONCLUSIONS:** This ratio has sensitivity to identify HFPDD children and could be useful in their child care.

### 3. Justification and Need for Study

"We attempted to derive a behavioral indicator connected to sociability based on comparing the behavioral characteristics of two groups of children, children who are socially challenged (with high functioning pervasive developmental disorders (HFPDD) and those who are not (children with typical development (TD)" (p.491).

### 4. Literature Review

The authors cited 45 references from the literature. Journals cited included *Journal of Epidemiology, Trends in Cognitive Science, Brain Imaging Behavior, Child Development, Science, Journal of Child Psychiatry and Psychology, Developmental Psychology, Perceptual and Motor Skills, Japanese Journal of Child Adolescent Psychiatry,* and *Early Development and Parent.* The majority of articles were published in the last ten years.

### 5. Research Hypothesis or Guiding Question

The authors sought evidence to demonstrate that children with high functioning pervasive developmental disorders (HFPDD) as compared to a normal typical group of children responded differently in their social behavior as observed in playing a Japanese game.

*continues*

> BOX 4-3
>
> ## Example of Developmental Observation *continued*
>
> ### 6. Methods
>
> Six video cameras, two microphones, and an optical motion capture system set up inside an observation room recorded the social interaction of the participants.
>
> ### 7. Results
>
> The results of the observations indicated that children with HFPDD have problems conveying their interests through movement and seemed to have difficulty in nonverbal communication.
>
> ### 8. Conclusions
>
> "Making the assumption that children with developmental disorders are creating communicative signals, if we make efforts to pick up those signals, and educate widely with this objective, we may be able to create a society where children with developmental disorders can live comfortably" (p. S497).
>
> ### 9. Limitations of the Study
>
> Further research is needed to replicate the study with another group of children with HFPDD to determine if the methodology is reliable and valid in observing children at play.
>
> ### 10. Major References Cited in the Study
>
> Frith, C. D., & Frith, U. (2006). The neuronal basis of mentalizing. *Neuron, 50*, 531–534.
>
> Ozonoff, S., & Miller, J. N. (1995). Teaching theory of mind: A new approach to social skills training for individuals with autism. *Journal of Autism and Developmental Disorders, 25*, 415–433.
>
> Rogers, S. J., Hepburn, S. L., Stackhouse, T., & Wehner, E. (2003). Imitation performance in toddlers with autism and those with other developmental disorders. *Journal of Child Psychiatry and Psychology, 44*, 763–781.
>
> Sallows, G. O., & Graupner, T. D. (2005). Intensive behavioral treatment for children with autism: Four-year outcome and predictors. *American Journal of Mental Retardation, 110*, 417–438.
>
> Yamamoto, J., Kakutani, A., & Terada, M. (2001). Establishing joint visual attention and pointing in autistic children with no functional language. *Perceptual Motor Skills, 92*, 755–770.

## 4.3.4 Longitudinal Research (Prospective Designs)

Are there developmental factors over a period of time that can cause changes in a person's anatomical and physiological processes, predisposing her to illness? Does prolonged exposure to smog cause lung cancer? How does exposure to radiation over a period of time cause leukemia? Do adults with obesity develop heart disease when they are middle-aged at a higher rate than adults who are not obese? Do children who have high IQs become leaders in the society when they are adults? What is the prognosis for high-risk children who come from socially disadvantaged environments? What is the relationship between occupational hazards and the later onset of disease? These problems are all affected by time factors.

**Longitudinal research** is a method used in observing the effects of independent variables on dependent variables over a determined period of time. The investigator uses longitudinal research to predict an outcome based on the presence of caus-ative factors. For example, a team of researchers may study groups of individuals over a period of 20 years from young adult to middle age and observe whether certain groups are more vulnerable to heart attacks than other groups. In occupational therapy, a researcher may examine the long-term effects of sensory integration on academic achievement in children with learning disabilities. Box 4–4 provides an example of longitudinal research relating cholesterol to coronary heart disease.

---

### BOX 4-4

## Example of Longitudinal Study

### 1. Bibliographic Notation

Sendroy-Terrill, M., Whiteneck, G. G., & Brooks, C. A. (2010). Aging with traumatic brain injury: Cross-sectional follow-up of people receiving inpatient rehabilitation over more than 3 decades. *Archives of Physical Medicine and Rehabilitation, 91,* 489–497.

### 2. Abstract

**OBJECTIVE:** To investigate aging with traumatic brain injury (TBI) by determining if long-term outcomes after TBI are predicted by years postinjury and age at injury after controlling for the severity of the injury and sex. **DESIGN:** Cross-sectional follow-up telephone survey. **SETTING:** Community residents who had received initial treatment in a comprehensive in-patient rehabilitation hospital. **PARTICIPANTS:** Survivors of TBI (N = 243) stratified by years postinjury (in seven 5-year cohorts ranging from 1 to over 30 years postinjury) and by age at injury (in 2 cohorts of people injured before or after age 30). **INTERVENTIONS:** None. **MAIN OUTCOME MEASURES:** Measures of postconcussive symptoms, major secondary conditions including fatigue (*Modified Fatigue Impact Scale*), physical and cognitive activity limitations (*FIM, Alertness Behavior Subscale of the Sickness Impact Profile, Medical Outcomes Study 12–Item Health Status Survey Short Form*), societal participation restrictions (*Craig Handicap Assessment and Reporting Technique*), environmental barriers (*Craig Hospital Inventory of Environmental Factors*), and perceived quality of life (*Satisfaction with Life Scale*). **RESULTS:** Most problems identified by the outcome measures were reported by one-fourth to one-half of the study participants. Increasing decade's postinjury predicted declines in physical and cognitive functioning, declines in societal participation, and increases in contractures. Increasing age at injury predicted declines in functional independence, increases in fatigue, declines in societal participation, and declines in perceived

*continues*

BOX 4-4

**Example of Longitudinal Study** *continued*

environmental barriers. **CONCLUSIONS:** This investigation has increased our understanding of the aging process after TBI by demonstrating that both components of aging (years postinjury and age at injury) are predictive of several outcomes after TBI.

**Key Words:** brain injuries, brain injury, chronic, follow-up studies, outcomes assessment (health care), rehabilitation

### 3. Justification and Need for Study

The purpose of this descriptive exploratory study was to determine whether age at injury is associated with progressive functional decline. This hypothesis has important intervention implications, particularly because the advent of neuroprotective therapies for dementia will make it important to identify people at risk for cognitive decline in late life.

### 4. Literature Review

The authors did an extensive review of the literature with 54 references cited. Examples of the journals cited included: *Archives of Physical Medicine and Rehabilitation, Brain Injury, Annals of Neurology, Journal of Head Rehabilitation Trauma, Archives in Neurology, NeuroRehabilitation, Journal of Neurology, Journal of Trauma,* and *Journal of the American Medical Association* (JAMA).

### 5. Research Hypothesis or Guiding Question

The primary hypothesis stated that older patients show greater decline in neurological function over the first 5 years after TBI than younger patients.

### 6. Methods

The study was identified as a longitudinal cohort study. It included participants who met the following criteria: (a) age of 16 years or older at the time of traumatic brain injury, (b) arrival at a hospital emergency department within 8 hours after injury, (c) receipt of acute and rehabilitation treatment at a traumatic brain injury model system (TBIMS) affiliated hospitals, (d) complete *Disability Rating Scale* (DRS) 25 scores taken at 1- and 5-year follow-up evaluations, and (e) provision of informed consent directly or by proxy. At the time of this investigation, 1127 patients were eligible to receive a 5-year post-TBI DRS evaluation specified in the TBIMS protocol, and 624 (55%) patients had complete DRS data 5 years post-TBI. Four hundred twenty-eight patients had complete DRS outcome data at both year 1 and year 5 (38%) and constituted the cohort analyzed here.

### 7. Results

All three age groups improved between admission and rehabilitation through year 5, and the magnitude, or slope, of improvement among the three age groups was similar through the first year post injury. Paired-sample *t*-test results show significant improvement in functioning over time among the youngest group as measured by the four outcome measures (i.e., DRS, *FIM*, cognitive domain of the *FIM*, *Extended Glasgow Outcome Scale* (GOS-E). In addition, the intermediate group showed significant improvement on the DRS, and the oldest did not show significant improvement on any of the outcome measures. Change scores for the outcome measures were examined as a marker of the magnitude of improvement between year 1 and year 5. The two younger groups showed greater change in DRS than the oldest group, and there were no differences in magnitude of change among the other outcome measures.

## 8. Conclusions

The study supported the primary hypothesis that older survivors of TBI show greater functional decline than younger survivors. Results from this study show that younger survivors of TBI showed significant improvement in disability ratings between the first and fifth years postinjury, whereas older counterparts did not show significant improvement in outcome measures over the same time period. Furthermore, the results suggest older survivors have a higher risk of functional decline than younger survivors, because patients 26 years or younger showed a lower rate of decline over a 4-year span than older patients.

## 9. Limitations of the study

One limitation of the study was the potential for systematic bias created by subjects lost to follow-up. Employment could be overestimated because of the loss of subjects with prior histories of substance abuse. Another limitation of the present investigation is that it is difficult to determine whether the decline in disability rating over time experienced by the oldest group is attributed to disabling effects of brain injury or simply decline associated with normative aging. Future studies may need to incorporate an orthopedic control group separated into age groups.

## 10. Major References Cited in the Study

Consensus Conference (1999). Rehabilitation of persons with traumatic brain injury (NIH Consensus Development Panel on Rehabilitation of Persons with Traumatic Brain Injury). *Journal of the American Medical Association, 282,* 974–983.

Flanagan, S. R., Hibbard, M. R., & Gordon, W. A. (2005). The impact of age on traumatic brain injury. *Physical Medicine and Rehabilitation Clinics of North America, 16,* 163–177.

Thurman, D. J., Alverson, C., Dunn, K. A., Guerrero, J., & Sniezek, J. E. (1999). Traumatic brain injury in the United States: A public health perspective. *Journal of Head Trauma Rehabilitation, 14,* 602–615.

Whitnall, L., McMillan, T. M., Murray, G. D., & Teasdale, G. M. (2006). Disability in young people and adults after head injury: 5–7 year follow up of a prospective cohort study. *Journal of Neurology, Neurosurgery, and Psychiatry, 77,* 640–645.

### 4.3.5 Field Observation (Ethnography)

About the same time that Gesell (1928) was experimenting with his photographic dome, cultural anthropologists developed scientific methods for collecting data describing the everyday lives of aboriginal people. Franz Boas, the noted anthropologist, wrote in the foreword to Margaret Mead's classic study *Coming of Age in Samoa* (1928) the following, which summarized field research:

> Through a comparative study of these data and through information that tells us of their growth and development, we endeavor to reconstruct, as well as may be, the history of each particular culture. Some anthropologists even hope that the comparative study will reveal some tendencies of development that recur so often that significant generalizations regarding the processes of cultural growth will be discovered. (p. xiii)

Mead attempted to answer the question "Are the disturbances which vex our adolescents due to the nature of adolescence itself or to the civilization?" (pp. 6–7). She lived in Samoa for six months, and there she analyzed the life and development of 68 girls between the ages of 8 and 20. She was particularly concerned with three villages on the island of Tau.

In her field study, Mead painted a vivid and complete picture of the island life of adolescent girls. She felt that certain characteristics, basically Samoan, enable adolescent girls to pass through puberty without the storms and crises that are part of living in Western society. Chiefly, a Samoan girl may leave her immediate household and go to live with another family at any time, especially if she feels put upon. Other characteristics concern life roles, absence of double standards, familiarity with disasters such as death, casual family relationships as opposed to intense ones, and a specific place in society for each member. Further, the author pointed to a tolerance for sexually diverse behavior and concomitant lack of guilt feelings about such behavior, absence of extreme poverty, and a less stressful environment as reasons for a more serene adolescence than that found elsewhere in the world.

Mead's pioneering research led to the field of **ethnography**: to reconstruct accurately a particular culture and to search for patterns that can be generalized to a specific population. The observations occur in a natural setting, such as in a primitive village, urban neighborhood, family home, playground, street corner, Israeli kibbutz, or a family coping with slum life in New York City. (See also Hall, 1966; Jessor, Colby, & Shweder, 1996).

Jules Henry's (1971) in-depth study of five families in which a child with psychosis was present is a bleak and brilliant example of field observation. He proposes that the main difference between "them and us" is "that they [families with a child with psychosis] seem to go to extremes and do too many things that are upsetting" (p. xx). Henry detailed communication patterns, physical interaction, and positions of power in each of the five families. He faithfully recorded the emotional content of the parents' communication patterns and their effects on their children. To record accurately, he lived with four of the five families for a short time and relied on a trained observer to supply similar observations about the fifth family. The five studies involved field visits to each family once a week. Rapport was established when the investigator informed each family that this kind of observation would perhaps aid other children with psychosis. He maintained confidentiality in the study by altering some of the details of family life and all of the names of the families.

A study entitled *Clinical Observation of Ghetto Four-Year-Olds: Organizational Involvement, Interpersonal Responsiveness and Psychosexual Content of Play* by Borowitz, Costello, and Hirsch (1971) is a good example of field observation methodology. In this study, children were observed while playing in semistructured settings. The play sessions were filmed on 16-mm silent movie film and tape-recorded simultaneously. Independent raters later analyzed the data using play behavior scales that the authors developed.

## The Application of Field Observation (Ethnography) to Occupational Therapy

What research problems are appropriate to field observations? Some possibilities are as follows:

- Research involving the culture of individuals with disabilities living in specialized environments such as halfway houses, forensic units, adult day care, psychiatric hospitals, communities for individuals with physical disabilities, and residential institutions for the individuals with profound intellectual disabilities (Gleason, 1990; McColl & Peterson, 1997)
- Client advocacy (Sachs & Linn, 1997)
- Occupational therapy practice (Fitzgerald, Mullavey–O'Byrne, & Clemson, 1997)
- Meaning of play (Gleason, 1990)
- Mental health day programs (Townsend, 1996)
- Inclusionary settings for individuals with special needs (Falk–Ross, 1996; Miller, 1990)
- Daily occupations of Orthodox Jewish couples (Frank et al., 1997)
- Cultural diversity (Adger, 1994; Klimidis, Minas, & Kokanovic, 2006; Luera, 1994; Malave & Duquette, 1991; Whiteford, 1995)
- Cultural competency of healthcare professionals (Nobel, Nobel, & Hand, 2009)
- Ethnogeriatric studies (McBride, & Lewis, 2004)
- Aging adult children with disabilities and their families (Barnhart, 2001)

## Advantages of Field Observation

The main purpose of field observation or ethnography is to describe accurately the social structure and social processes engaged in by a group of people. The investigator observes the interactions between members of a group, records their responses, and describes their formal codes for communications and the unwritten rules that guide their behaviors (Frederick, 1928; Mead, 1928). In the field study, the investigator structures observations while being as unobtrusive as possible in the environment to minimize the influence of one's presence on those being observed. One major advantage of the field observation is that data obtained from this method are not affected by artificial laboratory conditions. Another advantage is that the investigator observes behavior directly rather than eliciting verbal responses, such as through group personality tests. A third advantage is that the observer, who is not a part of the culture, will recognize patterns and behaviors differently from the way that these are acknowledged by those within the culture. Indeed, the "outsider" assists in bringing to the forefront patterns that, being embedded in "insider" behavior, are not readily described or easily recognized by members of the group.

Which research method would be appropriate for examining the interactions in a residential school for individuals with profound intellectual disabilities? It is not possible to construct experimental conditions or control for all of the possible variables that could affect the dependent variable, which is, in this example, the rate of development in the child who is profoundly retarded. The most appropriate method would be qualitative research, where the investigator observes, like an ethnographer in a natural setting, the structures and processes of the institution and the transactions and interactions among all the participants in the institutional setting.

## Methods of Field Observation

The investigator using field observation research is initially guided by research questions that focus on the important issues in social structures and social processes, such as education, vocational preparation, health care, child-rearing practices, sexual expression, ethical standards, peer relationships, leisure patterns, and recreation (see Box 4–5). Broad areas selected for field observation are decided before the investigator collects data. The preparation for field observation is detailed in the Research Design section. Here the investigator decides:

- The total time period for field observation
- The methods used in establishing rapport with the group
- The broad areas in a social structure to be investigated
- The observational recording devices to be used (e.g., camcorders, audio tapes)
- Methods for preserving the confidentiality of group and obtaining informed consent
- Test instructions for collecting data (e.g., rating scales, questionnaires, and attitude surveys)

BOX 4-5

## Example of Ethnographic Research

### 1. Bibliographic Notation

Berinstein, S., & Magalhaes, L. (2009). A study of the essence of play experience to children living in Zanzibar, Tanzania. *Occupational Therapy International, 16,* 89–106.

### 2. Abstract

This study aimed to gain an understanding of the essence of play experience to children in Zanzibar, Tanzania. A phenomenological approach using the Photovoice method was adopted. The study was carried out over four weeks, with 12 boys and 4 girls. Four key themes emerged from the analysis of 116 photographs: creative play, physical play/games, football and equipment play. The findings suggest that play experience in Zanzibar has aspects of creativity and resourcefulness and influences from tradition, culture and poverty. Furthermore, that opportunity for play may differ for children in Tanzania, compared with children in Western countries. Unequal boy and girl participants, and the lack of representation of children with a disability, were some limitations of this study. The occupational therapy profession may want to further investigate the opportunities for play for children living in developing countries. Additionally, it may be valuable to look at different aspects of play, such as its meaning to children from different cultures and its potential restorative value for children who have experienced traumatic events.

### 3. Justification and Need for Study

Play is recognized to be universal in nature, but influenced by its cultural context. The context and culture of Tanzania will influence how children living in poverty experience play. This study aimed to gain an understanding of the essence of play experience to children living in Zanzibar, Tanzania.

### 4. Literature Review

Forty-two references were cited in this study. The journals selected included: *American Journal of Occupational Therapy, Australian Journal of Occupational Therapy, Child: Care, Health and Development, Canadian Journal of Occupational Therapy, Archives of Pediatrics and Adolescent Medicine, Pediatrics, Journal of Children and Poverty, Journal of Community Practice, Health, Education and Behavior,* and *Journal of Advanced Nursing.*

### 5. Research Hypothesis or Guiding Question

Does the opportunity for play, as well as the meaning of play, differ in Tanzania as compared to Western countries?

### 6. Methods

A phenomenological approach using the Photovoice method was used, in order to explore the essence of play experience to children living in Zanzibar, Tanzania. The participants were students, ranging from 10 to 13 years old, from a school in Zanzibar, Tanzania. This school has students from varying socioeconomic backgrounds who are predominantly of the Muslim religion and speak Swahili as their first language.

## 7. Results

Four categories emerged from the Photovoice process that included creative play, physical play/games, football, and equipment play. Children seemed to view play as about just having fun, about getting fit, strengthening the body, and about social interaction. In Zanzibar, play seems to have aspects of creativity, resourcefulness, differences between boys and girls, and influences from tradition and culture.

## 8. Conclusions

Play seems to be self-driven, outside the relationship of the family, a social endeavour, and about waking the body up and occupying free time, as opposed to being about developing social, physical, and cognitive skills. Furthermore, despite the lack of adult encouragement and available resources to play, children find ways to engage in play together.

## 9. Limitations of the Study

The available time to carry out this research was limited to the duration of the first author's (researcher's) occupational therapy placement in Zanzibar. Second of all, assistance was limited to the researcher's supervisor in Canada. Thirdly, financial assistance was limited to what the researcher could afford. More support may have allowed for opportunity to work more closely with the participants. Moreover, financial support would have allowed the researcher to hire a translator for the duration of the four weeks and purchase more disposable cameras to permit more opportunity to practice. Other factors limiting this study were the researcher's lack of previous experience in carrying out Photovoice and the language barrier that existed.

## 10. Major References in the Study

Burdette, H. L., & Whitaker, R. C. (2005). Resurrecting free play in young children. *Archives of Pediatrics & Adolescent Medicine, 159*, 46–50.

Ginsburg, K. R. (2007). The importance of play in promoting healthy child development and maintaining strong parent-child bonds. *Pediatrics, 119*, 182–191.

McArdle, P. (2001). Children's play. *Child: Care, Health and Development, 27*, 509–514.

Simo-Algado, S., Mehta, N., Kronenberg, F., Cockburn, L., & Kirsh, B. (2002). Occupational therapy intervention with children survivors of war. *Canadian Journal of Occupational Therapy, 69*, 205–217.

### 4.3.6 Historical Research

#### Definition

**Historical research** is a systematic method for reconstructing events that happened in the past to describe and understand them. As applied to occupational therapy, historical research pertains to (a) the chronology of events in occupational therapy, (b) the interrelationship among these events, and (c) the critical factors influencing them. For example, one might want to describe the events and identify the individuals that led to the formation of the discipline of occupational therapy in 1917. In studying historical data in occupational therapy, the investigator examines the individuals who were significant in shaping events and creating change and the institutions or organizations that were part of the historical process. The scientific approach to collecting historical data is similar to all methods of research in that the investigator proposes a research problem, states guiding questions, collects data, interprets the results, and arrives at conclusions and implications. The main differences between historical research and other types of research models are in the format of guiding questions and in the use of related literature. In historical research, the guiding questions serve as the generating rationale for collecting data, and the literature review provides the data; whereas the literature review generates guiding questions in other qualitative methods.

#### Purposes

Fraenkel and Wallen (1990) suggested five purposes for historical research:

1. "To make people aware of what has happened in the past so they may learn from past failures and successes" (p. 411): For example, cone stacking has been used rather than craft activities to increase fine motor coordination. The craft activity is client-centered and increases motivation, whereas the cone stacking is a nonmeaningful repetitive activity.
2. "To learn how things were done in the past to see if they might be applicable to the present day problems and concerns" (p. 411): The model used in adult day centers from the 1950s and 1960s was successful in treating individuals with psychosocial illnesses. Adult day care centers now use this model in caring for individuals with Alzheimer's disease.
3. "To assist in prediction" (p. 412): Special education has alternated between placing students with special needs into self-contained classrooms and into the general education program. Examination of mainstreaming in the 1980s demonstrated that these students may not succeed in the general education program without support from special educators, occupational therapists, and other allied health personnel.
4. "To test hypotheses concerning relationships or trends" (p. 412): Over the last 80 years, an examination of trends of employment settings has shown a change for occupational therapists from primarily hospital-based settings to schools and home health care.
5. "To understand present educational practices and policies more fully" (p. 412): To understand Medicare reimbursement, occupational therapists study previous legislation and litigation leading to the present policies.

#### Historical Research Related to Occupational Therapy

- Bockoven, J. S. (1971). Occupational therapy–A historical perspective. Legacy of moral treatment–1800s to 1910. *American Journal of Occupational Therapy, 25*, 223–225.
- Cockburn, L. (2005). Canadian occupational therapists' contributions to prisoners of war in World War II. *Canadian Journal of Occupational Therapy, 72*, 183–188.
- Frank, G. (1992). Opening feminist histories of occupational therapy. *American Journal of Occupational Therapy, 46*, 989–999.
- Friedland, J., & Silva, J. (2008). Evolving identities: Thomas Bessell Kidner and occupational therapy in the United States. *American Journal of Occupational Therapy, 62*, 349–360.
- Gutman, S. A. (1995). Influence of the U.S. military and occupational therapy reconstruction

aides in World War I on the development of occupational therapy. *American Journal of Occupational Therapy, 49,* 256–262.

- Hamlin, R. B. (1992). Embracing our past, informing our future: A feminist revision of health care. *American Journal of Occupational Therapy, 46,* 1028–1035.
- Horghagen, S., Josephsson, S., & Alsaker, S. (2007). The use of craft activities as an occupational therapy treatment modality in Norway during 1952–1960. *Occupational Therapy International, 14,* 42–56.
- Newton, S. (2007, Jan–Mar). The growth of the profession of occupational therapy. *US Army Medical Department Journal,* 51–58.
- Peloquin, S. M. (1991). Occupational therapy service: Individual and collective understandings of the founders, Part 2. *American Journal of Occupational Therapy, 45,* 733–744.
- Reitz, S. M. (1992). A historical review of occupational therapy's role in preventive health and wellness. *American Journal of Occupational Therapy, 46,* 50–55.
- Stecco, C., & Aldegheri, R. (2008). Historical review of carpal tunnel syndrome. *La Chirurgia degli Organi di Movimento, 92,* 7–10.
- Woodside, H. H. (1971). Occupational therapy—A historical perspective. The development of occupational therapy 1910–1929. *American Journal of Occupational Therapy, 25,* 226–230.

## Hypothetical Questions Examined in Occupational Therapy

- How did occupational therapists treat individuals with polio during the 1950s?
- What treatment techniques did occupational therapists use in large mental hospitals during the 1930s?
- What are some of the experiences and education of noted individuals in occupational therapy?
- How is occupational therapy treated in the literature by individuals who write about their disability experiences?

- How have different philosophical viewpoints in occupational therapy influenced treatment in the schools?
- What is the history of the use of arts and crafts in occupational therapy?
- What are the major theories that impact on clinical treatment?

### Format of Historical Research

The outline of historical research is as follows:

*Part I:* The statement of problem and significance of the study (e.g., how the study impacts on occupational therapy)

*Part II:* Guiding questions and methods for collecting data

*Part III:* The results, including the collection of data from primary and secondary sources

*Part IV:* A discussion of the results based on previous data from other studies

*Part V:* Conclusions, implications of results, and recommendations for further study

***Part I: The Statement of Problem and Significance of the Study.*** What are potential areas for historical research in occupational therapy? How does one determine its significance? These are issues of concern for the historical researcher or historiographer planning a study. Jacques Barzun (1974), in a discussion of psychohistory, stated that the primary purpose of the new history is explanation, and the ulterior motive is action. He stated, "The type of explanation sought is the scientific; that is, showing a connection ('durable link') between the facts and a definable cause. Classification, then analysis, then prediction is the sequence that leads naturally to action" (p. 60).

Barzun suggested that the historiographer's main motive is to obtain evidence in support of a cause. In effect, the historical researcher is a tool for change. This approach to medicine and health care can lead to research supporting causes that advocate change in the delivery of health care, public health education, the training and preparation of health professionals, and the training of special educators. The vulnerability of this approach is that the researcher could subjectively determine what evidence to cite. The historiographer should start with a relevant problem and objectively collect data. Table 4–7 outlines the relationship between the researcher's motive and the problem being investing using the historical research model.

***Part II: Guiding Questions and Methods for Collecting Data.*** After narrowing the area of investigation to a researchable question, the researcher states any assumptions underlying the study. These assumptions are the researcher's preliminary opinions, attitudes, and knowledge in the area. For example, if interested in what factors led to the development of the rehabilitation movement in the twentieth century, the researcher could propose tentative assumptions. These are:

- The rehabilitation movement developed in response to the health needs of the individual who is chronically disabled.
- Governmental legislation related to Social Security facilitated the rehabilitation movement.
- The industrialized countries were first to educate specialized rehabilitation workers.
- World War I and World War II generated the need for developing a technology for restoring function in soldiers who were severely wounded.

- The first leaders in the rehabilitation movement were social reformers.

Continuing with the above examples, the researcher generates the following questions:

- What was the historical chronology of the rehabilitation movement?
- How did social welfare programs influence rehabilitation legislation?
- How did advances in medical treatment influence rehabilitation of individuals with chronic disabilities?
- When did the allied health professions emerge and start the rehabilitation movement?
- What scientific technology facilitated advances in rehabilitation medicine?
- Who are the leaders and supporters of the rehabilitation movement?

These guiding questions provide the content areas for the literature search and collection of data. The plan for collecting the data should be carefully formulated. The **research plan** is the outline of primary and secondary sources to be used in the data collection procedure. These sources include the following:

- Published books, periodicals, newspapers, and pamphlets

## TABLE 4-7

**Relationships between Researcher's Motive and Investigated Problem**

| Motive of Researcher | Statement of Problem |
| --- | --- |
| Establishing the occupational therapist as an independent practitioner | How did the independent health practitioner evolve historically? |
| Integrating the individual with intellectual disabilities into the community | What factors led to the institutionalization of individuals with intellectual disabilities from 1900 to 1950? |
| Incorporating wellness in health education of public schools | What is the history of health education in public schools? |
| Assuring the right of access to primary health for every individual | Historically what are the determining factors regarding access to health care? |
| Gaining parity in health insurance coverage for psychosocial disabilities | Why have insurance companies typically restricted reimbursement for psychosocial disabilities? |

- Unpublished conference proceedings and minutes of meetings
- Official records and vital statistics
- Governmental documents, archives, and publications
- Personal letters, diaries, and memoirs
- Collateral interviews of eyewitnesses
- Tape recordings and films

***Part III: Data Collection.*** The essential task of the historical researcher is to collect reliable and valid data. By obtaining various sources of information, one is able to crosscheck the data, thereby substantiating one's conclusions. This procedure is called **triangulation**. **Primary sources** that represent "firsthand" data, such as eyewitnesses and contemporary documents, are the best evidence for the historical researcher. In comparison, **secondary sources** are the interpretations and critiques of historical evidence based on primary data. Primary sources are the raw data for historical research, whereas secondary sources serve as supportive evidence. In researching a problem, the investigator should seek evidence that is direct, objective, and verifiable. It should be clear that one unit of datum is not conclusive. The "personal equation," which is the observer's effect on what is being observed and measured, must be controlled by the investigator's substantiating evidence from more than one primary source as eyewitness account.

Secondary sources such as encyclopedias, textbooks, and critical essays are useful in initially obtaining an overview of a historical problem. These sources represent the generally accepted versions of historical events that have been "retold" in a reductive manner. The critical historiographer need not accept any evidence until primary data can substantiate the facts.

***Part IV: Discussion of Results,*** and ***Part V: Conclusions and Recommendations.*** Before making any conclusions or generalizations, the investigator must critically analyze the raw data of a historical study for its validity. The historical researcher must examine every document and piece of evidence with a skeptical eye, seeking substantiating proof for the authorship and the accuracy of its contents. *External criticism* of a document is a testimony of its authenticity. The Hippocratic writings are an example of unknown authorship and unknown copyright date. It is important for the historical researcher to substantiate the author of every document, the date it was written, and the place of origination or presentation, as evidence for external validity. Historians frequently use indirect means for collecting evidence. These methods include archeology and paleography (e.g., study of ancient manuscripts and examination of art objects). Ancient medical instruments used in surgery were discovered through archeological evidence. Questions that might be asked when examining external validity are (Fraenkel & Wallen, 1990):

- Did the purported author actually write the document or report the event?
- Do we know the exact the date that the document was written?
- Do we know where the document was written or where the observation took place?
- Are we sure that external events or individuals did not influence the writing of the document or observation data?
- Are we sure the document is genuine?

The next step of the historical researcher is to establish the validity or truth contained in a document. This process is called *internal criticism.* The purpose of this process is to establish as near as possible the actuality of an event. Fraenkel and Wallen (1990) suggested the following types of questions:

- Was the author an eyewitness to the event?
- Did the author participate in the event?
- What expertise did the author have to discuss or report the event?
- Was the author biased or subjective in the observation, or did the author have a vested interest in the event?

Historical surveys of medical progress are frequently filled with interpretative statements that go beyond the evidence and selective omissions that fail to give a true perspective of events or individuals who had an impact on treatment. It is left to the historical researcher in occupational therapy to carefully evaluate the biases of the authors when interpreting evidence. Generalizations and synthesizing statements should be carefully documented. In examining the causes of events, the historiographer takes a multidimensional point of view looking at the influences of contemporary practices of treatment, discoveries, patterns of dysfunction, governmental and community intervention, war, and natural disasters. One variable rarely changes the course of history.

A good example of historical research is a scholarly manuscript by Saul Benison (1972), "The History of Polio Research in the United States: Appraisal and Lessons." In this article, Benison documented the chronological events that led to a safe and effective vaccine for preventing polio. He analyzed the problem from three perspectives: (a) time

of events, (b) settings where research took place, and (c) individuals and scientists who had an impact on the problem and facilitated progress in the development of a vaccine. These three factors are detailed in Table 4–8.

In documenting the chronology of events and the individuals who made important contributions to the development of a successful polio vaccine, Benison used the following primary sources:

- Contemporary accounts of the early polio epidemics from 1894 to 1910
- Autobiographical notes
- History of the Rockefeller Institute

## TABLE 4-8

**History of Polio Research in the United States**

| Time | Event | Setting | Contributors |
|------|-------|---------|--------------|
| 1884 | Polio epidemics identified in U.S. | | |
| 1907 | Initial research in polio | Rockefeller Institute | Flexner |
| 1910–1913 | Poliovirus implicated | Rockefeller Institute | Flexner and associates |
| 1920–1930 | Transmission of polio | Rockefeller Institute | Olitsky et al. |
| 1938 | Warm Springs Foundation | Georgia | Roosevelt et al. |
| 1938 | Electron microscope | Germany | Borries |
| 1946 | Immunization of monkeys | Johns Hopkins | Morgan |
| 1948–1951 | Identification of poliovirus | U. California | Kessel |
| | | Johns Hopkins | Bodian |
| | | U. of Pittsburgh | Salk |
| 1949 | Cultivation of poliovirus | Harvard | Enders et al. |
| 1952 | Salk vaccine (dead intramuscular [i.m.] vaccine) | U. Pittsburgh | Salk |
| 1954 | Mass vaccinations | U. Michigan | Francis |
| 1958 | Sabin Vaccine (oral live vaccine) | U. Cincinnati | Sabin |

**Note:** Adapted from "The History of Polio Research in the United States: Appraisal and Lessons" by S. Benison. In *The Twentieth-Century Sciences: Studies in the Biography of Ideas*, pp. 308–343, by G. Holton, New York: W. Norton. Copyright 1972 by W. Norton.

- Foreign journals
- Scholarly articles by Flexner (1910) and associates
- Conference proceedings
- Research articles
- *Bulletin of the History of Medicine*
- National Foundation Archives
- History of Warm Springs
- Private communication
- Minutes of committees
- Files from the National Foundation
- Biographical essays
- Final reports of research grants
- Congressional hearings

In total, Benison used 117 citations to document his article. He concluded that the development of a successful polio vaccine was a cooperative effort by researchers in major universities funded by two private organizations—The Rockefeller Foundation and the National Foundation—with external support from the United States Public Health Service. Benison's lesson in the article was that modern medical progress is a cooperative effort where researchers from diverse settings are supported by the federal government, private foundations, and voluntary health agencies.

The historical research article by Benison is an example of rigorous documentation providing strong external validity. Benison's article should serve as a model for research in occupational therapy. (See Box 4–6 for another example of historical research.)

---

## BOX 4-6

### Example of Historical Research

#### 1. Bibliographical Notation

Sachs, D., & Sussman, N. (1995). Historical research: The first decade of occupational therapy in Israel: 1946–1956. *Occupational Therapy International, 2,* 241–256.

#### 2. Abstract

The present study examined the first decade of the development of occupational therapy in Israel: 1946–1956. The structural-functional approach to the study of professions, which provided the theoretical framework for this study, identifies three formal organizations in the professions: the practice, the educational system, and the association. The purpose of this article was to follow the development of occupational therapy and to examine the interrelations of the profession's three formal organizations in the reviewed period. The methodology of the study was based on qualitative historical methods. Data collection included oral histories and published and unpublished written material. Data organization and analysis were within the framework of the structural-functional approach. Data analysis indicated that "expansion" was a major theme affecting the development of occupational therapy, the reason for which lies within the historical background of the period under investigation. In addition, data indicated that the practice was the strongest and most active organization in occupational therapy and that expansion in practice was beyond the capacity of both the educational system and the professional association. The interrelations of the three formal organizations, and the rapid expansion of occupational therapy practice, had a lasting effect on the development of occupational therapy in Israel (p. 241).

*continues*

BOX 4-6

## Example of Historical Research *continued*

### 3. Justification and Need for Study

Because "historical research sheds light on present behaviors and practices," (p. 242) this study was completed to "understand current theories and practices more accurately, and to plan intelligently for the future" (p. 242).

### 4. Literature Review

Forty-two references were cited in the study. Articles came from a wide variety of sources, including files at the Occupational Therapy School at the Hebrew University from 1947 to 1954; archives of Hadassah 1941–1949; *Israeli Journal of Occupational Therapy; Health Services in Israel: A Ten Year Survey 1948–1958*; and *Trade Unions in Israel.*

### 5. Research Hypothesis or Guiding Questions

The guiding questions explicitly stated were: (a) "How did the practice [in occupational therapy] develop and how did it adapt itself to the growing needs of the healthcare services?" (b) "How did the educational system cope with practice needs?" and (c) "How did the association [Israeli Occupational Therapy Association] meet the needs of the profession?"

### 6. Methods

Interviews were held with nine female occupational therapists who had been practicing between 1946 and 1956 and who were considered prominent leaders in the development of occupational therapy in Israel. Primary documents, including memoirs and archived materials, were accessed by the investigators. These materials were analyzed using the structural-functional approach (Parsons, 1939). The credibility of the data was obtained by validating oral testimonies with contemporary documents.

### 7. Results

The historical development was organized into three periods, each covering the practice, the education system, and the professional association: (a) Preliminary Period, 1941–1945; (b) The Formative Years, 1946–1948; and (c) Expansion: 1949–1956.

### 8. Conclusions

"Analysis of the data indicates that the practice was the strongest and most active organization [as compared with education and professional association] in the function of occupational therapy. Expansion in the practice was beyond the capacity of the education and the association—By employing historical research methods and a conceptual framework to the study of professions, this study exposed the origin of some of the problems faced by occupational therapy in Israel" (pp. 254–255).

### 9. Limitations of the Study

The study only interviewed nine individuals when collecting the bulk of the data. Also, some contemporary documents were not available and presumed to have been lost as a result of war conditions.

### 10. Major References Cited in the Study

Archives of Hadassah (1941–1949). *Occupational therapy correspondence services* (RQ, 1 HMO, Box 51), New York: Hadassah.

Files at the occupational therapy school, 1st class. (1947–1949). Jerusalem: Hebrew University.

Files at the occupational therapy school, 2nd class. (1949–1951). Jerusalem: Hebrew University.

Files at the occupational therapy school, 3rd class. (1952–1954). Jerusalem: Hebrew University.

Grushka, T. (1959). *Health services in Israel: A ten year survey 1948–1958*. Jerusalem: Ministry of Health.

Grushka, T. (1968). *Health services in Israel*. Jerusalem: Ministry of Health.

Sussman, N. (1989). *The history of occupational therapy in Israel: The first decade—1946–1956*. Unpublished master's thesis: New York University: New York.

Potential areas for historical research in occupational therapy include:

- Biographies of founders of the discipline of occupational therapy
- Development of innovative assistive technology
- Development of social attitude toward psychosocial illness
- Chronological analysis of the treatment of a disability
- History of the occupational therapy discipline
- History of a hospital, health facility, organization, or institution
- History of reimbursement practices
- History of movements in occupational therapy (e.g., rehabilitation and normalization)

## 4.4  Collecting Qualitative Data

There are many ways to collect qualitative data. Table 4–9 gives some examples. These are more fully explained in the following paragraphs.

### 4.4.1  Interviewing

The most common data collection method in qualitative research is interviewing. Using interviews as a research method rests on the assumption that "the perspective of others is meaningful, knowable, and able to be made explicit" (Patton, 1990, p. 270). In short, researchers conduct interviews to find out about things that cannot be directly observed. Everyday familiarity with conversational or therapeutic interviews can lead novice researchers to regard interviewing for research purposes as quite straightforward; but to effectively use interviewing as a research method requires knowledge of, and practice with, available techniques.

Research interviews take several forms. Interviews can be done face-to-face, over the telephone, or in a group. The format may be structured, semistructured, or open-ended. Interviewing may be used to collect personal experiences, to understand particular phenomena, or to identify the perspective of a particular group of people. Interviews may be brief or lengthy, they may be "one-off," or part of a series.

**TABLE 4-9**

**Methods of Collecting Data in Qualitative Research**

| Type | Definition | Research Example |
|------|------------|------------------|
| Interviewing | Data collection method for obtaining information through face-to-face verbal exchange or mailed or through telephone surveys. Interviews can occur in a single session or over multiple sessions. Interviews can be group or individually obtained and can be structured, semi-structured, or unstructured. Structured interviews have specific questions that are answered by the interviewee, whereas unstructured interviews have no specific questions but may have general areas of discussion. Semi-structured interviews are a combination of both (Fontana & Frey, 1994). | *Focus groups: Semi-structured group interview*<br>Lau, A., Chi, I., & McKenna, K. (1998). Self-perceived quality of life of Chinese elderly people in Hong Kong. *Occupational Therapy International, 5,* 118–139. |
| Naturalistic observational techniques | "The act of noting a phenomenon, often with instruments, and recording it for scientific or other purposes" (Morris, 1973, p. 906). Qualitative observation occurs in the natural setting among the targeted population without intervention by the observer. The focus of naturalistic observation is to examine "trends, patterns, and styles of behavior" (Adler & Adler, 1994, p. 378).<br><br>Naturalistic observation occurs through videotaping, audiotaping, photography, or through participant observation. | *Observational case study*<br>Henry, J. (1971). *Pathways to madness.* New York: Random House. |
| Mute evidence | Primary sources, such as field notes, diaries, memos, letters, and official records (e.g., marriage licenses, banking statements, driving records), but not audiotapes or videotapes that can be heard or viewed. | *Historiography*<br>Benison, S. (1972). The history of polio research in the United States: Appraisal and lessons. *The twentieth-century sciences: Studies in the biography of ideas* (pp. 308–343). New York: W. Norton.<br><br>Jonsson, H. (1998). Ernst Westerlund—A Swedish doctor of occupation. *Occupational Therapy International 5,* 155–171. |
| Personal experience | Understanding of someone's life story through questioning who we are through the narrator, through our relationship to the text, and the way we interpret the text (Clandinin & Connelly, 1994). The life stories told by an individual become a means of educating self and others. Autobiography, case histories, and life stories are all part of personal experience. | *Personal journals*<br>Jung, B., & Tryssenaar, J. (1998). Supervising students: Exploring the experience through reflective journals. *Occupational Therapy International, 5,* 35–48. |

Oftentimes investigators will employ a combination of interviewing approaches if this suits the purpose of the research and the research questions. For example, an interview may begin with a standardized, structured format, followed by sections made up of semi-structured questions. Alternatively, the interview may begin with an unstructured, open-ended format and conclude with a set of standardized questions. The type of interview that will best suit the research purpose needs particular care and thought.

### Structured Interviewing

In this type of interview, the interviewer uses a pre-established set of questions in a uniform manner. Although the questions may be open-ended, the interviewer cannot alter the predetermined format. The aim of this structured approach is to achieve as close as possible a standard format across interviewers and respondents. One disadvantage of this approach is that the interviewer is not able to pursue topics of interest that arise during the interview.

### Semi-structured Interviewing

This type of interviewing utilizes a general interview guide. The issues to be covered in the interview are predetermined; however, question format and exact content are not prespecified. Rather, the interviewer uses a guide that can be adapted, as necessary, during the interview. Semistructured interviewing is an effective use of time while still allowing the interviewer to build rapport and conduct the interview in a flexible way. This approach is particularly appropriate for group interviews where it can be used to encourage all participants to contribute to the topic under discussion.

### Unstructured Interviewing

Unstructured interviews are sometimes referred to as "informal conversational interviews" or "in-depth interviews." The purpose of this approach is to interview respondents without imposing any a priori categories on the content or format of the interview. The emphasis is on listening and on understanding each interviewee's individual point of view, not on explaining interviewees' perspectives within a predetermined interpretive framework (Holstein & Gubrium, 1995).

Unstructured interviews often occur as part of observation in field research. They may also be used with a specific purpose in mind, such as exploring one or more issues in depth. In unstructured interviewing, most of the questions flow from the immediate interview context. Specific questioning techniques are used to elicit, as clearly as possible, the way that each interviewee constructs meaning. For example, Spradley (1979) suggested three types of questions: descriptive, contrast, and structural. Patton (1990) also listed a number of alternative questioning formats. Whichever techniques are used, the researcher's primary task is to understand as fully as possible the interviewee's point of view.

Unstructured interviews are particularly useful for interviewing individuals over a period of time. Later interviews can be used to elaborate information gathered in earlier interviews to help build a comprehensive picture of the topic being investigated. One disadvantage of unstructured interviewing is the time involved. Another is the resources needed to analyze the quantity and variety of information gained.

### Group Interviews

Interviewing people in groups is gaining popularity in allied health research. Group interviews are commonly called "focus groups," which may be structured, semi-structured, or unstructured. Group interviews are a cost-effective and efficient way to gather information. Interviewers need to be experienced in managing group processes, however. For example, aspects of group interaction, such as the tendency of one or more members to dominate the group or the group members sliding into "group think," may impede the interview process (Frey & Fontana, 1995).

### Attentive Listening

The role of self is critical in interviewing. Interviewing requires a commitment to, and an interest in, understanding another's point of view. Developing skills as an attentive listener are as important, if not more so, than becoming a skilled questioner. To resist the temptation to fit individuals into predetermined response categories requires careful listening and skillful questioning. Questions need to be as unambiguous, focused, and value-free as is humanly possible. Compiling such questions and learning how to create a context in which interviewees are willing to answer openly and honestly require effort and practice. The rewards are well worth the time spent.

### Using a Tape Recorder

Using a tape recorder is an efficient and accurate method to record an interview, although this needs to be done unobtrusively so as not to inhibit interviewees' responses. As an ethical issue, client consent should be obtained before tape-recording. Researchers can easily become dependent on using a tape recorder, and disaster strikes if for any reason a taped account is not possible. Not using a tape recorder requires a methodical approach and self-discipline to make sure that the researcher's notes are adequate. This is essential if the researcher is to gather the richest possible information in as many situations as possible.

There are instances in which tape recording is not a suitable means of documenting information. Using a tape recorder may invade the privacy of the participant by drawing attention to the interviewee. Circumstances may mitigate against adequate sound recording, particularly in open and crowded public places such as a shopping center. Tape recording may be inappropriate when the aim is to keep interviews as informal as possible.

Experience suggests that interviewees frequently share valuable information when tape recording is not possible, for example, on the sidewalk or just after the machine is turned off. No matter how relaxed interviewees become with a tape recorder, occasions still occur when information is withheld for privacy reasons or because of personal embarrassment. It is, therefore, most unwise to rely on taped interviews. Alternative procedures are described in the section on field notes (Section 4.4.3) discussed later in the chapter.

### 4.4.2 Observation

Observation is essential to understanding human and natural phenomena. As Adler and Adler (1994) noted, "as long as people have been interested in studying the social and natural world around them, observation has served as the bedrock source of human knowledge" (p. 377). Observation in qualitative inquiry goes by several terms: "participant observation," "direct observation," "field research," or "qualitative observation." Whatever the term employed, the essence of observation "lies in the prolonged and unobtrusive presence of a *sensitive* and *trained* observer among the people being studied" (Edgerton & Langness, 1978, p. 339, italics added). All observational methods require disciplined training and rigorous preparation.

The primary purpose of observation in qualitative research is to describe. Description includes the setting, the activities taking place, the participants, and the meaning of the setting and its activities from the participants' perspective. Observing activities as they take place provides the researcher with direct first-hand experience. This is essential to a full understanding of the phenomena under investigation. There are a number of sources of data in fieldwork settings. These include the physical setting, social interactions and activities (both planned and informal), the language used, nonverbal communication, unobtrusive indicators, program documents and "notable nonoccurrences" (Patton, 1990). In any setting, however, there is far more happening than can be accurately observed and documented. Therefore, qualitative researchers usually employ a framework to guide their fieldwork observations.

Several dimensions to observing need careful consideration in the research design phase. These are the role of the observer, portrayal of role and purpose, and duration and focus of observation.

### Role of the Observer

The first dimension relates to the extent to which the observer not only observes, but also participates in the setting. There are several typologies of observer involvement in research settings. For example, Gold (1958) outlined four modes: the complete participant, the participant-as-observer, the observer-as-participant, and the complete observer. The latter is rarely used now owing to the ethical concerns about covert observation.

Adler and Adler (1994) suggested three roles for researchers as observers: the complete-member-researcher, the active-member-researcher, and the peripheral-member-researcher. These roles fall along a continuum. The role chosen will depend on the purpose and nature of the research study. The peripheral-member-researcher is part of a setting while remaining removed from the core activities. The active-member-researcher participates in the core activities of the setting. The complete-member-researcher is one who already has full membership in the setting or converts to genuine membership during the study.

### Portrayal of Role and Purpose

Researchers may explicitly explain their observer role and purpose, may choose not to disclose any information about their observational role, or may portray their role somewhere in between these two extremes. The nature of the research questions and the access the researcher has to the setting and their position within that setting will influence how much others are told about the researcher role. For example, in primarily evaluative research, there will usually be full and complete explanation of the observational component. As Patton (1990) succinctly noted, "People are seldom deceived or reassured by false or partial explanations—at least not for long" (p. 212). By contrast, in research of a more public nature, there may be little need to describe exactly what will be observed, or when, how, and why it will be observed.

### Duration and Focus of Observation

Observation may occur once only, happen for a limited period, or be of varying duration carried out multiple times over an extended period. The duration of the observational period relies heavily on the purpose of the research. For example, research investigating complex processes that change over time, such as adaptation to acquired disability, require prolonged observation. In contrast, the timeliness and resources available for evaluation research often determine how much—or how little—observation occurs.

Not everything in a single research project warrants observation. The focus and scope of the observation need to be considered when framing the research question. Decisions will need to be made, for example, about whether to observe a small number of occasions in great depth or many occasions in less depth.

## 4.4.3 Field Notes

Field notes are the basic tool of the qualitative researcher. As Patton noted, "There are many options in the mechanics of taking field notes.... *What is not optional is the taking of field notes*" (Patton, 1990, p. 239, italics in original). Taking field notes can be used to substitute for tape-recording interviews. Note taking can also be used to expand the taped account, for example, with enriching descriptions of visual "pictures" of participants' facial expressions, gestures, and other nonverbal behaviors. Taking notes also expands the opportunities to collect data. For example, note taking can provide a documented account of participants' reactions and interactions.

As noted above, researchers need to learn to observe methodically. Similarly, learning to systematically document observations requires the researcher to develop disciplined methods. The first step in this process is to decide on a format. Field notes can be in one notebook or can be contained in a file system. The second step is to organize the different types of field notes according to their content, which will vary according to their purpose. The purposes of field notes include maintaining a transcript file, a personal log, or an analytical log (Minichiello, Aroni, Timewell, & Alexander, 1995).

The transcript file contains descriptive data about the observation or interview setting. This includes where the observation took place, who was present, and what social interactions and activities took place. This file may also contain a diagram of the setting. The transcript file also contains either a transcription of the interview or a written account of the observation. The secret of making good field notes for the transcript file is to be descriptive, concrete, and detailed. The researcher needs to avoid interpretation or judgment, loosely defined comparisons, and abbreviations that, although making sense at the time of documenting, may mean nothing at all when reviewing the file. This file should also contain direct quotations of what the research participants say. The quotations may be documented in the actual transcript of a recorded interview. If not, it is critical that the researcher record relevant information in the participants' own words. Participants' words can be differentiated from the researcher's descriptions by using quotation marks.

The personal log is the repository for the researcher's thoughts on the field research. This log includes personal feelings, reactions to the fieldwork experience, and personal and methodological reflections during the study. Writing this log needs to be done as soon as possible after each encounter in the field. It is not possible at the end of a study to go back and capture the feelings, reactions, and reflections that occurred during fieldwork. Keeping the personal log in the form of a journal may be helpful. Using headings and subheadings will help to organize the material and make it easier to review the contents in the analysis stage. The headings will vary according to research focus. For example, headings can be used to organize the material according to the sequence of events.

The analytical log contains the researcher's insights and reflections on data collection and analysis in the context of the theoretical framework of the study. Minichiello et al. (1995) suggested that this is where the researcher asks and answers questions such as: What is it that I know so far? What do I not know? What do I need to know? How do I collect this information? This log also provides a record or audit trail of the analysis and theoretical propositions as these develop throughout the study.

## 4.4.4 Political and Ethical Context for Research

The political context sets the background for any research project. This context ranges from the micropolitical of personal relationships to the macropolitical of government sponsorship of research. Feminist research and research about race and ethnicity have highlighted the potential nature of research as a political activity. Grappling with the political context may seem overwhelmingly daunting to the beginning researcher. This is more so because little is written about how experienced researchers understand and deal with the political dimensions of the

contexts in which they are working (Shaffir & Stebbins, 1991). Consideration of the political context is crucial in the research design phase.

Much has been written about the stages of fieldwork, particularly strategies for entering and leaving the field (see, for example, Schatzman & Strauss, 1973, and Shaffir & Stebbins, 1991). Personal factors such as age, race, and gender of both the researcher and the research participants affect fieldwork. Other influences on fieldwork include the nature and status of the researcher's institution and the institution where the research occurs, for example, a prestigious teaching hospital compared to a community health center. "Gate-keeping"—the term used to describe institutional power holders blocking access to people served by their institution—does occur in the health and welfare fields. For example, family workers may be unwilling to inform client families about a proposed research project or may tell only some families and not others. This may be done on the grounds that some families are more likely to be willing to participate, are more articulate, or are more able to withstand yet another intrusion into their lives. Frequently, however, those families not informed are less well educated, are from minority ethnic groups, or are disadvantaged parents. Professional gate-keeping of these families may result in nonrepresentative samples for the research.

Professional associations, academic institutions, funding bodies, and medical facilities have ethical standards and convene human ethics committees. These have a mandate to permit or disallow proposed research according to federal and state regulations. Traditionally, the ethical precepts of biomedical research have been applied to social science research, although this research is more likely to be of a qualitative nature. These regulations, although providing a useful framework, may offer little guidance for the proper and ethical conduct of research in the field. Of primary interest to field researchers are issues of consent, privacy, confidentiality, trust, and betrayal (Bulmer, 1982).

Gaining the informed consent of research participants is essential to the ethical conduct of any research. Informed consent, however, is not as straightforward as it first appears. What happens, for example, to individuals' behaviors if they are informed a priori that they will be observed? What constitutes "informed" consent under circumstances such as mental illness, cognitive limitations, extreme youth, and extreme age? Research in the medical, rehabilitation, and allied health fields is often carried out with individuals identified as vulnerable subjects on ethics clearance forms. Obtaining informed consent from research participants in these groups may require special procedures (Booth & Booth, 1994; Llewellyn, 1995).

A major aim for ethical researchers is to protect the privacy and confidentiality of research participants. Typical ways that this is done include keeping data in locked storage, destroying identifying material, and using pseudonyms in research reports. Safeguards also need to be in place against less obvious intrusions on participant privacy and confidentiality. For example, the researcher's institutional affiliation, the description of the research context, or the bibliography of the research report may give away the research location and the likely participants.

Finishing a field research study presents a further ethical concern. At the beginning of a research study, intense effort, possibly over weeks, months, or even years will have gone into building trust with the research participants. At the end of the study, the researcher leaves while the participants remain. After a period of engagement, the participants may feel betrayed or, at the very least, let down. There are no simple rules to deal with this possibility. Each researcher must find a way to leave the field in an acceptably ethical manner. Fontana and Frey (1994) suggested a three-point guide to exercising moral responsibility toward research participants: "to our subjects first, to the study next and to ourselves last" (Fontana & Frey, 1994, p. 373).

## 4.5 Analyzing Qualitative Data

A diverse variety of methods exist for analyzing qualitative data (for example, see Barnard, McCosker, & Gerber, 1999; Bryman & Burgess, 1994; Miles & Huberman, 1994; Strauss & Corbin, 1998;

Van Manen, 1990). Qualitative data analysis methods are based on the following general principles.

### 4.5.1 Principles of Qualitative Data Analysis

The first principle is that the analysis is conducted concurrently with data collection. This means that as analysis occurs, the researcher develops further questions that guide ongoing data collection. The researcher analyzes the data, proposes new questions or tentative propositions, and then "checks these out" by returning to the data. This proposing and verifying process illustrates the movement between inductive and deductive procedures typical of qualitative analysis procedures.

The second principle is that the analysis process is systematic. Methods vary according to schools of thought and the researcher's interpretive framework. All methods make use of systems that involve reflection, are open to examination, and can be applied to more than one researcher. Miles and Huberman (1994) described their system as follows: "Margin notes are made on the field notes, more reflective passages are reviewed carefully, and some kind of summary sheet is drafted. At the next level are coding and memo writing" (p. 432). These memos are analytic in nature and result from reflection on the data. Memos help the process of generating an increasingly more abstract conceptualization from the concrete field data (Miles & Huberman, 1994).

The third principle is that, during the analytic process, the data are "divided" into segments. These segments of data, however, remain part of the whole. Dividing the data into segments is carried out by using content analysis procedures. The researcher reviews the data from transcribed interviews or questionnaire responses or field notes and gives a name or code to each unit of meaning. This process is called *open coding* (Strauss & Corbin, 1998). The names or codes given to these units of meaning are developed directly from the text data or are generated from previous studies, from the relevant literature, or from a combination of all these sources.

The fourth principle is that comparison is the main intellectual tool that the researcher employs in doing the analysis. Comparison is used to "discern conceptual similarities, to refine the discriminative power of categories, and to discover patterns" (Tesch, 1990, p. 96). Glaser and Strauss (1967) developed the term *constant comparative analysis* to describe the process whereby the researcher compares and contrasts elements of data in a search for recurring regularities. These regularities are further compared and contrasted to develop concepts. These concepts are then compared and contrasted to form internally consistent and mutually exclusive categories.

The fifth principle is that the researcher refines the category organizing system as familiarity with the data develops. Using the comparative process, the researcher clusters together categories that are alike. The organizing system remains flexible, becoming more conceptually sound and parsimonious as the researcher develops a deeper understanding of the phenomena under study. This occurs as the categories are expanded and elaborated, which occurs by building on existing information, making links between items of information, and proposing and verifying new information. Category organization is continually refined until "theoretical saturation" is reached (Glaser & Strauss, 1967). Theoretical saturation is said to occur when new data lead to redundancy and the categories appear to be conceptually sound.

The sixth and final principle is that the goal of qualitative analysis is synthesis of the data into a higher level of conceptualization. In this process, a qualitative researcher has dual roles. The first is to describe phenomena as they exist—the what, how, when, and where. The second is to interpret and explain these phenomena as concepts. Patton (1990) suggested that this involves "discovering" and "uncovering:"

- *Discovering* involves elaborating concepts that are obvious to participant and researcher alike.
- *Uncovering* requires clarifying or elaborating already existing sociological concepts or building new concepts from the research setting.

In summary, the aim in qualitative research designs is not casual determination, prediction, or generalization as in quantitative research. Rather, qualitative researchers aim to elucidate relationships, investigate and interpret connections and, by so doing, develop an understanding about particular phenomena and their place within existing theoretical knowledge about the social world.

### 4.5.2 Practice

Qualitative data is, most frequently, text derived from interview transcripts, questionnaire responses, field notes, and documents such as case records. The researcher may also use photographs and video (Harper, 1989). The volume of text data gathered can create a data management challenge. Miles and Huberman (1994) provided a useful summary of storage and retrieval requirements (Table 4–10).

Qualitative researchers need to develop a data management system that suits their own style or that of the research team and the purpose of the research. Traditional methods for organizing data are notebooks, file folders, card systems, filing cabinets, and the like. Newer methods include word-processing programs, databases, spreadsheets, and other computer-based programs. Storage and retrieval of data can be done quickly and efficiently using computer software.

Recent developments in computer software mean that researchers can also get help with data analysis. Several computer-based text analysis programs, known as Computer Assisted/Aided Qualitative Data Analysis (CAQDAS; 2010) aids in qualitative analysis such as transcription analysis, coding and text interpretation, recursive abstraction, content analysis, discourse analysis, and grounded theory methodology (Baugh, Hallcom, & Harrison, 2010). When choosing a software package, the researcher needs to be aware of the assumptions underlying the design of the software and to decide whether such assumptions are congruent with the research purpose and design. For example, a common assumption is that concepts are of a hierarchical nature (such that *A* is an instance of a higher order concept *B,* and so on). Three widely known qualitative data analysis (QDA) programs are Nvivo (http://www.qsrinternational.com//default.aspx), Ethnograph (http://www.qualisresearch.com/default.htm), and

---

**TABLE 4-10**

**What to Store, Retrieve from, and Retain**

---

- Raw material: field notes, tapes, site documents

- Partially processed data: write-ups, transcriptions. Initial version and subsequent corrected, "cleaned," "commented-on" versions

- Coded data: write-ups with specific codes attached

- The coding scheme or thesaurus, in its successive iterations

- Memos or other analytic material: the researcher's reflections on the conceptual meaning of the data

- Search and retrieval records: information showing which coded chunks or data segments the researcher looked for during analysis and the retrieved material; records of links made among segments

- Data displays: matrices or networks used to display retrieved information, along with the associated analytic text; revised versions of these

- Analysis episodes: documenting of what was done, step by step, to assemble the displays and write the analytic text

- Report text: successive drafts of what is written on the design, methods, and findings of the study

- General chronological log or documentation of data collection and analytic work

- Index of all the above material

**Note:** Adapted from *Designing Qualitative Research*, (4th ed.), by C. Marshall, 2006, Thousand Oaks, CA: Sage.

---

ATLAS/ti (http://www.atlasti.com/). Reviews of available programs, their functions, advantages, and shortcomings are available at the CAQDAS Networking Project (http://caqdas.soc.surrey.ac.uk/) and Qual Page (http://www.qualitativeresearch.uga.edu/QualPage/).

## 4.6 Credibility in Qualitative Research

In qualitative research designs, the aim is to make sense of the meanings that people bring to phenomena in the social world. Qualitative researchers therefore want to make sure that their research findings are credible in the everyday sense of being plausible, believable, and trustworthy (Morse, 1994). Researchers using experimental designs and quantitative methods for collecting and analyzing data use constructs of reliability and validity. Many investigators have written on ways to address credibility in qualitative research. These range from applying the experimental concepts of reliability and validity to suggesting alternative concepts better suited to qualitative designs (see, for example, Kirk & Miller, 1986, and Lincoln & Guba, 1985). Among these writers, there is general agreement that three elements of the inquiry process must be addressed. These are the research techniques used, the researcher's credibility, and the assumptions underpinning the study.

Credibility of the research techniques can be checked by testing rival explanations, by searching for negative cases, and by triangulation. The first, testing rival explanations, requires the researcher to consider and "test out" alternative explanations to that proposed and then to report the results. Searching for negative cases is a related process.

In this instance, the researcher searches for cases that do not fit the proposed patterns or themes identified from the data. Identifying negative or outlier cases increases understanding of the commonly occurring cases and, therefore, the totality of the phenomenon under investigation. The last way to check credibility is by a process called "triangulation."

*Triangulation* has come to mean the use of multiple methods, sources, analysts, or theoretical perspectives to verify the information gained in different arenas. The aim of triangulation is "to guard against the accusation that a study's findings are simply an artifact of a single method, a single source, or a single investigator's bias" (Patton, 1990, p. 470). Triangulation of methods may involve collecting both quantitative and qualitative data for comparison and potential reconciliation. This helps to expand and elaborate the quality of information gained by one method alone.

Triangulation of sources involves comparing the consistency of information derived from varying sources, for example, comparing the data gathered from interviews and observations, from public and private documents, or from informants making the same claim independently. Triangulation across analysts is becoming more common. This can take the form of agreement between the field notes of one observer and the observations made by another, for example. Lastly, some investigators have suggested triangulation of theoretical perspectives. This means applying more than one theoretical perspective to the research findings to reveal any differences and similarities (Patton, 2001).

As mentioned at the beginning of this chapter, the researcher is an integral part of the qualitative research process. Concern for researcher credibility is therefore an inherent part of the verification process. Researcher credibility is dependent on training, experience, and acknowledgment of the researcher role in the research process. Most of all, credibility requires a clear and concise explanation of the researcher role and contribution to the study findings. It is the researcher's responsibility to explain the extent of possible researcher effect on the study and whether changes in perceptions or responses occurred during the study or whether any predispositions or biases influenced the study findings. Describing the researcher's interpretive framework allows the reader to understand exactly how the researcher framed the research question and collected and analyzed the data.

The final element is the need for concise clarification by the researcher of the philosophical orientation underpinning the study. For example, there is continuing debate about the place of objectivity in scientific inquiry. This often takes the form of competition between the two paradigms of quantitative and qualitative research (Guba, 1990). Clear explanation by the researcher of the philosophical orientation of the study helps to place the study findings within a particular interpretive framework and allows readers to judge the authenticity of the study results for themselves. Frank and open explanation in reporting research enhances credibility (Linkov, Loney, Cormier, Satterstrom, & Bridges, 2009).

Readers of qualitative research need a method to evaluate study credibility and the contribution to knowledge of the study findings. Frost et al. (2007) in an article "What Is Sufficient Evidence for The Reliability and Validity of Patient-Reported Outcome Measures?" concluded that "Various qualitative (e.g., focus groups, behavioral coding, cognitive interviews) and quantitative approaches (e.g., differential item functioning testing) are useful in evaluating the reliability and validity of PRO [patient reported outcomes] instruments" (p. s94). Some tests deal specifically with evaluating qualitative studies (e.g., Higgs, 1998). The following questions proposed by Schwandt and Halpern (1988) and cited in Miles and Huberman (1994, p. 439) provide useful criteria for readers in the medical and rehabilitation research literature:

- Are findings grounded in the data? (Is sampling appropriate? Are data weighted correctly?)
- Are inferences logical? (Are analytic strategies applied correctly? Are alternative explanations accounted for?)
- Is the category structure appropriate?
- Can inquiry decisions and methodological shifts be justified? (Were sampling decisions linked to working hypotheses?)

- What is the degree of researcher bias (premature disclosure, unexplored data in field notes, lack of search for negative cases, feelings of empathy)?
- What strategies were used for increasing credibility (second readers, feedback to informants, peer review, adequate time in the field)?

## 4.7 Summary

In summary, qualitative research offers a diversity of methods well suited to the interests of researchers in the medical and rehabilitation fields. The increasing popularity of these methods in these fields is evident in the growing number of qualitative studies reported in the occupational therapy literature and the appearance of journals devoted specifically to qualitative research studies.

Until recently, however, the positivist experimental tradition (quantitative research) was predominant in the medical profession and in rehabilitation and related health professions. As this text makes clear, both quantitative and qualitative research approaches contribute to the development of scientific inquiry in clinical research. The challenge for researchers in occupational therapy is to incorporate qualitative and quantitative approaches into their research studies. A recent example of integrating both qualitative and quantitative research was carried out in a study by Uhlig et al. (Uhlig, Fongen, Steen, Christie, & Ødegård, 2010) exploring the effectiveness of Tai Chi with patients diagnosed with rheumatoid arthritis. Quantitative analysis was used to measure muscle function in the lower extremities, and qualitative measures were applied in measuring subjective aspects in the study. They concluded that "the combination of qualitative and quantitative research methods shows that Tai Chi has beneficial effects on health not related to disease activity and standardised health status assessment, and may contribute to an understanding of how Tai Chi exerts its effects" (p.43).

## CHAPTER 5

# The Research Problem

*The great working hypotheses in the past have often originated in the minds of the pioneers as a result of mental processes which can best be described by such words as "inspired guess," "intuitive hunch," or "brilliant flash of imagination."*

—J. B. Conant, 1951, *Science and Common Sense* (p. 48)

## Operational Learning Objectives

By the end of this chapter, the learner will:

- Identity a significant research topic in an area of clinical practice, administration, or education.
- Write a paragraph justifying the need for a research study.
- Identity a feasible research problem.

- Formulate relevant questions pertaining to a research problem.
- Identify possible psychological blocks and flaws in research designs that could potentially deter the research.
- Outline a general plan for data collection.

## 5.1 The Need for Problem-Oriented Research in the Health Professions

Since the middle of the twentieth century, health research in the United States has multiplied beyond the volume that could have been predicted a century earlier. During the nineteenth century, a medical scientist could easily have read most of the published research in a wide range of health specialties. A scholar in the sciences in the nineteenth century would also be familiar with the literary and artistic worlds. Today it is impossible. C. P. Snow (1964), in his discussion of the two worlds of science and humanities, was one of the first to recognize the isolating effect of specialization in the twentieth century. Scientists and humanists now live in two cultures, deprived of the sharing and communication that existed in the eighteenth and nineteenth centuries. Specialization and the narrowing of interest in scientific topics have led to a multiplicity of professional associations and published journals.

Currently, there are thousands of scientific journals published monthly, semimonthly, and quarterly. There is also a growing trend toward electronic publication where scholars can read articles directly from the Internet. A gap exists between the methods used in social science research and research in the biological and physical sciences. Quantitative research is more prevalent in the biological and physical sciences, whereas the social sciences apply relatively more qualitative research methods for collecting data. Research in the social sciences is most vulnerable to criticism because of the subjective nature of qualitative research. On the other hand, there is a pressing need for social progress (e.g., the reduction of alcoholism, drug addiction, juvenile crime, and mental illness).

The gap between research in the social sciences and that gap's impact on social problems has led to criticism of applied research. Yet one need only examine the history of medical progress to realize the tremendous gains science has made through applied research, such as in the reduction of heart disease, the survivor rates for cancer patients, and surgery for cataracts. There is also a strong need for basic research in areas that may not seem relevant at the moment, as with cellular research and microbiology, where theory and basic research carried out 60 years ago have led to practical results in understanding the immune system and how it impacts AIDS. There is a need for basic research into life processes, such as in DNA, muscle metabolism, and neurological and cognitive areas of human development. The need exists for problem-oriented research that can be applied in the areas of health, medicine, occupational therapy, and special education. A research study begins with establishing the need, significance, and implications of the results.

## 5.2 Selecting a Significant Research Problem

How does a researcher select a significant area for investigation? What factors in an individual's personal life, education, or clinical experience generate a research interest? William Harvey in the introduction of his book *On the Motion of the Heart and Blood in Animals*, written in 1628, described his purpose in investigating the problem of circulation of blood in the following quotation:

> Since, therefore, from the foregoing considerations and many others to the same effect, it is plain that what has ... been said concerning the motion and function of the heart and arteries must appear obscure, inconsistent, or even impossible to him who carefully considers the entire subject, it would be proper to look more narrowly into the matter to contemplate the motion of the heart and arteries, not only in man, but in all animals that have hearts; and also by frequent appeals to vivisection, and much ocular inspection, to investigate and discuss the truth. (p. 73)

Harvey selected the problem of investigating the circulatory system after he evaluated the previous studies as contradictory and inconclusive. His motivation to study the problem was based on his desire to bring clarity to an area of medicine that is vital to human survival. This desire to clarify is an important motivating force in the researcher. There are numerous examples in the history of scientific research of individuals seeking to understand the basic anatomical and physiological processes of humans.

Other motivating forces can also generate research. Individuals can pursue a research area because they seek insight into a disease or disability that has touched their own life or the life of a family member or close friend. In 1847, Ignaz Semmelweis, a relentless investigator, pursued the causes of puerperal fever (i.e., blood poisoning associated with childbirth) after the death of a friend (Sinclair, 1909). Louis Braille, blinded at the age of four, became a teacher of the blind and in 1824 devised a reading method for the blind (Mellor, 2006). Some situations that may motivate an individual to pursue an area of research include:

- A clinician becomes a researcher after becoming aware of the need for more effective treatment methods or diagnostic instruments. There are many instances in the history of medicine where practitioners became part-time researchers and made notable contributions through their efforts. For instance, A. R. Luria (1980), a Russian neuroscientist, became interested in the way the brain worked after evaluating neurological injuries occurring in soldiers. He used case study research to explore neurological disorders and from this developed a concept of how an undamaged brain works.
- A dramatic increase in the incidence of a disease produces national priorities for research. In the United States during the last 60 years, there has been a significant amount of research effort directed at cancer, cardiovascular disease, and AIDS. These areas have received added attention from researchers partly because of the dramatic increases in the incidence of these illnesses and partly because of the availability of federal grant support. It is no secret that

national politics and priorities can determine a research investigator's career. On the other hand, the abuse of federal grant support in the opportunism of research can also become an overriding problem in neglecting research areas that are significant, yet receive little interest from the granting foundations and governmental agencies.

- An inspiring teacher can generate an interest in a content area. There is no doubt that universities are an ideal place for research because they can play an active, yet neutral, role in facilitating research efforts. Universities need not be caught in political decisions.
- A student develops an interest in a research area through intellectual curiosity spurred by intense reading and study. As the student gains more understanding in a specific area, more questions are raised, which motivate research.

From these motivating forces and others, the researcher selects an area of investigation. From this point, how does one maintain momentum and nurture research interests sometimes in the face of insignificant results and tedious, laborious work?

The story of Fleming's discovery of penicillin in 1929 is an example of persistence (Brown, 2004). The impetus for Fleming's investigation was the catastrophic rate of death that occurred during World War I from infected wounds. Fleming sought a chemical substance that would destroy the pathogenic germs entering the body from an open flesh wound. After 10 years of painstaking laboratory work that involved growing bacterial colonies and observing the reactions of chemicals, he was successful in discovering a powerful therapeutic agent that would eventually change the course of medical practice.

There were two landmark events in Fleming's work. The first occurred in 1922 when he noticed that a foreign chemical substance prevented a bacterial colony from growing. At this point in his work, Fleming was unable to isolate or identify the chemical substance. In 1928, he noticed that a bacterial culture of staphylococci had accidentally become contaminated by mold. He found that the mold produced a substance that retarded the growth of the bacteria. The chemical substance was later identified by an American mycologist, Thom, as *Pénicillium notatum*. After the substance was identified, Fleming was able to produce penicillin in the laboratory and experiment with its effect on bacteria and on normal human tissues. It was not until 1943, about 20 years after Fleming's original investigations, that penicillin was mass produced in Great Britain and the United States.

In analyzing Fleming's discovery, a combination of persistence and responsiveness to accidental discovery was the key factor. Fleming first asked a researchable question: Is there a chemical substance that can stop the growth of harmful bacteria in the bloodstream without destroying normal human tissue? He persisted in his efforts to solve the problem over a period of 25 years until his successful discovery of penicillin.

Compared to medicine, research originating from occupational therapy is in the beginning stages of development. Potential directions for research abound in the areas of evaluation and treatment and in the areas of professional education and administration. Research originates out of the relationship between the evaluation and treatment of a specific disability. By analyzing a disability, the clinical researcher tries to determine where the major gaps in knowledge exist. For example, in evaluating and treating the client with arthritis, are there effective evaluative instruments? What treatment methods have been demonstrated to be effective? What factors in the client's life affect the course of the illness? From this analysis, the researcher can identify a research problem.

This same process of generating research also is evident in analyzing the educational and administrative aspects of occupational therapy in addressing such questions as the admission of students into a program, effective supervision and evaluation of staff, maintenance of morale in job satisfaction, and design of the curriculum. The need for research is justified when a researcher can establish the significance of the results. For example, the researcher should ask, "If I collect this data, what impact will the results have on treatment, education, or admin-

istration?" A researcher should clearly state the implications of the study, relating it to the evaluation or treatment of a specified disability or the educational or administrative practices that the results could affect. Before data are collected, the researcher should be able to think through the impact of the results. An *if* (results positive or negative)... *then* (recommendations and options taken) contingency is the initial strategy that the researcher proposes.

## 5.3 Identifying Problems Resulting from a Disability

In selecting a disability area for research, investigators can be guided by their own clinical experience in an area of specialization. For example, the significance of a problem can be gauged by the leading causes of death and the leading causes of hospitalization. The 15 leading causes of death in the United States in 2007 are shown in Table 5–1.

For the researcher, these disabilities and diseases represent significant health problems. Evaluation and diagnosis are ongoing concerns for the therapist. Methodological research such as in diagnostic hardware, clinical observational methods, screening procedures, and objective tests can become the focal point of an investigation. The development of specific treatment techniques or protocols that can be generalized to a population with disabilities represents another fertile direction for researchers. Treatment techniques such as sensory-integration therapy (SI), neurodevelopmental therapy (NDT), aquatic therapy, hippo therapy, stress management, and biofeedback are a few examples of research areas generated from examining the needs of people with disabilities.

## 5.4 Identifying Significant Issues in Professional Education

Who should become occupational therapists? Are there specific abilities, personalities, intellectual potentials, or academic achievements necessary before entering a professional preparatory program? What is the rationale for each characteristic? How

## TABLE 5-1

**Fifteen Leading Causes of Death in 2007**

| Cause | 2007 |
| --- | --- |
| All causes | 2,423,712 |
| Diseases of heart | 616,067 |
| Malignant neoplasms | 562,875 |
| Cerebrovascular diseases | 135,952 |
| Chronic lower respiratory diseases | 127,924 |
| Accidents (unintentional injuries) | 123,706 |
| Alzheimer's disease | 74,632 |
| Diabetes mellitus | 71,382 |
| Influenza and pneumonia | 52,717 |
| Nephritis, nephrotic syndrome and nephrosis | 46,448 |
| Septicemia | 34,828 |
| Intentional self-harm (suicide) | 34,598 |
| Chronic liver disease and cirrhosis | 29,165 |
| Essential hypertension and renal disease | 23,965 |
| Parkinson's disease | 20,058 |
| Assault (homicide) | 18,361 |
| All other causes (residual) | 451,034 |

**Note:** The table shows the number and rank for the top causes of death in the United States in 2007. The data include all races and were obtained from page 3 of the *National Vital Statistics Report, 58*(19), May, 2010, published by the Centers for Disease Control and Prevention. Retrieved from http://www.cdc.gov/nchs/data/nvsr/nvsr58/nvsr58_19.pdf

are admission requirements for entrance to an occupational therapy program determined? Who among the faculty and staff in the occupational therapy departments determines policy for admission? These questions examine the assumptions underlying the education of occupational therapists. For the occupational therapy educator, the recruitment, screening, and selection of students pose realistic problems that should provide significant areas for investigation.

Along with the admission process, the curriculum is a potential area for research. The educational curriculum includes the classroom teaching methods, curricular content, audiovisual aids, clinical education, problem-based learning, and student evaluation. Examples of these potential areas of research in educating occupational therapy students are listed in Table 5–2.

Administration of clinical programs, personnel policies, budgetary planning, physical plant layouts, and job satisfaction are often neglected areas of research, although the effect of administrative policies sometimes have more impact on the course of a client's disability than do the direct effects of treatment. Public health policies to mass vaccinate a population, access to health care, and staff morale are all critical areas of concern that have important implications in the total health needs. These are all potential areas for research.

TABLE 5-2

**Methods and Content of Professional Programs in Occupational Therapy**

| Classroom Teaching Methods | Curricula Content | Presentation Methods | Clinical Education | Student Evaluation |
|---|---|---|---|---|
| • Case studies | • Basic sciences | • Audiovisual methods | Level 1 | • Grades: number and letter grades |
| • Laboratory experiences (e.g., testing or intervention) | • Dynamics of interactions | • Computer-assisted instruction | • Short-term experiences with or without supervision | • Grades: pass/fail |
| • Lecture | • Evaluation and intervention techniques | • Distance learning | • Observations (single day) | • Individual counseling |
| • Problem-based learning | • Practice areas (e.g., geriatrics, mental health, pediatrics, physical disabilities) | • Internet | • Clerkships (weekly) | • Observation of students in clinical settings |
| • Role playing | | • Presentation software (e.g., PowerPoint) | Level 2 | • Competency-based evaluation |
| • Seminar | | • Videos | • Two 3-month affiliations with supervision | |
| • Student-oriented group projects | • Research design | | • Internships or affiliations | |
| | • Supervision and administration | | • Optional experience | |
| | | | • Optional affiliations in a specialty area | |

© Cengage Learning 2013

## 5.5 Justifying the Research Problem

Once the investigator identifies a research area, statistical data indicating the extent of the problem should be cited. (See Table 5–3 as an example of statistical data). A problem involving one of the 15 leading causes of death or hospitalization is obviously significant. Nonetheless, how does one justify investigating a rare disease, such as amyotrophic lateral sclerosis (ALS), that affects proportionately few people? On the other hand, should an investigator's freedom be restricted by governmental agencies deciding which areas to fund research? The question of research significance does touch on societal values. Nations establish priorities in areas of health that realistically affect research efforts.

It is assumed that the individual scientist should have the freedom to pursue any area of investigation as long as it does not endanger the lives of the subjects.

Yet, research should not be isolated from the pressing needs of a society. If, for example, osteoarthritis becomes a problem of epidemic proportions in the United States during the twenty-first century, then society should justly allocate a large percentage of its health resources to those researchers seeking means to reduce the incidence of osteoarthritis. Establishing research priorities in a democratic society involves the participation of a broad spectrum of groups who represent the policy makers, clinicians, consumers, and researchers. Governmental agencies, universities, pharmaceutical companies, and private foundations are the primary sources for the financial support of research and, thus, the policy makers for research. The recipients of research grants are those clinical practitioners, students, educators, and administrators who have convinced policy makers of the significance and validity of their research proposals.

In summary, the researcher justifies an investigation by establishing the need for a study based on an analysis of a health problem and the implications

## TABLE 5-3

**Prevalence of Selected Chronic Conditions in Adults in the United States in 2008**

| Chronic Condition | Percent of Adults over 18 |
|---|---|
| Arthritis | 22.2 |
| Chronic Joint Symptoms | 26.7 |
| Emphysema | 1.6 |
| Feelings of Sadness, Hopelessness, Worthlessness | 12.0 |
| Hearing Problems | 15.0 |
| Hypertension | 24.2 |
| Low Back Pain | 13.8 |
| Physical Function Difficulties (e.g. climbing 10 steps without resting) | 14.0 |
| Vision | 11.0 |

**Note:** Table adapted from the "Summary Health Statistics for U. S. Adults: National Health Interview Survey, 2008: Provisional Report" by J. R. Pleis, J. W. Lucas, and B. W. Ward, 2009, in *Vital Health Statistics*, Volume 10, Number 242. Retrieved from http://www.cdc.gov/nchs/data/series/sr_10/sr10_242.pdf

of the results. The need for an investigation is documented by the following statistical data:

- The **incidence rate** (initial occurrences) and **prevalence rate** (existing cases in the population) of a disability, derived from primary statistical data;
- The leading causes of death as reported by national and international centers for health statistics (e.g., World Health Organization);
- The number of first admissions and readmissions to a hospital caused by a disability, obtained from national and state public health agencies;
- The number of physician and outpatient visits reported as the result of a disability;
- The days lost at work because of specific health problems, compiled from Department of Labor Statistics and Workers' Compensation;
- The incidence of social disabilities (i.e., alcoholism, drug addiction, adult crime, juvenile delinquency, and child abuse) available through the national and state public health agencies and the state attorney general's office;
- The number of occupational therapists employed in the United States as provided by professional organizations, the *Occupational Outlook Handbook* (published by the United States Department of Labor), and state employment agencies; and
- Statistics on the number of hospitals, outpatient clinics, state institutions for individuals with intellectual disabilities and mental illness, rehabilitation centers, and other patient care facilities, usually available from public health agencies or through directories published by municipal and state organizations and private social service agencies.

## 5.6  Narrowing the Investigation

**Problem-oriented research** is a process of asking questions and gathering data. The investigator generates a question and intellectually ponders the possible outcomes. This ability to formulate research questions and to predict outcomes is an essential part of the research process. The Socratic method of teaching is based on this principle of questions and answers that invariably lead to other questions and answers until a topic is exhausted. This method is also used in problem-based learning where students examine a case study by asking relevant questions and developing hypotheses.

Brainstorming a problem is another method for generating questions by creative free association. The researcher must be able to freely generate questions that on initial examination may seem unrelated or unfeasible. Many great discoveries, when they were first reported publicly, seemed like "hair-brained" ideas that would never work. Roentgen, a physicist, accidentally discovered X-rays when examining the results of passing electricity through a vacuum tube (Glasser, 1933). He then proceeded to ask himself questions regarding its applicability to medical diagnosis. On hearing of Roentgen's discovery in 1895, people in the streets were incredulous. Many felt that X-rays would be used like a camera to spy on people or to expose them. Later, medical scientists raised questions regarding the potential of X-rays in the diagnosis and treatment of cancerous growths.

This process of asking questions and observing the outcome is the essential part of research. At first, the question may be general, ill-conceived, unclear, and incongruous. As the researcher explores and defines what is actually being asked, the research question becomes sharper until, as Graham Wallas (1926) stated:

> Our mind is not likely to give us a clear answer to any particular problem unless we set it a clear question, and we are more likely to notice the significance of any new piece of evidence, or new association of ideas, if we have formed a definite conception of a case to be proved or disproved. (p. 84)

The persistent effort on the researcher's part to brainstorm a problem, to think it through, to ponder silently, or to discuss it with a colleague brings the researcher closer to a solution. For some investigators, the problem incubates; whereas for others, the problem stirs. Whatever the style is, the researcher must be able to stay with a problem while trying to overcome the apparent pitfalls and cul-de-sacs that

are created. Many a researcher is stymied by the assumption of others that the problem is too complex or impossible to solve or by the knowledge that others have failed to find a solution. The investigator must persist in working through the problem. For example, low back pain is a significant health problem that affects a large number of sedentary and manual workers. It directly affects industrial production, psychological well-being, and participation in sports and leisure activities.

Although low back pain is widespread in the population and has significant implications, practitioners have been only partially successful in treating this disability. Experienced occupational therapists observe that low back pain is an elusive syndrome that is difficult to diagnose and sometimes difficult to separate from malingering or psychosomatic effects. Other clinicians are hesitant to investigate the problem because of the subjective nature of measuring pain. Others state that the neurophysiology is too complex to investigate. These reactions to low back pain should not deter research. Investigators entering into an area of research can become overwhelmed by the immensity of a problem, but they need not try to solve all aspects of the problem, including objective diagnosis and successful treatment. Researchers should instead attempt to "slice off" a portion of a research problem that is feasible within the limitations of time and resources available. The process of formulating a research problem by a clinician is summarized in Figure 5–1.

Let us examine hypothetical examples of research questions derived from significant health problems (Table 5–4). These research questions are derived directly from an analysis of a health problem. The specificity of the question depends on the uniqueness of the investigator's interests. After researchers identify an area of investigation and document the significance of the study, they are faced with the task of narrowing the area of investigation into a feasible chunk within a designated time span. Some researchers devote their entire professional life to a specific area of research; others drastically change their research areas as they broaden their interests.

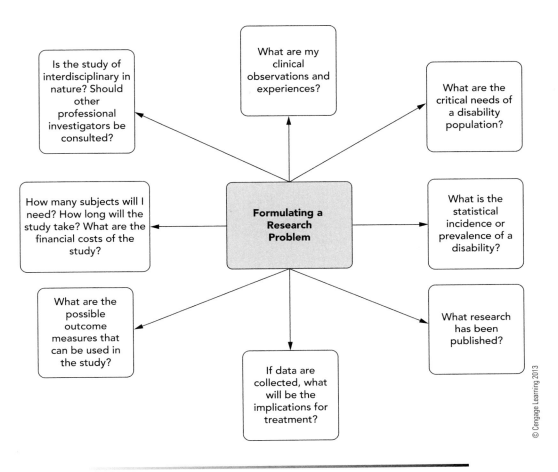

**FIGURE 5-1** Clinical Formulation of a Research Problem

## 5.6.1 Determining Feasibility

In the process of narrowing the investigation to a feasible study, the investigator should, as a preliminary procedure, carefully examine the following questions:

1. How long will data collection take?
    a. Laboratory experiments—the length of time required for preparing and collecting data for each participant
    b. Travel time—the length of time required to get to and from the data collection site
    c. Interview time—time for each subject multiplied by total number of subjects equal total interview time
    d. Mail survey—researcher must account for response time and possibly a second mailing
    e. Correlational study—individual or group testing time periods
    f. Methodological—consideration of time for constructing instrument and obtaining reliability and validity data
2. What measuring instruments are available for testing constructs and variables?
    a. Cost—expenses incurred to obtain test instruments
    b. Expertise—level of competency or experience needed to administer and interpret test results

TABLE 5-4

**Hypothetical Research Questions Related to Disability**

| Disability | Research Question |
|---|---|
| AIDS | How can prescriptive exercise help in reducing symptoms? |
| Cerebral palsy | Is development sequential and hierarchical in children with motor lesions in the cerebral cortex? |
| Depression | What is the role of exercise in increasing serotonin? |
| Hypertension | Can blood pressure rates be self-regulated through biofeedback techniques? |
| Learning disability | What are significant factors in facilitating handwriting? |
| Intellectual disability | How does the environment facilitate or restrict learning? |
| Multiple sclerosis | What are the effects of stress on "triggering" episodes? |
| Schizophrenia | Can relaxation therapy help the individual to manage stress? |
| Social deprivation | How does a parent affect language acquisition when talking or reading with the child? |
| Stroke | How does client motivation significantly affect recovery of function? |
| Traumatic brain injury | What issues need to be addressed if school reentry is to be successful? |

© Cengage Learning 2013

3. Are participants readily available? Where can participants be obtained?
   a. Screening criteria—used to determine participant inclusion
   b. Incentives for the participants—Will payment or some other incentive be given to the participants?
4. What expertise is needed to carry out the intervention?
   a. Investigator skill: Does the researcher have the skills to implement the intervention?
   b. Assistant: What training will be required for the assistant, if one is needed?
5. Finance:
   a. Cost: What are the total financial costs of the research, and who will finance them?
   b. Funding Source: Who will finance the costs?
6. Institutional Review Board:
   a. How long will it take for approval?
   b. Ethical standards: What are the ethical standards set by the investigator or institution? (See Section 7.12)
7. Operational definitions of variables (See Section 7.3)

## 5.7 Psychological Blocks in Selection of a Research Problem

Frequently, graduate students confronted with the task of completing a thesis, dissertation, or study that involves collecting primary data are stymied in selecting a researchable topic. Students often belabor the process and frequently change their research area. In the process of selecting a feasible research problem, the student can become frustrated and blocked. In overcoming these psychological blocks, the student should examine the consequences of a research study and its potential significance. The following examples are typical of the psychological blocks that interfere with selecting a research problem.

- A research topic is dropped prematurely because the investigator fails to locate enough published studies related to the topic.
- The investigator is overwhelmed by the multiplicity of studies published in an area and concludes that further research is not necessary because the area has already been researched sufficiently. The investigator drops the topic without rigorously evaluating the validity and conclusiveness of results.
- The research topic selected is too broad, considering the time constraints of an investigator. Instead of narrowing the research topic to a feasible study, the investigator terminates the study.
- A preliminary investigation of a research area reveals difficulty in measuring an outcome variable. The investigator drops the study without seeking to construct an instrument that could reliably and validly measure the outcome.

- An investigator is motivated to explore a research area with the goal of making an important and original contribution to the body of knowledge. The investigator refuses to delimit a study after realizing the amount of time necessary to complete the study and subsequently terminates the investigation.

Selecting a researchable problem should be an ongoing process where the investigator explores the relevance, feasibility, applicability, and significance of a study. The worksheet guide in Box 5–1 lists the areas that a researcher should be aware of in the process of selecting and narrowing a researchable problem.

## 5.8 Worksheet Guide for Selecting a Research Problem

Box 5–1 provides a worksheet that can be used to select a research problem.

---

### BOX 5-1

#### Worksheet Guide for Selecting a Research Problem

**1. What is the target population?** (e.g., group with disabilities, or student or clinician from the allied health profession)

**2. What are the perceived needs of the population?** (e.g., investigating causes of disability; evaluation and diagnostic methods; student performance; evaluation of therapists' effectiveness; investigation of treatment techniques; evaluation of personnel factors)

**3. What are the primary and secondary sources relevant to responses 1 and 2?**

- journal articles

| 1. |
|----|
| 2. |
| 3. |
| 4. |
| 5. |

*continues*

BOX 5-1

## Worksheet Guide for Selecting a Research Problem *continued*

| | |
|---|---|
| • textbooks | 1. |
| | 2. |
| | 3. |
| | 4. |
| | 5. |
| • statistical compendiums | 1. |
| | 2. |
| | 3. |

### 4. Are independent and dependent variables identifiable?

| | |
|---|---|
| • independent variables: (presumed causes) | 1. |
| | 2. |
| | 3. |
| • dependent variables: (presumed effects) | 1. |
| | 2. |
| | 3. |
| | 4. |

### 5. How can the research impact on...

| | |
|---|---|
| • treatment? | |
| • education? | |
| • administration? | |

### 6. Can research variables be operationally defined?

### 7. What explanation or theory accounts for the presumed relationship between variables?

### 8. What research design(s) are relevant to the study? Identify model and state research question relative to research model.

| *Quantitative* | |
|---|---|
| • Experimental (pretest/posttest) | |
| • Methodological (construction of instrument) | |
| • Evaluation (evaluation of health care system) | |
| • Correlation (relationship between variables) | |

| | |
|---|---|
| *Qualitative* | |
| • Survey (description of population) | |
| • Historical (reconstruction of events) | |
| • Clinical or naturalistic observation (dynamic analysis of subject) | |
| • Heuristic (discovery of relationships) | |

**9. Research problem/question**

| | |
|---|---|
| • State the research problem. | |
| • State the hypothesis in null or directional form. | |
| • State the guiding question. | |

**10. To which groups are the research findings directed?** (e.g., clinicians, individuals with disabilities, students, academicians, program administrators)

**11. Feasibility check**

| | |
|---|---|
| • Where can participants be obtained? | |
| • How many participants are necessary? | |
| • What tests, instruments, or apparatuses will be necessary to measure outcome? | |

**12. What are financial costs?**

| | |
|---|---|
| • travel | |
| • mailings | |
| • tests and apparatus | 1. |
| | 2. |
| | 3. |
| | 4. |
| • protocols | 1. |
| | 2. |
| | 3. |
| | 4. |
| • clinical time | |
| • computer analysis | |
| • books and duplicating | |
| • clerical and typing | |
| • laboratory analysis of findings | |

*continues*

| BOX 5-1 | **Worksheet Guide for Selecting a Research Problem** *continued* |
|---|---|

**13. Analysis of Time** (List the projected time sequence or dates for completion of research phases.)

| Initiation of study | Review of literature | Preparation for data collection | Approval from IRB | Collection of results | Writing discussion chapter | Completion of study |
|---|---|---|---|---|---|---|
| | | | | | | |

© Cengage Learning 2013

## 5.9 Why Research Proposals Are Disapproved

The following list of major reasons for the disapproval of research proposals is based on the authors' experiences as raters on governmental and university committees. The list is summarized in Table 5–5.

- **The research problem is insignificant, and the results will have little impact on clinical practice currently or in the future.** An example of an insignificant problem is an investigation of the relationship of low birth weight with the incidence of cerebral palsy. A literature search in this area already confirms that low birth weight is one among many risk factors for cerebral palsy. Nonetheless, not all infants with cerebral palsy are born prematurely, nor are all infants with low birth weight destined to have cerebral palsy. This study will have little impact on our understanding of the causes of cerebral palsy and will not provide insight into the prevention and treatment. The projected results from this type of study would have a splintering effect where one variable is linked to a disability that has already been found to have multiple causes. A better study in a related area would

be to examine the effects of low birth weight on one area of development, such as motor function. In this way, the investigator can narrow the research and control for extraneous variables that could have a potential effect on the results.

- **The hypothesis presented is not supported by scientific evidence and seems speculative.** As a hypothetical example, a researcher proposes that a computer software program in cognitive rehabilitation is effective in treating individuals with brain injuries. The investigator equates improvement with the client's ability to learn a computer game. The investigator does not demonstrate through a literature review that there is a carryover of this computer skill to the learning of functional skills in independent living. A better study is to investigate the types of skills that are facilitated while learning with a computer.

- **The research problem is more complex than the investigator presents, and it needs to be narrowed down.** For example, a researcher proposes to examine the effects of sensory-integration therapy on children with Attention-Deficit/Hyperactivity Disorder (ADHD). Both variables are complex and must be operationally defined. Sensory-integration therapy

## TABLE 5-5

**Reasons Why Research Proposals are Denied**

| | |
|---|---|
| 1. | The research problem is insignificant, and the results will have little impact on clinical practice currently or in the future. |
| 2. | The hypothesis presented is not supported by scientific evidence and seems speculative. |
| 3. | The research problem is more complex than the investigator presents, and it needs to be narrowed down. |
| 4. | The anticipated results from the study will be of only local significance and will lack external validity or generalizability. |
| 5. | The research proposed has too many uncontrolled elements. |
| 6. | The research methodology seems overly complex and difficult to replicate. |
| 7. | The proposed outcome measures are inappropriate, unstandardized, unreliable, or invalid. |
| 8. | Extraneous variables are left uncontrolled and may have an influence on the results. |
| 9. | Overall design of the study seems incomplete and not well conceived. |
| 10. | The statistical tests suggested for analyzing the data are not appropriate. |
| 11. | Selection of subjects for the study is not representative of a target population. |
| 12. | The treatment procedure under investigation has not been adequately defined in enough detail to replicate. |
| 13. | The literature review seems outdated and lacks landmark studies in the area of investigation. |
| 14. | The equipment identified in the study is outmoded or unsuitable. |
| 15. | The investigator has not proposed adequate time for completion of the study. |
| 16. | Resources are inadequate to complete the study. |
| 17. | The setting and environment for the study are unsuitable. |
| 18. | The investigator has not considered the ethical nature of the study, such as stating the potential physical and psychological risks to participants in an informed consent form, or has not received approval from an institutional review board (IRB) regarding human subjects. |

includes a number of components in treatment, whereas ADHD is a complex disorder with multiple causes. A better study is to identify one aspect of sensory-integration therapy, such as vestibular stimulation, and evaluate its effectiveness with a measurable variable, such as motor proficiency, as assessed by the *Miller Assessment for Preschoolers* (MAP; Miller, 1988).

- **The anticipated results from the study will be of only local significance and will lack external validity or generalizability.** An example of a flawed proposal is when a researcher designs a survey of job satisfaction for occupational therapists in a local school district without con-

sidering the generalizability to a larger sample or population. The data collected from this study would have only local interest and could not be generalized to teachers in other schools. In a better study of job satisfaction among occupational therapists, the researcher would determine first the demographics of an average occupational therapist, considering age, gender, and educational level. These variables could be used to determine if the occupational therapists are representative of a larger population. The survey would be designed with the intention of applying it to a more general sample. Questions would be generated that examine the broad issues of job satisfaction among occupational therapists in general, rather than looking at local issues that affect job satisfaction in that particular school district.

- **The research proposed has too many uncontrolled elements.** For example, a researcher wants to study the effects of in utero exposure to alcohol on children born with fetal alcohol syndrome (FAS). The amount of alcohol exposure is unknown and is dependent on the mother's self-report, which is often unreliable. In addition, the home environment and genetic makeup are variables that may play a part in the child's behavior. These variables are difficult to measure, and the researcher often neglects them. A better approach is a retrospective case study analysis of an infant with FAS and the child's mother, exploring the dynamics of the case.

- **The research methodology seems overly complex and difficult to replicate.** For example, a researcher wants to examine the relationship between the onset of a depressive episode and an individual who is vulnerable. The interaction among family relationships, work situations, and personal attitudes are complex and make it difficult to identify the interactive factors that result in depression. Because of the individuality of each episode, replication of the study using a group method or survey would be difficult and might distort results. A better study would include a qualitative research method using an in-depth case study approach to identify within each individual the interactive effects that trigger depression.

- **The proposed outcome measures are inappropriate, unstandardized, unreliable, or invalid.** A researcher investigating the effects of exercise on depression creates a scale for depression without testing for its reliability or validity. A better approach to measurement is to use more than one instrument to measure outcome (triangulation). For example, the investigator can use a physiological measure, a standardized test, and a client self-report. These three measures will increase the internal validity of the study in assessing outcome.

- **Extraneous variables are left uncontrolled and may have an influence on the results.** For example, a researcher wants to examine the effect of a specific treatment method on improving motor skills. Although the researcher is careful to administer pre- and posttests, extraneous variables, such as practice at home, additional interventions, or sessions per week, are not included in the analysis. These variables will most certainly affect the results. A better study would be to take frequent measures of performance, perhaps at the beginning and end of each therapy session, to determine changes in skill level. Another possibility is to have the client and researcher keep a log describing motor performance.

- **Overall design of the study seems incomplete and not well conceived.** In this example, elements of the research proposal are missing, such as controlling for extraneous variables that could possibly influence the results, or omitting a large section of the literature review. It is important for the researcher to work with an outline that lists the essential components of a research proposal.

- **The statistical tests suggested for analyzing the data are not appropriate.** An investigator has collected ordinal data, such as ranking of students on an achievement test. Rather than using a nonparametric test, such as the Spearman rank correlation used for ordinal type data, the researcher inappropriately applies a parametric test, such as the Pearson product-moment correlation statistical test used for interval scale data. The statistical test applied should be based on the measurement scale of data. The assumptions of parametric statistics, such as normality of data distribution, should be followed. The appropriate statistics are based on the assumptions underlying the statistical tests. (See Chapter 8.)

- **Selection of subjects for the study is not representative of a target population.** If it is known that the incidence of traumatic brain injuries (TBI) is higher for males than females by more than 2 to 1 and that more than 50 percent of clients with TBI are between the ages of 15 and 24, then the investigator should try to select participants who reflect these statistics. This is especially true for studies where the investigator intends to generalize results to a representative sample. Nonetheless, there are studies in which the investigator is interested in examining a nonrepresentative sample that is a portion of the target population, such as females or children with TBI. Then the investigator must delineate clearly the target population in the title of the study.

- **The treatment procedure under investigation has not been adequately defined in enough detail to replicate.** An investigator identifies the independent variable as counseling; however, not enough detail is given regarding the type, frequency, and duration of counseling. Therefore, this study cannot be replicated.

- **The literature review seems outdated and lacks landmark studies in the area of investigation.** In reviewing the literature, it is wise to first examine current secondary texts or to survey articles in the area to identify the major landmark studies that are cited frequently. An up-to-date literature review also can be found by scanning the current journals in a subject area and by looking at the journal's yearly index.

- **The equipment identified in the study is outmoded or unsuitable.** For example, a test that has been standardized for adults is used for children. This is inappropriate and unsuitable for the study.

- **The investigator has not proposed adequate time for completion of the study.** In outlining the proposal for a study, the researcher should set up a timeline graph that breaks down the components of the study into time periods. (See Box 5–1: Worksheet Guide in Section 5.8.)

- **Resources are inadequate to complete the study.** For example, a research plan includes a request for funds to pay assistants to collect data. The funds requested for support are insufficient to complete the study.

- **The setting and environment for the study are unsuitable.** In this instance, the investigator attempts to complete a complex study without securing an appropriate environment for the study, such as a fully equipped laboratory or testing area that is free from distracting noise.

- **The investigator has not considered the ethical nature of the study, such as stating the potential physical and psychological risks to subjects in an informed consent form, or has not received approval from an institutional review board (IRB) regarding human subjects.** For example, a researcher begins to collect data for a study on apraxia and its relationship to students with learning disabilities before the **institutional review board (IRB)** has approved the research design. This is unethical, and data collected cannot be used in the final analysis.

## 5.10 Summary

How does one create a research project? Where do research ideas come from? What are the essential variables in formulating a research problem? Occupational therapy is an applied health profession, meaning that the focus in the profession is in problem solving and clinical reasoning as applied to helping the client become independent in his or her everyday occupation. Research in occupational therapy is problem-oriented and focused on developing the assessments and interventions to assist clients. In this chapter, the emphasis is on helping the researcher to select a significant research project related to occupational therapy practice. Education in the preparation of becoming an occupational therapist, administration related to occupational therapy, and client intervention are the three major areas of research in occupational therapy. This chapter is the transition from formulating a significant research question to implementing the project. In the next chapters, the reader is introduced to the "nuts and bolts" of research, literature review, methodology, statistics, selection of a test instrument, and scientific writing.

## CHAPTER 6

# Review of the Literature

*That "the library" as yet unspecified—is the repository of by far the largest part of our recorded knowledge needs no demonstration. The author of an active article on West Africa who reports that the annual rainfall in Fernando, PA, is 100 inches found this information in the library—in a book. It is most unlikely that he measured the rain himself.*

—Jacques Barzun and Henry Graff, 1970,
*The Modern Researcher* (p. 63)

## Operational Learning Objectives

By the end of this chapter, the learner will:

- Identify the main purpose of a literature review.
- Initiate a computer-based library search, such as OT Search, MEDLINE®, PubMed®, CINAHL, ERIC, HealthStar, and Google Scholar.
- Compare and contrast referral and primary sources.

- Initiate a search of the literature identifying relevant research articles.
- Critically evaluate the validity of research studies.
- Outline a comprehensive search of the related literature.

## 6.1 The Need for a Literature Review

Good research is part of a cumulative process in which information expands in many directions. Breakthroughs in knowledge do not occur suddenly. The scientist exploring solutions to problems first masters the previous literature to determine (a) what has been accomplished, (b) where the cul-de-sacs are, and (c) what research is in the forefront of knowledge. A search of the literature involving the location of relevant studies is a critical part of the research process. It is impossible to conceive of a researcher devising a research plan without first examining previous findings. The literature search is not only a method of uncovering; it is also a way for the researcher to attain a historical perspective and overview of a problem.

Scientific research is a force that advances knowledge. For many scientists, discovery of new information or technology is a process of juxtaposing research from diverse fields in relation to an identifiable problem. Norbert Wiener (1948) in his work on cybernetics, which eventually led to the invention of the computer, attained success by brainstorming with engineers, psychiatrists, educators, and physicists. These specialists were able to share their ideas, and their collaboration stimulated the examination of a problem from many perspectives. Wiener, from this experience, developed a theory of thinking based on the integration of physical science theory with behavioral observations. The lesson from Wiener's careful research is that investigators exploring the literature should not only examine studies directly related to a problem, but should also try to find studies from other fields that have an indirect or implied relationship to their question.

If, for example, researchers are interested in examining the relationship between staff morale and treatment effectiveness, they would need to search the literature in management psychology if a preliminary search reveals a lack of studies in occupational therapy. The diversity of findings adds strength to a study, especially if corroboration of data appears from different professions.

The Hawthorne effect, which was first noted in factory workers, is now widely accepted as a factor in clinical treatment. Spinoffs from research in the space programs, such as the advances in nutrition, computer programming, temperature control, and monitoring of vital bodily functions, are examples of applying data generated from a seemingly unrelated field.

The investigator's main goals in searching the literature are to:

- Make an exhaustive search for related studies
- Identify the landmark studies that have an important impact in the area investigated
- Evaluate the validity of the research findings
- Integrate and synthesize the results into subject areas
- Summarize the findings from previous studies, highlighting areas where results are either inconclusive or controversial

These goals are part of the overall preliminary process of research that precedes data collection.

## 6.2 Conceptual View of a Literature Search

The steps involved in a conceptual view of the literature search are shown in Figure 6–1. Each of these steps is described below.

1. **The first step in initiating a literature search is to identify the key words in the study.** The **key words** may be identified through (a) reading a secondary source, (b) having experience with a particular population, (c) reviewing a journal article, or (d) examining a thesaurus of terms such as MeSH (http://www.ncbi.nlm.nih.gov/mesh). Use the MeSH database to find Medical Subject Heading Terms to build a literature search strategy. ERIC (Education and Resources Information Center; http://www.eric.ed.gov/) is another database that publishes a thesaurus. These key words can be linked to the independent variable (e.g., intervention technique), dependent variable (e.g., desired outcome), outcome measure (e.g., ACL), target population (e.g., individu-

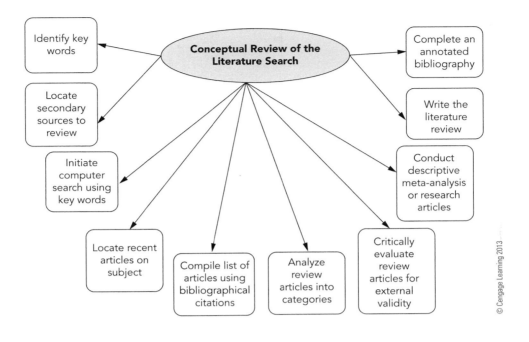

**FIGURE 6-1** Conceptual Review of the Literature Search

als with spinal cord injury), contextual setting (e.g., assisted living center), age range (e.g., older adults), or frame of reference (e.g., occupational behavior). Key words are important for researchers when initiating a computer search because they help to differentiate between similar materials. For example, if a researcher wants to examine the literature on sensory integration, use of the key words "sensory integration" will eliminate studies that examine NDT.

2. **The next step in a literature search is to locate a textbook or review article in which the researcher can obtain an overall summary of the major research in the specific area.** For example, a researcher may be interested in the effectiveness of occupational therapy on the achievement of students with learning disabilities. The researcher would examine a recent textbook or review article on pediatric occupational therapy to gain an overall view of treatment and to identify recent references. The textbook or review

article may help in the identification of key words and in narrowing the focus of the study.

3. **Next, the researcher is ready to do a computer search of recent articles in the field.** PubMed®, Google Scholar, MEDLINE®, CINAHL, or ERIC are examples of databases that can be used. Another way to examine recent articles is to look at the article in current issues or the cumulative yearly index in the journals. The *American Journal of Occupational Therapy* (AJOT) and *Occupational Therapy International* (OTI) are two examples of referral sources. Examining the bibliography in relevant articles may also help to locate other articles. After the researcher has identified relevant articles, it is important to file the bibliographic citations and abstract for later use. (See discussion of bibliographic citations later in this chapter.)

4. **The next step is the categorization of the articles into types of publications, such as review, research, or theoretical papers.** (See Table 6–1.)

## TABLE 6-1

**Categorization of Publications**

| Types of Publications | Examples of Publications |
| --- | --- |
| Primary Data Research | Journal articles<br>Dissertations<br>Theses<br>Conference proceedings<br>Government documents<br>Statistical surveys |
| Review Articles | Journal articles<br>Monographs |
| Evaluation Findings | Joint Commission on Accreditation Results<br>Special commissions |
| Conceptual or Theoretical Papers | Journal articles<br>Monographs<br>Conference proceedings |
| Position Papers | Journal articles<br>Associational and organizational statements<br>Monographs<br>Editorials |
| Secondary and Tertiary Information | Popular magazines<br>Scientific American<br>Encyclopedias<br>College texts |
| Other Publications | Test manuals<br>Reference books for test instruments<br>Book reviews<br>Software programs and reviews<br>Manuals for self-help devices |
| Bibliographic References | Books in Print<br>Information retrieval system<br>Directories of reference |

© Cengage Learning 2013

Articles can also be categorized into subject areas for easier review.

5. **The researcher must critically evaluate each article for external (i.e., generalization of results) and internal validity (i.e., rigor of the methodology).** The researcher examines how the variables were controlled, the subject selection, the randomness of the selection, reliability and validity of the outcome measures, and the operational definition of the independent variable.

6. **A descriptive tabulation of research studies identified by the literature review is the next step.** The researcher designs a table that includes the title of the study, the date of publication, the authors or researchers, number of subjects, treatment methodology, outcome measures, statistical results, and conclusions (Table 6–2).

7. **The researcher is now ready to write the literature review from an outline.** The review should include an integrated summary of the various articles.

## TABLE 6-2

### Effect of Exercise on Depression: Example of Descriptive Tabulation

| Study | Subjects | Treatment Technique | Outcome Measures | Results |
|---|---|---|---|---|
| Blue (1979). Aerobic running as a treatment of moderate depression. | 2 adult patients with chronic depression | Aerobic running program 3 times per week, for 9 weeks | Zung Self-Rating Depression Scale (SDS; Zung, 1965) | Significant reduction of depression. |
| Bosscher (1993). Running and mixed physical exercises with psychiatric patients who are depressed. | 24 men and women diagnosed with depression and hospitalized in psychiatric hospital | E[a]: short-term running therapy, 3 times a week for 8 weeks<br><br>C: Mixed physical and relaxation exercises, 3 times a week for 8 weeks | Zung Self-Rating Depression Scale (SDS; Zung, 1965) | Significant improvement for running group; no significant improvement for mixed physical and exercise group. |
| Brollier et al. (1994). Aerobic exercises: A potential occupational therapy modality for adolescents with depression. | 4 adolescent boys from a private psychiatric hospital with diagnosis of depression | Brisk walking and running 3 times a week for 1 hour over 65-day period | Beck Depression Inventory (BDI; Beck et al., 1961) | Results showed a general decrease in depression scores of all subjects. |
| Doyne et al. (1983). Aerobic exercise as a treatment of depression in women. | 4 women with major depressive disorder (MDD) | Aerobic exercise for 6 weeks | Beck Depression Inventory (BDI; Beck et al., 1961) Depression Adjective Check-Lists (DACL; Lubin, 1981) | Significant reduction in depression scores compared with pre-exercise screening phase. |
| Doyne et al. (1987). Running versus weight lifting in the treatment of depression. | 40 women diagnosed with depression | E$_1$: walked/ran on indoor track in 7-minute intervals for 8 weeks<br><br>E$_2$: used weight-lifting machine for 8 weeks<br><br>C: no treatment | Beck Depression Inventory (BDI; Beck et al., 1961); Hamilton Rating Scale for Depression (HRDS; Hamilton, 1960); Depression Adjective Check-Lists (DACL; Lubin, 1981) | Both aerobic and weight-lifting groups showed significant improvement in depression; no change in control group. |
| Greist et al. (1979). Running as a treatment for depression. | 13 men, 15 women, aged 18 to 30 | E: 10 patients ran 3 to 4 times/week<br><br>C: 18 in psychotherapy | Response Symptom Checklist (Greist et al., 1979) | Running as treatment for moderate depression was as effective as psychotherapy. |

*continues*

## TABLE 6-2

### Effect of Exercise on Depression: Example of Descriptive Tabulation *continued*

| | | | | |
|---|---|---|---|---|
| Kaplan et al. (1983). The effect of a jogging program on psychiatric inpatients with symptoms of depression. | 12 women, 6 men, aged 15 to 38, patients in acute care psychiatric ward | Warm-up and cool-down exercises; 20 minutes of graded walking/jogging on indoor track; short discussion of exercise and health-related topics | Self-report questionnaire (5-point Likert scale); observation by co-leaders | Decreased sleep disturbances and increased self-esteem. |
| Martinsen et al. (1985). Effects of aerobic exercise on depression: A controlled study. | 43 subjects, ages 17 to 60 with MDD | $E_1$: 9 patients receiving tricyclic antidepressants (TCAs) and aerobic exercise for 1 hour 3 times week for 9 weeks<br><br>$E_2$: 15 patients receiving aerobic exercise but no TCAs<br><br>$C_1$: 14 patients receiving TCAs and OT 3 times a week for 9 weeks<br><br>$C_2$: 5 patients receiving OT but not TCAs | *Psychopathological Rating Scale* (CPRS; Åsberg et al., 1978); *Beck Depression Inventory* (BDI; Beck et al., 1961) | Significantly lower depression scores for those participating in aerobic exercises than others; maximum oxygen uptake noted in aerobic training groups resulted in greater antidepressive effects. |
| Martinsen et al. (1989). Comparing aerobic with nonaerobic forms of exercise in the treatment of clinical depression: A randomized trial. | 90 inpatients in a psychiatric hospital with diagnosis of depression | E: 43 patients, brisk walks and jogging 3 times a week for 8 weeks<br><br>C: 47 patients; muscular strength, flexibility and relaxation, exercises 3 times week for 8 weeks | *Beck Depression Inventory* (BDI; Beck et al., 1961); *Montgomery and Åsberg Depression Rating Scale* (MADRS; Montgomery & Åsberg, 1979) | Depressed scores in both groups were reduced significantly, but no significant difference between groups. |
| Rape (1987). Running and depression. | 21 Caucasian males running 15 or more miles per week; 21 Caucasian males, non-exercisers | Matched two-group design comparing runners with non-exercisers | *Beck Depression Inventory* (BDI; Beck et al., 1961) | Runners were significantly less depressed than were non-exercisers. |

**Note:** *E* refers to the experimental group. *C* refers to the control group.

8. **Finally, the researcher should develop an annotated bibliography.** Articles should be organized by subject heading, with research articles listed separately from theoretical articles. The **annotated bibliography** includes the published **abstract**. The purpose of the abstract is to provide the reader with a quick overview of the problem under investigation, the methods used in data collection, the results reported, and the conclusions. The abstract is an intermediary step between the bibliographical citation and the complete journal article. Because the abstract is a self-contained summary, it can provide the researcher with all the information desired in a specific research area. The annotated bibliography serves as a primary data source for the research study. It also helps the reader gain an overview of the research study.

## 6.3 Locating Sources of Related Literature

More than 4,000 periodicals are currently published every year in medical and health-related areas. The task of searching the literature would be enormous if the investigator had to review each and every periodical individually. How can the investigator quickly obtain a list of studies that are relevant so as to narrow the search and reduce the number of hours examining the online catalog and library stacks? For the persevering investigator seeking to identify every study conceivable, the task could be endless. Realistically, the investigator accepts the limitation that some published and unpublished studies will not be located. For example, studies published in foreign journals that have not been translated, recent unpublished papers presented at conferences and institutes, ongoing research where the investigator has not published the findings, and research studies by students presented in unpublished theses, dissertations, or special studies may not be found. These are realistic limitations to every study. Nonetheless, with the availability of the Internet and computer systems for information retrieval, the present-day investigator is able to locate a vast portion of the literature.

The literature search is divided into two areas: referral sources and primary sources of data. These two areas are outlined in Table 6–3.

The first step in searching the literature is to locate where the relevant studies are reported, that is, in which journal, source book, or dissertation. The **referral source** supplies bibliographical information locating a specific study. The use of key words allows the student or researcher to

---

### TABLE 6-3

**Sources for Literature Search in Occupational Therapy**

| Referral Sources | Primary Sources of Data |
| --- | --- |
| • Information retrieval systems | • Journals |
| • Abstracting periodicals and bibliographic indexes | • Theses |
| • Directory of references | • Conference proceedings |
| • Annual reviews | • Government documents |
| | • Statistical compendiums |
| | • Unpublished studies |

*Ethical Dilemmas in School-Based Therapy: Implications for Occupational Therapy*

**Josephine Mae Smith**

**Key Words:** adolescence, learning disabilities, school-based ethics, occupational therapy, decision making

*Abstract:* An analysis…

© Cengage Learning 2013

**FIGURE 6-2**   An Example of Key Words Listed before the Abstract and Journal Article: The use of these key words will lead the reader to other related articles.

identify more easily those studies that cover a particular topic. Frequently, the key words for a specific article are listed immediately before or after the abstract. This is illustrated in Figure 6–2, in which the key words (adolescence, learning disabilities, school-based, ethics, occupational therapy, decision making) have been listed before the abstract. A student or researcher looking for related articles would use one or more of these key words in the computer search.

Each database has its own thesaurus that contains key words or concepts by using a controlled vocabulary. The controlled vocabulary provides a structure for classifying articles into given topics. Most databases are accessed online through library websites. Many of these searchable databases have, as a search option a "tick box" to search subject terms. If this option is selected, then based on the words entered into the search text box, a list of subject terms comes up. This list of subject terms can provide a more focused search strategy. For more specialized words, such as names of tests, specific intervention theories (e.g., sensory integration, cognitive-behavioral, or NDT), the exact term will suffice to locate the articles. As noted previously, MEDLINE® uses MeSH subject headings.

### The Thesaurus

MeSH is the National Library of Medicine's (NLMs) controlled vocabulary thesaurus. It consists of sets of terms naming descriptors in a hierarchical structure that permits searching at various levels of specificity.

MeSH descriptors are arranged in both an alphabetic and a hierarchical structure. At the most general level of the hierarchical structure are very broad headings such as "Anatomy" or "Mental Disorders." More specific headings are found at more narrow levels of the eleven-level hierarchy, such as "Ankle" and "Conduct Disorder." There are 25,588 descriptors in 2010 MeSH. There are also over 172,000 entry terms that assist in finding the most appropriate MeSH Heading, for example, "Vitamin C" is an entry term to "Ascorbic Acid." In addition to these headings, there are more than 190,000 headings called Supplementary Concept Records (formerly Supplementary Chemical Records) within a separate thesaurus.

### MeSH Applications

The MeSH thesaurus is used by NLM for indexing articles from 5,400 of the world's leading biomedical journals for the MEDLINE/PubMED® database. It is also used for the NLM-produced database that includes cataloging of books, documents, and audiovisuals acquired by the library. Each bibliographic reference is associated with a set of MeSH terms that describe the content of the item. Similarly, search queries use MeSH vocabulary to find items on a desired topic.

### Establishing and Updating MeSH

The Medical Subject Headings Section staff continually revise and update the MeSH vocabulary. Staff subject specialists are responsible for areas of the health sciences in which they have knowledge and expertise. In addition to receiving suggestions from indexers and others, the staff collect new terms as they appear in the scientific literature or in emerging areas of research; define these terms within the context of existing vocabulary; and recommend their addition to MeSH. Professionals in various disciplines are also consulted regarding broad organizational changes and close coordination is maintained with various specialized vocabularies.

### MeSH Data

MeSH, in machine-readable form, is provided at no charge via electronic means. The MeSH web site (http://www.nlm.nih.gov/mesh) is the central access point for additional information about MeSH and for obtaining MeSH in electronic form. (NLM, 2010a, para. 1-5)

Most information retrieval systems use **Boolean logic** as the strategy to build search statements. Boolean logic uses the logical operators *and, or,* and *not* to represent relationships between topics in a symbolic manner (see Figure 6–3). Some systems also use the search operators of *with* and *in*. The use of the term *with* identifies those articles in which the connected terms are used in the same field (e.g., "traumatic brain injury with cognitive-behavior therapy"), whereas the use of the term *in* specifies the particular field ("traumatic brain injury in title"). By combing search terms with these logical operators, the researcher can limit or enlarge the search.

For example, if a researcher is looking for articles regarding the treatment of traumatic brain injury using cognitive-behavior therapy in

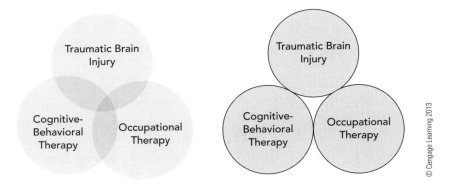

© Cengage Learning 2013

**FIGURE 6-3** An Example of Boolean Thinking: In the first example (the left diagram), the researcher is interested in information about *traumatic brain injury* AND *cognitive-behavior therapy* AND *occupational therapy*. The articles retrieved from the search will be found in the intersection that contains all three terms. In the second example (the right diagram), articles about *traumatic brain injury*, OR *cognitive-behavior therapy*, OR *occupational therapy* will be found. The first example is a more specific search that yields a smaller number of articles.

occupational therapy settings, the search term would be written as:

> traffic *traumatic brain injury and cognitive-behavior therapy and occupational therapy*

Use of these terms, as well as the delimiter *and*, would limit the search to only those articles in occupational therapy in which both traumatic brain injury and cognitive-behavior therapy have been discussed. Articles that contain only etiology or only treatment will not be obtained.

If, on the other hand, the researcher is interested in articles that describe either traumatic brain injury or cognitive-behavior therapy, the search statement is written as:

> *(Traumatic brain injury and occupational therapy) or (cognitive-behavior therapy and occupational therapy)*

Articles that examine either traumatic brain injury or cognitive-behavior therapy *and* occupational therapy, or both traumatic brain injury and cognitive-behavior therapy will be obtained. Thus, this search statement produces a larger list of citations, including the citations from the first search statement. Because each system uses a slightly different search technique, it will be necessary to obtain specific information about search strategies for the system used (e.g., OT Search, MEDLINE®, or ERIC).

## 6.3.1 Information Retrieval Systems

Automated systems for storing and retrieving information have revolutionized libraries. Though print-only journals still exist, many involve an online version, and many journals now are exclusively online. Through computer and Internet technology, persons seeking information have access to an enormous amount of information available through these electronic, online journals. Many of these online journals can be accessed through the journal's publisher for free or through a fee-based system. Many hospital and university libraries subscribe to various searchable database conglomerates and provide access to databases and electronic online journals for clinicians, faculty, staff, and students. The particular type of searchable database(s) offered by any given institution is determined by the type of subscription with which the institution has contracted. The major information retrieval systems relevant to research in medicine, rehabilitation, health care, and education are described in this section. Additionally, there are a few databases that are free to the public and can be accessed through any computer connected to the Internet, for example, PubMed® and Google Scholar.

**PubMed®** (http://www.ncbi.nlm.nih.gov/pubmed/)
PubMed® comprises more than 19 million citations for biomedical literature from MEDLINE®, life science journals, and online books. Citations may include links to full-text content from PubMed® Central and publisher web sites (http://www.ncbi.nlm.nih.gov/sites/entrez). PubMed® is accessible through any computer that is connected to the Internet.

**MEDLINE®** (Medical Literature Analysis and Retrieval System Online)
MEDLINE® is a database focused on biomedical literature. It has a fascinating history as a product of MEDLARS, which was developed during the Cold War as a repository of biomedical information.

> MEDLINE is the largest component of PubMed® (http://pubmed.gov), the freely accessible online database of biomedical journal citations and abstracts created by the U.S. National Library of Medicine (NLM®). Approximately 5,400 journals published in the United States and more than 80 other countries have

been selected and are currently indexed for MEDLINE. A distinctive feature of MEDLINE is that the records are indexed with NLM's controlled vocabulary, the Medical Subject Headings. (MeSH; NLM, 2010c, para. 1)

The National Network of Libraries of Medicine is composed of eight U.S. regional medical libraries that provide searches for health scientists. These federally designated regional medical libraries also provide consultative services and interlibrary loan privileges to other medical libraries within their region. Contact information for the National Library of Medicine Regional Offices (NN/LM) is listed in Table 6-4.

The National Library of Medicine houses a National Information Center on Health Services Research and Health Care Technology (NICHSR; see Box 6-1).

---

## TABLE 6-4

### National Library of Medicine Regional Offices

**Toll-Free Phone Number for all Regional Medical Libraries: (800) 338–7657**

| | |
|---|---|
| For general information, contact National Network of Libraries of Medicine (NN/LM)<br><br>National Network Office<br>National Library of Medicine<br>8600 Rockville Pike, Room B1–E03<br>Bethesda, MD 20894 | **Phone**: (301) 496–4777<br>**Fax**: (301) 480–1467<br>**URL**: http://nnlm.gov/ |
| **1. _Middle Atlantic Region_** (MAR; States served: DE, NJ, NY, PA)<br><br>NN/LM Middle Atlantic Region<br>New York University Medical Center<br>423 East 23rd Street, Floor 15 South<br>New York, NY 10010 | **Telephone within the MAR Region**: (800) 338–7657<br>**Outside of MAR Region**: (212) 263–2030<br>**Fax**: : (212) 263–4258<br>**URL**: http://nnlm.gov/mar/<br>**E-mail**: rml@library.med.nyu.edu |
| **2. _Southeastern/Atlantic Region_** ( SE/A; States served: AL, FL, GA, MD, MS, NC, SC, TN, VA, WV, the District of Columbia, Puerto Rico, and the U.S. Virgin Islands)<br><br>NN/LM SE/A Region<br>University of Maryland, Baltimore<br>Health Sciences and Human Services Library<br>601 W. Lombard Street<br>Baltimore, MD 21201–1512 | **Telephone within the SE/A Region**: (800) 338–7657, choice #1 on menu<br>**Outside of SE/A Region**: (410) 706–2855<br>**Fax**: (410) 706–0099<br>**URL**: http://nnlm.gov/sea/<br>**E-mail**: HSHSLNLMsea@hshsl.umaryland.edu |
| **3. _Greater Midwest Region_** (GMR; States served: IA, IL, IN, KY, MI, MN, ND, OH, SD, WI)<br><br>National Network of Libraries of Medicine<br>Greater Midwest Region<br>1750 W. Polk St. M/C 763<br>Chicago, IL 60612–4330 | **Telephone within the GMR Region**: (800) 338–7657 and option #1<br>**Outside of GMR Region**: (312) 996–2464<br>**Fax**: (312) 996–2226<br>**URL**: http://nnlm.gov/gmr/<br>**E-mail**: gmr4u@uic.edu |

*continues*

## TABLE 6-4

**National Library of Medicine Regional Offices** *continued*

**Toll-Free Phone Number for all Regional Medical Libraries: (800) 338–7657**

| | |
|---|---|
| **4. *Midcontinental Region*** (MCR; States served: CO, KS, MO, NE, UT, WY)<br><br>National Network of Libraries of Medicine/MidContinental Region (NN/LM-MCR)<br>University of Utah<br>Spencer S. Eccles Health Sciences Library<br>10 North 1900 East<br>Salt Lake City, UT 84112–5890 | **Telephone within the MCR Region**: (800) 338–7657<br>**Outside of MCR Region**: (801) 587–3412<br>**Fax**: (801) 581–5410<br>**URL**: http://nnlm.gov/mcr/<br>**E-mail**: rml4@rml4.utah.edu |
| **5. *South Central Region*** (SCR; States served: AR, LA, NM, OK, TX)<br><br>NN/LM South Central Region (NN/LM SCR)<br>Houston Academy of Medicine–Texas Medical Center (HAM–TMC) Library<br>1133 John Freeman Blvd.<br>Houston, TX 77030–2809 | **Telephone within the SCR Region**: (800) 338–7657<br>**Outside of SCR Region**: (713) 799–7880<br>**Fax**: (713) 790–7030<br>**URL**: http://nnlm.gov/scr/<br>**E-mail**: nnlm-scr@exch.library.tmc.edu |
| **6. *Pacific Northwest Region*** (PNR; States served: AK, ID, MT, OR, WA)<br><br>Regional Medical Library<br>University of Washington<br>Box 357155<br>1959 NE Pacific St.<br>Seattle, WA 98195–7155 | **Telephone within the PNR Region**: (800) 338–7657 (800 DEV ROKS)<br>**Outside of PNR Region**: (206) 543–8262<br>**Fax**: (206) 543–2469<br>**URL**: http://nnlm.gov/pnr/<br>**E-mail**: nnlm@u.washington.edu |
| **7. *Pacific Southwest Region*** (PSR; States served: AZ, CA, HI, NV, and U.S. Territories in the Pacific Basin)<br><br>University of California, Los Angeles (UCLA)<br>Louise Darling Biomedical Library<br>12-077 Center for the Health Sciences<br>Box 951798<br>Los Angeles, CA 90095–1798 | **Telephone within the PSR Region**: (800) 338–7657<br>**Outside of PSR Region**: (310) 825–1200<br>**Fax**: (310) 825–5389<br>**URL**: http://nnlm.gov/psr/<br>**E-mail**: psr-nnlm@library.ucla.edu |
| **8. *New England Region*** (NER; States served: CT, MA, ME, NH, RI, VT)<br><br>National Network of Libraries of Medicine, New England Region (NN/LM NER)<br>University of Massachusetts Medical School<br>222 Maple Ave.<br>Shrewsbury, MA 01545–2732 | **Telephone within the NER Region**: (800) 338–7657<br>**Outside of NER Region**: (508) 856–5979<br>**Fax**: (508) 856–5977<br>**URL**: http://nnlm.gov/ner/<br>**E-mail**: nnlm-ner@umassmed.edu |

BOX 6-1

## National Information Center on Health Services Research and Health Care Technology (NICHSR)

The 1993 NIH Revitalization Act created a National Information Center on Health Services Research and Health Care Technology (NICHSR) at the National Library of Medicine to improve "the collection, storage, analysis, retrieval, and dissemination of information on health services research, clinical practice guidelines, and on health care technology, including the assessment of such technology."

The Center works closely with the Agency for Healthcare Research and Quality (AHRQ), formerly the Agency for Health Care Policy and Research (AHCPR), to improve the dissemination of the results of health services research, with special emphasis on the growing body of evidence reports and technology assessments which provide organizations with comprehensive, science-based information on common, costly medical conditions and new health care technologies.

The overall goals of the NICHSR are: to make the results of health services research, including practice guidelines and technology assessments, readily available to health practitioners, health care administrators, health policy makers, payers, and the information professionals who serve these groups; to improve access to data and information needed by the creators of health services research; and to contribute to the information infrastructure needed to foster patient record systems that can produce useful health services research data as a by-product of providing health care.

### Products and Services

NICHSR coordinates the development of information products and services related to health services research.

- HealthSTAR (Health Services Technology, Administration, and Research) was an online bibliographic information service that resided as a separate database available from the National Library of Medicine from February 1994 (originally called HSTAR) to December 2000. Materials that comprised HealthSTAR, have now migrated to other NLM online web-based environments: (1) journal citations are being added weekly to NLM's PubMed (http://pubmed.gov/) (2) books, book chapters, technical reports, and conference papers are added regularly to NLM's online catalog, LocatorPlus (http://locatorplus.gov), and (3) meeting abstracts from AcademyHealth (formerly Academy for Health Services Research and Health Policy and the Association for Health Services Research), Health Technology Assessment International (HTAi) (formerly International Society of Technology Assessment in Health Care), and the Cochrane Colloquium annual conferences have moved to the NLM Gateway (http://gateway.nlm.nih.gov/). Users can go to these specific environments to search for HSR literature, or they can use the NLM Gateway to simultaneously search across all information services.

*continues*

- HSRProj (http://www.nlm.nih.gov/hsrproj/) and the NLM Gateway (http://gateway.nlm.nih.gov, under the Other Collections category), a database of citations to research-in-progress funded by federal and foundation grants and contracts, became available in 1995. HSRProj builds upon a database developed in prototype by staff of AcademyHealth and the Cecil Sheps Center at the University of North Carolina with funding from the Pew Charitable Trust. It includes over 5,000 citations to ongoing or recently completed research funded since 2000.
- HSRR (Health Services and Sciences Research Resources; http://www.nlm.nih.gov/nichsr/hsrr_search/), is a free searchable catalog of research datasets, instruments, and software relevant to health services research, behavioral and social sciences, and public health.
- HSTAT (Health Services/Technology Assessment Text; http://hstat.nlm.nih.gov), is a free, Web-based resource of full-text documents that provide health information and support health care decision making. HSTAT's audience includes health care providers, health service researchers, policy makers, payers, consumers, and the information professionals who serve these groups. It includes Agency for Healthcare Research and Quality (AHRQ) evidence reports, guideline documents, and technology assessments, NIH Consensus Development Conference Statements and Technology Assessment Workshop Reports, the U.S. Task Force on Preventive Services' Guide to Clinical Preventive Services, HIV/AIDS Treatment Information Service (ATIS) approved guidelines, and Substance Abuse and Mental Health Services Administration (SAMHSA) treatment improvement protocols.
- DIRLINE®, (available from NLM Gateway, http://gateway.nlm.nih.gov, under the Consumer Health category) NLM's Directory of Information Resources onLINE, has a special subfile covering health services research organizations including those involved in technology assessment and development of practice guidelines.

In addition to its online databases, NICHSR and other NLM staff develop guides, fact sheets, bibliographies, and other products targeted to health services researchers. To find many of these, go to the Health Services Research and Public Health Information Programs Web page at http://www.nlm.nih.gov/hsrph.html

### Outreach and Training

NICHSR collaborates with other NLM components and with members of the National Network of Libraries of Medicine® (NN/LM) to exhibit NLM products and services and to present specially focused training classes at national meetings of HSR-related organizations. NICHSR also provides training programs for medical librarians to improve their ability to respond to health services research questions and to support the conduct of such research, and training activities directed toward producers and users of health services research.

## Research and Development

NICHSR supports a number of intramural and extramural research and development projects designed to improve access to useful health services research data. Current efforts include: expansion of the Unified Medical Language System® (UMLS®) Metathesaurus® to improve its utility in creating and retrieving computer-based patient records; and funding of extramural research and evaluation involving the creation and use of computer-based patient records.

**For more information on NICHSR, contact:**

**National Information Center on Health Services Research and Health Care Technology (NICHSR)**

**National Library of Medicine**

**8600 Rockville Pike**

**Building 38A, Room 4S-410, Mail Stop 20**

**Bethesda, MD 20894**

Voice: (301) 496–0176; Fax: (301) 402–3193

E-mail: nichsr@nlm.nih.gov; Internet: http://www.nlm.nih.gov/nichsr/

NLM's home page is: http://www.nlm.nih.gov.

For a complete list of NLM Fact Sheets visit: http://www.nlm.nih.gov/pubs/factsheets/factsheets. html Or, write to: Office of Communications and Public Liaison, National Library of Medicine, 8600 Rockville Pike, Bethesda, Maryland 20894. Fax: (301) 496-4450: E-mail: publicinfo@nlm. nih.gov

(This material was obtained from the NICHSR fact sheet, available at http://www.nlm.nih.gov/pubs/factsheets/nichsr_ fs.html)

*OT Search* (http://www1.aota.org/otsearch/ index.asp)

OT Search, formerly called OT BibSys, is a bibliographic database that requires payment of a yearly fee. The American Occupational Therapy Association developed the database and owns it. Many occupational therapy programs pay the site fee so that their students and faculty can have access to the database. The database covers literature in the disciplines of occupational therapy and related subject areas, such as rehabilitation, education, psychiatry or psychology, and health care delivery or administration. Information that identifies the material and the abstract necessary for obtaining the full text of the indexed resources is available on the website (American Occupational Therapy Association, 1999–2011).

The repository for the official documents for AOTA along with OT search is located in the Wilma L. West Library.

AOTF's Wilma L. West (WLW) Library is home to a unique collection of resources that help to advance research, education, and leadership in occupational therapy and raise public awareness of the vital link between everyday living and health.

The collection includes monographs, journals, dissertations, theses, conference proceedings, and audio-visual materials covering the literature of occupational therapy and related subject areas, including rehabilitation, education, psychiatry or psychology, and health care delivery/ administration.

The contents of the WLW Library are indexed in OT SEARCH [which] is an online bibliographic database with over 39,400 bibliographic records. Drawing from this database, the library operates as a national clearinghouse of occupational therapy information for AOTA members and occupational therapy professionals. Librarians can assist in performing literature searches, obtain factual information for specific queries, provide guidance on additional sources of information, or send photocopies of documents in compliance with copyright laws. [Nominal] charges apply for literature searches and document delivery services. …

The WLW Library also houses a variety of resources related to research, education, and occupational therapy practice. These resources include:

- WLW Library Resource Notes
- Research Competencies for Occupational Therapy
- Responsible Conduct of Research
- Research Priorities and Parameters of Practice for Occupational Therapy
- Research Across the Curriculum Archives of the American Occupational Therapy Association (AOTA), which are housed in the WLW Library. (American Occupational Therapy Foundation, 1998–2011, para. 1–5)

### CINAHL (Cumulative Index to Nursing & Allied Health; http://www.cinahl.com)

This database, updated monthly, covers English-language journals and literature from 1982 to the present in the disciplines of nursing and allied health, including emergency services, health education, and social services in health care. Publications from the following allied health fields are indexed:

- Athletic Training
- Audiology
- Cardiopulmonary Technology
- Dental Hygiene
- Emergency Services
- Health Information Management
- Medical Assisting
- Medical/Laboratory Technology
- Nutrition & Dietetics
- Occupational Therapy
- Physical Therapy and Rehabilitation
- Physician Assistants
- Radiologic Technology
- Respiratory Therapy
- Social Service in Health Care
- Speech-Language Pathology
- Surgical Technology

Selected journals are also indexed in the areas of consumer health, biomedicine, and health sciences librarianship, to just name a few. In total, more than 2,980 journals are regularly indexed; of these, more than 600 provide full-text articles. CINAHL maintains more than 2 million records. The database also provides access to healthcare books, nursing dissertations, selected conference proceedings, standards of professional practice, educational software, and audiovisual materials in nursing and other health-related fields. CINAHL uses nearly 13,000 subject headings. More information about CINAHL can be found at http://www.ebscohost.com/cinahl/.

### ERIC (Educational Resources Information Center; http://eric.ed.gov/)

ERIC is a database of materials used by educators, researchers, and the general public. It is sponsored by the Institute of Education Sciences (IES) in the U.S. Department of Education and provides access to more than 1.3 million bibliographic records of journal and non-journal literature from 1966 to the present. Full-text materials in ADOBE PDF format, as well as bibliographic sources, are available. Materials include journal articles, books, research syntheses, conference papers, technical reports, and policy papers.

### PsychINFO (http://www.apa.org/pubs/databases/psycinfo/index.aspx)

PsychINFO is an online database with over 2.8 million records that covers the disciplines of psychology and related fields, including psychiatry, sociology, anthropology, education, pharmacology, physiology, linguistics, psychopharmacology, and other areas as well. PsychINFO indexes records published from the 1800s with some material being originally published in the seventeenth and eighteenth centuries. The records include journal articles, books, dissertations, and other secondary publications.

### REHABDATA

(http://www.naric.com/research/rehab/default.cfm)

With over 75,000 records, this database, sponsored by the National Rehabilitation Information Center, lists citations of research, reports, monographs, and other material that focus on rehabilitation of individuals with physical or intellectual disabilities. The database, funded by the National Institute on Disability and Rehabilitation Research (NIDRR), is to provide information to anyone who has an interest in learning more about the issues related to and surrounding disabilities.

### ABLEDATA (http://www.abledata.com)

ABLEDATA, also funded by NIDRR, provides information in the area of assistive technology and rehabilitation equipment.

> AbleData's most significant resource is the AbleData database of assistive technology, which contains objective information on more than 35,000 assistive products (over 22,000 of which are currently available). For each product, we provide a detailed description of the product's functions and features, price information (when available), and contact information for the product's manufacturer and/or distributors. We also offer information on non-commercial prototypes, customized and one-of-a-kind products, and do-it-yourself designs. (AbleData, n.d., para. 3)

### OTseeker

(http://www.otseeker.com/default.aspx)

> OTseeker is a database that contains abstracts of systematic reviews and randomised controlled trials relevant to occupational therapy. Trials have been critically appraised and rated to assist you to evaluate their validity and interpretability. These ratings will help you to judge the quality and usefulness of trials for informing clinical interventions. In one database, OTseeker provides you with fast and easy access to trials from a wide range of sources. (OTseeker, n.d., para. 1)

Using the search window, users can determine the internal validity, as well as the statistical integrity, of the study. The database was initiated in 2003 and is updated on a regular basis.

### Other Databases

*OTDBase* (http://www.otdbase.org/) is provided for a modest fee and contains abstracts from about 20 international occupational therapy journals. The system is user-friendly and cross-indexes articles.

*OVID* (http://www.ovid.com) accesses several databases (e.g., MEDLINE® and CINAHL). Because additional databases are being developed, the reader may want to explore library sources and online services for additional information.

*Embase*, or the *Excerpta Medica Database* (http://embase.com) is a comprehensive biomedical and pharmacological database produced by Elsevier. Over 20 million indexed records from more than 7,000 peer-reviewed journals are available.

*Internet Mental Health* (http://www.mentalhealth.com/) is a free web database that provides information on the 54 most common mental disorders.

*Health Education Research* (http://her.oxfordjournals.org/) publishes original, refereed papers that are germane to vital issues in health education, as well as the promotion of health education from around the world. In so doing, the journal provides a valuable link between research and practice.

*Health Administration Press* (http://www.ache.org/pubs/abouthap.cfm).

*Health Administration Press* is a division of the Foundation of the American College of Healthcare Executives (ACHE). Founded in 1972 with support from the W. K. Kellogg Foundation, Health Administration Press has grown from a small office on the campus of the University of Michigan to one of the largest publishers of books and journals on all aspects of health services management, including textbooks for use in undergraduate and graduate courses. (American College of Healthcare Executives, 2008, para. 1)

*CSA Sociological Abstracts* (http://www.csa.com/factsheets/socioabs-set-c.php), managed by ProQuest, formerly Sociological Abstracts, provides abstracts from more than 1,800 serials published in sociology and related disciplines. The database also provides abstracts of books, book chapters, dissertations, and conference papers. Records are available from 1952 to the present.

*Social Work Abstracts* (http://www.naswpress.org/publications/journals/swab.html), formerly *Social Work Research and Abstracts*, is published in print format four times a year. It is also available online through the OVID or EBSCO databases. The journal focuses on social work and social welfare using over 500 national and international journals. Approximately 900 abstracts are published each quarter.

*Dissertation Abstracts Online* (http://library.dialog.com/bluesheets/html/bl0035.html)

> *Dissertation Abstracts Online* is a definitive subject, title, and author guide to virtually every American dissertation accepted at an accredited institution since 1861. Selected Masters theses have been included since 1962. In addition, since 1988, the database includes citations for dissertations from 50 British universities that have been collected by and filmed at The British Document Supply Centre. (ProQuest Information and Learning, 2000, p. 1)

*Biological Abstracts* (http://www.ovid.com/site/catalog/DataBase/24.pdf) report the world's bioscience research. This database contains more than 11.3 million records with more than 250,000 being added every year. Indexed are journal records in areas of life science, genetics, anatomy, physiology, environmental pollutants, nutrition, psychiatry, public health, as well as other biology related records.

*Science Citation Index Expanded* (http://thomsonreuters.com/products_services/science/science_products/a-z/science_citation_index_expanded//) and *Social Science Citation Index* (http://thomsonreuters.com/products_services/science/science_products/a-z/social_sciences_citation_index). These databases provide "researchers, administrators, faculty, and students with quick, powerful access to the bibliographic and citation information they need to find research data, analyze trends, journals and researchers, and share their findings" (Thomson Reuters, 2011b, para. 1). Additionally, one can retrieve information about published works that have cited specific authors or published materials.

*Current Contents Connect*® (http://thomsonreuters.com/products_services/science/science_products/a-z/current_contents_connect/) is a:

> current awareness database that provides easy Web access to complete tables of contents, abstracts, bibliographic information, and abstracts from the most recently published issues of leading scholarly journals, as well as from more than 7,000 relevant, evaluated websites. Also included is full bibliographic information from some electronic journals before they are published. (Thomson Reuters, 2011a, para. 1)

*NIH Office of Extramural Research* (http://grants.nih.gov/grants/oer.htm) is an online database that contains information about health research currently supported by various agencies of the National Institutes of Health, thereby allowing scientists and administrators of science programs to identify current research activities in areas relating to their own endeavors.

*Annual Reviews* (http://www.annualreviews.org/) "publishes authoritative reviews in 40 focused disciplines within the Biomedical, Life, Physical, and Social Sciences. Among the most highly cited in scientific literature, they are available online and in print to individuals, institutions, and consortia worldwide" (Annual Reviews, 2010, para. 1).

*Google Scholar* (http://scholar.google.com/intl/en/scholar/about.html).

> *Google Scholar* provides a simple way to broadly search for scholarly literature. From one place, you can search across many disciplines and sources: articles, theses, books, abstracts and court opinions, from academic publishers, professional societies, online repositories, universities and other web sites. Google Scholar helps you find relevant work across the world of scholarly research. (Google Scholar, 2010, para. 1) Similar to the Science Citation Index database, records in Google Scholar are linked to other published work that has cited that record. Google Scholar can be accessed by any computer that has Internet access.

*The Cochrane Library* (http://www.thecochranelibrary.com/view/0/index.html) "is a collection of six databases that contain different types of high-quality, independent evidence to inform health-care decision-making, and a seventh database that provides information about groups in The Cochrane Collaboration" (The Cochrane Library, 2010a, para. 1). Associated with the Cochrane Library is the Cochrane Systematic Reviews of randomized control trials. These systematic reviews attempt:

> to identify, appraise and synthesize all the empirical evidence that meets pre-specified eligibility criteria to answer

a given research question. Researchers conducting systematic reviews use explicit methods aimed at minimizing bias, in order to produce more reliable findings that can be used to inform decision making. (The Cochrane Library, 2010b, para. 1)

### 6.3.2 Sources for Health Statistics

Statistical information is an essential part of the literature search. The incidence of diseases, hospitalization rates, occupational accidents, infant mortality rates, and the leading causes of death are examples of data compiled by government agencies and published in periodicals available to researchers. A common source of primary statistical information, located at http://www.cdc.gov/nchs/Default.htm, is the National Center for Health Statistics.

FEDSTATS, available at http://www.fedstats.gov/, provides additional information.

> **FedStats**, which has been available to the public since 1997, provides access to the full range of official statistical information produced by the Federal Government without having to know in advance which Federal agency produces which particular statistic. With convenient searching and linking capabilities to more than 100 agencies that provide data and trend information on such topics as economic and population trends, crime, education, health care, aviation safety, energy use, farm production and more, FedStats is your one location for access to the full breadth of Federal statistical information. (FedStats, 2007, para. 1)

Statistical reports are issued periodically. The Vital and Health Statistic Series, complied by the National Center for Health Statistics, may be useful to health care researchers. The complete list of this series is available at http://www.cdc.gov/nchs/products/series.htm.

- *Series 1: Programs and collection procedures:* Reports that describe the general programs of the National Center for Health Statistics and its offices and divisions, data collection methods used, definitions, and other material necessary for understanding the data.
- *Series 2: Data evaluation and methods of research:* Studies of new statistical methodology including experimental tests of new survey methods, studies of vital statistics collection methods, new analytical techniques, objective evaluations of reliability of collected data, and contributions to statistical theory.
- *Series 3: Analytical and epidemiological studies:* Reports presenting analytical or interpretive studies based on vital and health statistics, carrying the analysis further than the expository types of reports in the other series.
- *Series 4: Documents and committee reports:* Final reports of major committees concerned with vital and health statistics and documents, such as recommended model vital registration laws and revised birth and death certificates.
- *Series 5: International vital and health statistics reports:* Analytical and descriptive reports comparing U.S. vital and health statistics with those of other countries.
- *Series 6: Cognition and survey measurement:* Measurement using methods of cognitive science to design, evaluate, and test survey instruments.
- *Series 10: Data from the National Health Interview Survey:* Statistics on illness, accidental injury, disability, use of hospital, medical, dental, and other services, and other health-related topics, based on data collected in a continuing national household interview survey.
- *Series 11: Data from the National Health Examination Survey; the National Health and Nutrition Examination Surveys, and the Hispanic Health and Nutrition Examination Survey:* Data from direct examination, testing, and measurement of national samples of the population provide the basis for two types of reports: (a) estimates of the medically defined prevalence of specific diseases in the United States and the distributions of the noninstitutionalized population with respect to physical, physiological, and psychological characteristics; and (b) analysis of relationships among the various measurements without reference to an explicit finite universe of persons.
- *Series 12: Data from the institutional population surveys:* Statistics relating to the health characteristics of persons in institutions and on medical, nursing, and personal care received, based on national samples of establishments providing these services and samples of the residents or patients. This series was discontinued after 1969. Information in this series appears in Series 13.
- *Series 13: Data from the National Health Care Survey:* Statistics on the utilization of health manpower and facilities providing long-term care, ambulatory care, and family planning services.
- *Series 14: Data on health resources: Manpower and facilities:* Statistics on the numbers, geographic distribution, and characteristics of health sources including physicians, dentists, nurses, other health manpower occupations, hospitals, nursing homes, outpatient and other inpatient facilities.
- *Series 15: Data from special surveys:* Statistics on health and health-related topics collected in special surveys that are not a part of the continuing data systems of the National Center for Health Statistics.
- *Series 16: Compilations of advance data from vital and health statistics:* These reports provide early release of data from the health and demographic surveys of the National Center for Health Statistics. Many of these releases are followed by detailed reports in the Vital and Health Statistics Series.
- *Series 20: Data on mortality:* Various statistics on mortality other than as included in regular annual or monthly reports. Special analyses by cause of death, age, and other demographic variables; geographic and time series analyses;

and statistics on characteristics of death not available from the vital records based on sample surveys of those records.

The Global Health Observatory (http://www.who.int/gho/en/) "is the WHO's portal providing access to data and analyses for monitoring the global health situation. It provides critical data and analyses for key health themes, as well as direct access to the full database" (World Health Organization, 2010, para. 1). Data from the WHO programs, including health-related databases, reports, and geographical maps and country profiles from WHO member nations, can be found here.

The *Demographic Yearbook* and other reports are published by the statistical office of the United Nations, Department of Economic and Social Affairs, New York (http://unstats.un.org/unsd/demographic/default.htm). Statistics compiled from 250 countries of the world are included. Topics include population rates, mortality rates by disease, life expectancy tables, and marriage, divorce, and migration statistics.

Other statistical compendiums include the following:

- *American Statistics Index* (ASI), published by Congressional Information Service, contains all data collected by the federal government in various subjects (http://library.lexisnexis.com/ws_display.asp?filter=CIS Executive Branch)
- U.S. Bureau of the Census (http://www.census.gov/)
- U.S. Bureau of Labor Statistics (http://www.bls.gov/)
- U.S. Department of Agriculture (http://www.usda.gov/wps/portal/usda/usdahome)

### 6.3.3 Directories of References

**Directories of references** are books that provide a comprehensive source for locating studies in specified fields. They provide lists and short reviews of available textbooks, journals, bibliographies, dictionaries, atlases, databases, and government documents. The following directories are a sample of the many reference resources available to the clinical researcher. The main limitation of directories is the rapidity with which new sources of information are created, which makes it almost impossible for a directory to be up to date. When using a directory, the researcher should be aware of the copyright date.

- Blake, J. B., & Roos, C. (Eds.). (1967). *Medical reference works 1679–1966: A selected bibliography*. Chicago: Medical Library Assoc. The purpose of the publication, as stated by the editors, is "To survey the world's bioscientific, medical, and allied health literature and select and organize from it an annotated list of the major works useful in gaining access to publications or frequently needed data" (p. iii). Indexes and abstracts, bibliographies, proceedings of Congress, dictionaries, periodicals, and directories related to such areas as medicine, anatomy, medical education, hospitals, neurology, psychiatry, nursing, nutrition, pediatrics, physical medicine and rehabilitation, psychology, public health research in progress, and sociology are listed in the publication.
- Bowker Company (2011; http://www.greyhouse.com/bowk_med.htm /), a leading source for national and international bibliographic information, in both printed material and digital material. The company provides information to consumers in such areas as books and serials in print. Typically used by librarians and book sellers, it can be a resource for finding specific books in the health sciences.
- Post, S. G. (Ed.). (2004). *Encyclopedia of bioethics: Volumes 1–5* (3rd ed.). New York: Gale Cengage Learning/Macmillan Reference USA. Also available in electronic format (eBook). The fifth volume may be of special interest, as it contains the appendices, including primary documents, numerous bibliographies, and a list of additional resources.
- Huber, J. T., Boorkman, J. A., & Blackwell, J. (2008). *Introduction to reference sources in the health sciences* (5th ed.). New York: Neal-Schuman Publishers. The book contains bibliographic and informational sources of monographs,

periodicals, abstracting services, databases, U.S. government documents and technical reports, conferences, medical and health statistics, and audiovisual reference sources.

- Walters, L., Kahn, T. J., & Goldstein, D. M. (Eds.). (2009). *Bibliography of bioethics* (Vol. 35). Washington, DC: Georgetown University, Kennedy Institute. This bibliography of bioethical topics has been published annually since 1975. It provides a comprehensive cross-disciplinary listing of journals, newspaper articles, monographs, essays, court decisions, and audiovisual materials. The bibliography is designed for anyone concerned with bioethics, including scientists, health professionals, and legal scholars. (http://bioethics. georgetown.edu/publications/biobib/index.html)

### 6.3.4 Current Research

Current research not included in computer retrieval systems or annual reviews can be found in most recently published periodicals. Most university and medical libraries have reading rooms where current scientific journals are placed on open shelves.

A perusal of newly published articles may be helpful in gaining an overview of a topic and establishing an up-to-date bibliography of related literature. Key words often will be listed under the abstract. Use of these key words to identify additional literature through databases and indexes may result in additional material. Current journals will also be helpful in locating individuals engaged in ongoing research, allowing researchers to request current reprints of articles, unpublished research, and conference papers. In general, most scholars will be flattered to receive requests from individuals genuinely interested in their work, and they will respond readily. The standard format in requesting reprints is to list the bibliographical citation (i.e., journal, volume, date, and title) as in the example in Figure 6-4.

### 6.3.5 Journals

A list of occupational therapy journals published around the world is supplied in Table 6–5. A list of biomedical journals that generally follow the manuscript requirements for the International Committee for Medical Journals is available at http://www.icmje.org/journals.html; whereas a list of biomedical journals, most of which are open access (e.g., immediately and permanently available online without charge) can be found at http://www.biomedcentral.com/browse/journals/.

Mary Johnson (mjohnson@yahoo.com)
Sent: Friday July 16, 2011 3:20 PM
To: John T. Clark

Dear Mr. Clark,
Please send me a reprint of your article Occupational Therapy for Adults with Alzheimer's published in Occupational Therapy for Adults (2010), volume 8, pp. 35-40.

If it is in electronic form, please send it to mjohnson@yahoo.com. If it is in print, please send it to Mary Johnson, 1927 Main Street, Anytown, ME 02217.

Thank you very much.

Mary Johnson

© Cengage Learning 2013

**FIGURE 6-4** An Example of an E-mail Request for an Article: Notice that the request includes the author, title of article, date of article, journal, and page numbers. If the article is unpublished, the request should state that.

## TABLE 6-5

**Compendium of Journals in Occupational Therapy**

### American Journal of Occupational Therapy (AJOT)

Website: http://www.aota.org/Pubs/AJOT_1.aspx

Editor-in-chief: Sharon Gutman

4720 Montgomery Lane

PO Box 31220

Bethesda, MD 20824-1220 USA

Phone: (301) 652–2682 ext. 2864

Fax: (301) 652–7711

### Australian Occupational Therapy Journal (AOJT)

Website: http://www.wiley.com/bw/journal.asp?ref=0045-0766&site=1

E-mail: cs-journals@wiley.com

Editor: Elspeth Froude

Journal Customer Services

John Wiley & Sons Inc.

350 Main Street

Malden MA 02148 USA

Tel (toll free): (800) 835–6770

### British Journal of Occupational Therapy (BJOT)

Website: http://www.cot.co.uk/bjot/

E-mail: Elizabeth.Thorogood@cot.co.uk

BJOT Editorial Assistant

106–114 Borough High Street

Southwark, London, SE1 1LB England

Phone: +020 7357 6480

### Canadian Journal of Occupational Therapy (CJOT)

Website: http://www.caot.ca/

E-mail: cjoteditor@caot.ca

Editor: Marcia Finlayson

CAOT

CTTC Bldg

3400–1125 Colonel By Dr.

Ottawa, ON K1S 5R1 Canada

Phone: (613) 523–2268

Fax: (613) 523–2552

*continues*

**TABLE 6-5**

**Compendium of Journals in Occupational Therapy** *continued*

### Ergotherapie & Rehabilitation (German Journal of OT) (E&R)

E-mail: dwolf@schulz-kirchner.de OR c.berting@et-reha.dve.info

Editor: Christa Berting-Huneke

Schulz-Kirchner Verlag GmbH

Frau Dagmar Wolf

Mollweg 2

D-65510 Idstein, Germany

Phone: +49 6126 9320-0

Fax: +49 6126 9320-50

### Ergoscience (ERGOS)

Ergoscience is produced by Editors from Germany, Switzerland, Austria, and the Netherlands.

Website: http://www.thieme-connect.de/ejournals/toc/ergoscience/

E-mail: helpdesk@thieme-connect.d

### ErgOThérapie (ErgOT)

Website: http://www.anfe.fr

E-mail: edition@technimediaservices.fr

Editor: editergo@yahoo.fr

Association Nationale Francais des Ergothérapeutes

Service Abonnements (Subscriptions)

B.P.1

59 361 AVESNES SUR HELPE CEDEX

Tel : 03 27 56 38 56 Fax: 03 27 61 22 52

### Hong Kong Journal of Occupational Therapy (HKOTA)

Website: http://www.hkjot-online.com/

Editor: Kenneth N.K. Fong

The *Hong Kong Journal of Occupational Therapy* is an official publication of the Hong Kong Occupational Therapy Association (HKOTA).

### Hand Therapy (HT)

E-mail: bahthandtherapy@googlemail.com

Publisher: The Royal Society of Medicine Press Ltd.

Published for The British Hand Therapists Ltd. and The European Federation of Societies for Hand Therapy

BAHT

PO Box 304

WOODBRIDGE

IP12 9EX

Telephone: +01 394610131

NOTE: Listed as British Journal of Hand Therapy (BJHT) thru 2009, then HT from 2009 to present.

### Israeli Journal of Occupational Therapy (IJOT)

Website: http://www.isot.org.il

E-mail: isot@barak-online.net

Israeli Society of Occupational Therapy

P.O. Box 24148

Tel Aviv 61241, Israel

Alternative Address: P.O. Box 101

Woodmere, NY 11598 USA

Phone & Fax: (516) 569–0830

### Indian Journal of Occupational Therapy for All India OT Association (IJOT[India])

For full free text copy go to:

Website: http://www.medind.nic.in/iba/ibam.shtml

E-mail: anilsrivastava20@hotmail.com

Editor, Anil K. Srivastava

93 Laxmanpuri Faizabad Road,

Lucknow 226016 (India)

Tel.: (0522) 2350482, (0522) 3958974

### Irish Journal of Occupational Therapy (IJOT)

Website: http://www.aoti.ie

E-mail: aoti@eircom.net

Association of Occupational Therapists of Ireland

P.O. Box 11555

Ground Floor Office, Bow Bridge House

Bow Lane

Kilmainham, Dublin 8 IRELAND

Phone/fax: +01 6337222

### Journal of Japanese Association of Occupational Therapists (JJAOT)

E-mail: dep.international@jaot.or.jp

Morimitsu-shinko Bldg., 1–5–9

Kotobuki, Taito-ku, Tokyo 111–0042 Japan

Phone: 03 5826 7871 (from abroad +81-3-5826-7871)

Fax: 03 5826 872 (from abroad 03-5826-7872)

### Journal of Occupational Science (JOS)

Website: http://www.jos.edu.au/

E-mail: JOSsecretary@unisa.edu.au

*continues*

> ## TABLE 6-5

**Compendium of Journals in Occupational Therapy** *continued*

School of Occupational Therapy

University of South Australia

North Terrace

Adelaide, South Australia, 5000 Australia

NOTE: Listed as Journal of Occupational Science Australia: JOSA thru 1998, then JOS from 1999 to present.

### New Zealand Journal of Occupational Therapy (NZJOT)

Website: http://www.nzaot.com/publications/journal/download.php#

E-mail: nzaot@nzaot.com

Level 9, 85 The Terrace

PO Box 10–493

Wellington 6143 New Zealand

Tel: +64 4 473-6510

Fax: +64 4 473-6513

### Occupational Therapy International (OTI)

Website: http://wileyonlinelibrary.com/journal/oti

Editor: Franklin Stein (fstein@usd.edu)

John Wiley & Sons, Inc.

Attn: Journals Admin Dept UK

111 River Street

Hoboken, NJ 07030 USA

Phone: (800) 385–6770 or (201) 748–6645

### OTJR: Occupation, Participation and Health (OTJR)

Website: http://www.otjronline.com

E-mail: OTJR@slackinc.com

Managing Editor

6900 Grove Road

Thorofare, NJ 08086–9447 USA

Telephone: (856) 848–1000

Fax: (856) 853–5991

NOTE: As of 2002, OTJR filed on library shelves under OTJR, NOT Occupational Therapy Journal of Research.

**Occupational Therapy in Mental Health (OTMH); Occupational Therapy in Health Care (OTHC); Physical and Occupational Therapy in Pediatrics (POTP); Physical and Occupational Therapy in Geriatrics (POTG)**

These four journals are from:

Website: http://www.TaylorandFrancis.com

Taylor & Francis Group

325 Chestnut Street, Philadelphia, PA, 19106 USA

Phone: (800) 354–1420

**Occupational Therapy Now/Actualités Ergothérapiques (OTNow)**

CAOT's Practice Magazine

Website: http://www.caot.ca

Full articles from 1997 online for CAOT members at CAOT

CAOT Publications ACE

Phone: (800) 434–2268

**Philippine Journal of Occupational Therapy (PJOT)**

E-mail: lyle_d5@yahoo.com

Editor: R. Lyle Duque, Program Director

Editor, Philippine Journal of Occupational Therapy

Life Skills Therapy Center

30 Earth St.

San Sebastian Village

Tarlac City 2300, Philippines

Phone: +63 919 3271720

**South African Journal of Occupational Therapy (SAJOT)**

Website: http://www.sajot.co.za/index.php/sajot

E-mail: sajot@mweb.co.za

Editor: Marj Concha

Occupational Therapy Association of South Africa

PO Box 11695

Hatfield, 0028, SOUTH AFRICA

Tel: + 0117832589

Fax: + 0117832589

**Scandinavian Journal of Occupational Therapy (SJOT)**

Website: http://informahealthcare.com/occ

Informa Healthcare

Box 3255

103 65 Stockholm, Sweden

Tel: +46-(0)8-440 80 40

Fax: +46-(0)8-440 80 50

*continues*

© Cengage Learning 2013

---

TABLE 6-5

**Compendium of Journals in Occupational Therapy** *continued*

---

**Revista Terapia Ocupacional Galicia (TOG)**

Website: http://www.revistatog.com

E-mail: miguelrevistatog@yahoo.es

Editor: Miguel Angel Talavera Valverde

Publisher Journal: The Galician Professional Association of Occupational Therapist (APGTO)

**World Federation of Occupational Therapy Bulletin (WFOT)**

Website: http://www.wfot.org

E-mail: admin@wfot.org.au

World Federation of Occupational Therapists

PO Box 30

Forrestfield

Western Australia

Australia 6058

Fax: 61 8 9453 9746

---

## 6.4 Recording Information from Research Articles

The beginning researcher should develop a system for recording, organizing, and storing information related to a content area. It is important to develop this system early in the process by recording bibliographic information from all sources at the time it is obtained, even if the researcher may not later use the material (Englehart, 1972). The reconstruction of bibliographic sources at a later time can be time-consuming and difficult. An effective method of organizing data is to use a letter-size folder for each subject heading or variable in a study. Some investigators photocopy studies from periodicals or newspapers that relate to a specific area. Using information obtained from each of these articles, researchers are able to compile an up-to-date annotated bibliography.

In recording notes from a study, 3 × 5 index cards are helpful when compiling a bibliography, whereas 5 × 8 index cards may be useful for more extensive information, such as long quotes or abstracts. An example of a card is shown in Figure 6–5. The card should contain the following information from each study:

1. A bibliographical notation that includes all information used in a citation (See Chapter 9 for examples of citations.)
2. Library call number or ERIC number can be helpful also, as this allows the researcher to find the publication quickly
3. Abstract of study, including number of subjects, data collection methodology, test instruments, results, and conclusions
4. Important quotations (including page numbers) that can be cited in the literature review
5. Any reactions to the article, such as evaluation of the validity of results or generalizations offered

By recording this information accurately, the researcher saves time and effort from having to return to the source of the information whether it be in the library or from an information site on the Internet. Researchers should obtain information from many different types of publications. Although original sources

Braverman, S. E., Spector, J., Warden, D. L., Wilson, B. C., Ellis, T. E., & Bamdad, M. J. (1999). Multidisciplinary TBI inpatient rehabilitation programme for active duty service members as part of a randomized, clinical trial. Brain Injury, 13(6), 405-415.

OBJECTIVE: To evaluate the effectiveness of a multidisciplinary rehabilitation program for military service members with moderate brain injury

DESIGN: Randomized control trial

SETTING: Impatient rehabilitation program in a U.S. military tertiary care hospital

PATIENTS: 67 active-duty individuals with moderate to severe TBI

INTERVENTION: "Eight week rehabilitation program combining group and individual therapies with an inpatient milieu-oriented neuropsychological focus. Group therapies included fitness, planning and organization, cognitive skills, work skills, medication, and milieu groups, and community re-entry outings. Individual therapy included neuropsychology, work therapy, occupational therapy, and speech and language pathology" (p. 405)

Continued

---

DESIRED OUTCOME: Successful return to work and return to duty.

RESULTS: At 1-year follow-up, 64 individuals returned to work (96%), and 66% (44/67) returned to duty.

CONCLUSION: The multidisiplinary rehabilitation program demonstrated an effective approach to rehabilitate military service members with TBI.

REACTION:
- may not be generalizable to nonmilitary personnel
- doesn't operationationally define outcome measures
- can the research design be replicated?

FIGURE 6-5   An Example of an Index Card Used in Collecting Information from Articles

should be used for citation, valuable information can be gleaned from secondary and tertiary sources.

## 6.5 Evaluating Validity of Research Findings

The finding and citing of research are not the final processes in reviewing literature. A critical analysis is a vital task of the investigator. One of the more difficult tasks in a literature review is the ability to review the articles in an integrated fashion. One cannot evaluate and critique each article separately; rather, the integration of the information must be done by synthesizing the information (Finley, 1989). One outcome of this type of evaluation is that the reader begins to build a conceptual framework, thereby allowing for a more mature evaluation of other literature in the field.

The quality of the research and the validity of the conclusions need to be evaluated before the research can be integrated with other results. When contradictory results arising from different studies occur, the investigator should seek to offer an explanation based on the research methodologies. Occasionally,

investigators reviewing literature cite the results and conclusions of previous research without determining the size of sample, data collection procedures, and measuring instruments used. It should be obvious to the reader that results of studies involving small samples and using tests that have low reliability are not as valid as large-scale studies in which rigorous methodology and reliable measuring instruments are used. In reporting previous literature, the investigator should consider the following factors in evaluating the validity of the research findings:

- The size of the sample, sampling procedure, and representativeness
- Control of extraneous variables that can potentially affect results
- Evidence of research bias in conclusions that are not consistent with results
- Selection of reliable and valid measuring instruments
- Data collection procedures
- Statistical techniques employed

In addition to these factors, the reader should ask a number of questions about the article. These questions are summarized in Table 6–6.

---

### TABLE 6-6

**Critically Reviewing a Research Article**

**Introduction**

- Does the introduction state the hypothesis directly, or is the hypothesis implied?
- Does the literature review support the hypothesis?
- Are the choices of outcome measures relevant to the study?
- Is the study feasible and does the study expand knowledge in the field?

**Methodology**

- Based on the information presented in the study, can the study be replicated?
- How were the participants chosen for the study?
- Are the demographics of the participants adequately described?
- Were unusual circumstances or extraneous variables (e.g., use of medication, time of testing) described?
- What were the reliability and validity of the outcome measures?
- Were appropriate tests used for the population studied?

- Were the measures free from external bias?
- Were appropriate statistics used?

**Results and Discussion**

- Were the results reported in an understandable and clear manner?
- Are the figures and tables clear and consistent with the text?
- Was the discussion related to the findings?
- Was there discussion regarding the acceptance or rejection of the null hypothesis?
- Did the investigator discuss limitations of the study and the need for future research?

**Note:** Adapted from material "A Reader's, Writer's, and Reviewer's Guide to Assessing Research Reports in Clinical Psychology," by Brendan A. Maher, 1978, *Journal of Clinical and Consulting Psychology, 46*, 835–838. Copyright 1978 by American Psychological Association.

## 6.6 Outlining the Literature Review Section

Whether the researcher is reporting results in a journal article or preparing a thesis, he or she must decide how much of the background literature should be cited. The *Publication Manual of the American Psychological Association* (2010) recommends that a writer of a journal article should:

> Discuss the literature but do not include an exhaustive historical review. Assume that the reader has knowledge in the field for which you are writing. ... A scholarly review of earlier work provides an appropriate history and recognizes the priority of the work of others. Citation of a specific credit to relevant earlier works is part of the author's scientific and scholarly responsibility. ... Cite and reference only works pertinent to the specific issue and not works of only tangential or general significance. If you summarize earlier works, avoid nonessential details; instead, emphasize pertinent findings, relevant methodological issues, and major conclusions. Refer the reader to general surveys or reviews of the topic if they are available. (p. 11)

In contrast to the journal article, the writer of a master's thesis or doctoral dissertation should include extensive background literature, which demonstrates to the reader that the researcher is cognizant of the important findings with which the present study rests. The researcher should document the continuity of findings. The literature review in a master's thesis or doctoral dissertation serves as a vehicle for presenting chronologically the progression of knowledge in a specific area. Thus, the literature review should reflect the development of a problem by first presenting general background findings and then gradually narrowing to the significant variables identified in the title of the study.

A search of the literature will result in identifying literature that is directly related to the topic at hand, literature less directly related but that should be read, and literature that is unrelated. Although it will be important to peruse all of these, only the articles directly related to the topic will be used in a literature review. Locke, Spirduso, and Silverman (1987) suggested that the literature review "is made to serve the reader's query by supporting, explicating, and illuminating the logic now implicit in the proposed investigation" (p. 59). A well-written literature review allows the reader to (a) understand the significance of the research question, (b) validate the connection between previously conducted research directly related to the present research question, and (c) grasp the reasons for the proposed methodology.

The plan for presenting previous literature should include a logical development that incorporates both a chronological sequence and a topical order. By using an outline, the researcher begins to organize the data found in reviewing the literature. The outline is a working tool. It should change to accommodate new ideas and evidence.

One way to develop an outline is by organizing the index cards into groups by topic, which makes the writing easier for a number of reasons. First, by examining and reviewing the cards, important themes and topics may emerge. Second, because the cards have been organized by subject, the writer does not waste time looking through the articles and other references for related material. Third, by placing them into groups, the cards can be further organized into a logical outline or sequence.

Although actually writing the literature review can be challenging, the completed product gives the researcher a sense of accomplishment. The literature review section of a study should represent an extensive process that is the basis for implementing the research design. The worksheet in Box 6–2 describes this process.

---

### BOX 6-2

## Worksheet for Literature Review

**1. State the research problem in question form**

**2. Identify variables in the study**

- Independent variables

| | |
|---|---|
| 1 | |
| 2 | |
| 3 | |

- Dependent variables

| | |
|---|---|
| 1 | |
| 2 | |
| 3 | |
| 4 | |

- Target populations

| | |
|---|---|
| 1 | |
| 2 | |
| 3 | |
| 4 | |
| 5 | |

- Specific setting for study (e.g., hospital, clinic)

| | |
|---|---|
| 1 | |
| 2 | |
| 3 | |
| 4 | |

### 3. Checklist for locating references (list titles)

- Information retrieval systems

| | |
|---|---|
| 1 | |
| 2 | |

- Directories of references

| | |
|---|---|
| 1 | |
| 2 | |

- Bibliographical indexes

| | |
|---|---|
| 1 | |
| 2 | |

- Annual reviews

| | |
|---|---|
| 1 | |
| 2 | |

- Abstracting periodicals

| | |
|---|---|
| 1 | |
| 2 | |

- Textbooks

| | |
|---|---|
| 1 | |
| 2 | |

- Personal communication from experts

| | |
|---|---|
| 1 | |
| 2 | |

### 4. Primary Sources Utilized (list)

- Journals

| | |
|---|---|
| 1 | |
| 2 | |

- Statistical compendium

| | |
|---|---|
| 1 | |
| 2 | |

- Conference proceedings

| | |
|---|---|
| 1 | |
| 2 | |

- Theses and dissertations

| | |
|---|---|
| 1 | |
| 2 | |

© Cengage Learning 2013

## 6.7   Summary

In this chapter, the authors discuss the importance of and the necessity for a thorough review of the literature as an integral part of a research project. In this process, the researcher needs to locate and retrieve the most important studies relevant to the research project and to evaluate the validity of the methods used in collecting data. Although online database searches such as PubMed.com® are particularly suited for identifying articles from published medical and health-related periodicals (both peer reviewed and non-peer reviewed), several other resources are identified for retrieving health statistics that are helpful in justifying the need for the study. An up-to-date list of the primary occupational therapy journals that are published internationally is provided in this chapter. The authors also discuss the different types of published literature such as research studies, review articles, and theoretical papers. A discussion of how to critically analyze a published research study is described. Finally, a summary worksheet for the literature review is included that can help the reader to organize a systematic search.

## CHAPTER 7

# Research Design and Methodology

*The quality of research depends not only upon the adequacy of the research design but also upon the fruitfulness of the data-collection techniques which are employed. The purpose of the various data-collection techniques is simply to produce precise and reliable evidence which is relevant to the research questions being asked. Fulfillment of this purpose, however is rarely simple.*

—M. Johoda, M. Deutsch, and S. W. Cook, 1951,
*Research Methods in Social Relations* (p. 92)

## Operational Learning Objectives

By the end of this chapter, the learner will:

- State a research hypothesis or guiding question.
- Operationally define a research variable.
- Identify any assumptions underlying a proposed research study.
- Diagram a research study.
- Identify the possible methodological limitations in a research study.
- State the theoretical rationale underlying a proposed research study.
- Design a procedure for selecting participants for a study.

- Design screening criteria for participant inclusion.
- Define and contrast the terms *random sampling, random assignment, convenience sampling, representative sampling*, and *target population*.
- Define *test reliability* and *test validity*.
- Evaluate the feasibility, reliability, and validity of a published test or measuring instrument.
- Compare and contrast the four scales of measurement.

- Understand the concept of internal validity.
- Design a data collection procedure for a proposed research study.
- Understand ethical principles underlying human research.
- Outline a research proposal including an informed consent protocol.
- Understand the concept of external validity.
- Describe the major research designs and methodological limitations of a study.

## 7.1 Proposing a Feasible Research Question

The initial step in research is asking the right questions. Science progresses along the continuum of knowledge by researchers seeking solutions to key problems. Historically, researchers gain advanced knowledge by posing feasible questions. For example:

- What are the basic anatomical structures and physiological functions of human beings?
- How are diseases transmitted?
- What chemical substances destroy specific microorganisms that cause diseases?
- How can we detect the presence of trace chemicals in food and blood?
- What are the causes of specific diseases?
- What effect does a child with disabilities have on the family?
- What is the effect of including a child with disabilities in a general education classroom?
- What are the most effective methods for rehabilitating individuals with traumatic brain injury?

Scientists have raised numerous questions that have guided research and led to solutions. In the research design section, the investigator raises specific testable or feasible questions that guide the data collection.

In proposing research, the investigator reviews the following six areas:

1. Statements of hypotheses or guiding questions
2. Operational definitions of variables
3. Underlying assumptions of the study
4. Diagrammatical relationship between variables
5. Methodological limitations of the study
6. Overall theoretical rationale guiding the study

## 7.2 Statement of Hypothesis

A **hypothesis** is a statement predicting the relationship between variables. In logic, it is stated as an **if–then contingency**. For example, consider the hypothesis: "There is a positive, statistically significant relationship between obesity and heart disease in sedentary workers." In this hypothesis, there is a predicted relationship between obesity and heart disease among sedentary workers expressed as "*if* obesity (in sedentary workers), *then* heart disease." The hypothesis contains the question and predicts a directional relationship. (A direction can be either positive or inverse.)

How does the investigator arrive at a hypothesis or guiding question? The review of literature as discussed in Chapter 6 serves as the generating force in guiding the proposed hypothesis or guiding question. The relationship among a research question, a guiding question, and a hypothesis is described in Table 7–1. The hypothesis is a specific statement that can be derived from a research question or guiding question. Table 7–2 shows the relationship between a research model and a statement of hypothesis or guiding question.

In quantitative research, the investigator needs to state a guiding question or hypothesis that leads to data collection. In qualitative research, the guiding question or hypothesis can arise during data collection. For example, a researcher who is initially interested in the problems associated with obtaining employment for individuals with schizophrenia may change his or her focus to an examination of the relationship between stress and employment. The qualitative researcher has more flexibility in stating guiding questions or hypotheses than does the quantitative researcher who must state the question prior to collecting data. Once the guiding question or hypothesis is stated, the researcher needs to operationally define the variables.

## TABLE 7-1

### The Relationship among a Research Question, a Guiding Question, and a Hypothesis

|  | Definition | Purpose | Example |
|---|---|---|---|
| **Research question** | A broad inquiry into a general area of investigation | Leads researcher into an extensive literature review | What is the relationship between repetitive motion and hand injuries? |
| **Guiding question** | A statement of inquiry that leads to data collection | Identifies factors that relate to a specific research question | What factors in repetitive motion injury are related to carpal tunnel syndrome? |
| **Hypothesis** | A detailed statement that can be tested through inferential statistics | Evaluates effectiveness or significant relationship between variables | There is no statistically significant difference in the use of biofeedback versus splinting in remediating the symptoms of carpal tunnel syndrome. |

© Cengage Learning 2013

## TABLE 7-2

### The Relationship between the Research Model and the Hypothesis

| | Quantitative Research Models | |
|---|---|---|
| | Statements | Examples of Research Questions |
| **Experimental (prospective research design)** | Hypothesis: directional or null | How effective is exercise in reducing symptoms of depression? |
| **Methodological** | Guiding question | What factors must be considered in designing a (specific) instrument or test for measuring pain? |
| **Evaluation** | Guiding question | How effective is the occupational therapy department in preventing rehospitalizations? |
| **Heuristic (retrospective research design)** | Guiding question | What risk factors are related to the etiology of multiple sclerosis? |
| **Correlational** | Hypothesis: directional or null | Is there a statistically significant positive relationship between perceptual motor abilities and reading? |
| **Survey** | Guiding question | What are the personality characteristics of the leaders in the field of occupational therapy? |

*continues*

TABLE 7-2

**The Relationship between the Research Model and the Hypothesis** *continued*

| | Qualitative Research Methods | |
|---|---|---|
| | Statements | Examples of Research Questions |
| Individual case study | Guiding question | What are the dynamic factors and processes underlying the cause of schizophrenia in a specific individual? |
| Operations research | Guiding question | What is the impact of the prospective payment system on the quality of home health care? |
| Child development studies | Guiding question | What are the sequential steps in a child's development of the palmer grasp? |
| Longitudinal research (prospective designs) | Guiding question | What are the long-term effects on children exposed to cocaine in utero? |
| Field observation (ethnography) | Guiding question | How do parents' attitudes toward a child with Down syndrome affect the child's development? |
| Historical | Guiding question | What are the historical roots of the concept of humanism in occupational therapy? |

© Cengage Learning 2013

## 7.3 Operationally Defining a Variable

Variables are operationally defined by stating or describing (a) the treatment procedure (presumed independent variable), (b) the outcome measure (dependent variable), and (c) the screening criteria for participant selection. Operational definitions make it possible for researchers to replicate a research study. Many differences arising from the inconsistent results of several investigators often can be traced to different operational definitions of the same stated conceptual variables. For example, the following variables could become ambiguous unless one describes in detail how they are measured or procedurally defined:

- Cognitive rehabilitation (treatment procedure)
- Intelligence (screening criterion for participant inclusion)
- Language disorder (dependent variable or screening criterion for participant inclusion)
- Muscle strength (dependent variable or screening criterion for participant inclusion)
- Spasticity (dependent variable or screening criterion for participant inclusion)
- Sensory-integration therapy (treatment procedure)
- Visual motor ability (dependent variable or screening criterion for participant inclusion)
- Work hardening (treatment intervention)
- Individuals with low back pain (screening criterion for participant inclusion)

Research became rigorous when researchers described experimental procedures in detail so that other investigators could duplicate the exact experiment or study. The rigor in operationally defining a variable is associated with *internal validity*. Results cannot be accepted unless it is known how the investigator defined the variables. Conflicts over the effectiveness of treatment techniques, descriptions of target populations, and measurements of outcome are caused by comparing seemingly similar variables, which are, in fact, different because of the way they are measured. How many definitions are there for "self-perception," "cognitive disability," "language therapy," "manual dexterity," "work capacity," and "low back pain"? The conceptualization of variables described by investigators may be entirely different if these variables are not operationally defined.

Ineffectual research is typified by the omission of operational definitions. The problem is compounded when investigators synthesize findings in an area by "lumping" studies. For example, if visual perception is defined operationally through group tests, individual tests, clinical observations, and functional performance, then conflicts will arise when examining the relationship between visual perception and a variable such as ADL. A researcher's often fallacious interpretation of the literature and subsequent invalid conclusions are a result of equating variables even though the operational definitions are different.

In operationally defining a variable, the investigator should consider the following questions:

- What is the theoretical rationale underlying the definition?
- What is the accepted definition of a variable as stated in a dictionary or occupational therapy textbook?
- How can the variable be measured?
- Does the investigator need to establish the screening criteria in defining a target population?
- Is the variable defined by a standardized procedure (e.g., employing a treatment technique)?
- Can a mathematical formula be employed in the definition (e.g., in ergonomics when defining work output)?

## 7.4 Stating Assumptions

A researcher undertaking an investigation may make certain assumptions that are usually unstated.

These assumptions can be on a general level, such as:

- All diseases have a cause.
- Intelligence is the result of the interaction between genetic structure and environmental opportunities.
- Obesity is the result of overeating and inactivity.
- Language development is maturational.
- Disengagement from social activity is a learned behavior, rather than a biological determinant.
- Learning is a complex variable that is not entirely based on external reinforcement.

Other assumptions can be more subtle, such as:

- Rehabilitation of individuals with severe disabilities should have a high priority in a society.
- People with alcohol dependency should be treated as persons with medical problems rather than as criminals.
- Individuals with intellectual disabilities should be integrated into community schools rather than isolated in large institutions.
- Home health care is more cost-effective than hospitalization.

In designing a research study, the investigator should be aware of all the assumptions underlying the study. Whether the assumptions are made explicit in reporting the results is at the discretion of the researcher. Nonetheless, in preparing a research proposal, the researcher must state all assumptions.

When distinguishing an assumption from established evidence, it should be clear from the previous examples that assumptions are controversial or inconclusive theory that can also reflect the investigator's values or biases. Many assumptions are tacitly implied by an investigator who assumes that all people accept certain beliefs or hold certain opinions. A researcher should try to identify all assumptions being made in the study as an indication of his or her own subjective biases and beliefs. Whenever possible, a reference should be used when stating assumptions. The reference could be either theoretical or supported by research.

## 7.5 Diagrammatical Relationships between Variables

In clarifying the research design, it is helpful for the investigator to diagram the study, especially in a proposal, showing the relationship among variables, populations sampled, and operational definitions.

## 7.5.1 Experimental Model

For example, a researcher is interested in testing two therapeutic interventions for students with moderate intellectual disabilities who have difficulty in self-care activities. The experimental model is used in this study. The diagrammatical relationship between variables is depicted in Figure 7–1.

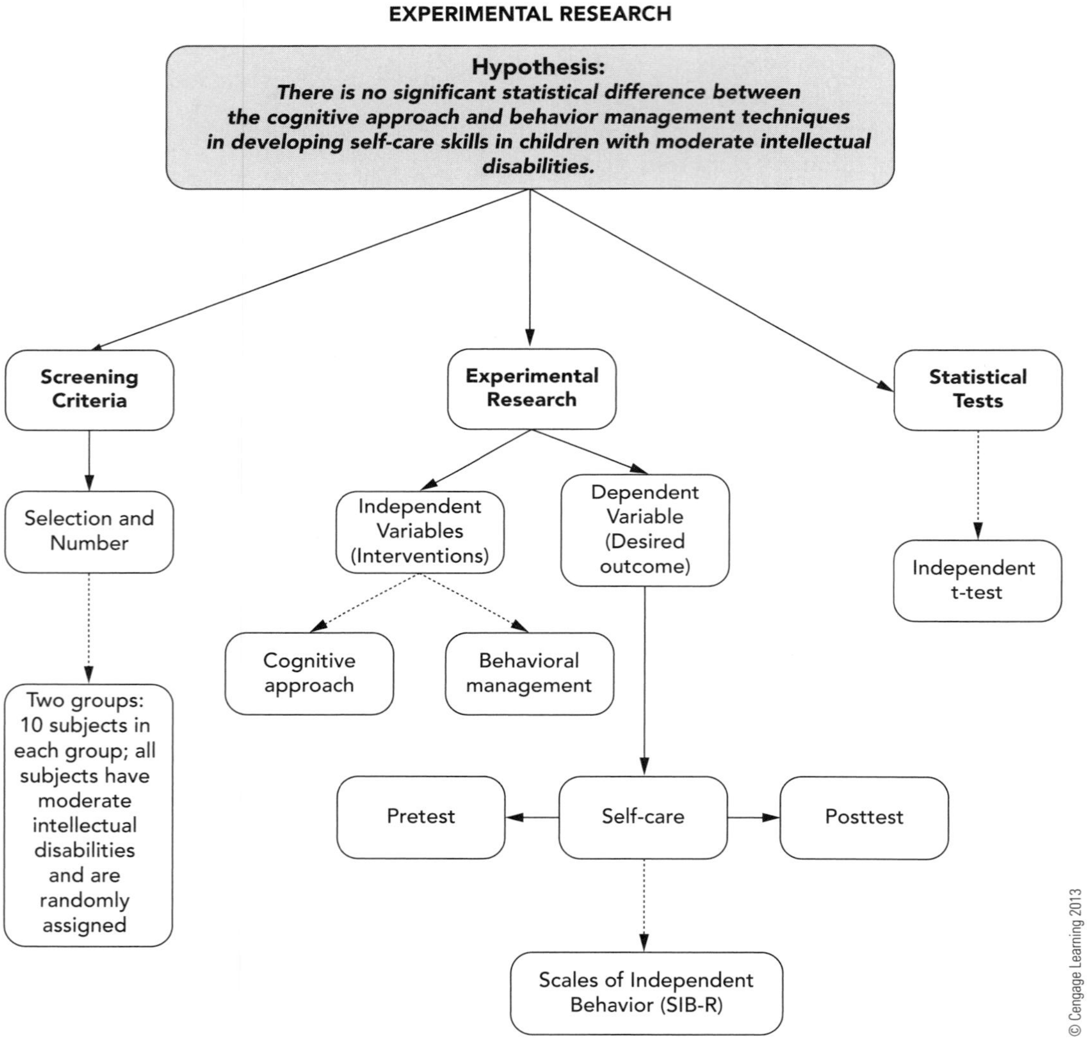

**EXPERIMENTAL RESEARCH**

**Hypothesis:**
*There is no significant statistical difference between the cognitive approach and behavior management techniques in developing self-care skills in children with moderate intellectual disabilities.*

© Cengage Learning 2013

**FIGURE 7-1** Diagrammatic Relationship among Variables in Experimental Research

- In this hypothetical example, the guiding question is, "Is the cognitive approach more effective than the behavioral approach in increasing self-care abilities among individuals with moderate intellectual disabilities?"
- An operational definition of "moderate intellectual disability" is required (IQ score obtained on an individual test between 40 and 55, subaverage adaptive behavior skills in two or more areas [e.g., leisure, communication, social skills] and occurrence in the developmental years). Age, gender, ethnicity, and socioeconomic status should be considered.

## 7.5.2 Correlational Model

A correlational model would be diagramed in a hypothetical study involving coma. The variables are now considered to have an associational or statistical relationship, not a cause-effect relationship. The hypothetical relationship among variables is diagrammed in Figure 7–2. In this model, the independent variable is not experimentally induced; therefore, it is considered to be presumed.

- In this model, the guiding question for the hypothetical example is, "Is there a statistically significant relationship between the number of days in a coma and the severity of cognitive deficits?"
- An operational definition of the "population" and the "severity of cognition deficits" are required. In the hypothetical example, the population is defined as those individuals who (a) have sustained a traumatic brain injury from a motor vehicle accident (MVA), (b) are participating in a

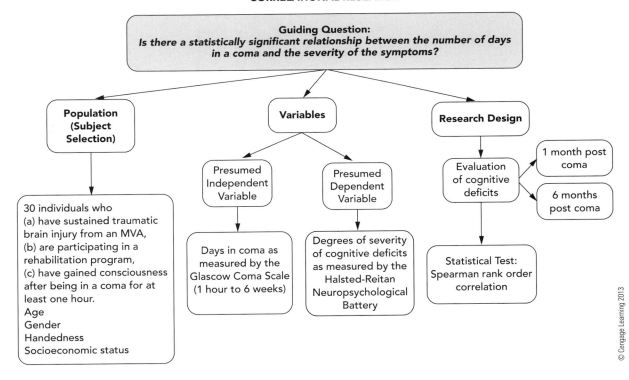

**FIGURE 7-2**  Diagrammatic Relationship among Variables in Correlational Research

rehabilitation program, and (c) have gained consciousness after being in a coma for at least one hour. Age, gender, socioeconomic status, and handedness must also be considered. Measurement tools include the *Glascow Coma Scale* and the *Halsted–Reitan Neuropsychological Battery*.

### 7.5.3 Methodological Model

Using methodological research, such as in developing a test, the researcher outlines the study by the diagram found in Figure 7–3. In this model, there is no hypothesis; rather, the researcher proposes a guiding question.

● In the hypothetical question, the researcher wants to design a reliable and valid instrument for assessing the ability to cope with stress.

The construct of "stress" needs to be defined based on theoretical concepts from a literature review. Individuals who deal well with stress and individuals with mental illness who have difficulty dealing with stress participate in obtaining normal values for the instrument. Stratification of age, gender, and socioeconomic status would occur by examining the differences that may occur because of these variables.

### 7.5.4 Evaluation Model

In evaluation research, the investigator determines the effectiveness of a health system in meeting the defined objects. This model is diagramed in Figure 7–4. As in methodological research, the researcher uses a guiding question to propose the

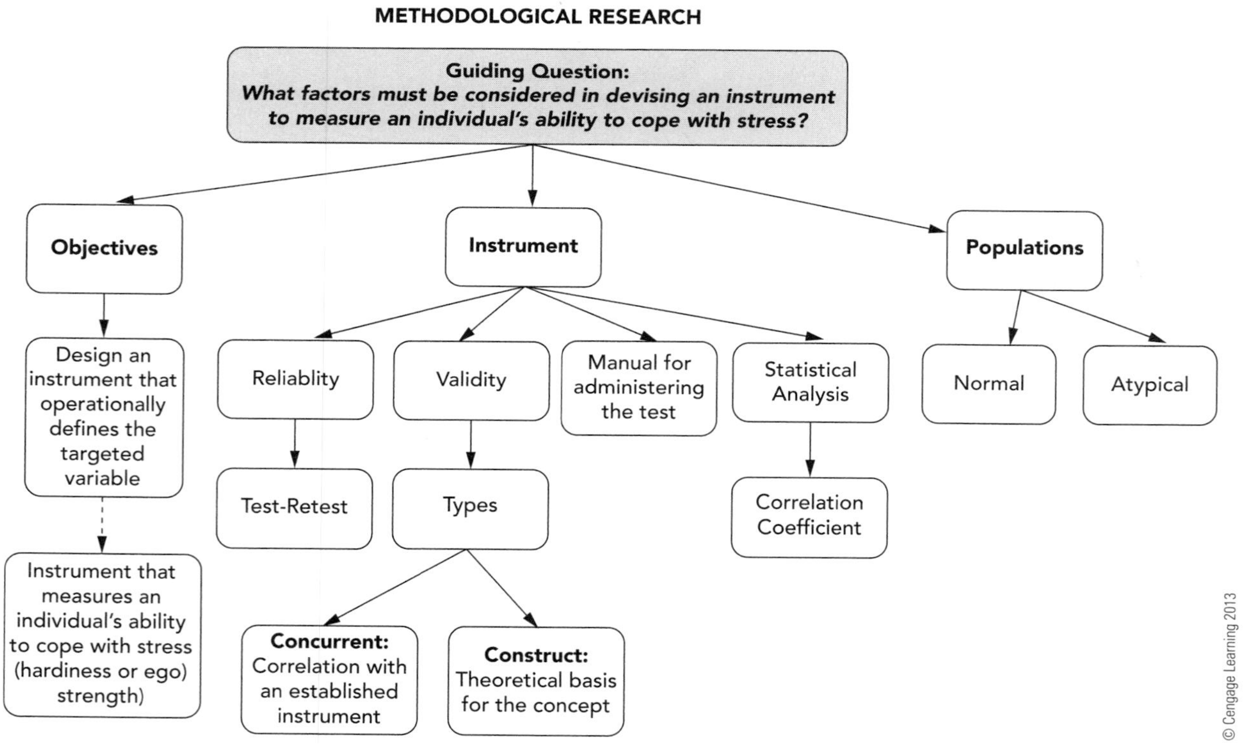

FIGURE 7-3 Diagrammatic Relationship among Variables in Methodological Research

© Cengage Learning 2013

**EVALUATIVE RESEARCH**

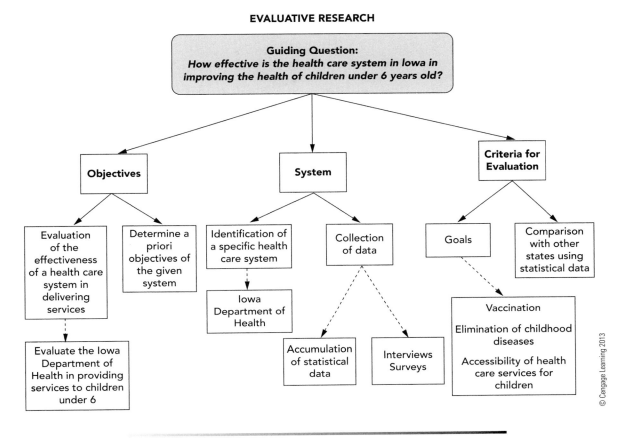

**FIGURE 7-4**   Diagrammatic Relationship among Variables in Evaluative Research

research. The researcher must determine the a priori objectives of the system. In the hypothetical example, the investigator would determine the mission statement and the objectives of the Iowa health care system, then would use these criteria to determine the effectiveness of the system. General criteria for comparison purposes also would be used. In the example, statistical information would be used to compare Iowa's health care system with those of other states.

### 7.5.5 Heuristic Model

A researcher using a heuristic model seeks to understand and discover the relationship among heuristic factors. In a hypothetical study, such as

discovering risk factors for a disease, the researcher seeks to identify the factors that are significantly related to the disability. The hypothetical example, using heart disease, is depicted in Figure 7–5. In this example, the risk factors for heart disease are identified through literature review. The population studied includes individuals with post-coronary heart disease. Control factors include age, gender, socioeconomic status, ethnicity, and severity of disease.

### 7.5.6 Survey Model

In this model, the researcher is interested in identifying characteristics of a homogeneous population. For example, in a hypothetical study, the researcher is interested in examining the level of job

**HEURISTIC RESEARCH**

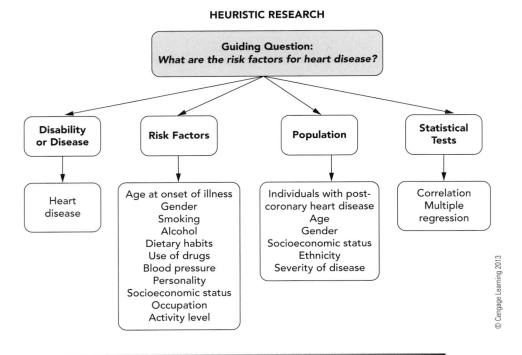

**FIGURE 7-5** Diagrammatic Relationship among Variables in Heuristic Research

satisfaction among occupational therapists in the United States (see Figure 7–6). After the survey is completed, the results can be compared with a similar study focusing on another professional group, such as nursing.

- The population is identified, but only a sample of the population receives the survey. Of those receiving the survey, it is expected that 50 percent will respond. Thus, in a population of 120,000 occupational therapists in the United States, only 12,000 will receive the survey, and only 6000 are expected to respond.
- The survey is sent to a striated sample of the population giving a representative sample of the distribution of occupational therapists in the United States. Although the striation is based only on geographical location, the statistical analysis from the results of the survey separates job description (e.g., pediatrics, physical dysfunction,

psychosocial) and demographics (e.g., age, gender, socioeconomic status, ethnicity).

- In the methodology, the researcher must design a valid and reliable questionnaire. Statistical analysis consists of descriptive statistics, including a frequency distribution table, a statistical pie, and histograms.

### 7.5.7 Qualitative Models

Qualitative research models include:

- Individual case study
- Operations research
- Child development studies
- Longitudinal research (prospective designs)
- Field observation (ethnography)
- Historical research

Figure 7–7 depicts a hypothetical study of a family in which a child has a bipolar disorder. In selecting

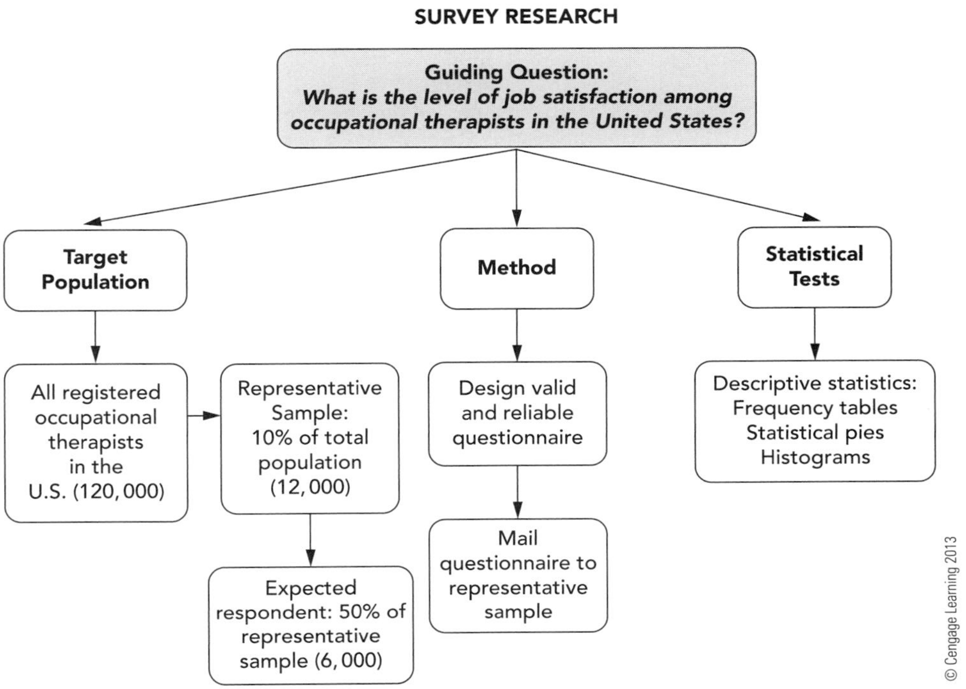

**SURVEY RESEARCH**

**FIGURE 7-6**   Diagrammatic Relationship among Variables in Survey Research

a family, the researcher would consider the child's diagnosis, severity of illness, family constellation, and cooperativeness of the family to participate in a study. Additional considerations include the research methods used for data collection and for analyzing the results.

## 7.6  Theoretical Rationale

Theory generates research, and research generates theory. Research should be a planned activity based on a theoretical rationale. Why are variables correlated? Why do we think this treatment will work? Why do we project these results? What factors justify the conclusions proposed? The researcher is not only interested in the questions *Does it work?* or *Is it curative?* but also *Why is the treatment effective? Why is there a relationship between causative factors and the onset of illness?* Theories in science are in a continual state of change. As knowledge progresses in an area, theory changes to accommodate the new information. Researchers do not assume that theories and knowledge are static. What currently is accepted as truth may be revised later when new research data are obtained.

The investigator needs to state the underlying theory from which the research design is generated, regardless of the theory's robustness or meagerness. Research is not justified if we collect meaningless bits of information for future analysis. For example, if a researcher working on techniques to improve motor skills in children with severe intellectual disabilities finds a statistically significant difference between behavior modification and a comparable method in motivating the children to use motor skills but does not explain why behavior modification is effective, the research is incomplete. If, in this example, the group that received behavior modification realized significantly improved motor skills more than the control group did, the reader is left to speculate the causes for the differences. Was the Hawthorne effect controlled? Are there other explanations? The absence of a theoretical explanation leaves

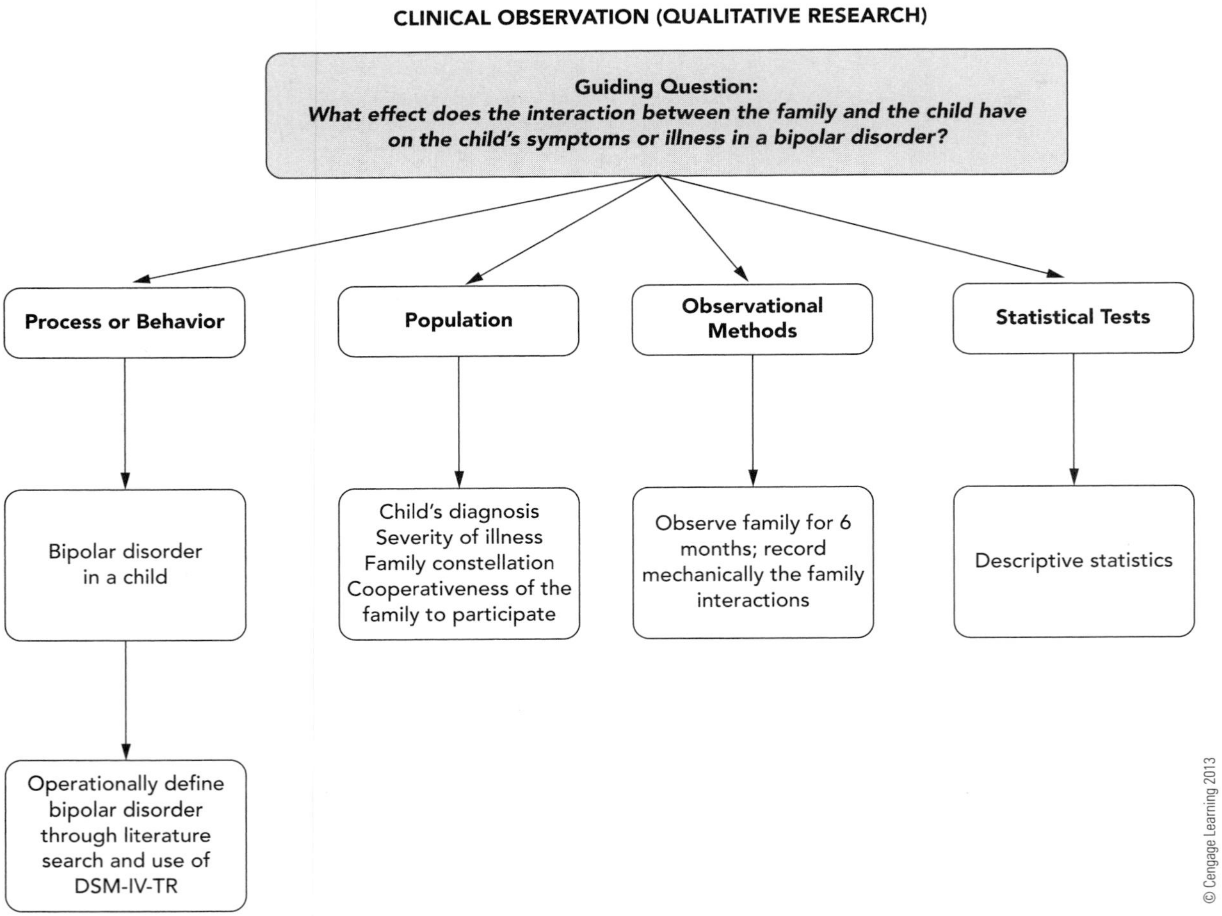

**CLINICAL OBSERVATION (QUALITATIVE RESEARCH)**

**FIGURE 7-7**  Diagrammatic Relationship among Variables in Qualitative Research, Using an Individual Case Study

a gap in the research and leaves it open to the reader to speculate why motor development was enhanced. Speculations are raised, such as:

- Interpersonal relationships influenced motor learning
- Treatment stimulated motor development
- Reinforcement used in behavior modification was more effective than that used in the comparable methods
- Tests selected were unreliable and inappropriate

The reader can make many speculations in the absence of a theoretical rationale. Research should be guided by theory and explanation, rather than merely presenting data that describe the relationships among variables.

## 7.7 Internal Validity

*Internal validity* is a theoretical concept that refers to the rigor in an experiment or research design. The degree of internal validity depends on the extent to which the investigator has controlled all variables that can potentially affect the results. If an experiment or research design is judged to have good internal validity, then the experimenter has been able to control for factors that could potentially distort the results. High internal validity is demonstrated by:

- A double-blind study in which the investigator eliminates researcher bias and subject influence
- Control of the placebo effect whereby the subject's suggestibility and personal influence are eliminated
- Inclusion of a control group to eliminate the Hawthorne effect
- Matching comparative groups to ensure that all groups compared are not different in variables such as age, gender, degree of disability, intelligence, and socioeconomic status
- Baseline measures of pretest to ensure that comparative groups are equivalent
- Posttest measures that are compared with pretest measures
- High reliability and validity of outcome measures or tests to ensure that variables are accurately measured
- Regard for maturational factors that could distort results
- Random selection of subjects to reduce bias in samples
- Standardization of administering test and research procedures
- Control for practice effect in test taking to ensure that gain in scores is not attributable to the participant's familiarity with test

Some ways to increase internal validity are listed in Table 7–3.

## TABLE 7-3

### Increasing Internal Validity

| Problem | Solution |
| --- | --- |
| Hawthorne effect | Ensure that control and experimental groups receive equal treatment time. |
| Honeymoon effect | Do a follow-up study. |
| Placebo effect | Use motivational techniques to help clients self-improve. |
| Bias of researcher | Have objective test administrator collect pre-post data. |
| Unreliability of test | Design new instrument with the goal of high reliability and validity. Use triangulation (e.g., clinical observation, client report, physiological measure). |
| Insensitivity of test to detecting changes in behavior | Use criterion-referenced testing. Use triangulation. |
| Unsubstantiated validity | Do a pilot study to test validity with an established test instrument. |
| Sample is not representative of target population | Use striated samples. Examine characteristics of sample group for similarities with target population (e.g., age, gender, severity of illness). |
| Maturational factors affect results | Use covariance in statistical analysis (ANCOVA) to control for differences in pre- and post-measures. |
| Differences in cognitive abilities of individuals | Use covariance (ANCOVA) to control for cognitive levels. |
| Comparative groups are not equal | Set up selection criteria for selection inclusion (e.g., age, gender, SES, intelligence, ethnicity). |
| Treatment method is not stated clearly | Operationalize treatment method so that it can be replicated. |

## 7.8 Methods Section

The methodology section of a study includes the following components: the method of selecting subjects, location of study, description of tests and apparatuses used in measuring variables, procedure for collecting data, statistical techniques used for analyzing data, computer use (if applicable), projection of time for completing the study, and the procedure of obtaining informed consent from human subjects. Pragmatic, as well as rational, considerations guide the investigator in finding the answers to the following questions:

- How many subjects should be included in the study?
- Should subjects be randomly selected, or should they be volunteers or a convenience sample?
- Where should the study take place?
- What tests, diagnostic procedures, questionnaires, or rating scales should be employed in the study?
- What are the procedures and time sequence for data collection?
- What are the costs of the study?

The process for the research methodology is shown in Figure 7–8.

## 7.9 Selection of Participants

One primary purpose of research is to discover relationships between variables in sample groups and to generalize these relationships to a larger population. The ability to generalize results establishes the *external validity* of a study. Because research usually involves sample groups from populations, rather than the total population, the selection of a representative sample is crucial when generalizing results.

In selecting a sample, the first step is to identify a **target population**. For example, individuals with spinal cord injury, individuals who are juvenile offenders, occupational therapists, graduate students, or administrators of rehabilitation programs are identifiable populations. The target population is narrowed considerably by establishing screening criteria. Screening criteria contain both *inclusion* and *exclusion* factors. For example, a researcher interested in cardiac rehabilitation may want to

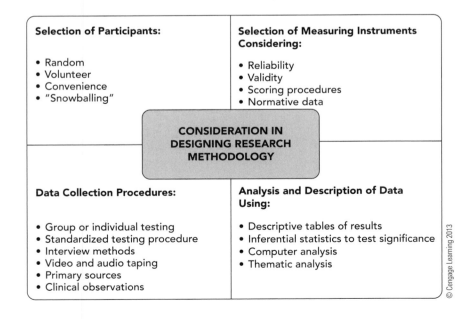

| Selection of Participants: | Selection of Measuring Instruments Considering: |
|---|---|
| • Random<br>• Volunteer<br>• Convenience<br>• "Snowballing" | • Reliability<br>• Validity<br>• Scoring procedures<br>• Normative data |

**CONSIDERATION IN DESIGNING RESEARCH METHODOLOGY**

| Data Collection Procedures: | Analysis and Description of Data Using: |
|---|---|
| • Group or individual testing<br>• Standardized testing procedure<br>• Interview methods<br>• Video and audio taping<br>• Primary sources<br>• Clinical observations | • Descriptive tables of results<br>• Inferential statistics to test significance<br>• Computer analysis<br>• Thematic analysis |

© Cengage Learning 2013

**FIGURE 7-8** Sequential Process of Research Methodology: Notice that there are four basic steps and, within those steps, questions that must be answered.

select a specific population within the area of cardiovascular disease (e.g., individuals who have had heart transplants). The screening criteria will enable the investigator to identify a specific population and to control the variables that could potentially affect the results. In setting up screening criteria for patients with cardiac disease, variables such as age, gender, socioeconomic status, occupation, body type (endomorph, ectomorph, and mesomorph), onset of illness, and range of cardiorespiratory function as indicated by pulse rate and blood pressure should be considered.

Refinement of these variables should narrow the population. An example of a target population obtained from a priori criteria is (inclusion variable): (a) individuals with coronary disease, (b) male, (c) middle-class, (d) living in urban areas, (e) between the ages of 55 and 65, (f) primarily sedentary, and (g) with resting pulse rates below 80. In considering exclusion factors, the researcher specifies variables that are screened out of the study. These variables could include the absence of secondary illnesses (as determined by clinical examination), intellectual disabilities, or psychosocial dysfunctions.

The example from a double case study by Kopolow and Jensen (1975) shows the extensiveness of criteria employed in selecting two participants with quadriplegia (see Table 7–4). Screening criteria are identified prior to subject selection. The investigator operationally defines the variables identified in the criteria. The rigor in specifying the population to be studied within a narrow domain enables other investigators to replicate the research design by isolating specific variables. By specifying the population and operationally defining the variables in the screening criteria, the investigator has identified a target population.

The next step in selecting participants for the study is to locate all of the units in the target population. Studies of the personality characteristics of allied health professionals, for example, would entail obtaining annual directories of members from professional associations, noting that not all practicing therapists are members of their professional associations. (See Appendix A–1 for a list of professional organizations and their Internet addresses.)

Location of populations with disabilities, such as individuals with paraplegia living in the

## TABLE 7-4

### Screening Criteria for Study Participant Inclusion (Quadriplegia)

1. The participants were individuals with $C_{5,6}$ traumatic quadriplegia.

2. The participants were male.

3. The participants were 18 to 26 years of age at onset of injury.

4. The participants had at least a high school education.

5. One participant was engaged in either full- or part-time employment, including student and/or homemaker, whereas the other participants were unemployed.

6. The participants were residing in nonmedical facilities.

7. The participants were 1 to 2 years post-injury.

8. The participants were Caucasian.

9. The participants were native, English-speaking Americans.

10. The participants had normal cognitive functioning.

11. The participants' medical records were available.

12. The participants were willing to participate in the study and signed an informed consent form.

community, may be obtained through consumer organizations that represent geographic areas. By geographically limiting the representativeness of the study, the investigator controls for social and environmental factors that could potentially affect the results. On the other hand, the investigator may want to guide the scope of the study by identifying **stratified samples**, that is, homogeneous subgroups of a population based on variables such as geography, educational level, and treatment setting (e.g., community vs. hospital or disability group). Stratified samples are usually determined by previous evidence implying that the variable identified has a significant effect on a dependent variable. For example, in examining the guiding question, *Does exercise prevent the recurrence of heart disease?* the investigator would control for the variable of smoking because previous evidence has related smoking to heart disease. In using stratified samples, the investigator would separate populations of smokers who exercise from nonsmokers who do not exercise.

Appendix A–2 provides a selected list of consumer health organizations and their Internet addresses. Additional ideas for obtaining participants can be obtained from the *Encyclopedia of Associations: International Organizations: An Associations Unlimited Reference* (Edition 50; Gale Group, 2011). This resource lists addresses and telephone numbers of nearly 21,000 national and international associations, including professional health associations.

### 7.9.1 External Validity

*External validity* refers to the researcher's ability to generalize the results of a research study from a sample to a total or target population. In general, researchers seek to generalize the results from a study to the population at large. For example, if a researcher found in a clinical study that aerobic exercise is effective in reducing depression in a particular sample, he or she would want to test whether the results could be generalized to all individuals with clinical depression. The extent to which an investigator can with confidence generalize the results of a study depends on the number of subjects in the study and whether the study has been replicated, confirming previous results. It is not unusual for government agencies to

sponsor extensive clinical trials using large numbers of subjects to test the effectiveness of a new vaccine. These types of studies have a high degree of external validity. The example of the development of the polio vaccine during the 1950s demonstrates the ability to obtain external validity from one extensive clinical trial. External validity is also dependent on internal validity, however. In other words, the results of a study cannot be generalized to a population if internal validity is weak.

### 7.9.2 Random Sampling

Researchers see *Random sampling* and **random assignment** as methodological virtues. If a study includes a random selection of subjects, it is assumed that the investigator has controlled for researcher bias when selecting a representative sample of the population. The concept of random sampling implies that in a population that includes all the components (e.g., all occupational therapists, all individuals with diagnoses of schizophrenia, all nursing homes), units of subjects or institutions are representative of the total population. Random sampling is a method to select a representative group from the population. Random sampling does not necessarily ensure a representative group; it serves to eliminate researcher bias in selecting a sample.

One method used in random sampling is to assign a number to each population unit and select a representative sample by choosing units from a list of random numbers. For example, an investigator wants to randomly select 40 graduate programs in occupational therapy that are representative of all the programs, totaling approximately 125 in the United States. The investigator would assign a number from 1 to 125 to each school and then from a list of random numbers select 40 schools. Because the schools are dispersed throughout the country, a representative sample of 40 should reflect the geographical distribution. If a check of the 40 schools reveals that the sample is biased in the direction of a single region, then repeated random selections would be obtained until a fair degree of geographical representativeness occurs.

At this point, the reader may ask, why bother with obtaining a sample from random numbers? Why not just merely select a school from each geographical region? The reason this is not valid is because the researcher may overtly or inadvertently select schools that are typical of an educational philosophy or teaching model. Random sampling is simply a method to ensure researcher objectivity. In clinical research on human subjects, this method is sometimes difficult because subjects have the option to participate in the study. Another difficulty is in applying random sampling techniques to potentially large populations of individuals with disabilities situated in a wide geographic area. Is it possible to randomly sample all children with spina bifida, all patients with coronary disease, all prison inmates, all adolescents with ADHD, or all individuals with spinal cord injury in the United States?

The complexities and problems in locating every subject in the population do not warrant the errors that will occur by the very nature of the process. If random sampling of large populations is not practical, are there other objective selection methods that a clinical researcher can use? The answer to this question is *yes*—if the researcher maintains objectivity by devising systematic methods to obtain subjects and by narrowing the study. By delimiting the population, the investigator can apply random sampling techniques. For example, instead of defining the population as all patients with arthritis in the United States, the researcher delimits the population to all patients with arthritis treated in a specific hospital. The title of the study should describe the population sampled. For example, consider these hypothetical titles:

- *Survey of Hand Function in the Patient with Arthritis*
- *Survey of the Hand Function of Individuals with Arthritis in a General Hospital in the Northeast*

In the first example, the investigator implies that the survey represents all patients with arthritis. In the second example, the investigator has delimited the population to those patients with arthritis receiving treatment in a specific hospital. For most investigators, it is almost impossible realistically to sample a nationwide population of patients with arthritis. The difficulty in locating every member of the population, the cost of the survey, and the extensive time involved in collecting data are practical considerations that would hinder such a study.

## 7.9.3 Convenience Sample and Volunteers

It is valid to randomly sample from a **convenience sample** (i.e., a population readily available to a researcher) as long as the researcher does not generalize the results to that portion of the population that was not sampled. In selecting a random sampling of patients with arthritis from an identified population, the researcher would consider the following factors:

- Diagnosis of arthritis operationalized by physician evaluation or by anatomical or physiological evidence
- Age groupings separated into designated units
- Differentiation of gender
- Occupational groupings, such as professional, skilled, unskilled
- Socioeconomic status
- Level of education
- Age of onset
- Presence of stress
- Other relevant variables that could potentially affect the onset and course of arthritis, such as exercise, diet, physical condition, obesity, and weather.

The variables above can be used to establish screening criteria for subject inclusion in the study or in setting up stratified samples that can be statistically analyzed later for differences.

Another method to counteract researcher bias in selecting subjects is *random assignment*. For instance, if an investigator is interested in comparing simultaneously two treatment methods for patients with stroke, random assignment would be applied after a population of patients with stroke in a specific rehabilitation center is identified through screening criteria. The investigator would establish two samples by randomly assigning participants to each group from a list of random numbers. In this hypothetical example, the selection of the specific rehabilitation center where the patients with stroke were treated actually provides a convenience sample.

Another frequently used method of obtaining subjects in clinical research is the use of **volunteers**. The limitation of using volunteers is that they are a

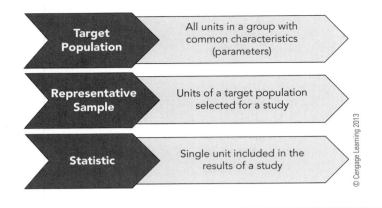

**FIGURE 7-9** Difference between population, representative sample, and statistic

self-selected group who may not be representative of a population. The use of screening criteria with volunteers is one method to determine if the volunteers are a representative group in a target population. In many studies, volunteers are used to assess normal physiological function, and it is important that the investigator establish criteria for normality, excluding individuals with above or below average vital capacities. In combination with an objective screening procedure, volunteers are acceptable samples in selected studies.

The relationship among the target population, representative sample, and statistic is shown in Figure 7–9.

The actual subject included in a study is called a **statistic**. Subjects can be lost in a study through attrition, such as death, change of residence, or voluntary dropout of the study. The characteristics of a population such as physiological capacities, personality factors, and demographic information (i.e., social and personal data) are parameters. These values are usually estimated or unknown because most populations are too large to measure in their entirety.

## 7.10 Size of Sample

Researchers are constantly plagued by the question: *How many subjects should I include in the study?* The often-repeated response is: *As many as possible because the higher percentage of subjects from a population, the more the likelihood that the sample is a true representation.* The problem of the sample size can also be analyzed from the statistical point of

view, which takes into account statistical significance at a confidence level. If one is familiar with statistical tables for the *t*-test, analysis of variance, and **correlation coefficient**, then it will become clear that in arriving at a statistically significant result, the number of subjects affects significance because the degrees of freedom are derived from the number of subjects in a study.

For example, in applying the **Pearson product-moment correlation** (commonly referred to as the "Pearson correlation") to a study, a small *r* of .20 can be statistically significant at the .05 level with samples sizes over 100. On the other hand, the researcher needs an *r* of .58 for a sample size of 10 subjects to obtain statistical significance at the .05 level. In summary, if an investigator is interested in using statistics to derive an adequate sample size, he or she must take into consideration the critical values needed at specific levels of statistical significance, such as the .05 or .01 levels, and the difference between means of groups that will be accepted as clinically significant.

Another consideration in determining sample size is the time length of the study and the financial resources available to collect data from participants. For example, if the researcher has only three months to collect data, the number of participants is limited to the time it takes within this period. If the researcher assumes that he or she needs as many subjects as possible, then the costs and the time for collecting data for each participant should be calculated as part of the research proposal. Many times these pragmatic considerations are the sole criteria for determining sample size, especially when one is awarded a grant for the research.

It is possible to either have too small of a sample size, which could possibly lead to a **Type I error**, or too large of a sample size, which could lead to a **Type II error**. A power analysis is a method by which an educated guess can be made regarding mustering an adequate sample size. Although there are different power analysis strategies based on the research design, one of the most common types is to calculate for a simple experimental design where there are two conditions. This type of power analysis will calculate the number of required persons within each condition. Care must be taken to consider the total number of required participants based on the number of conditions within the study. It is important to keep in mind, when determining the sample size, the following concepts: *Type I error*, which is the probability of concluding that there was a difference in the dependent variable(s) across conditions when in truth there wasn't, or *Type II error*, which is the probability of concluding that there was no difference in the dependent variable(s) across conditions when in truth there was. Type I error is associated with the Greek letter alpha (i.e., $\alpha$), whereas Type II error, with the Greek letter beta (i.e., $\beta$). **Statistical power** has to do with the probability that a Type II error will not occur and is associated with the formula $1-\beta$. Traditionally, $\alpha$ is set at .05, and $\beta$ is set at .2. (See Chapter 8 for more information.)

## 7.11 Selection of Measuring Instrument

### 7.11.1 Selecting a Specific Test for a Research Study

The decision whether to select a published test (i.e., publisher or article) or to construct a new test is a frequent dilemma for the researcher. Figure 7–10 describes this process. Further discussion on this topic is in Chapter 9.

The conceptual definition of a variable should lead the investigator to a specific test that is the most appropriate one when operationally defining a variable. In clinical research, it is critical for the investigator to select a measuring instrument that has high reliability and is a valid measure of outcome. Measuring improvement or change in such areas as cognition, psychosocial, self-care, motor, vocational skills, and leisure interests depends directly on the adequacy and sensitivity of the instrument. A crude measuring instrument that does not have the capacity to detect subtle changes in an individual's functioning or behavior is of limited value to the researcher.

### 7.11.2 Concept of Measurement and Numbers: Data

Data in statistics are derived from empirical observations. These observations are the result of a standardized measurement procedure, such as simple counting, interviews, psychometrics, or machine monitoring of physiological functions. *Measurement* is the assignment of numbers to objects, persons, or events according to rules. Measurement transforms certain attributes of the world into numbers, which can then be summarized, organized, and analyzed by statistical procedures.

The properties or characteristics of objects, persons, or events are called *variables* (e.g., height, weight, intelligence). A variable will typically assume two or more different values, reflecting the fact that objects, persons, or events vary in characteristics. This concept of *individual differences* is central to most scientific disciplines. One of the purposes of statistics is to reflect and summarize such individual differences in the values of variables.

### 7.11.3 Measurement Scales

Measurement scales are a system for the numerical representation of the values of a variable. Four basic types of measurement scales are distinguished in statistics:

#### Nominal Scale

**Nominal scale** is the most discrete and simplest level of measurement. With nominal scale measurement, observations are arranged into various classes or categories. Observations falling into the same class or category are considered qualitatively equivalent, whereas observations in different classes are considered qualitatively different. The classification of eye color, for example, into blue,

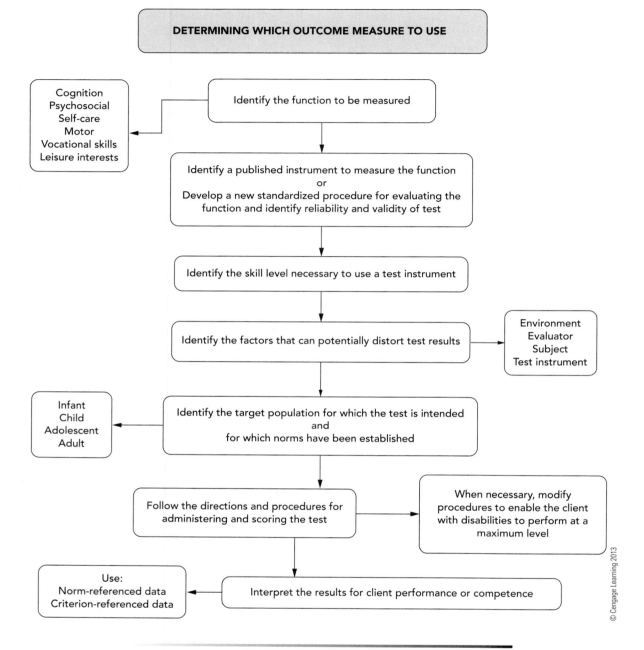

**FIGURE 7-10** Steps in Choosing a Test Instrument and the Process of Deciding What to Use as the Outcome Measure: The researcher must decide whether to construct a new test or use a previously published test based on a number of factors.

brown, hazel, or grey, is an example of nominal scale data.

Numbers are assigned usually to each class or category, but these numbers merely reflect differences among the classes. The numbers do not reflect magnitude or order; they only distinguish one class or category from another.

With nominal scale measurement, categories and classes are determined, and a count is made of the number of observations in each category. Because nominal data constitute the most elementary level of measurement, the only arithmetic operation that can be performed on the numbers is counting the number of observations in a category and then analyzing proportional differences among categories. Examples of nominal scale data in health research include diagnostic categories, subspecialization areas, geographic locations, leisure interests, and health care environments (e.g., hospitals, nursing homes, or rehabilitation clinics).

### Ordinal Scale

**Ordinal scale** is the next level of measurement where objects or individuals are not only distinguished from one another, but also are arranged in order or rank. The numerical values of a variable are arranged in a meaningful order to indicate a hierarchy of the levels of the variable or to show relative position. Examples of ordinal scale data are birth order among siblings, the order of finish in a race, or the relative academic standing of university students in a class. The numbers assigned in the above examples not only distinguish between individuals, but also indicate the order or rank of the individuals relative to one another.

The major limitation of ordinal scales is the inability to make inferences about the degree of difference between values on the scale. Numbers assigned in ordinal scale measurement have the properties of both distinctness and order, but the difference between the numbers may not be equal. For example, the difference between 1st and 3rd place in a race may not be equivalent to the difference between 25th and 27th place in the race. There

may be wide or narrow differences between each rank. With ordinal scale data, it is only possible to state that one individual or object ranks above or below another. Examples in health care include percentile rank, the degree of improvement, muscle strength categories (e.g., good or fair), self-care index, the severity of illness or injury, and the degree of pain.

### Interval Scale

**Interval scale** extends ordinal scales by adding the principle that equal differences between scale values have equal meaning. Thus, the difference between each variable score is equivalent. With interval measurement, numbers serve two purposes: (a) to convey the order of the observations and (b) to indicate the distance or degree of differences between observations. Numbers are assigned so that equal differences in the numbers correspond to equal differences in the property or attribute measured. However, the zero point of the interval scale can be placed arbitrarily and does not indicate absence of the property measured.

Examples of interval scale data are calendar years and the temperature scales of Celsius and Fahrenheit. In a temperature scale, the difference between 10 and 15°C is the same quantitative difference as between 20 and 25°C, but 20°C is not twice as warm as 10°C because there is no true zero point.

Interval scales are important in scientific research. Many human characteristics and attributes, such as intelligence scores, range of motion, dexterity, coordination, and standard scores, are scales with approximately equal intervals. In addition, more sophisticated inferential statistical procedures may be performed with interval scale data compared with the lower-level nominal and ordinal data.

### Ratio Scale

**Ratio scale** is the highest level of measurement and includes the maximum amount of information. The ratio scale is named as such because the ratio of numbers on the scale is meaningful. Because there is a genuine zero point, equal ratios between scale values have equal meaning (i.e., the ratio 40:20 is equivalent to 100:50 or 120:60). The zero point on a ratio scale indicates total absence of the property measured. With ratio scale data, all arithmetic operations (addition, subtraction, multiplication, and division) are possible. Measurement of such variables as height, weight, heart rate, and respiratory rate are all ratio scaled. Figure 7–11 illustrates the differences between the four basic types of measurement scales, and Table 7–5 illustrates their characteristics and properties.

Progress in scientific research gained momentum with the design of tests and instruments that measured and recorded human functioning accurately. The measuring instrument is the sine qua non of research. Without an adequate measuring instrument, a problem remains unresearchable. The adequacy of a measuring instrument is determined by its reliability (i.e., consistency in measurement) and validity (i.e., soundness in measurement).

Various examples of measurable variables in health and education research are described in Table 7–6. "In its broadest sense, measurement is the assignment of numerals to objects or parts according to rule" (Stevens, 1951, p. 1).

In the foregoing example (Table 7–6) of measurable variables, numbers can be assigned to indicate the degree of improvement, strength, perceptual ability, and quality of life. Rating scales can also be devised using a continuum of measurement, equal intervals, or item ranking. Likert-type scales using descriptor adjectives is another alternative. In this scale, it is not assumed that there are equal intervals between numbers (e.g., 1 to 2 is not assumed to be the same distance as 2 to 3) or that there is an absolute zero. Nonetheless, measurement at this level is an improvement over a clinician subjectively stating, on the basis of treatment, that the patient has either improved or not improved. Measurement enables the clinical researcher to operationally define and objectively evaluate an outcome variable. Without objective measurement, clinicians have no criteria or standards to compare the effects of various treatment modalities.

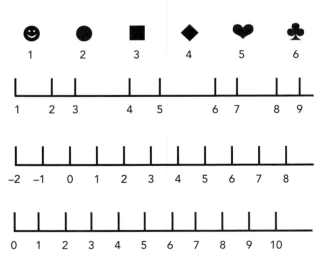

**Nominal scale:** Numbers act as labels only, indicating differences in kind (e.g., identification numbers).

**Ordinal scale:** Numbers represent rank ordering. Differences between rank are not equidistant (e.g., grade levels).

**Interval scale:** Equal differences between values represent equal amounts, but ratios have no meaning because of the arbitrary location of the zero point (e.g., temperature).

**Ratio scale:** Equal differences between values represent equal amounts. Equal ratios of values are also equivalent because of a genuine zero point (e.g., weight scale).

© Cengage Learning 2013

**FIGURE 7-11** Differences among the Four Measurement Scales Illustrated

## TABLE 7-5

### Classification of Measurement Scales

| Measurement Scale | Type of Variable | Researcher Application | Purposes | Examples |
|---|---|---|---|---|
| Nominal | Discrete | Sorting of items | Establishing mutually exclusive groups | Occupations, diagnostic groups |
| Ordinal | Discrete | Rank ordering of items | Determination of greater or lesser | Patient improvement, clinical performance of students |
| Interval | Continuous | Equal ordering of items | Establishing equal intervals on a continuum | Intelligence, perceptual-motor abilities, work capacities |
| Ratio | Continuous | Equal ordering of items with an absolute zero point | Establishing continuous measurement with zero point | Range of motion, muscle strength, weight, height, auditory and visual acuity |

© Cengage Learning 2013

## TABLE 7-6

### Measurable Variables

| Variable to Be Tested | Examples of Measuring Instruments |
|---|---|
| Hand strength: | Dynamometer |
| Range of motion: | Goniometer |
| Attitudes toward individuals with disabilities: | Attitudes Toward Disabled Persons Scale |
| Clinical performance of students: | AOTA's Clinical Rating Scale |
| Psychological improvement: | Tennessee Test of Self Concept (TTSC) |
| Social values and life goals: | Life Satisfaction Index (LSI) |
| Stress management: | Stress Management Questionnaire (SMQ) |
| Sensory integration: | Sensory Integration and Praxis Tests (SIPT) |
| Cognitive functioning: | Allen's Cognitive Level (ACL) |
| Self-care: | Functional Independence Measure (FIM) |
| Developmental levels: | Miller Assessment for Preschoolers (MAP) |
| Eye-hand coordination: | Beery-Buktenica Developmental Test of Visual-Motor Integration, (6th ed.; VMI-6) |
| Perceptual ability: | Test of Visual Perceptual Scales (non-motor; 3rd ed.; TVPS-3) |
| Social skills: | Kohlman Evaluation of Living Skills (KELS) |
| Hand function: | Jebsen-Taylor Hand-Function Test (JTHFT) |

© Cengage Learning 2013

For example, an investigator is interested in comparing two methods of increasing self-care skills in patients who have experienced a stroke. After establishing two groups on the basis of screening criteria and random assignment, the researcher operationally defines self-care skills, such as independence in dressing. The operational definition includes the test and procedure in measuring the dependent variable, *self-care*. In another example involving retrospective research, an investigator is interested in correlating the relationship between disengagement in social decision making and choice of housing for individuals who are older (e.g., nursing home care or independent community living). The presumed independent variables, *housing arrangements*, are hypothesized to affect social decision making. Screening criteria are established in operationally defining the two housing arrangements. The researcher would then select the settings, and subjects would be selected randomly from each institution. The crux of the research is in operationally defining the concept of social decision making by selecting an objective standardized test.

In selecting a measuring instrument the researcher is faced with two basic questions with regard to psychometric properties:

1. Does the instrument measure a variable consistently?
2. Is the instrument a true measure of the variable?

The first question seeks a reliability index, and the second question raises the issues of validity.

## 7.11.4 Reliability

If one assumes that a specific characteristic of an individual remains stable over time, then a reliable measuring instrument should reflect the stable characteristics through repeated trials. For example, an electron microscope, sensitive enough to enlarge chromosomes so that a researcher can perceive them, maintains a consistency in measurement. In the physical sciences, where comparison dictates the foundation of measurement, the reliability of instruments has evolved progressively. Nonetheless, the individual using a sensitive measuring

instrument can affect what is being measured (Heisenberg Uncertainty Principle). For example, astronomers observed that the individual's reaction time in viewing the movement of stars affects calculation of determining distances between the stars. In response to this human factor, astronomers developed automatic means to record distances between celestial objects. The control of the personal equation in measurement is an important factor to consider in every research study where there is an interaction between the object observed and the investigator. This is especially true in qualitative research, such as in interviewing subjects where the investigator's presence affects the behavior of the interviewee.

Researchers strive to reduce the error factor in measurement by increasing the reliability of an objective test or instrument and reducing the variability of extraneous factors in the individual. Instruments, such as the electrocardiograph (EKG or ECG), electroencephalograph (EEG), X-ray, electromyograph (EMG), positron emission tomography (PET scan), magnetic resonance imaging (MRI), and single-photon emission computed tomography (SPECT) are usually reliable indicators of bodily functions. On the other hand, questionnaires, surveys, rating scales, attitude inventories, interest tests, and objective psychological tests may be less reliable. The nature of the test affects the reliability index.

Automatic instruments that record bodily functions need to be mechanically sound or calibrated to be reliable. In devising a reliable instrument, the investigator is concerned with eliminating items that are ambiguous or that can be answered in more than one way. Reliability is not a simple concept that merely reflects the consistency of the instrument. In any test administered to subjects, individual differences—such as level of reading ability, need to conform, desire to please the examiner, motivation, and test anxiety—are important factors that could potentially increase the error variance and decrease the consistency of response. Because human beings are constantly reacting to internal and external factors, reliability must be interpreted in a relative degree when considering psychological tests, questionnaires, and attitude scales. Most researchers with human subjects accept a reliability coefficient of approximately $r = .80$ or above to be an acceptable level of a test's consistency in measuring a variable.

### Techniques for Measuring Test Reliability

Test reliability is usually measured by correlating two sets of scores and arriving at a correlation coefficient. For example, an investigator is interested in devising a test of perceptual-motor ability with school-age children from 8 to 11 years old. In the process of devising the test, the investigator constructs 50 items that measure perceptual-motor ability. The items are screened for clarity in a pilot study with 24 children as subjects. The investigator seeks to determine **split half reliability** and **test-retest reliability**. In split half reliability, the test is broken into two equal parts (in this example, 25 items each) and correlated with each other. In test-retest reliability, a test is given twice within a short period of time (usually within 2 weeks) and the scores on the two tests are correlated.

In the hypothetical example shown in Table 7–7, there is a perfect positive correlation ($+1.00$) between the scores on the first and second tests. The scores reflect also a **practice effect**, which is typical of test-retest reliability. A practice effect exists when scores increase consistently as a function of the subject's familiarity with the content of the test and his or her reduced anxiety. In many published tests, the practice effect is controlled when developing normative data.

### 7.11.5 Item Analysis

When devising a test or assessing students, a researcher may be interested in the effectiveness of individual test items that differentiate between high and low achievers. The researcher may also be interested in eliminating those items that are ambiguous and have a low discriminative level. Item analysis is a method of gauging the difficulty value and ambiguity of each item. In item analysis, the percentage of passes and failures are calculated for each item. For example, if items 1, 2, and 3 are passed respectively by 80, 60, and 40 percent of the subjects, we can infer that item 3 is either more difficult or more ambiguous than item 1 or item 2. Another method

### TABLE 7-7

**Hypothetical Data for Testing Reliability**

| | Test-Retest Reliability | |
|---|---|---|
| Subject | Test 1 | Test 2 |
| 01 | 69 | 72 |
| 02 | 34 | 37 |
| 03 | 71 | 74 |
| 04 | 20 | 23 |
| 05 | 95 | 98 |
| 06 | 10 | 13 |
| 07 | 99 | 102 |
| 08 | 81 | 84 |
| 09 | 92 | 95 |
| 10 | 49 | 52 |
| 11 | 97 | 100 |
| 12 | 63 | 66 |
| 13 | 86 | 89 |
| 14 | 9 | 12 |
| 15 | 96 | 99 |
| 16 | 81 | 84 |
| 17 | 20 | 23 |
| 18 | 69 | 72 |
| 19 | 81 | 84 |
| 20 | 24 | 27 |
| 21 | 97 | 100 |
| 22 | 55 | 58 |
| 23 | 54 | 57 |
| 24 | 97 | 100 |
| 25 | 68 | 71 |

© Cengage Learning 2013

is analyzing items to determine which items were passed by high scorers and failed by low scorers. This analysis will enable the researcher to separate those items that have discriminative value. Items that are passed in all cases have little discriminative value but may indicate the level at which all members of the group are functioning. This may be particularly important in criterion-reference tests where the test administrator is most concerned with issues related to competency.

## 7.11.6 Validity

Validity reflects the authenticity of a test. Does the test measure what it purports to measure? A test may measure a concept consistently but it may not, in fact, measure what the researcher identifies as the intent of the test. Psychological tests purporting to measure general intelligence, self-image, body defensiveness, and attitude toward individuals with disabilities may be measuring other concepts. The degree to which a test is valid is the degree of empirical evidence that corroborates the results of a test. Tests or instruments that collect primary data, such as an EMG, X-ray, goniometer, ergometer, and MRI are easily verified and corroborated. By contrast, tests that collect secondary data derived from multiple factors in the individual, such as visual perception, are more difficult to validate. Personality, attitude, values, perception, and interests are complex variables derived from many facets of the individual's life that are related to genetic, social learning, cultural identification, and physiological factors. The researcher seeking to validate a visual-perceptual test is limited by the ability to corroborate the findings. Traditionally, validity is established on the following bases:

- **Content or face validity**: the degree to which the test appears to measure a concept by a logical analysis of the items. Does each item appear to relate to the content being tested?
- **Concurrent validity**: the degree of correlation with another standardized instrument. A new test may be developed because it is less time-consuming and less expensive than another established validated instrument. What is the correlation between the established test and the new test?
- **Predictive validity**: the degree to which a test can predict success or accuracy over a period of time (longitudinally). For example, a test devised to predict success in a graduate program

for occupational therapists or success in a rehabilitation program for patients with stroke are examples of predictive validity. In the examples, follow-up data from longitudinal studies would determine the correlation between the initial test predictor score and subsequent success in a program.

- **Construct validity**: considered to be the highest form of empirical evidence that scientific researchers seek. Construct validity assumes a theoretical rationale underlying the test instrument. In testing an instrument for construct validity, the researcher seeks behavioral data to substantiate the position that the test is in fact measuring a defined variable. For example, an investigator devising a test to measure self-image would first construct a theory that underlies the concept. The theory would include developmental factors, relationships with other variables, and behavioral observations supporting the evidence for construct validity. In another example, the electroencephalogram, which records brain waves and is used indirectly for diagnosing brain damage, can be checked for construct validity through dissection of an animal brain or through postmortem examination.

## 7.12 Ethical Principles Guiding Human Research

Boxes 7–1 through 7–5 give examples of documents related to ethical issues guiding clinical research.

### 7.12.1 The Declaration of Helsinki

The Declaration of Helsinki, which offers recommendations for conducting experiments using human subjects, was adopted in 1962 and revised by the 18th World Medical Assembly (WMA), Helsinki, Finland, in 1964. There have been several subsequent revisions with the latest (at the time of this printing) being adopted at the General Assembly WMA meeting in Seoul, October 2008. The 2008 version, reprinted in Box 7-1, is available on the Internet at http://www.wma.net/en/30publications/10policies/b3/index.html

BOX 7-1

## Declaration of Helsinki[1]

### WORLD MEDICAL ASSOCIATION DECLARATION OF HELSINKI

### Ethical Principles for Medical Research Involving Human Subjects

*Adopted by the 18th WMA General Assembly, Helsinki, Finland, June 1964, and amended by the:*
*29th WMA General Assembly, Tokyo, Japan, October 1975*
*35th WMA General Assembly, Venice, Italy, October 1983*
*41st WMA General Assembly, Hong Kong, September 1989*
*48th WMA General Assembly, Somerset West, Republic of South Africa, October 1996*
*52nd WMA General Assembly, Edinburgh, Scotland, October 2000*
*53rd WMA General Assembly, Washington 2002 (Note of Clarification on paragraph 29 added)*
*55th WMA General Assembly, Tokyo 2004 (Note of Clarification on Paragraph 30 added)*
*59th WMA General Assembly, Seoul, October 2008*

### A. INTRODUCTION

1. The World Medical Association (WMA) has developed the Declaration of Helsinki as a statement of ethical principles for medical research involving human subjects, including research on identifiable human material and data. The Declaration is intended to be read as a whole and each of its constituent paragraphs should not be applied without consideration of all other relevant paragraphs.

2. Although the Declaration is addressed primarily to physicians, the WMA encourages other participants in medical research involving human subjects to adopt these principles.

3. It is the duty of the physician to promote and safeguard the health of patients, including those who are involved in medical research. The physician's knowledge and conscience are dedicated to the fulfillment of this duty.

4. The Declaration of Geneva of the WMA binds the physician with the words, "The health of my patient will be my first consideration," and the International Code of Medical Ethics declares that, "A physician shall act in the patient's best interest when providing medical care."

---

[1]This document, amended from the original Declaration of Helsinki, is available on the Internet at http://www.wma.net/en/30publications/10policies/b3/index.html. Copyright, World Medical Association. All Rights Reserved.

*continues*

BOX 7-1

## Declaration of Helsinki *continued*

5. Medical progress is based on research that ultimately must include studies involving human subjects. Populations that are underrepresented in medical research should be provided appropriate access to participation in research.

6. In medical research involving human subjects, the well-being of the individual research subject must take precedence over all other interests.

7. The primary purpose of medical research involving human subjects is to understand the causes, development and effects of diseases and improve preventive, diagnostic and therapeutic interventions (methods, procedures and treatments). Even the best current interventions must be evaluated continually through research for their safety, effectiveness, efficiency, accessibility and quality.

8. In medical practice and in medical research, most interventions involve risks and burdens.

9. Medical research is subject to ethical standards that promote respect for all human subjects and protect their health and rights. Some research populations are particularly vulnerable and need special protection. These include those who cannot give or refuse consent for themselves and those who may be vulnerable to coercion or undue influence.

10. Physicians should consider the ethical, legal and regulatory norms and standards for research involving human subjects in their own countries as well as applicable international norms and standards. No national or international ethical, legal or regulatory requirement should reduce or eliminate any of the protections for research subjects set forth in this Declaration.

### B. PRINCIPLES FOR ALL MEDICAL RESEARCH

11. It is the duty of physicians who participate in medical research to protect the life, health, dignity, integrity, right to self-determination, privacy, and confidentiality of personal information of research subjects.

12. Medical research involving human subjects must conform to generally accepted scientific principles, be based on a thorough knowledge of the scientific literature, other relevant sources of information, and adequate laboratory and, as appropriate, animal experimentation. The welfare of animals used for research must be respected.

13. Appropriate caution must be exercised in the conduct of medical research that may harm the environment.

14. The design and performance of each research study involving human subjects must be clearly described in a research protocol. The protocol should contain a statement of the ethical considerations involved and should indicate how the principles in this Declaration have been addressed. The protocol should include information regarding funding,

sponsors, institutional affiliations, other potential conflicts of interest, incentives for subjects and provisions for treating and/or compensating subjects who are harmed as a consequence of participation in the research study. The protocol should describe arrangements for post-study access by study subjects to interventions identified as beneficial in the study or access to other appropriate care or benefits.

15. The research protocol must be submitted for consideration, comment, guidance and approval to a research ethics committee before the study begins. This committee must be independent of the researcher, the sponsor and any other undue influence. It must take into consideration the laws and regulations of the country or countries in which the research is to be performed as well as applicable international norms and standards but these must not be allowed to reduce or eliminate any of the protections for research subjects set forth in this Declaration. The committee must have the right to monitor ongoing studies. The researcher must provide monitoring information to the committee, especially information about any serious adverse events. No change to the protocol may be made without consideration and approval by the committee.

16. Medical research involving human subjects must be conducted only by individuals with the appropriate scientific training and qualifications. Research on patients or healthy volunteers requires the supervision of a competent and appropriately qualified physician or other health care professional. The responsibility for the protection of research subjects must always rest with the physician or other health care professional and never the research subjects, even though they have given consent.

17. Medical research involving a disadvantaged or vulnerable population or community is only justified if the research is responsive to the health needs and priorities of this population or community and if there is a reasonable likelihood that this population or community stands to benefit from the results of the research.

18. Every medical research study involving human subjects must be preceded by careful assessment of predictable risks and burdens to the individuals and communities involved in the research in comparison with foreseeable benefits to them and to other individuals or communities affected by the condition under investigation.

19. Every clinical trial must be registered in a publicly accessible database before recruitment of the first subject.

20. Physicians may not participate in a research study involving human subjects unless they are confident that the risks involved have been adequately assessed and can be satisfactorily managed. Physicians must immediately stop a study when the risks are found to outweigh the potential benefits or when there is conclusive proof of positive and beneficial results.

21. Medical research involving human subjects may only be conducted if the importance of the objective outweighs the inherent risks and burdens to the research subjects.

*continues*

BOX 7-1

## Declaration of Helsinki *continued*

22. Participation by competent individuals as subjects in medical research must be voluntary. Although it may be appropriate to consult family members or community leaders, no competent individual may be enrolled in a research study unless he or she freely agrees.

23. Every precaution must be taken to protect the privacy of research subjects and the confidentiality of their personal information and to minimize the impact of the study on their physical, mental and social integrity.

24. In medical research involving competent human subjects, each potential subject must be adequately informed of the aims, methods, sources of funding, any possible conflicts of interest, institutional affiliations of the researcher, the anticipated benefits and potential risks of the study and the discomfort it may entail, and any other relevant aspects of the study. The potential subject must be informed of the right to refuse to participate in the study or to withdraw consent to participate at any time without reprisal. Special attention should be given to the specific information needs of individual potential subjects as well as to the methods used to deliver the information. After ensuring that the potential subject has understood the information, the physician or another appropriately qualified individual must then seek the potential subject's freely-given informed consent, preferably in writing. If the consent cannot be expressed in writing, the non-written consent must be formally documented and witnessed.

25. For medical research using identifiable human material or data, physicians must normally seek consent for the collection, analysis, storage and/or reuse. There may be situations where consent would be impossible or impractical to obtain for such research or would pose a threat to the validity of the research. In such situations the research may be done only after consideration and approval of a research ethics committee.

26. When seeking informed consent for participation in a research study the physician should be particularly cautious if the potential subject is in a dependent relationship with the physician or may consent under duress. In such situations the informed consent should be sought by an appropriately qualified individual who is completely independent of this relationship.

27. For a potential research subject who is incompetent, the physician must seek informed consent from the legally authorized representative. These individuals must not be included in a research study that has no likelihood of benefit for them unless it is intended to promote the health of the population represented by the potential subject, the research cannot instead be performed with competent persons, and the research entails only minimal risk and minimal burden.

28. When a potential research subject who is deemed incompetent is able to give assent to decisions about participation in research, the physician must seek that assent in addition to

the consent of the legally authorized representative. The potential subject's dissent should be respected.

29. Research involving subjects who are physically or mentally incapable of giving consent, for example, unconscious patients, may be done only if the physical or mental condition that prevents giving informed consent is a necessary characteristic of the research population. In such circumstances the physician should seek informed consent from the legally authorized representative. If no such representative is available and if the research cannot be delayed, the study may proceed without informed consent provided that the specific reasons for involving subjects with a condition that renders them unable to give informed consent have been stated in the research protocol and the study has been approved by a research ethics committee. Consent to remain in the research should be obtained as soon as possible from the subject or a legally authorized representative.

30. Authors, editors, and publishers all have ethical obligations with regard to the publication of the results of research. Authors have a duty to make publicly available the results of their research on human subjects and are accountable for the completeness and accuracy of their reports. They should adhere to accepted guidelines for ethical reporting. Negative and inconclusive as well as positive results should be published or otherwise made publicly available. Sources of funding, institutional affiliations and conflicts of interest should be declared in the publication. Reports of research not in accordance with the principles of this Declaration should not be accepted for publication.

## C. ADDITIONAL PRINCIPLES FOR MEDICAL RESEARCH COMBINED WITH MEDICAL CARE

31. The physician may combine medical research with medical care only to the extent that the research is justified by its potential preventive, diagnostic or therapeutic value and if the physician has good reason to believe that participation in the research study will not adversely affect the health of the patients who serve as research subjects.

32. The benefits, risks, burdens and effectiveness of a new intervention must be tested against those of the best current proven intervention, except in the following circumstances:
    - The use of placebo, or no treatment, is acceptable in studies where no current proven intervention exists; or
    - Where for compelling and scientifically sound methodological reasons the use of placebo is necessary to determine the efficacy or safety of an intervention and the patients who receive placebo or no treatment will not be subject to any risk of serious or irreversible harm. Extreme care must be taken to avoid abuse of this option.

33. At the conclusion of the study, patients entered into the study are entitled to be informed about the outcome of the study and to share any benefits that result from it, for example, access to interventions identified as beneficial in the study or to other appropriate care or benefits.

*continues*

## Declaration of Helsinki *continued*

34. The physician must fully inform the patient which aspects of the care are related to the research. The refusal of a patient to participate in a study or the patient's decision to withdraw from the study must never interfere with the patient-physician relationship.

35. In the treatment of a patient, where proven interventions do not exist or have been ineffective, the physician, after seeking expert advice, with informed consent from the patient or a legally authorized representative, may use an unproven intervention if in the physician's judgment it offers hope of saving life, re-establishing health or alleviating suffering. Where possible, this intervention should be made the object of research, designed to evaluate its safety and efficacy. In all cases, new information should be recorded and, where appropriate, made publicly available.

### 7.12.2 Harvard University Medical School

The guidelines reproduced in Box 7–2 "outline principles that should be followed at Harvard Medical School when conducting research." They are a supplement to the *Guidelines for Investigators in Scientific Research*, first issued in February 1988 (Harvard Medical School, 1996). The full document, *Faculty Policies on Integrity in Science*, is available in hard copy from the Office for Research Issues, Harvard Medical School (1991).

BOX 7-2

## Guidelines for Investigators in Clinical Research[2]

### Introduction

These guidelines outline principles that should be followed at Harvard Medical School when conducting research. They are a supplement to the Guidelines for Investigators in Scientific Research, first issued in February 1988. Clinical research may be defined as investigations involving human subjects or the use of patient samples. The scientific practices described here are generally accepted by investigators conducting both multi-center and single-institution clinical studies and help ensure both the quality and integrity of scientific findings in clinical research. The guidelines are not intended to relieve investigators of any ethical obligations that may be imposed by individual Institutional Review Boards overseeing the rights of study subjects in clinical research.

[2]Reprinted with permission from the Office for Research Issues, Harvard Medical School. Copyright 1996, Harvard Medical School. This document is available at http://www.hms.harvard.edu/integrity/clinical.html

A major component of clinical research consists of either prospective clinical trials or retrospective studies based on medical or administrative records. Of these two types of studies, prospective trials contain fewer chances for investigator bias and for lost or incomplete data than do retrospective studies, and are to be preferred whenever they are feasible. Some phenomena, however, such as rare diseases or diseases requiring exceptionally long follow-up, can only be studied from a case series assembled from medical records. These guidelines address issues that arise in both types of studies.

The implementation of these guidelines rests within each of the affiliated institutions and the department in which the research is conducted. Whenever research is carried out by non-faculty, such as a student or fellow, the supervisor of that individual is responsible for ensuring that these guidelines are followed.

## I. EXPERIMENTAL DESIGN

Successful clinical studies acknowledge the complexity of conducting scientific research with human subjects, and are based both on the principles of experimental design and on respect for the rights of study subjects. Experiments in human subjects generally have highly variable outcomes, and efficient designs that lead to unbiased conclusions are critical.

### Recommendations

1. Each study, whether it be observations on one or more patients, a randomized trial, or a population based study, should have clearly articulated research objectives that can be achieved from a successful execution of the study design.

2. Whenever some aspects of a study involve clinical or scientific specialties outside the expertise of the investigator, drafts of the protocol or research plan should be circulated to specialists in those areas for review and comment.

3. Every prospective or retrospective clinical study should have a written protocol or research plan that states the goals of the study, provides a background and rationale for the study, specifies the criteria for inclusion or exclusion of cases, outlines the methods and timings of follow-up, gives a precise definition of the types of anticipated outcome measures, and gives the details of the statistical design. The study design should minimize the possibility for investigator bias in the interpretation of the results. The design specification may range from a description of anticipated measurements in an exploratory study to a precise specification of the number of cases that will be registered in a phase III randomized trial. In the case of prospective trials, the protocol should describe in detail how patients are to be treated or managed. Any substantial changes to the conduct of the study, including modifications of the sample size, eligibility criteria, or treatment regimens, should be reflected in amendments made to the protocol or research plan and approved by co-investigators and the Institutional Review Board.

4. In randomized clinical trials, the sequence of treatment assignments should be prepared by a statistician or other experienced investigator associated with the trial and kept confidential. In no instance should an investigator treating patients on the trial know the sequence of potential treatment assignments.

*continues*

BOX 7-2

## Guidelines for Investigators in Clinical Research *continued*

5. Clinical studies all require approval of local Institutional Review Boards. Every prospective clinical study should contain an Informed Consent form that explains in clear, non-technical terms the possible risks and benefits for subjects participating in the trial.

## II. DATA MANAGEMENT AND TRIAL MONITORING

Complete and accurate data are an essential part of the record of any clinical research. Since serious problems can occur when data are missing or are not consistent with source medical records, each study should include a plan for the keeping of accurate and well documented data not subject to loss through computer failure or insecure storage.

### Recommendations

1. In prospective trials, data should be abstracted from source medical records as the trial proceeds, using data collection forms designed at the outset of the study. Data collection forms should also be used in retrospective record studies.

2. The criteria for the evaluation of study subjects (including the classification of outcome and any treatment side effects) should be specified in the protocol or research plan.

3. Interim review of the data from an ongoing trial should make use of statistical methods that guard against increased false-positive or false-negative reporting rates caused by inappropriate conclusions from preliminary analyses.

4. For research involving primary data collection, the principle investigator should retain original data for as long as practically possible, but never for less than five years from the first major publication or from the completion of an unpublished study. All data should be kept in the research unit responsible for conducting the study. Copies of computer programs and the results from statistical calculations used in research involving nationally gathered survey data should also be kept by research units for a minimum of five years from publication based on these results. After notification to responsible departmental officials, principal investigators may make copies of original data or computer programs for personal use or when moving to another research unit or institution.

5. If primary data are kept on a computer file, backup files should be maintained, preferably at a second site, to prevent loss from computer failure.

## III. SCIENTIFIC REPORTING

Writing a manuscript reporting the results of a clinical study is a complex and demanding task. Unclear or ambiguous reports reduce the value of a study and may lead to a discrediting of the research.

### Recommendations

1. The statistical analysis used in reporting the results should coincide with the planned analysis used to design the study. Reasons should be given in the manuscript for any different analyses that are used.

2. All cases registered in a clinical trial or records reviewed in a retrospective study must be accounted for in any manuscript reporting the results. Any case not used in the analysis of outcome data should be identified (by case number) and the reason for exclusion noted.

## IV. AUTHORSHIP

Clinical studies often involve investigators from several subspecialties, and it may not always be possible for a single investigator to confirm each piece of data used in the report of a trial. While each participating investigator must be actively involved in verifying the sections of a manuscript that discuss his/ her specialty area, there must nevertheless be a primary author who is responsible for the validity of the entire manuscript.

### Recommendations

1. Criteria for authorship of a manuscript should be determined and announced by each department or research unit. The committee considers the only reasonable criterion to be that the co-author has made a significant intellectual or practical contribution. The concept of "honorary authorship" is deplorable.

2. The first author should assure the head of the research unit or department chairperson that he/she has reviewed all primary data on which the report is based and provide a brief description of the role of each co-author. (In multi-institutional collaborations, the senior investigator in each institution should prepare such statements.)

3. Appended to the final draft of the manuscript should be a signed statement from each co-author indicating that he/she has reviewed and approved the manuscript to the extent possible, given individual expertise.

The *Code of Federal Regulations*, published by the Department of Health and Human Services (2009) provides additional information concerning the use of human research. This information is available at http://www.hhs.gov/ohrp/humansubjects/guidance/45cfr46.html#46.101(b) Other federal regulations can be found at the Code of Federal Regulations website (http://www.gpoaccess.gov/cfr/index.html)

### 7.12.3 Human Subjects Review Protocol (HSRP)

Any institution actively involved with research involving human subjects needs to establish an institutional review board (IRB) as outlined in the U.S. Federal Policy 45 CFR 46. Research involving human subjects falls into one of three categories: convened, expedited, or exempt. The determination is based on the risk to human subjects. A basic rule of thumb is that research protocols that have more than minimal risk are required to be assigned to the convened application process. Minimal risk is defined as "the probability and magnitude of harm or discomfort anticipated in the research are not greater in and of themselves than those ordinarily encountered in daily life or during the performance of routine physical or psychological examinations or tests" (United States Department of Health and Human Services, 2009, §46.102 Definitions, para. i.). If there is risk associated with the research protocol, but the risk is no more than minimal, then the protocol will be assigned to an expedited review. In protocols where there is no risk involved, then the IRB review designation will be exempt.

Convened reviews require more effort by the entire IRB and are thus more carefully scrutinized than the other two types of review. Whereas, the expedited review generally involves less scrutiny, it still requires a thorough review by one or more IRB member(s) for approval. The exempt review usually involves fewer IRB members than the other two types of review, but still requires a thorough IRB review. The IRB application process usually includes an application (see Box 7–3), an informed consent (see Box 7–5), the research protocol, and a financial disclosure and conflict of interest form, as well as any supporting data collection tools, instruments, advertisement flyers/brochures, and letters of support. A full IRB application is a thoughtful process and also requires that all persons associated with the research protocol have documented training in the following:

- Health Insurance Portability and Accountability Act (HIPAA) (http://www.hhs.gov/ohrp/humansubjects/assurance/filasurt.htm)
- Federal wide assurance for the protection of human subjects (http://www.hhs.gov/ohrp/humansubjects/guidance/belmont.htm)
- Protecting Human Research Participants Online Course (http://phrp.nihtraining.com/users/overview.php)

Box 7–3 is an example of an application for an expedited review used by The University of Toledo, whereas Box 7–4 is an example of a checklist from The University of Toledo that can be used by the research to conform to IRB guidelines. It is important, however, for researchers to follow the guidelines established by the IRB in which they are affiliated.

## 7.13 Data Collection Procedures

The time schedule for collecting data, the costs of the study, the setting for administering group or individual tests, a cover letter to prospective subjects explaining the nature of the study, an individual data collection sheet recording descriptive information and test scores, an informed consent agreement between the researcher and subject, and the statistical techniques used to analyze the data are all factors for the investigator to consider in the prospectus for the study.

The checklist in Table 7–8 should guide the investigator in preparing a data collection procedure. The reader should review this frequently to ensure that all parts of the data collection have been considered.

### 7.13.1 Informed Consent and Forms

The **informed consent form** is a legal document that informs participants about the procedures that are to occur, the place in which the data collection will occur, the amount of time required for participation, and the potential risks or hazards of the study. Informed consent must be documented (United States Department of Health and Human Services, 2009). A copy of the signed informed consent form must be obtained for the principal investigator's files from each participant, or in the case of a minor, the parent, guardian, or surrogate parent. A copy should be given to each participant. The participant's copy should include the name, address, telephone number, and e-mail address of the person to whom requests for information or results may be addressed. It must also include the name, address, telephone number, and e-mail address of the person to whom complaints may be addressed. The informed consent form should be written in language that is easily understood by all participants.

BOX 7-3

## The University of Toledo Expedited Research Application

**INSTRUCTIONS:**

All UT research using living human subjects, or samples or data obtained from them, directly or indirectly, with or without their consent, must either be approved in advance by the UT Institutional Review Board (IRB), or be found to meet narrow criteria for exemption from IRB oversight by the IRB office. This Form will help the PI to determine if the project is likely to meet the criteria for expedited review and to document the decision on this request.

**Expedited review** procedures are described in 45 CFR 46.110 (OHHS) and 21 CFR 56.110 (FDA). In short, the IRB Chair or one or more experienced reviewers, designated by the Chair from among members of the IRB, review the research and approve it or refer it to the convened IRB for full IRB review. The criteria for Expedited Review can be found on the UT DHRP/IRB forms page and the **Federal Register 63 FR 60364-60367, November 9, 1998**.

For a research project to qualify for expedited review, the following must apply:

**The University of Toledo**
**Department for Human Research Protections**
**Biomedical Institutional Review Board**
CCE Building – Room 0106
3025 Arlington Avenue, Toledo, Ohio 43614-2570
Phone: 419-383-6796   Fax: 419-383-3248
(FWA00010686)

### EXPEDITED RESEARCH
### INSTRUCTIONS, CATEGORIES & APPLICATION

*For designation as a new research project involving no more than minimal risk to human subjects.*

(A)   Research activities that **(1) present no more than minimal risk to human subjects\*, and (2) involve only procedures listed in one or more of the following categories, may be reviewed by the IRB through the expedited review procedure authorized by 45 CFR 46.110 and 21 CFR 56.110**. The activities listed should not be deemed to be of minimal risk simply because they are included on this list. Inclusion on this list merely means that the activity is eligible for review through the expedited review procedure when the specific circumstances of the proposed research involve no more than minimal risk to human subjects.

(B)   The categories in this list apply regardless of the age of subjects, except as noted.

*continues*

(C)    The expedited review procedure may not be used where identification of the subjects and/ or their responses would reasonably place them at risk of criminal or civil liability or be damaging to the subject's financial standing, employability, insurability, reputation, or be stigmatizing, unless reasonable and appropriate protections will be implemented so that risks related to invasion of privacy and breach of confidentiality are no greater than minimal.

(D)    The expedited review procedure may not be used for classified research involving human subjects.

(E)    The standard requirements for informed consent (or its waiver, alteration, or exception) apply regardless of the type of review--expedited or convened--utilized by the IRB.

(F)    Expedited categories one (1) through seven (7) pertain to both initial and continuing IRB review.

*Minimal Risk* is defined as "the risk of harm anticipated in the proposed research that is not greater, considering the probability and magnitude, than those ordinarily encountered in daily life or during the performance of routine physical or psychological examinations or tests."

## INSTRUCTIONS:

1.    Review the Expedited Categories below and mark the appropriate checkbox(es).
2.    Complete the entire Expedited Research Application form that follows on pages 4 - 11.
3.    Access the Expedited Checklist via the hyperlink or DHRP web page and submit with application.
4.    You may not begin your research project until you receive a written approval document from the UT IRB. This is especially important if you are seeking approval from more than one IRB.

## EXPEDITED RESEARCH CATEGORIES 63 FR 60364-60367, November 9, 1998

**Please identify all that apply to your research (check applicable boxes)**

| ☐ 1. | Clinical studies of drugs and medical devices only when condition (a) or (b) is met. | |
|---|---|---|
| | ☐ 1a | Research on drugs for which an investigational new drug application (21 CFR Part 312) is not required. (Note: Research on marketed drugs that significantly increases the risks or decreases the acceptability of the risks associated with the use of the product is not eligible for expedited review.) |
| | ☐ 1b | Research on medical devices for which (i) an investigational device exemption application (21 CFR Part 812) is not required; or (ii) the medical device is cleared/approved for marketing and the medical device is being used in accordance with its cleared/approved labeling. |

| ☐ 2. | Collection of blood samples by finger stick, heel stick, ear stick, or veni-puncture as follows: | |
|---|---|---|
| | ☐ 2a | from healthy, non-pregnant adults who weigh at least 110 pounds. For these subjects, the amounts drawn may not exceed 550 ml in an 8 week period and collection may not occur more frequently than 2 times per week; or |
| | ☐ 2b | from other adults and children (17 years old or younger) considering the age, weight, and health of the subjects, the collection procedure, the amount of blood to be collected, and the frequency with which it will be collected. For these subjects, the amount drawn may not exceed the lesser of 50 ml or 3 ml per kg in an 8 week period and collection may not occur more frequently than 2 times per week. |
| ☐ 3. | Prospective collection of biological specimens for research purposes by non-invasive means. <br><br> <u>Examples:</u> <br> a. hair and nail clippings in a non-disfiguring manner; <br> b. deciduous teeth at time of exfoliation or if routine patient care indicates a need for extraction; <br> c. permanent teeth if routine patient care indicates a need for extraction; <br> d. excreta and external secretions (including sweat); <br> e. un-cannulated saliva collected either in an un-stimulated fashion or stimulated by chewing gum-base or wax or by applying a dilute citric solution to the tongue; <br> f. placenta removed at delivery; <br> g. amniotic fluid obtained at the time of rupture of the membrane prior to or during labor; <br> h. supra- and sub-gingival dental plaque and calculus, provided the collection procedure is not more invasive than routine prophylactic scaling of the teeth and the process is accomplished in accordance with accepted prophylactic techniques; <br> i. mucosal and skin cells collected by buccal scraping or swab, skin swab, or mouth washings; <br> j. sputum collected after saline mist nebulization. | |
| ☐ 4. | Collection of data through noninvasive procedures (not involving general anesthesia or sedation) routinely employed in clinical practice, excluding procedures involving x-rays or microwaves. Where medical devices are employed, they must be cleared/approved for marketing. (Studies intended to evaluate the safety and effectiveness of the medical device are not generally eligible for expedited review, including studies of cleared medical devices for new indications.) <br><br> <u>Examples:</u> <br> a. physical sensors that are applied either to the surface of the body or at a distance and do not involve input of significant amounts of energy into the subject or an invasion of the subject's privacy; <br> b. weighing or testing sensory acuity; | |

*continues*

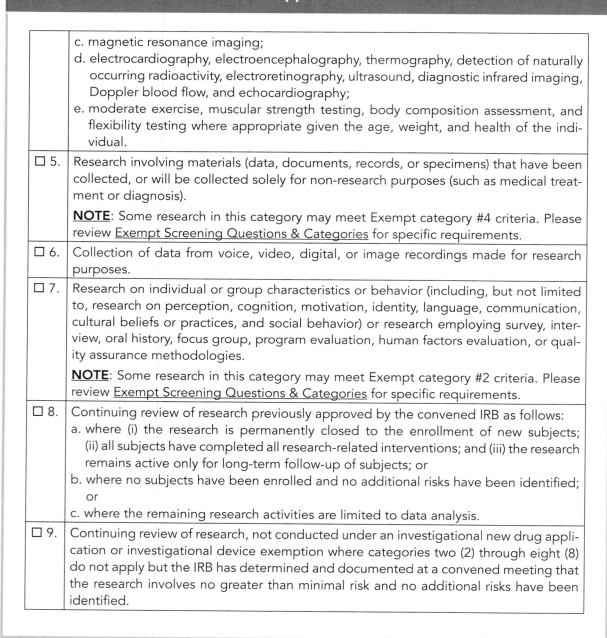

BOX 7-3

## The University of Toledo Expedited Research Application *continued*

|  |  |  |
|---|---|---|
|  |  | c. magnetic resonance imaging; |
|  |  | d. electrocardiography, electroencephalography, thermography, detection of naturally occurring radioactivity, electroretinography, ultrasound, diagnostic infrared imaging, Doppler blood flow, and echocardiography; |
|  |  | e. moderate exercise, muscular strength testing, body composition assessment, and flexibility testing where appropriate given the age, weight, and health of the individual. |
| ☐ | 5. | Research involving materials (data, documents, records, or specimens) that have been collected, or will be collected solely for non-research purposes (such as medical treatment or diagnosis). **NOTE**: Some research in this category may meet Exempt category #4 criteria. Please review <u>Exempt Screening Questions & Categories</u> for specific requirements. |
| ☐ | 6. | Collection of data from voice, video, digital, or image recordings made for research purposes. |
| ☐ | 7. | Research on individual or group characteristics or behavior (including, but not limited to, research on perception, cognition, motivation, identity, language, communication, cultural beliefs or practices, and social behavior) or research employing survey, interview, oral history, focus group, program evaluation, human factors evaluation, or quality assurance methodologies. **NOTE**: Some research in this category may meet Exempt category #2 criteria. Please review <u>Exempt Screening Questions & Categories</u> for specific requirements. |
| ☐ | 8. | Continuing review of research previously approved by the convened IRB as follows: a. where (i) the research is permanently closed to the enrollment of new subjects; (ii) all subjects have completed all research-related interventions; and (iii) the research remains active only for long-term follow-up of subjects; or b. where no subjects have been enrolled and no additional risks have been identified; or c. where the remaining research activities are limited to data analysis. |
| ☐ | 9. | Continuing review of research, not conducted under an investigational new drug application or investigational device exemption where categories two (2) through eight (8) do not apply but the IRB has determined and documented at a convened meeting that the research involves no greater than minimal risk and no additional risks have been identified. |

## A. STUDY INFORMATION

| | | | |
|---|---|---|---|
| **Date** | | **IRB Number:**<br>(Assigned by IRB office) | |
| **Study Title:** | | | |
| **Principal Investigator or Faculty Advisor:** | | **Rocket ID #<br>or S.S. #** | |
| **Department:** | | | |
| **Contact Person:**<br>(If applicable) | | | |
| **Contact Person's Role on Project:** | | **Pager:** | |
| **Contact Person's Phone:**<br>**Contact Person's Fax:** | | **Email:** | |
| **Is this a student project?** | ☐ Yes   ☐ No | | |

## B. STUDY PERSONNEL

Please list all study personnel involved in the conduct of this study. Anyone who is "engaged in research" must be listed below. This includes those personnel who interact or intervene with subjects and/or have access to subjects' identifiable private information. This list may be different (usually longer) than the key personnel list included in a federal grant.

**All study personnel must complete human subject research training and submit the certification documents to the IRB office. IRB review of the study will not begin without verifying completion of this requirement.**

**Only UT faculty, staff, students, or registered volunteers are considered "UT-affiliated" and thus covered by the UT IRB review. All non-affiliated study personnel must have their participation reviewed by their institution's IRB, or complete an Individual Investigator Agreement with The University of Toledo.**

| Study Personnel's First/Last Name | UT Affiliated | UT I.D. # | Role in Protocol | Role in the Consent Process | | Research Training Completed? | |
|---|---|---|---|---|---|---|---|
| | | | | Explain Only | Explain & Obtain | Yes | No |
| *John Smith | ☐ | | *Principal Investigator | ☐ | ☐ | ☐ | ☐ |
| *Jane Doe | ☐ | | *Coordinator | ☐ | ☐ | ☐ | ☐ |
| *Ann Jones | ☐ | | *Co-Investigator | ☐ | ☐ | ☐ | ☐ |
| | ☐ | | | ☐ | ☐ | ☐ | ☐ |
| | ☐ | | | ☐ | ☐ | ☐ | ☐ |
| | ☐ | | | ☐ | ☐ | ☐ | ☐ |
| | ☐ | | | ☐ | ☐ | ☐ | ☐ |
| | ☐ | | | ☐ | ☐ | ☐ | ☐ |
| | ☐ | | | ☐ | ☐ | ☐ | ☐ |

*Example of required information; please delete examples when filling in table.*

*continues*

BOX 7-3

**The University of Toledo Expedited Research Application** *continued*

| C. STUDY FUNDING | | | |
|---|---|---|---|
| ☐ Unfunded | ☐ Funded | ☐ Intramural | ☐ *Extramural |
| Amount: $ | ☐ Per subject | ☐ Total | |
| If Intramural, please provide UT Institutional Account number: | | | |
| If *Extramural, please provide the following information: | | | |
| Agency/Company Name: | | Agency ID No./Protocol #: | |
| Agency/Company Address: | | | |
| Agency/Company Contact: | | | |
| Agency/Company Contact Phone: | | | |
| Contact E-Mail: | | | |
| Extramural Funding Status: | ☐ Pending | ☐ Funded | ☐ Planned |
| Contract Status: | ☐ Pending | ☐ Finalized | |
| Grant or Company Protocol Title: *(If different than study title)* | | | |
| *GRANT PROPOSAL - If the research protocol is currently supported by a grant proposal, **OR** if support for the research protocol has been requested under a grant proposal, attach the research proposal/protocol that <u>was sent</u> to the agency, committee or sponsor. | | | |

**ALL** UT Faculty and staff members listed as study personnel must submit an RSP Conflict-of-Interest Disclosure Form. Please see section J. Conflict-of-Interest, for an explanation of potential conflicts and a link to the form.

| D. PERFORMANCE SITE(S) |
|---|
| List all performance sites for this study. Attach permission letters and/or current IRB approval memos (on the site's official letterhead) for off-campus sites. **Check box if site is "engaged in research."** A site becomes "engaged" in human subjects research when its employees or agents: (i) intervene or interact with living individuals for research purposes; or (ii) obtain individually identifiable private information for research purposes [45 CFR 46.102(d),(f)]. (Do not list non-UT sites in industry-sponsored multi-center studies.) |

| Performance site Name | Address | Engaged in research? Yes | No |
|---|---|---|---|
| | | ☐ | ☐ |
| | | ☐ | ☐ |
| | | ☐ | ☐ |
| | | ☐ | ☐ |
| | | ☐ | ☐ |
| | | ☐ | ☐ |

### E. STUDY SUMMARY

Please provide summary statements to answer the questions below in non-technical, layman's terms. A separate, complete Protocol document explaining the elements of the project should also accompany this application. The following hyperlinked guidance document can be used as an outline. <u>The Elements of a Research Protocol</u>

1. What is the objective of the study?

2. Provide a brief background and significance of the proposed research.

3. Describe the study procedures and information to be collected. Clearly denote the procedures which are standard-of-care and those which are research specific.

4. Describe any risks to the subject including the potential for loss of confidentiality, if any.

5. Describe how risks will be minimized.

6. For use of medical records:
   Will you have ongoing contact with the subjects?
   Will you be recording identifiers or using codes that can be linked to subject's records?
   What is the date timeframe of charts that you plan to review? (e.g., 02/01/1999 – 02/01/2001)

<u>IMPORTANT NOTE:</u> *Retrospective* chart review involves medical records that were in place <u>BEFORE</u> you received IRB approval. Any chart information that comes into existence <u>AFTER</u> IRB approval is granted would be considered *Prospective.*

7. In addition to the attached research protocol, provide a 1-2 sentence description of the proposed research. *(All research approved by expedited review must be reported to the convened IRB. This brief description will be reported on the IRB agenda.)*

*continues*

BOX 7-3

## The University of Toledo Expedited Research Application *continued*

### F. HUMAN RESEARCH SUBJECTS

**Subject Population:**

Maximum number to be enrolled at this institution:

If multi-site, total number of subjects for entire project:

What is the gender of the subjects?  ☐ Male  ☐ Female  ☐ Both

What is the age range of the subjects?

**1. To what health/disease category will the human subjects belong?**

**2. What will be the total duration of involvement of each subject in the study?**

**3. Is the research limited to any particular age, gender, ethnic, or racial group?** *(If an equitable recruitment from among all populations is not anticipated, please provide justification. If research is not limited to any particular group, be sure to check the appropriate boxes in #4 if any of the listed vulnerable populations may possibly be included in the study population.)*

**4. Will any of the following vulnerable populations be included?**

☐ Minors            ☐ Minorities                  ☐ Fetuses         ☐ Pregnant women
☐ Prisoners         ☐ Mentally incapacitated      ☐ Terminally ill  ☐ non-English speaking
☐ Elderly           ☐ Severe Psychological        ☐ UT's students or staff
                      Disorders

**5. What additional safeguards are in place to protect vulnerable populations involved with the proposed research to avoid coercion or undue influence?**

**6. Please outline the criteria for selection and exclusion of subjects.**

7. **Will subjects receive compensation for their participation, monetary or otherwise?**
YES ☐   NO ☐
If YES, specify.
Describe any conditions under which a subject would receive partial or no payment:

8. **What financial obligations will subjects incur as a result of participating in the research study?** Identify expenses such as travel costs, drugs, devices, lab tests, etc. Be as specific as possible. *(Itemize the procedures not covered by research funds and approximate their cumulative cost.)*

## G. RECRUITMENT PROCEDURES

1. What method(s) will be used to identify and recruit prospective subjects? Please specify the source of potential subjects.

2. Check all types of recruitment material that will be utilized in the study. Attach copies of this material to the application.

☐ Advertisements     ☐ Newsletters     ☐ Internet
☐ Brochures          ☐ Radio           ☐ Contact letters to patients or physician
☐ Flyers/posters     ☐ Other (Describe)

3. Will you access stored medical records, data, or specimens for research use? If yes, specify the source.

## H. THE CONSENT PROCESS – *Please complete the applicable section(s).*
    H-1. <u>Written Informed Consent</u>    H-2. <u>Alteration or Waiver of Informed Consent</u>
    H-3. <u>Waiver of *Written* Consent</u>    H-4. <u>Waiver of HIPAA/PHI for Research Purposes</u>

## H-1. WRITTEN AND SIGNED INFORMED CONSENT

*Per Federal regulations, (45 CFR 46.117), informed consent shall be documented by the use of a <u>written</u> consent form <u>approved by the IRB</u> and signed by the subject or the subject's legally authorized representative. A copy shall be given to the person signing the form.*

*Please attach a copy of all Consent/Assent forms for this study.*

*continues*

**BOX 7-3**

## The University of Toledo Expedited
## Research Application *continued*

1. **How and where will informed consent be obtained?** (e.g., in the clinic, PI's private office, subject's home, etc.)

2. **When will the potential subjects or their legally authorized representatives initially be approached for consent and by whom?**

3. **Will there be an opportunity for potential subject to take consent form home to consider the options and to discuss participation with family members. If not, explain why.**

4. **If subjects are minors or mentally disabled, describe how and by whom permission will be granted?**

5. **How and by whom will it be determined that the subjects or their legally authorized representatives understand the research project and their rights as participants?**

6. **Where will the record of consent be stored?** *Please note: If the subject is a patient, a copy must be kept in the subject's permanent medical record.*

7. **Please list all study personnel who will obtain consent.**

### H-2. ALTERATION OR WAIVER OF CONSENT

*The IRB may waive the requirements to obtain informed consent provided the IRB finds and documents the following four items. If you are requesting a waiver of the consent requirement, please provide justification in the space below that each of the four conditions have been met.*

*If this project involves Protected Health Information (PHI), you must __also__ complete the H-4 section and a* Waiver of HIPAA Authorization for Use and Disclosure of PHI for Purposes of Research *request form and submit it with this application.*

(1) the research involves no more than minimal risk to the subjects;

(2) the waiver or alteration will not adversely affect the rights and welfare of the subjects;

(3) the research could not practicably be carried out without the waiver or alteration; and

(4) whenever appropriate, the subjects will be provided with additional pertinent information after their participation.

## H-3. WAIVER OF WRITTEN INFORMED CONSENT
*(Waiver of the documentation requirement.)*

*The IRB may waive the requirement for the investigator to obtain a <u>signed</u> consent form for some or all subjects if it finds the following two requirements. If you are requesting a waiver of <u>written</u> consent, please provide justification in the space below that both of the conditions have been met. The informed consent process must still occur and an altered (short form) explanation of the research is required.*

*Please attach a copy of the cover memo or information sheet that will be distributed to subjects.*

(1) The only record linking the subject and the research would be the consent document and the principal risk would be potential harm resulting from a breach of confidentiality. Each subject will be asked whether the subject wants documentation linking the subject with the research, and the subject's wishes will govern;
*Justification:*

**OR**

(2) That the research presents no more than minimal risk of harm to subjects and involves no procedures for which written consent is normally required outside of the research context.
*Justification:*

*continues*

BOX 7-3

## The University of Toledo Expedited
## Research Application *continued*

### H-4. WAIVER OF HIPAA AUTHORIZATION FOR USE AND DISCLOSURE OF PROTECTED HEALTH INFORMATION (PHI) FOR PURPOSES OF RESEARCH

☐ Please check here if you are requesting a Waiver of HIPAA Authorization for Use and Disclosure of Protected Health Information (PHI) for Purposes of Research. Complete the *Waiver of HIPAA Authorization* request form and submit it with this application.

### I. CONFIDENTIALITY

Data include not only paper documents, but also blood samples, tissues, etc.

1. What methods will be employed to ensure the confidentiality of participation and data?

2. How will data be collected and recorded?

3. If a key or code will be used for recording dates, please describe how this will be used.

4. Where will data be stored during the study and how will it be secured?

5. Who will have access to the data and/or to the codes?

6. If data with identifiers will be released, specify the person(s) or agency to which this information will be released?

7. What will happen to the data when the research is complete? *(All study records should be kept a minimum of three years after the completion of the study. PHI data/records must be kept for six years.)*

## J. CONFLICT OF INTEREST

Please print and attach the <u>RSP Conflict of Interest Disclosure Form</u> for each individual listed on this application. If submitted to RSP during the contract process, please attach a <u>copy</u> to this application.

Is there any real or apparent conflict of interest on the part of any study personnel (e.g., stock or stock options, interest in technology, consultant to sponsor)?    Yes ☐   No ☐

If Yes, please explain:

Please check the appropriate response for this study:

☐ The RSP Conflict of Interest Disclosure Forms are attached to this application.

☐ The RSP Conflict of Interest Disclosure Forms have been submitted to RSP as part of the contract process for this research study.

## K. ASSURANCES

### Principal Investigator's Assurance Statement:

- I certify that the information provided in this application is complete and accurate.

- I understand that as Principal Investigator, I have the ultimate responsibility for the protection of the rights and welfare of human subjects, and the strict adherence to any study-specific requirements imposed by the IRB.

- I agree to comply with all IRB and Institutional policies and procedures, as well as with all applicable Federal, State, and local laws and regulations regarding the protection of human subjects in research and the conduct of clinical research.

- I also agree to the following:
  1. to accept responsibility for the scientific and ethical conduct of this research study,
  2. to obtain prior approval from the Institutional Review Board before amending or altering the research protocol or implementing changes in the approved consent form, study sites or study personnel, recruitment procedures,
  3. to immediately report to the IRB any serious adverse reactions and/or unanticipated effects on subjects which may occur as a result of this study,
  4. to train study personnel in the proper conduct of human subjects research,
  5. to assure that the personnel approved to explain and obtain consent have read the protocol, understand the study, and are fully knowledgeable of ALL details of the protocol and are able to answer ALL questions from research subjects such as risks and alternative treatments and therapies.

*continues*

Reprinted by permission of The University of Toledo

> **BOX 7-3**
>
> ## The University of Toledo Expedited Research Application *continued*
>
> 6. to complete the Continuing Review and Final Report Forms required by the UT IRB,
> 7. to adhere to the standards of Good Clinical Practice (GCP)*, developed by the International Conference on Harmonization (ICH).
>
> _____     _____
> Signature of Principal Investigator          Date
>
> _____
> Printed name of Principal Investigator
>
> For information regarding Good Clinical Practices (GCPs), please access the following link:
> http://www.fda.gov/ScienceResearch/SpecialTopics/RunningClinicalTrials/default.htm
>
> ### L. DEPARTMENTAL CHAIR OR DEAN'S ASSURANCE STATEMENT
>
> My signature certifies that:
> 1. I have reviewed this application, and I believe that the benefits of the proposed research outweigh the risks to the study subjects.
> 2. The Principal Investigator has appropriate training, experience, and expertise to conduct this study.
> 3. The Principal Investigator has adequate staff and facilities to conduct the project.
> 4. If I become aware of any factors which have the potential to adversely affect the risk/benefit ratio for study subjects, or any issues that may reflect noncompliance with UT policies, or FDA and OHRP regulations regarding research with human subjects, I will immediately report these to the UT IRB.
>
> _____     _____
> Signature of Chair/Dean                       Date
>
> _____
> Printed name of Chair/Dean
>
> *Note: If the Principal Investigator is the Chair of a Department, the appropriate Dean's signature is required.*

BOX 7-4

## The University of Toledo
## Checklist for Complying with IRB Standards

**Department for Human Research Protections**
**UT Institutional Review Boards**
Center for Creative Education Building, Rooms 0106
3025 Arlington Avenue, Toledo, Ohio 43614-5804
Phone: 419-383-6796   Fax: 419-383-3248

### EXPEDITED REVIEW CHECKLIST

Please obtain all required signatures; Applicant(s), Faculty Advisor, Department Chair or Dean. Use the following checklist to ensure you are submitting a complete application to prevent delays in the review process. <u>Incomplete applications will be returned</u>.

| | Please submit the following items to the IRB office: |
|---|---|
| ☐ | <u>**One (1) original of the application with all pertinent attachments.**</u> |
| ☐ | **A disc or CD of the entire packet <u>or</u> an electronic version to** IRB.Biomed@utoledo.edu |
| | **Please include the following items:** |
| ☐ | The research protocol. Please submit a complete Protocol. The following guidance document outlines all required elements, <u>The Elements of a Research Protocol</u> |
| ☐ | The consent/authorization/assent form(s). |
| ☐ | A request for Waiver of Authorization for Use and Disclosure of Protected Health Information (PHI) for Purposes of Research. If the research project involves patient's records. |
| ☐ | A Literature Review – Please submit a list of the current, pertinent literature, summarize relevant conclusions from the literature cited, and provide your assessment of the risk-benefit ratio. |
| ☐ | A copy of all Data collection tools such as Excel spreadsheets, data forms, etc. |
| ☐ | A copy of all Survey instruments, questionnaires, other such study materials. |
| ☐ | A copy of all recruitment materials such as fliers, brochures, posters and proposed newspaper articles. All recruitment materials must be stamped APPROVED by the IRB <u>prior to use</u>. |
| ☐ | Permission letters from each performance site on their official letterhead. |
| ☐ | Original Training Verification forms, with completion certificates attached, for all study personnel. Applications are not processed until <u>all</u> research training has been completed. |
| ☐ | The grant application(s) if applying for grant funding. |

*continues*

### BOX 7-4

## The University of Toledo
## Checklist for Complying with IRB Standards *continued*

| | |
|---|---|
| ☐ | A copy of the Potential Conflict of Interest form for each individual listed as study personnel. |
| ☐ | Any other materials the P.I. believes are important for IRB review (e.g., IRB approval letters and/or correspondence from other performance sites, etc.) |

**All IRB submission forms can be found on the DHRP home page:**
http://utoledo.edu/research/RC/HumanSubs_Menu.html

### TABLE 7-8

**Checklist for Guiding Data Collection**

**Time Schedule**

- Have you determined the length of time needed for administering individual or group testing?
- Have you considered travel time and time for interviewing?
- Have you determined the length of time for scoring tests?

**Informed Consent**

- Have you prepared a form describing to the subject the procedure, tests, information, and length of time involved?
- Have you informed the participant that he/she may decline from the study without any implied penalty?
- Does the participant have a signed form in his/her possession?

**Data Collection Sheet**

- Have you prepared a data collection sheet for each subject, coding the name to guarantee anonymity and providing room for every datum item collected?

**Computer Analysis**

- Have you considered using computer time in analyzing the data?

**Statistical Techniques**

- Does the study meet the assumptions of a parametric statistic?
- If not, what specific nonparametric statistics will be used to analyze the data?
- Have you done a statistical analysis of the hypothetical data?

| Cost Analysis |
| --- |
| • Have you considered costs of purchasing tests or instruments? |
| • Have you considered costs of postage, address labels, and mailings? |
| • Have you considered costs of analyzing data? |
| • Have you considered costs of travel? |
| • Have you considered costs of telephone calls? |
| • Have you considered payment for participants? |

The following is described in detail in the informed consent form:

- The procedure for obtaining informed consent
- A brief statement regarding the objectives of the study
- The amount of time each subject will be asked to participate in the study
- The compensation, remuneration, or other awards, if any, to be received by the subjects
- A description of any expected benefits that may be obtained by the participant
- A description of the procedures and methods to be used in the study
- The identification of potential risks or hazards that might occur during the study
- The identification of any costs to the participant
- The procedures that will minimize any identified risks or hazards
- The procedures that will ensure confidentiality of the participants.

When children are used in research, additional procedures must be used. According to the *Code of Federal Regulations* (United States Department of Health and Human Services, 2009), permission must be obtained from the parents, guardians, or surrogate parents to use the child and assent must be obtained from the child:

> when in the judgment of the IRB the children are capable of providing assent. In determining whether children are capable of assenting, the IRB shall take into account the ages, maturity, and psychological state of the children involved. This judgment may be made for all children to be involved in research under a particular protocol, or for each child, as the IRB deems appropriate. If the IRB determines that the capability of some or all of the children is so limited that they cannot reasonably be consulted or that the intervention or procedure involved in the research holds out a prospect of direct benefit that is important to the health or well-being of the children and is available only in the context of the research, the assent of the children is not a necessary condition for proceeding with the research. Even where the IRB determines that the subjects are capable of assenting, the IRB may still waive the assent requirement under circumstances in which consent may be waived in accord with Sec. 46.116 of Subpart A. (§46.408 Requirements for permission by parents or guardians and for assent by children, para. a)

Although not required, the investigator may want to develop a written assent for children rather than just asking the child to verbalize assent. Care should be taken to ensure that the reading level is appropriate for the age and ability level.

Box 7–5 depicts a model for an informed consent form that was developed by the Department of Human Research Protections at The University of Toledo and is online at http://www.utoledo.edu/research/RC/HumanSubs/bioforms.html When examining this form, note that the italicized portion is to be replaced with appropriate statements.

BOX 7-5

## The University of Toledo Informed Consent Form

*Department Name*
*Department Address*
*Toledo, Ohio 43614*
*Phone #*
*Fax #*

*After following the instructions, please delete all items in red print.*
*If your Consent/Authorization form has an odd number of pages, please remember to include an additional page labeled "NO TEXT THIS PAGE" as page two of the form before copying the entire form double-sided. Please be sure to assign the "NO TEXT THIS PAGE" a page number and include the IRB number.*

*Use one of the following Consent title options:*

### ADULT RESEARCH SUBJECT INFORMATION AND CONSENT FORM

*(If a waiver for authorization of use and disclosure of PHI is being requested or research does not involve subjects for whom protected health information is available to the researchers.)* OR

### ADULT RESEARCH SUBJECT INFORMATION AND CONSENT FORM and AUTHORIZATION FOR USE AND DISCLOSURE OF PROTECTED HEALTH INFORMATION

### RESEARCH PROJECT TITLE

*(Capitalized and bolded, must match the title on the IRB application)*

Principal Investigator:                      *, [M.D., Ph.D., etc.]*
Other Staff (identified by role):            *, [M.D., Ph.D., etc.]*
Contact Phone number(s):        (419)

*(Please add the following seven bulleted items to all consent/authorization forms that are more than (4) single-sided pages long before the addition of this paragraph).*

### What you should know about this research study:

- We give you this consent/authorization form so that you may read about the purpose, risks, and benefits of this research study. All information in this form will be communicated to you verbally by the research staff as well.

- Routine clinical care is based upon the best-known treatment and is provided with the main goal of helping the individual patient. The main goal of research studies is to gain knowledge that may help future patients.

- We cannot promise that this research will benefit you. Just like routine care, this research can have side effects that can be serious or minor.

- You have the right to refuse to take part in this research, or agree to take part now and change your mind later.

- If you decide to take part in this research or not, or if you decide to take part now but change your mind later, your decision will not affect your routine care.

- Please review this form carefully. Ask any questions before you make a decision about whether or not you want to take part in this research. If you decide to take part in this research, you may ask any additional questions at any time.

- Your participation in this research is voluntary.

### PURPOSE (WHY THIS RESEARCH IS BEING DONE)

You are being asked to take part in a research study of **state what is being studied.** *The purpose of the study is to* **state what the study is designed to discover or test (if the study is for an investigational drug, you should indicate that the study is to test effectiveness and safety of the drug when appropriate in addition to including the sentence:** An investigational drug is one which has not been approved by the U.S. Food and Drug Administration (FDA).

You were selected as someone who may want to take part in this study because **state why the subject was selected and include the approximate (maximum) number of subjects in the study at UT and elsewhere.**

### DESCRIPTION OF THE RESEARCH PROCEDURES AND DURATION OF YOUR INVOLVEMENT

If you decide to take part in this study, you will be asked to **describe the procedures to be followed, including the purposes of the procedures, how long they will take, and their frequency. In describing the procedures involved in the study, you should list and describe standard treatment procedures as well as experimental procedures. Please clearly distinguish which procedures are experimental and which are approved standard of care. For approved standard of care procedures, please indicate which of these are being done solely for the purposes of this research. Include the expected duration of the subject's participation. Please list these procedures in an organized manner (e.g., in the order that the participant will be asked to complete them.) A format using bullet points is recommended for research involving multiple procedures and/or visits.**

### RISKS AND DISCOMFORTS YOU MAY EXPERIENCE IF YOU TAKE PART IN THIS RESEARCH

*Describe reasonably foreseeable risks, discomforts or inconveniences to persons choosing to take part in this research that are associated with the procedure (experimental or non-experimental) that is being done solely for the purpose of this research. This includes health, legal, economic, psychological, privacy, confidentiality and security risks. When there are multiple risks or discomforts, these should be listed in a bullet point or table format. Be sure to state the likelihood and seriousness of the risks. If this is a treatment study, add this statement:* Your condition may not get better or may become worse while you are in this study.

*continues*

> ## BOX 7-5
>
> ### The University of Toledo Informed
> ### Consent Form *continued*
>
> *State and explain risks, if any, to pregnant women. If the risk is significant, add the following section (i.e. Risks to Unborn Children). If there is no known additional risk to pregnant women, please state this.*
>
> *NOTE: The following section is required if there is a known risk or a potential for risk to unborn children.*
>
> #### RISKS TO UNBORN CHILDREN
> This research represents a significant risk to unborn children. Therefore, if you are a female of childbearing potential, you will be given a pregnancy test prior to the start of this research. If this test is positive, you will not be able to take part in this research. If your pregnancy test is negative at present and you choose to take part in this research, you will be given information on birth control procedures that must be used while you are taking part in this research so that you can avoid getting pregnant. You also will be told about the danger to the fetus (unborn child) should you become pregnant.
>
> *If applicable, add:* Males who are sexually active must take precautions while participating in this research so that that their female partners do not become pregnant. If you are a sexually active male and wish to take part in this research, you will be offered information on birth control procedures that you and your partner must use while taking part in this research so that your female partner does not become pregnant. You also will be advised as to the danger to the fetus should your partner become pregnant.
>
> Please be sure to ask the researcher any questions that you may have about acceptable methods of birth control and the risk to you, your partner or your unborn child at any time before or, if you decide to enroll, while you are taking part in this research.
>
> #### POSSIBLE BENEFIT TO YOU IF YOU DECIDE TO TAKE PART IN THIS RESEARCH
> *Describe any non-financial benefits to the subject or to others that may reasonably be expected from the research. Clearly state if the benefit is expected to be primarily for others. If benefits are mentioned, add:* We cannot and do not guarantee or promise that you will receive any benefits from this research.
>
> #### COST TO YOU FOR TAKING PART IN THIS STUDY
> *Specify what costs are the responsibility of the study sponsor and/or Principal Investigator and which are the responsibility of the subject. If there is a possibility of additional costs to the subject because of participation, this must be disclosed. Please note that billing of third-party payors for costs that a subject would <u>not</u> incur if he/she was not taking part in this research is not allowed according to <u>UT's policy pertaining to subject injury</u> (unless*

*otherwise allowed by written authorization of the Federal government (as with some special uses of devices/drugs). Billing of third party payors for <u>routine medical care</u> is allowed <u>only</u> if the cost of the care is <u>not</u> covered by a grant or through a contract with the sponsor. If your research is sponsored, please refer to the approved grant application or executed contract if you have any questions about this.*

## PAYMENT OR OTHER COMPENSATION TO YOU FOR TAKING PART IN THIS RESEARCH

If you decide to take part in this research you will receive *If the subject will receive any compensation for their participation, describe the amount or nature. Compensation may include money, free treatment, free medications, or free transportation. Money may be offered to reimburse expenses, time, inconvenience and transportation. However, money may not be used as an inducement to assume risks. Pro-rated subject payment based on how much of the study the participant completes <u>must</u> be stated and the method of pro-rating explained.*

*NOTE: The following section must be included for industry-sponsored research in which the institution is being reimbursed for all or some of the costs of the research.*

## PAYMENT OR OTHER COMPENSATION TO THE RESEARCH SITE

The University of Toledo is receiving money or other benefits from the sponsor of this research as reimbursement for conducting the research.

## ALTERNATIVE(S) TO TAKING PART IN THIS RESEARCH

*Indicate appropriate alternative procedures or courses of treatment, which may be advantageous to the subject, if any treatment is required. Any standard treatment that is being withheld must be disclosed. Include a statement that one alternative is no further therapy. <u>Palliative care should be included as an alternative if appropriate.</u> IF APPLICABLE, state that a potential participant will receive standard care whether or not he/she participates in the research study.*

## CONFIDENTIALITY - (USE AND DISCLOSURE OF YOUR PROTECTED HEALTH INFORMATION)

By agreeing to take part in this research study, you give to The University of Toledo (UT), the Principal Investigator and all personnel associated with this research study your permission to use or disclose health information that can be identified with you that we obtain in connection with this study. We will use this information to *describe the use of the information or purpose for disclosing the information, or delete the word "to" and state "for the purpose of conducting the research study as described in the research consent/authorization form".*

The information that we will use or disclose includes *describe the information or nature of information in a specific and meaningful manner, including the source or location of the information.* We may use this information ourselves, or we may disclose or provide access to the information to *[state the name or other specific identification of the persons, class of persons, or agencies that could receive the information (e.g., Food and Drug Administration*

*continues*

BOX 7-5

**The University of Toledo Informed
Consent Form** *continued*

*or other applicable governmental agencies) (for the purpose of safety, efficacy and compliance reports), study sponsor and its designees (for study oversight and monitoring), coordinating center (for data collection and study monitoring), outside laboratories (for processing of specimens), other sites participating in this research (for multi-institutional studies), statistician (for analysis of data), etc.]* as part of the research study. Under some circumstances, the Institutional Review Board and Research and Sponsored Programs of the University of Toledo may review your information for compliance audits. We may also disclose your protected health information when required by law, such as in response to judicial orders.

The University of Toledo is required by law to protect the privacy of your health information, and to use or disclose the information we obtain about you in connection with this research study only as authorized by you in this form. There is a possibility that the information we disclose may be re-disclosed by the persons we give it to, and no longer protected. However, we will encourage any person who receives your information from us to continue to protect and not re-disclose the information.

Your permission for us to use or disclose your protected health information as described in this section is voluntary. However, you will not be allowed to participate in the research study unless you give us your permission to use or disclose your protected health information by signing this document.

*Optional paragraph when subjects' access to their protected health information is suspended during a research study that includes treatment:*

Your access to your own protected health information *[or describe with particularity so much of the record that is restricted]* may be denied during the term of the research study, but you can access your information once the research study is completed.

You have the right to revoke (cancel) the permission you have given to us to use or disclose your protected health information at any time by giving written notice to *[list the name and address of the research study personnel that should receive the revocation]*. However, a cancellation will not apply if we have acted with your permission, for example, information that already has been used or disclosed prior to the cancellation. Also, a cancellation will not prevent us from continuing to use and disclose information that was obtained prior to the cancellation as necessary to maintain the integrity of the research study.

Except as noted in the above paragraph, your permission for us to use and disclose your protected health information *[state an expiration date or expiration event that relates to the individual or the purpose of the use or disclosure of information. "Will stop at the end of the research study" or "has no expiration date" may be appropriate, especially if the study involves the creation or maintenance of a research database or repository.]*

A more complete statement of University of Toledo's Privacy Practices is set forth in its Joint Notice of Privacy Practices. If you have not already received this Notice, a member of the research team will provide this to you. If you have any further questions concerning privacy, you may contact the University of Toledo's Privacy Officer at 419-383-3413.

*Note for sponsored research: Following review and approval by the sponsor and the UT Research and Sponsored Programs Administration, the UT IRB may request modifications to the indemnification language contained in the "In the Event of a Research Related Injury" section of the Consent/Authorization form.*

## IN THE EVENT OF A RESEARCH-RELATED INJURY

In the event of injury resulting from your taking part in this study, treatment can be obtained at a health care facility of your choice. You should understand that unless compensation is available from the sponsor as described below, the costs of such treatment will be your responsibility. Financial compensation is not available through The University of Toledo or The University of Toledo Medical Center.

*If the sponsoring agency has made a provision for payment of medical treatment for research-related injuries, include that information in this section. Please note that UT policy (#03-001) does not allow sponsors to restrict its responsibility for payment of costs associated with research-related injuries to immediate or emergency care for those injuries, nor does this policy allow the sponsor to require that third party payors be billed for the cost of these injuries in place of the sponsor directly paying for these costs*. By signing this form you are not giving up any of your legal rights as a research subject.

In the event of an injury, contact *If there is any risk of injury, you must provide the name and phone number of an appropriate contact person(s) who is(are) available 24 hours a day and their phone number(s) including area code. Please be sure to separate this statement from the rest of the sentence so that it can be easily identified.*

## VOLUNTARY PARTICIPATION

Taking part in this study is <u>voluntary</u>. You may refuse to participate or discontinue participation at any time without penalty or a loss of benefits to which you are otherwise entitled. If you decide not to participate or to discontinue participation, your decision will not affect your future relations with the University of Toledo or The University of Toledo Medical Center.

## NEW FINDINGS

You will be notified of new information that might change your decision to be in this study if any becomes available.

## OTHER IMPORTANT INFORMATION

*If the research involves a study drug or placebo that is being taken home, include:* It is important that you are the only one that takes the study drug or placebo that you are given as part of this research. *(NOTE: Delete "placebo" if not applicable)* It is very important that you keep it (these) out of the reach of children and persons who may not be able to read or understand the label.

*continues*

BOX 7-5

## The University of Toledo Informed
## Consent Form *continued*

### ADDITIONAL ELEMENTS
*Include this section when information that does not apply to the other sections needs to be included in this document.*

*When appropriate, include a statement of the consequences of a subject's decision to withdraw from the research and procedures for orderly termination of participation by the subject.*

*When appropriate, include anticipated circumstances under which the subject's participation may be terminated by the investigator without regard to the subject's consent/authorization and procedures for orderly termination of participation by the subject.*

*Note: All of the information in the following table (from "Offer to Answer Questions" to the end of the document) is an integral part of the consent form and cannot be divided between two pages. Please remember to insert an additional page in this document (as the 2nd single sided page) with "NO TEXT THIS PAGE" typed on it when appropriate (see instructions on top of first page) if this document has an odd number of single-sided pages. If there is a large gap in text between "Offer to Answer Section" and the section prior to it, please type "CONTINUED NEXT PAGE" in the gap.*

### OFFER TO ANSWER QUESTIONS
Before you sign this form, please ask any questions on any aspect of this study that is unclear to you. You may take as much time as necessary to think it over. If you have questions regarding the research at any time before, during or after the study, you may contact *[insert name of one or more researchers and their telephone number(s)]*.

If you have questions beyond those answered by the research team or your rights as a research subject or research-related injuries, please feel free to contact the Chairperson of the University of Toledo Biomedical Institutional Review Board at 419-383-6796.

### SIGNATURE SECTION (Please read carefully)

**YOU ARE MAKING A DECISION WHETHER OR NOT TO PARTICIPATE IN THIS RESEARCH STUDY. YOUR SIGNATURE INDICATES THAT YOU HAVE READ THE INFORMATION PROVIDED ABOVE, YOU HAVE HAD ALL YOUR QUESTIONS ANSWERED, AND YOU HAVE DECIDED TO TAKE PART IN THIS RESEARCH.**

**BY SIGNING THIS DOCUMENT YOU AUTHORIZE US TO USE OR DISCLOSE YOUR PROTECTED HEALTH INFORMATION AS DESCRIBED IN THIS FORM.**

The date you sign this document to enroll in this study, that is, today's date, MUST fall between the dates indicated on the approval stamp affixed to the bottom of each page. These dates indicate that this form is valid when you enroll in the study but do not reflect how long you may participate in the study. Each page of this Consent/Authorization Form is stamped to indicate the form's validity as approved by the UT Biomedical Institutional Review Board (IRB).

| | | |
|---|---|---|
| _____ | _____ | _____ |
| Name of Subject (please print) | Signature of Subject or Person Authorized to Consent | Date |

| | | | |
|---|---|---|---|
| _____ | _____ | _____ | a.m. |
| Relationship to the Subject (Healthcare Power of Attorney authority or Legal Guardian) | | Time | p.m. |

| | | |
|---|---|---|
| _____ | _____ | _____ |
| Name of Person Obtaining Consent (please print) | Signature of Person Obtaining Consent | Date |

| | | |
|---|---|---|
| _____ | _____ | _____ |
| Name of Witness to Consent Process (when required by ICH Guidelines) | Signature of Witness to Consent Process (when required by ICH Guidelines) | Date |

**YOU WILL BE GIVEN A <u>SIGNED</u> COPY OF THIS FORM TO KEEP.**

## 7.14 Methodological Limitations of a Study

Researchers can assume that most studies have limitations in selecting a sample, using a measuring instrument, collecting data, or analyzing results. A section devoted to the limitations of a study is an objective means for discussing flaws in research methods. This section is not meant to be an excuse or rationalization for not obtaining acceptable results or confirming predicted hypotheses, but rather an unbiased analysis of shortcomings in the research. These flaws in methodology do not necessarily mean that the research is worthless or inadequate; on the contrary, it serves to guide future researchers in avoiding the same mistakes when the research is replicated or another research design is proposed. Research often involves trial-and-error methods with factors of risk and uncertainty. Results are significant if the researcher has been objective and unbiased. The researcher's honesty and integrity are enhanced when both the merits and deficiencies of a study are objectively reported. Likewise, the limitations of a study can serve as the basis for recommending further research.

## 7.15 Summary

After the researcher selects a significant problem, the next step is to narrow the focus of the research into a feasible study. This chapter on research and methodology describes the step-by-step procedures in implementing a study from stating a testable hypothesis, operationally defining the independent and dependent variables, diagramming the study by showing the relationship among variables in the research models, and discussing the theoretical rationale underlying the study. All of these steps should be well-thought through before the researcher can actually collect data. It is the foundation for the study and it is the preparatory work that must be done before the study is carried forth. The next part of planning a research study is the methods section, which comprises selection of the participants, location of where data will be collected, the assessment tools that will be used in the study, and the strategy in increasing the internal validity of the study such as controlling for extraneous variables that can affect the outcome and results. The ethics of carrying out research is discussed in detail and an example of an informed consent procedure is included. This chapter is a pragmatic approach that delineates the essential factors in planning a research study.

# CHAPTER 8

# Data Analysis and Statistics

*Statistical interpretation depends not only on statistical ideas, but also on "ordinary" thinking. Clear thinking is not only indispensable in interpreting statistics, but is often sufficient even in the absence of specific statistical knowledge.*

—W. A. Wallis and H. V. Roberts, 1962,
*The Nature of Statistics* (p. 29)

## Operational Learning Objectives

At the end of this chapter, the learner will:
- Define statistics.
- Describe the importance of statistics in contemporary society.
- Understand the difference between descriptive and inferential statistics.
- Understand the concept of measurement and data.
- Understand the difference between discrete and continuous data.
- Identify seven statistical models for analyzing clinical research data.
- Distinguish between parametric and nonparametric statistical tests.
- Understand when to apply specific statistical tests to clinical research designs.

## 8.1 Definition and Meaning of Statistics

**Statistics**, as a practical discipline, is defined as the application of statistical tests and procedures for organizing, analyzing, and interpreting results or data according to mathematical formulas. Statistics is taught in almost every university and college in the United States. Although statistics is derived from mathematics, it is taught in many academic departments with application to economics; agriculture; medicine; natural, physical, and social science; nursing; the allied health professions; and education. The rapid development of mainframe and personal computers has expanded the role of statistics to almost every aspect of our lives including banking, retailing, education, manufacturing, farming, politics, communication, transportation, and health care. Through the availability of the Internet and e-mail, statistical programs and databases are easily accessible to researchers. Computer programs using sophisticated statistical models have enabled pollsters to predict election results based on representative sampling procedures and insurance companies to set up actuarial tables based on the presence or absence of risk factors for morbidity and mortality.

Statistics is also an essential component of clinical research, enabling the investigator to objectively describe and infer logical conclusions from the results. In general, statistical analysis of the data strengthens the impact of the results and allows the investigator to compare current findings with previous research. The researcher in occupational therapy should have a basic understanding of descriptive statistics and the most frequently used inferential statistical tests and procedures. For example, common inferential statistics include *t*-test and **analysis of variance (ANOVA)** for comparing sample means, Pearson product-moment correlation and **Spearman rank correlation** for testing relationships between variables, and **Chi-square** for testing the differences between observed and expected frequencies. The researcher should be able to calculate the incidence (initial occurrences) and prevalence (prevailing rates) of diseases and be able to read and interpret vital statistics related to morbidity and mortality. Quantifiable or measurable data are counted as statistics. For example, the total number of individuals with a spinal cord injury, the number of workers with disabilities, and the number of occupational therapists working in public schools are identifiable statistics.

Historically, the earliest statistics that local authorities amassed were census counts. Statistical occurrences also replaced subjective descriptions of populations, such as "abundant," "flourishing," and "enormous," to describe epidemics and population density. The first use of statistics recorded factual information, such as the annual rate of births, deaths, and marriages. During periods of epidemics, such as the "black death" (bubonic plague) in Europe during the sixteenth and seventeenth centuries, statistics were used to tabulate the number of deaths and their presumed causes. Also, tax collectors used statistics in Europe before the Middle Ages to assess wealth and agricultural holdings. In the latter half of the eighteenth century, census taking became a systematic governmental function. The U.S. Constitution of 1790 includes provision for a regular population census every 10 years. The application of probability theory to the prediction of death rates (actuarial tables among populations) and the use of sampling procedures advanced the science of statistics. In the mid-nineteenth century, statistical societies were founded (e.g., the American Statistical Association was organized in Boston in 1839). Vital statistics became more accurate, and methods were developed to analyze health data and to correlate injuries and diseases with occupation and social class.

The emergence of modern statistics based on probability theory led to the application of statistical methods in laboratory and clinical research. R. A. Fisher, a geneticist, extended statistics from small samples where inferences were made to large populations. The work of Fisher and his colleagues in the early part of the 1900s led the way to quantifiable analysis of research data in the biological, physical, and social sciences. Currently, hundreds of textbooks are published on the application and theory of statistics in a wide range of professional disciplines. In spite of this, the field of statistics is as much of an art as it is an empirical science. There are many points of disagreement on the correctness of applying specific statistical tests to research data. The student who is learning and applying statistics must decide which statistical tests are most appropriate for analyzing the results. How the variable is measured (e.g., continuous or discrete), the probability level required, and the direction of the hypothesis stated will help the researcher to select a specific statistical test.

The material presented in this chapter is organized to aid the student in reading and understanding statistics presented in research articles and to follow a step-by-step procedure in calculating statistical results. Each step in the process of deciding on the statistical test to be employed, the analysis of the raw data, and the interpretation of the statistical results should be carried through in a problem-solving, reflective manner.

## 8.2 Relationship of Statistics to Clinical Practice

Statistics as a methodology enables the researcher to organize, analyze, and interpret data. In the context of a research design, statistical application does not change the quality of the data or influence the validity of the results. In conducting research, the investigator should have an overall concept of the meaning of the projected results and how a statistical test will be used to accept or reject a hypothesis. For example, an investigator wishes to compare attitudes of health professionals and nonhealth professionals toward individuals with disabilities utilizing a survey questionnaire. The researcher has hypothesized that health professionals will have more positive, realistic attitudes toward individuals with disabilities than will nonhealth professionals. Then the researcher would apply a statistical test, such as an analysis of variance, to accept or reject the hypothesis.

The process of statistical analysis and its relationship to clinical practice is illustrated in Figure 8–1. In this example, a clinician proposes to test the effectiveness of a specific treatment method. Six stages may be distinguished in this process:

1. A hypothesis is conceived and postulated.
2. A research plan is devised to study the effects of a treatment method or procedure traditionally used by clinicians.
3. Quantifiable data are collected from a patient group.

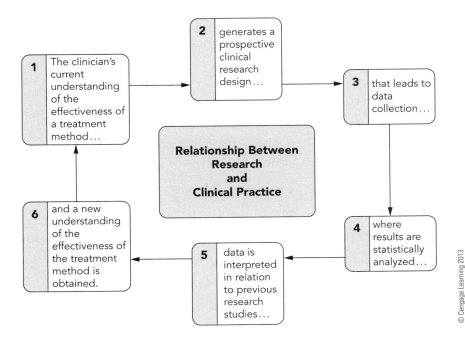

**FIGURE 8-1** Relationship between Research and Clinical Practice: Notice that the relationship is continuous. The completion of Step 6 leads back to Step 1. A clinician should be continually involved in practices that lead to research that can be applied to clinical practice.

4. The data are statistically processed and analyzed.
5. The results are interpreted.
6. Conclusions are drawn, and the information is disseminated back to the scientific community and clinical practitioners.

The cycle continues with new treatment methods introduced and ineffective methods discarded. Hopefully, the process leads to the evolution of clinical efficacy. This example demonstrates the importance of statistics to clinical research. What are the most common statistical procedures employed in clinical research?

Statistical procedures employed in clinical research are based on descriptive and inferential statistics. Figure 8–2 outlines the specific descriptive and inferential statistical tests.

- **Descriptive statistics** are procedures for reducing, summarizing, and describing results or data. In descriptive statistics, for example, a large set of data is reduced to summary values, graphs, frequency polygons and scatter diagrams, measures of central tendency (mode, median, and mean), measures of variability (range, standard deviation, and variance), and incidence and prevalence rates.
- **Inferential statistics** are methods for generalizing data collected from a representative sample to a larger target population that includes all subjects or observations. The essence of inferential statistics is to sample a representative portion of a population to infer information representative of the whole population. Inferential statistics are applied for two main purposes: (a) to estimate the characteristics of a population (parameters) and (b) to test hypotheses about populations. In inferential statistics, a sample is drawn from the target population, the characteristics of this sample are measured, and inferences or estimates about the corresponding characteristics are made to the population at large.
- A **parameter** is a descriptive value attributed to the sample population. Parameters are usually unknown. For example, in the population of individuals with spinal cord injury in North America, the parameter value of age would be inferred or estimated because it would be almost impossible to survey all individuals in North America who have spinal cord injury. The parameter value is usually estimated through descriptive studies of representative samples in more than one geographical area. The data from a representative

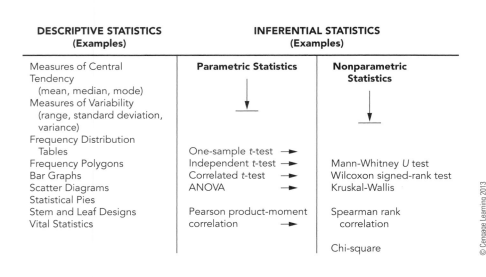

**FIGURE 8-2** Statistical Procedures and Tests Used in the Analysis of Data

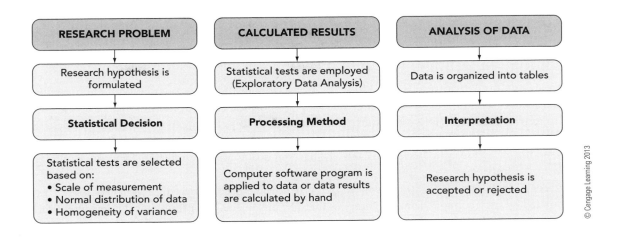

**FIGURE 8-3** The Process of Statistical Analysis

sample are extrapolated to the target population. The reliability of the estimate increases with the number of descriptive studies that show concurrence.

- A **statistic** is a quantitative measure of a sample. For example, the average heart rate of a sample of college students is 72 beats per minute. This is a statistic with a summary value representing the average heart rate in the sample. When a total population is available and every individual is measured, a parameter value may be computed directly. Population data usually are not available, so that researchers use a representative sample drawn from a population to compute a statistic and employ inferential statistics to estimate or extrapolate parameter values. Vital statistics are used to estimate the incidence or prevalence rates of a specific disability in a population. For example, if interested in determining the number of individuals with a diagnosis of muscular dystrophy in the United States, an investigator can carry out epidemiological studies with representative samples in specified geographic areas such as in the Midwestern states. Frequently, epidemiological studies are replicated in other geographical areas to test the validity of previous results and to monitor trends in the incidence and prevalence rates of specific diseases.

## 8.2.1 The Process of Statistical Analysis

The important steps for researchers are to develop a hypothesis, select the appropriate statistical test, calculate the results, and finally interpret the data. The decision process in applying statistics and interpreting the results is shown diagrammatically in Figure 8–3.

## 8.3 Key Definitions of Statistical Concepts

The first step in understanding statistics is to understand the definitions of statistical terms. With a conceptual understanding of statistics, one can critically understand published studies that use statistical designs. The bases on which hypotheses are substantiated or rejected and on which conclusions are generated are derived from a statistical analysis of the results. The following definitions are essential to understand statistics. They are listed alphabetically and are intended to be used as a reference aid.

- **Continuous variables** are examples of interval or ratio scale measurement. Weight, height, age, muscle strength, blood pressure, and hearing acuity are all examples of continuous variables. It is assumed that, in measuring continuous variables, there are an infinite number of values between each pair of scores.
- **Data** are the numerical results of a study. In a descriptive study of a population, data are enumerated totals, such as the number of emergency patients in a hospital clinic or the number of health care workers in a rural area. Descriptive statistics of populations, such as the mean and median, are data. In small sample research in which inferential (probability) statistics are used, data represent comparative results derived from the research. These results are the bases of discussion and interpretation. The singular of data is *datum* or *statistic*.
- **Degrees of freedom (*df*)** is a mathematically derived value used in reading statistical tables. It is *usually* calculated by subtracting 1 from the total number (*N*) of subjects in a group. It is defined as the number of observations in the calculation of a statistic that are free to vary.
- **Dichotomous variables** contain only two subsets, such as male and female subjects, improvement or no improvement, experimental and control group, or any other two variable sets created by the investigator or found naturally.
- **Discrete variables** identify separate categories, such as diagnostic groups, allied health professions, occupations, vitamins, pharmaceutical drugs, and treatment methods. Discrete variables belong to a set of objects sharing some trait or characteristic. They are examples of nominal scale measurements.
- A **directional hypothesis** predicts that:

  1. There will be a statistically significant difference in a specified direction between two groups after applying a treatment in experimental research, or
  2. There will be a statistically significant relationship (positive or inverse) between two variables.

- **Frequency** is the number of times that a result occurs. A frequency distribution table of results describes the number of times a variable falls into a discrete category.
- **Measures of central tendency** are descriptive statistics—such as the **mean**, **median**, and **mode**—that measure the center location of a data distribution.
- **Measures of dispersion or variability** are descriptive statistics that indicate the spread of scores in a data distribution. The **range, variance**, and **standard deviation (*SD*)** scores are measures of dispersion. Factors such as the difference between the highest and lowest scores and the number of scores that deviate from the mean influence measures of dispersion.
- **Nonparametric statistics** are sometimes referred to as "distribution-free" statistical tests because they are applied to data for which no assumptions are made regarding the normal distribution of the population and interval scale measurement. The advantages of nonparametric statistics are that they can be applied to small sample data without having to meet the stringent assumptions of parametric statistics. Examples of nonparametric tests include Chi-square, Spearman rank correlation, Mann-Whitney *U* test, Wilcoxon signed-rank test for correlated samples, and Kruskal-Wallis test.
- The **normal (bell-shaped) curve** represents a theoretical distribution that approximates the range and frequency of many human functions and anatomical descriptions, such as blood pressure, lung capacity, height, and weight. This theoretical distribution is also referred to as a Gaussian distribution. The major assumption underlying the concept of a normal curve is that variables are distributed along a continuum with the greatest frequency in the middle and the least frequency at the outer edges of the distribution. Figure 8–4 indicates the percentage of cases found within each area of the normal curve. For example, 68 percent of cases are distributed toward the center of the curve in a symmetrical pattern. The basis of inferential parametric statistics rests on the assumption that the sample data are derived from a population that is normally distributed.

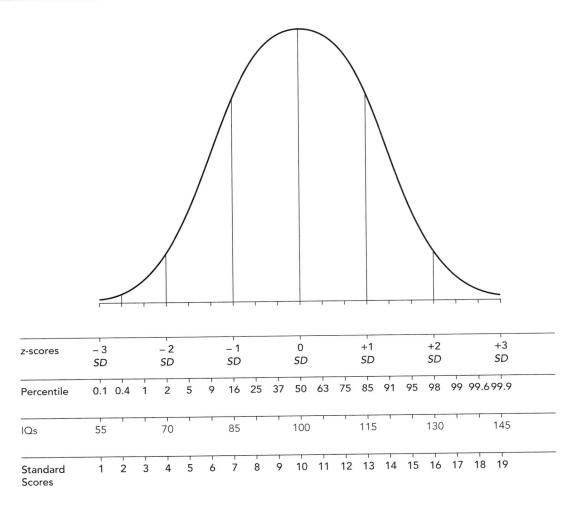

| z-scores | −3 SD | | −2 SD | | −1 SD | | 0 SD | | +1 SD | | +2 SD | | +3 SD |
|---|---|---|---|---|---|---|---|---|---|---|---|---|---|

| Percentile | 0.1 | 0.4 | 1 | 2 | 5 | 9 | 16 | 25 | 37 | 50 | 63 | 75 | 85 | 91 | 95 | 98 | 99 | 99.6 | 99.9 |
|---|---|---|---|---|---|---|---|---|---|---|---|---|---|---|---|---|---|---|---|

| IQs | 55 | 70 | 85 | 100 | 115 | 130 | 145 |
|---|---|---|---|---|---|---|---|

| Standard Scores | 1 | 2 | 3 | 4 | 5 | 6 | 7 | 8 | 9 | 10 | 11 | 12 | 13 | 14 | 15 | 16 | 17 | 18 | 19 |
|---|---|---|---|---|---|---|---|---|---|---|---|---|---|---|---|---|---|---|---|

Based on Wechsler's Scales

**FIGURE 8-4**   The Bell-Shaped Curve, which Illustrates the Percentage of Population at Each Level: Included in this figure are the relationships among the standard deviations (z-scores), percentiles, IQ scores, and standard scores.

- A **null hypothesis** predicts that there will be no statistically significant difference or correlation between two or more specified groups, that is, after experimentally manipulating a variable or when testing the relationships between variables.
- **Parametric statistics** are applied to data in which certain underlying assumptions have been made. These are:

  1. The variables measured approximate a normal distribution curve in the target population sampled.
  2. The sample is a random selection or is representative of the target population.
  3. The variables are measured by an interval scale; that is, there is equal arithmetical distance between each value or score.
  4. The variance, such as the standard deviation, within the compared groups is approximately the same.

Examples of parametric statistics are *t*-test, analysis of variance (ANOVA), and Pearson product-moment correlation.

● A **research hypothesis** is a prediction of results.

● **Standard deviation (*SD*)** is a statistical measure of the dispersion of scores from the mean.

● **Standard error of measurement (*SEM*)** is a statistical value that indicates the band of error surrounding a test score. For example, a raw score of 90 with a *SEM* of 4 represents a score ranging from 86 to 94.

● **Statistical assumptions** are preconditions that are required before a specific statistical test can be applied. These assumptions usually involve the following factors:

   a. The variable distributed in a population approximates the normal curve. For example, muscle strength, intelligence, systolic blood pressure, and height are variables that are assumed to approximate a normal curve in a standard population.

   b. The data collected are measurable. Some statistical tests require interval scale data, whereas other tests allow for ordinal or nominal data.

   c. There is homogeneity of variance within the group scores. Large differences in standard deviations of two groups present some difficulty, although it is unclear what constitutes a large difference. Some statisticians (Welkoitz, Ewen, & Cohen, 1971) have recommended ignoring this assumption of two sample sizes that are equal (and there is no vast differences between the standard deviations) when applying the *t*-test.

   d. The sample is randomly selected from a population. The object of random sampling is to obtain an unbiased sample that is to be truly representative of a population. The difficulty in obtaining a true random sample when applied to clinical research is that it is almost impossible to identify and locate a population (e.g., all individuals diagnosed with diabetes, arthritis, or schizophrenia) and then select a random sample from this population. The most prevalent sample in clinical research is the convenient sample accessible to the researcher, such as in a teaching hospital, university, public school, or outpatient clinic. It is possible, however, to assign random samples from a convenient population, such as hospital patients, who can be randomly assigned to experimental and control groups.

   e. The groups compared are independent of each other.

● **Statistical tables** contain critical levels and values of probability for accepting or rejecting a hypothesis. By using a statistical table, the investigator determines whether the statistical value obtained is significant compared with the critical value. Using statistical tables, the investigator decides the level of significance, such as .05 or .01.

● **Statistically significant** results means that differences between two or more groups are not due to chance. In every statistically significant result, there is a comparison between the effects on two or more groups.

   **Experimental Clinical Research**: In **clinical observation research**, statistically significant results are traditionally accepted at the .05 level or .01 level, which means that the results are not due to chance in 95 out of 100 cases or 99 out of 100 cases. In using the concept of statistical significance, the investigator performing experimental clinical research assumes an explanation that is sometimes confusing to students who think that statistics is an exact science that can be used to determine cause-and-effect relationships. Conclusive cause-and-effect relationships are only meaningful when an investigator can control every variable that may affect the results. The closest that medical research comes to the control of extraneous variables is in experimental animal research where environmental and sometimes genetic factors can be rigorously controlled. In clinical research with human subjects, it is almost impossible to attain results that are 100 percent conclusive because of the interactional effects among the therapist, patient, treatment method, and environment. Inferential statistics, which are based on probability theory, are applied to data derived from samples of populations so that everyone in a population is not tested or measured. Samples per se indicate inconclusive data and an uncertainty even if a representative sample has been selected. In summary, a statistically significant result in experimental clinical research implies the following:

   a.  Probability theory is assumed in interpreting the data.
   b.  A sample of population is used rather than the entire population.
   c.  There is an allowance for error based on a researcher's inability to control all variables that may possibly influence the results.
   d.  Conclusiveness of results is not assumed, and the investigator can only suggest that a cause-effect relationship exists.

●  **Test of statistical significance** is based on the characteristics of the normal curve and probability theory.

   a.  **Two-tailed tests of statistical significance** are used in analyzing data if the researcher has stated the hypothesis in a nondirectional or null form.
   b.  **One-tailed tests of statistical significance** imply that the researcher has predicted a directional hypothesis, and there is prior evidence, either through a literature review or clinical observation, that there will be a statistically significant difference between the groups or a statistically positive correlation between variables.

●  **Variables** are factors that can be operationally defined, categorized, and measured. Variables can be homogeneous groups, such as undergraduate university students, patients with hemiplegia, or hospital administrators. Variables are also conditions or behavior such as group therapy, cardiovascular disease, or ADL training. In experimental research, the **independent variable (IV)**, which is manipulated by the investigator, is the direct cause of the **dependent variable (DV)**, which is the resultant effect. Variables can be discrete, dichotomous, rank order, or continuous. (Also refer to Chapter 7 "Research Design and Methodology" for further discussion about variables.)
●  **Variance** is a measure of the average of each score's deviation from the mean. Variance is an intermediate value used in calculating the standard deviation ($SD$).

## 8.3.1  Universal Symbols Used in Statistics

| | |
|---|---|
| $\alpha$ | alpha, associated with hypothesis testing, the probability of a Type I error |
| $\beta$ | beta, associated with hypothesis testing and the chance of a Type II error |
| $\chi^2$ | Chi-square statistical test |
| $df$ | degrees of freedom |
| $f$ | frequency of cases in a distribution |
| $F$ | statistic associated with analysis of variance (ANOVA) |
| $\mu$ | mu, the population or parameter mean; oftentimes, this value is unknown and estimated by the mean |
| $H_0$ | null hypothesis or the concept that there is no statistically significant relationship between two or more variables (e.g., $\mu_1 = \mu_2$) |
| $H_1$ | alternative hypothesis, opposite of null hypothesis (e.g., $\mu_1 \neq \mu_2$) |
| $n$ | number of subjects within a designated sample |
| $N$ | total of number of subjects in a group or population |
| $p$ | probability of a chance occurrence |
| $p$-value | obtained or observed significance value; for example, if $p < \alpha$, $H_0$ is rejected |
| $r$ | the Pearson product-moment correlation coefficient indicating the degree of relationship between two variables or two sets of data |
| $r_s$ | the Spearman rank correlation coefficient for ordinal data (formerly $rho$ [$\rho$]) |
| $s$ | the standard deviation of a sample ($SD$) |

| | |
|---|---|
| $\sigma$ | lowercase sigma, the standard deviation of a population, usually estimated by $s$ |
| $\Sigma$ | uppercase sigma, sum of an arithmetic calculation |
| $t$ | $t$-test statistic |
| $t_{obs}$ | $t$ observed, $t$-value derived from the $t$-test |
| $t_{crit}$ | $t$ critical, the value derived from a statistical table of values found through $\alpha$ levels |
| $z$ | standard score measured in standard deviation units |
| $\neq$ | not equal to |
| $\geq$ | more than or equal to |
| $\leq$ | less than or equal to |
| $\overline{X}$ | the mean value of a sample |

## 8.4 Seven Statistical Models for Clinical Research

Seven statistical models for analyzing data are outlined in Table 8–1. These models represent the most frequently used statistical tests for clinical researchers. The format in presenting each model is to define the model and the statistical tests that the models represent, analyze an example of the statistical test from the literature, outline sequential steps in calculating the statistical results, and follow through with a hypothetical stepwise example. Many statistical tests are not covered in these models. References to textbooks on statistics are provided throughout the chapter as a guide for those researchers inspired to further explore the world of statistics. As one becomes adept in using statistical software programs for personal computers, the options for selecting statistical tests broaden. First, it is important for the clinical researcher to understand the concepts underlying the statistical applications, however. Doing statistical tests with a hand calculator and doing exploratory data analysis aids the researcher to better understand statistical processes that are done later through computer software programs.

### TABLE 8-1

**Seven Statistical Models**

| | Statistical Model | Purpose | Examples of Statistical Tests or Procedures |
|---|---|---|---|
| I. | Descriptive Statistics | Describe the statistical characteristics in samples or populations | Measures of central tendency (mean, mode, median) |
| | | | Measures of variability (range, standard deviation, variance) |
| | | | Frequency distribution table, frequency graph, scatter diagram, statistical pie, stem and leaf, vital statistics |
| **Inferential Statistics** | | | |
| II. | One-sample | Test the difference between a sample mean and a parameter mean | One-sample $t$-test |
| III. | Two independent samples | Test the differences between sample means from two independent groups | Independent $t$-test (parametric statistic) |
| | | | Mann-Whitney $U$ test (nonparametric statistic) |
| IV. | Paired-data sample | Test the differences between two conditions (means) in the same sample | Correlated $t$-test (parametric statistic) |
| | | | Wilcoxon signed-rank test (nonparametric statistic) |

## TABLE 8-1

**Seven Statistical Models** *continued*

| | Statistical Model | Purpose | Examples of Statistical Tests or Procedures |
|---|---|---|---|
| **V.** | *k*-independent samples | Test the differences between means from two or more independent groups | ANOVA (parametric statistic) Kruskal-Wallis (nonparametric statistic) |
| **VI.** | Correlation | Test the relationship between two variables | Pearson product-moment correlation (parametric statistic) Spearman rank correlation (nonparametric statistic) Regression line, correlation matrix |
| **VII.** | Observed frequencies | Test the differences between observed minus expected frequencies | Chi-square (nonparametric statistic) |

**Note:** Adapted from *Statistics for the Allied Health Sciences* by R. J. Larson, 1975, Columbus, OH: Merrill Publishing. Copyright 1975 by Merrill Publishing.

## 8.4.1 Model I: Descriptive Statistics

In this model, the researcher calculates descriptive statistics based on data collected from a representative sample or the total population. The statistical procedures include:

- Frequency distribution tables
- Frequency polygons
- Histograms and bar graphs
- Scatter diagrams
- Statistical pies
- Stem and leaf
- Measures of central tendency
- Measures of variability
- Vital statistics

## 8.4.2 Model II: One-Sample Problems

The purpose of this statistical model is to compare data collected from a representative sample of a population and then to compare the obtained value with a parameter value that is known or estimated or to a standard value. Examples include comparing air samples from a metropolitan area to a standard accepted for clean air. The research question that this model answers is whether the mean of the representative sample and the established parameter mean value are statistically significantly different. The statistical procedure for this model is the one-sample *t*-test.

## 8.4.3 Model III: Two Independent Samples

The purpose of this statistical model is to test whether the means for two representative samples are statistically significantly different. An example in clinical research is determining whether one treatment method (such as sensory-integration therapy) is more effective in reducing hyperactivity than a comparable treatment method (such as relaxation therapy) in two independent groups. The statistical test (independent *t*-test) is applied to determine whether there is a statistically significant difference between the two treatment methods. The **Mann-Whitney *U* test**, a nonparametric test, is another example used to evaluate data using this model.

### 8.4.4 Model IV: Paired-Data Sample

The primary purpose of this statistical model is to examine the difference between mean values in one sample group with two data points, such as pretest and posttest. This statistical model employs the correlated *t*-test to test whether there will be a statistically significant difference between the means in two conditions. This statistical model is frequently used in clinical research to determine if a treatment method is effective when compared to a baseline measure of a dependent variable. The **Wilcoxon signed-rank test**, a nonparametric statistical test, is an alternative to the parametric one-sample correlated *t*-test.

### 8.4.5 Model V: Independent Samples

If comparing the means of more than two independent samples, then the researcher applies an analysis of variance (ANOVA). The ANOVA is similar to the independent *t*-test when two independent samples are compared. If the results of the ANOVA are statistically significant, then the researcher employs post-hoc tests to determine which groups are statistically different from each other. These post-hoc tests (similar to *t*-tests) include the Scheffé, Duncan multiple analysis, or Tukey tests. The nonparametric alternative to ANOVA is the **Kruskal-Wallis test**.

### 8.4.6 Model VI: Correlational Sample

In this statistical model, the researcher measures the degree of relationship between two variables, such as in a study examining the relationship between perceptual motor skills and functional abilities in self-care. The relationship can range from zero, indicating that the two variables are completely independent and do not affect each other, to 1.00, indicating a perfect relationship between two variables. An example of a perfect correlation is the effect of temperature on the expansion of the chemical element mercury. As the temperature goes up, mercury expands; as the temperature goes down, mercury contracts. A perfect correlation can be positive (i.e., +1.00) when both variables change in the same direction, or it can be negative or inverse (i.e., −1.00) when the variables change in inverse directions (i.e., as one variable goes up, the other variable goes down). An example of an inverse relationship is the presence of serotonin, a neurotransmitter, and symptoms of depression. As serotonin is depleted in the blood, the symptoms of depression increase.

The relationship between two variables can be described in a scatter diagram. The Pearson product-moment correlation for interval scale data and the Spearman rank correlation for ordinal scale data are applied to evaluate the degree of relationship (*r*) between two variables. A regression line can be calculated when there is a high correlation between two variables. The regression line is calculated by using the results of the Pearson product-moment correlation coefficient and plugging the values into a formula for the regression line. In this formula, variable values are estimated from known *X* variable values. This is illustrated in Figure 8–5.

### 8.4.7 Model VII: Observed Minus Expected Frequencies

In this model, the investigator compares groups or conditions on the basis of frequency or nominal data. Chi-square is the statistical test used when comparing the differences between observed frequencies and expected frequencies based on probability. Chi-square is used frequently, for example, in drug research to compare the differences in the number of patients who have improved with an experimental drug as compared with the number of patients taking a placebo who have improved.

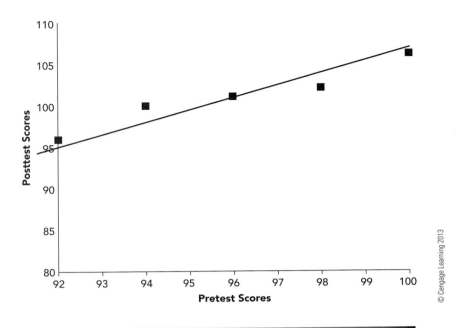

© Cengage Learning 2013

**FIGURE 8-5**  Example of a Scattergram Showing the Relationship between Two Variables: When the value of *X* is known, then the value of *Y* can be predicted by the use of the regression line.

## 8.5  Model I: Descriptive Statistics: Organization and Tabulation of Descriptive Data

### 8.5.1  Table of Percentage

Statistical analysis begins with organizing data into summary tables and diagrams. In descriptive studies, as in survey research, tabular summaries of data provide the results. For example, Table 8–2 summarizes data from interviews with 115 elderly residents in a nursing home regarding their risk for falling. The table reports the percentage of the 115 residents who replied "yes" to the interview questions. An alternative way of describing data is to list the actual frequency of responses, rather than convert the frequency to percentages. For example, 96 percent or 110 of the residents use eyeglasses, and only 6 percent or 7 of the subjects always or most of the time are dizzy on arising.

Another method of displaying data is to compare results between periods of time, distances, or events. For example, Table 8–3 lists cancer sites and the frequency of distribution in percentage across categories of cancer stages. When examining the data, the reader can note that some types of cancer are evenly distributed across the various stages (e.g., digestive system and liver, intrahepatic bile duct, and lung and bronchus), whereas other frequencies are clustered within one or two stages (e.g., melanoma of the skin, brain and other nervous system, and myeloma).

The above examples demonstrate the importance of descriptive statistics in summarizing results from a research study. The above examples demonstrate the importance of descriptive statistics in summarizing results from research studies or from data banks such as the Surveillance Epidemiology and End Results (SEER) which is maintained by the National Cancer Institute.

A number of methods can be used to describe data. The most frequently used descriptive methods for organizing data are discussed in the following section.

## TABLE 8-2

**Subjects' Reported Fall Risk Factors**

| Fall Risk Factor | % of Subjects Reporting |
|---|---|
| Health compared with peers | |
| • Excellent | 1 |
| • Good | 57 |
| • Fair | 28 |
| • Poor | 8 |
| Use eyeglasses | 96 |
| • Always/Most of the time | 55 |
| Use walking aid | 38 |
| • Always/Most of the time | 20 |
| Dizzy on arising | 31 |
| • Always/Most of the time | 6 |
| Pain in muscles, bones, joints | 80 |
| • Always/Most of the time | 45 |
| Hold on for support | 30 |
| • Always/Most of the time | 13 |
| Difficult to get in and out of bed | 16 |
| • Always/Most of the time | 4 |
| Use prescription medication | 80 |
| Use alcohol | 43 |
| • One a week or more | 7 |
| Stand on chair to reach | 56 |
| Have grab bars in bathroom | 85 |
| Breathless | 54 |
| • Always/Most of the time | 23 |

**Note:** From "Falls and Fear of Falling among Elderly Persons Living in the Community" by J. E. Walker and J. Howland, 1991, *American Journal of Occupational Therapy, 45*, p. 120. Copyright 1991 by *American Journal of Occupational Therapy*. Reprinted with permission.

## 8.5.2 Frequency Distribution Table

A *frequency distribution table* is organized into columns of data that include the number or frequency of cases (and the equivalent percentages) that fall into a designated category. In the research study in Table 8–4, a frequency distribution table describes the age and diagnosis group of the total population sampled in the study.

TABLE 8-3

**State Distribution (SEER Summary Stage 2000) by Cancer Site, All Ages, All Races, Both Sexes, 2000–2007**

| Cancer Site | Localized | Regional | Distant | Unstaged |
|---|---|---|---|---|
| Digestive System | 31.9 | 32.7 | 25.6 | 9.8 |
| Liver and Intrahepatic Bile Duct | 37.7 | 25.0 | 18.0 | 19.4 |
| Lung and Bronchus | 16.4 | 21.9 | 52.9 | 8.8 |
| Melanoma of the Skin | 83.8 | 8.3 | 3.7 | 4.2 |
| Brain and Other Nervous System | 72.9 | 15.8 | 2.2 | 9.0 |
| Myeloma | 4.7 | 0.0 | 94.2 | 1.0 |

**Note:** Cancer sites include invasive cases only unless otherwise noted. *Localized* means the cancer is only located at the organ where it began with no spreading. *Regional* means the cancer has spread beyond the primary site to nearby lymph nodes or organs and tissues. *Distant* means the cancer has spread from the primary site to distant organs or distant lymph nodes and *unstaged* means cancer for which there is not enough information to indicate a stage.

Young JL Jr, Roffers SD, Ries LAG, Fritz AG, Hurlbut AA (eds). SEER Summary Staging Manual - 2000: Codes and Coding Instructions, National Cancer Institute, NIH Pub. No. 01-4969, Bethesda, MD. 2001.

TABLE 8-4

**Distribution of Age and Group Assignment Based on Diagnosis**

| Age Group (Years) | Hemiplegic Group | | Control Group | | Total | |
|---|---|---|---|---|---|---|
| | No. | % | No. | % | No. | % |
| 45–49 | 3 | 17 | 2 | 11 | 5 | 14 |
| 50–54 | 0 | 0 | 2 | 11 | 2 | 6 |
| 55–59 | 2 | 11 | 1 | 6 | 3 | 8 |
| 60–64 | 2 | 11 | 1 | 6 | 3 | 8 |
| 65–69 | 5 | 28 | 6 | 33 | 11 | 31 |
| 70–74 | 5 | 28 | 5 | 28 | 10 | 28 |
| 75 + | 1 | 6 | 1 | 6 | 2 | 6 |
| Total | 18 | 100 | 18 | 100 | 36 | 100 |

Adapted from "Bimanual Upper Extremity Movements In Persons With Left Hemiplegia Due To Stroke" by M. S. Rice and K. M. Newell, 2004, *Archives of Physical Medicine and Rehabilitation, 85,* 629–634.

The first column of a frequency distribution table includes the class intervals (in this example, age group by years). It could also represent data such as range of motion in degrees, scores on perceptual tests, or diastolic blood pressure. The class intervals are separated into equal 5-year intervals in the above example (e.g., 45–49 and 50–54). The second column of a frequency distribution includes the number of classes tallied within the class intervals (e.g., 3 people between the ages of 45 and 49 years).

The third column includes the percentage of cases within a class interval. For example, there are 6 people in the control group within the class interval of 60 to 64. This represents 6 over a total of 18 people in the control group, or 33.33 percent which is rounded to 33 percent. We can also determine the *cumulative frequency* of each class interval and the *cumulative relative frequency* with the data provided in the study. The following data are reorganized into a frequency distribution table to include relative frequency and cumulative relative frequency for males only:

| Frequency Distribution Table for Males | | | | |
|---|---|---|---|---|
| **Class Interval** | **Frequency (f)** | **Relative f (%)** | **Cumulative f** | **Cumulative rf (%)** |
| 5 – 14 | 36 | 6 | 36 | 6 |
| 15 – 24 | 147 | 24 | 183 | 30 |
| 25 – 34 | 200 | 33 | 383 | 63 |
| 35 – 44 | 105 | 17 | 488 | 80 |
| 45 – 54 | 60 | 10 | 548 | 90 |
| 55 – 64 | 41 | 7 | 589 | 97 |
| > 65 | 21 | 3 | 610 | 100 |
| Unknown | 4 | 0.006 | 614 | 100 |
| **Total** | **614** | **100%** | **614** | **100%** |

**In summary:**

- Class *interval* is the category of score values in a distribution. The number of class intervals is determined by the number of subjects in the study and the range of values or scores.
- Frequency of cases includes the total number of cases within an assigned class interval.
- *Relative frequency* or *percentage* is the percentage of cases falling within the class interval and is calculated by dividing the number of cases within the class interval by the total number of cases in the distribution.
- *Cumulative frequency* represents the total number of scores within a class interval that is added cumulatively from the lowest to the highest class interval. The grand total of the cumulative frequency equals the total number of scores or cases in the distribution.
- *Cumulative relative frequency* or *cumulative percentage* is the percentage of cases added from the lowest class interval through the highest class interval. The percentage should total 100 percent.

The following table displays hypothetical ungrouped raw scores on resting heart rate for 50 healthy young adults.

## Constructing a Frequency Distribution Table

| Subject | Score | Subject | Score | Subject | Score | Subject | Score |
|---------|-------|---------|-------|---------|-------|---------|-------|
| 01 | 54 | 14 | 67 | 27 | 54 | 40 | 79 |
| 02 | 72 | 15 | 74 | 28 | 73 | 41 | 85 |
| 03 | 80 | 16 | 76 | 29 | 72 | 42 | 52 |
| 04 | 53 | 17 | 79 | 30 | 78 | 43 | 56 |
| 05 | 75 | 18 | 77 | 31 | 78 | 44 | 67 |
| 06 | 53 | 19 | 48 | 32 | 56 | 45 | 55 |
| 07 | 78 | 20 | 76 | 33 | 80 | 46 | 79 |
| 08 | 47 | 21 | 47 | 34 | 84 | 47 | 81 |
| 09 | 72 | 22 | 50 | 35 | 72 | 48 | 72 |
| 10 | 54 | 23 | 65 | 36 | 68 | 49 | 67 |
| 11 | 66 | 24 | 83 | 37 | 57 | 50 | 71 |
| 12 | 68 | 25 | 55 | 38 | 57 | | |
| 13 | 68 | 26 | 76 | 39 | 63 | | |

**Step 1.** *Record raw scores from ungrouped data.*

**Step 2.** *Identify the highest and lowest values in the distribution.* Subjects 08 and 21 have heart rate scores of 47 (lowest score). Subject 41 has a heart rate score of 85 (highest score).

**Step 3.** *Calculate the range (highest score to lowest score).* In our example, the range is 85 − 47 = 38.

**Step 4.** *Determine the number of class intervals.* The determination of the number of class intervals depends on the number of scores in the frequency distribution and the range of scores. Too many or too few class intervals may not give adequate information to describe the distribution. Determining the number of class intervals is a trial-and-error process. For example, compare the three frequency distributions using the same scores but with class intervals of too many, too few, and approximately correct. These data are shown in Table 8–5. Most researchers constructing frequency distributions establish 6 to 15 class intervals as a general rule.

## TABLE 8-5

### Intervals for Class Data

| Number of Class Intervals (CI) | | |
|---|---|---|
| Too Many (20 CI) | Too Few (4 CI) | Approximate Correct (13 CI) |
| 84–85 | 75–85 | 83–85 |
| 82–83 | 65–74 | 80–82 |
| 80–81 | 55–64 | 77–79 |
| 78–79 | 45–54 | 74–76 |
| 76–77 | | 71–73 |
| 74–75 | | 68–70 |

*continues*

TABLE 8-5

**Intervals for Class Data** *continued*

| Too Many (20 CI) | Number of Class Intervals (CI) Too Few (4 CI) | Approximate Correct (13 CI) |
|---|---|---|
| 72–73 | | 65–67 |
| 70–71 | | 62–64 |
| 68–69 | | 59–61 |
| 66–67 | | 56–58 |
| 64–65 | | 53–55 |
| 62–63 | | 50–52 |
| 60–61 | | 47–49 |
| 58–59 | | |
| 56–57 | | |
| 54–55 | | |
| 52–53 | | |
| 50–51 | | |
| 48–49 | | |
| 46–47 | | |

© Cengage Learning 2013

***Step 5.*** *Determine the size of a class interval.* The size of the class interval is determined through estimation by dividing the range of scores by the number of class intervals. Using the same example, the range of 38 is divided by 13 (the number of class intervals) to yield a class interval size of 3. It is recommended that an odd number be selected for the class interval so that the midpoint of the class interval is a whole number. For example, the midpoint of the class interval of 83 – 85 is 84. Later, in calculating group means from a frequency distribution table, the reader will find that it is easier to work with whole numbers than with fractions in calculating values.

On the other hand, if we determine that the size of a class interval in the previous example is 5, how many class intervals would be established? In this case, the range of scores (38) is divided by the size of the class intervals (5) to arrive at 8 class intervals.

| CI | Midpoint |
|---|---|
| 81 – 85 | 83 |
| 76 – 80 | 78 |
| 71 – 75 | 73 |
| 66 – 70 | 68 |
| 61 – 65 | 63 |
| 56 – 60 | 58 |
| 51 – 55 | 53 |
| 46 – 50 | 48 |

**Step 6.** *Tally the number of scores within each class interval.* Check to determine if the number of tallies total to the number of scores in the frequency distribution.

| Class Interval | Real Limits* | Midpoint | Tally | f | Cf |
|---|---|---|---|---|---|
| 83 – 85 | 82.5 – 85.5 | 84 | ||| | 3 | 50 |
| 80 – 82 | 79.5 – 82.5 | 81 | ||| | 3 | 47 |
| 77 – 79 | 76.5 – 79.5 | 78 | ||||||| | 7 | 44 |
| 74 – 76 | 73.5 – 76.5 | 75 | ||||| | 5 | 37 |
| 71 – 73 | 70.5 – 73.5 | 72 | ||||||| | 7 | 32 |
| 68 – 70 | 67.5 – 70.5 | 69 | ||| | 3 | 25 |
| 65 – 67 | 64.5 – 67.5 | 66 | ||||| | 5 | 22 |
| 62 – 64 | 61.5 – 64.5 | 63 | | | 1 | 17 |
| 59 – 61 | 58.5 – 61.5 | 60 | 0 | 0 | 16 |
| 56 – 58 | 55.5 – 58.5 | 57 | |||| | 4 | 16 |
| 53 – 55 | 52.5 – 55.5 | 54 | ||||||| | 7 | 12 |
| 50 – 52 | 49.5 – 52.5 | 51 | || | 2 | 5 |
| 47 – 49 | 46.5 – 49.5 | 48 | ||| | 3 | 3 |
| **Total** | | | **50** | | **50** |

*Defining the upper and lower real limits of the class intervals is described below.

The upper real limit of a class interval is the highest value contained in the interval. Conversely, the lower real limit of a class interval is the lowest value contained in the interval. In dealing with numbers having at least two decimals, round the number up to include it in the nearest class interval. For example, 82.50 or above would be tallied in the class interval 83–85. On the other hand, 82.44 would be tallied into the class interval 80–82 as shown in the example.

**Step 7.** *Determine the relative frequency or percentage.* Calculate the relative frequency of the scores in each class interval by dividing the number of cases or scores in the class interval by the number of cases in the frequency distribution. This is illustrated in Table 8–6.

Percentage = frequency of cases in the class interval / total cases in the frequency distribution

**TABLE 8-6**

**Calculation of Cumulative Frequency**

| Class Interval | Frequency | Percentage | Cumulative Percentage |
|---|---|---|---|
| 84 | 3 | 3/50 = 6% | 100% |
| 81 | 3 | 3/50 = 6% | 94% |
| 78 | 7 | 7/50 = 14% | 88% |
| 75 | 5 | 5/50 = 10% | 74% |
| 72 | 7 | 7/50 = 14% | 64% |

*continues*

TABLE 8-6

**Calculation of Cumulative Frequency** *continued*

| Class Interval | Frequency | Percentage | Cumulative Percentage |
|---|---|---|---|
| 69 | 3 | 3/50 = 6% | 50% |
| 66 | 5 | 5/50 = 10% | 44% |
| 63 | 1 | 1/50 = 2% | 34% |
| 60 | 0 | 0/50 = 0% | 32% |
| 57 | 4 | 4/50 = 8% | 32% |
| 54 | 7 | 7/50 = 14% | 24% |
| 51 | 2 | 2/50 = 4% | 10% |
| 48 | 3 | 3/50 = 6% | 6% |
| Total | 50 | 50/50 = 100% | 100% |

*Step 8.* *Determine cumulative frequency.* Calculate the cumulative frequency by adding the total frequency in each class interval consecutively from the highest class interval to the lowest. In the previous example, the number of cases in the class interval 83–85 is 3. This number is added to the number of cases in the class interval 80–82, which is also 3, giving a cumulative frequency of 6. The completed frequency distribution table is shown in Table 8–7.

TABLE 8-7

**Frequency Distribution of Heart Rate Scores for Hypothetical Population**

| CI | Midpoint | f | Cf | RF% | CRF% |
|---|---|---|---|---|---|
| 83 – 85 | 84 | 3 | 50 | 6 | 100 |
| 80 – 82 | 81 | 3 | 47 | 6 | 94 |
| 77 – 79 | 78 | 7 | 44 | 14 | 88 |
| 74 – 76 | 75 | 5 | 37 | 10 | 74 |
| 71 – 73 | 72 | 7 | 32 | 14 | 64 |
| 68 – 70 | 69 | 3 | 25 | 6 | 50 |
| 65 – 67 | 66 | 5 | 23 | 10 | 44 |
| 62 – 64 | 63 | 1 | 17 | 2 | 34 |
| 59 – 61 | 60 | 0 | 16 | 0 | 32 |
| 56 – 58 | 57 | 4 | 16 | 8 | 32 |
| 53 – 55 | 54 | 7 | 12 | 14 | 24 |
| 50 – 52 | 51 | 2 | 5 | 4 | 10 |
| 47 – 49 | 48 | 3 | 3 | 6 | 6 |

Summary of Construction of Frequency Distribution Table

1. Organize raw scores from ungrouped data by arranging values from the lowest to the highest scores.
2. Identify the lowest and highest scores in the distribution.
3. Calculate the range, which is the difference or distance from the lowest to the highest scores in the distribution.
4. Determine the number of class intervals, using the rule of thumb of selecting within a range of 6 to 15 categories of intervals.
5. Determine the size of each class interval. First, estimate the size of class intervals by dividing the range by the number of class intervals. Try to select an odd number so that the midpoint of the class interval will be a whole number.
6. Count or tally the number of scores within each class interval.
7. Calculate the relative frequency or percentage of scores in each class interval.
8. Calculate the cumulative frequency by adding in succession the frequencies in each class interval. Check that the number of cases counted in succession is equal to the total number of cases or scores in the distribution.
9. Determine the cumulative relative frequency, which is the percentage of cumulative frequency sitting in each class interval. It is customary to start from the lowest class interval when calculating cumulative values.

### 8.5.3 Graphs and Other Pictorial Representations

In addition to presenting data in tables, many researchers use pictorial presentations to display results and describe data. These presentations can be in the form of frequency polygons, histographs, bar graphs, pie graphs, and stem and leaf.

### 8.5.4 Frequency Polygon

A **frequency polygon** is a line graph displaying the frequency of data by categories. The categories compared are on the horizontal axis (abscissa), and the frequencies of occurrences are on the vertical axis (ordinate).

The frequency polygon in Figure 8–6 shows the percentage of U.S. males with a body mass index of 30 or greater by age group across a 10-year period. The biannual year groupings are listed on the X axis, the **abscissa**, and the percentage of males with obesity are on the Y axis, the **ordinate**. Note that usually the midpoint of the category is used as a reference point for plotting the frequencies within each category. In this example, the interval between percentages is 5 and the range on the ordinate is from 15 through 45. The creator of this graph collapsed the graph to eliminate the intervals between 0 and 15. This was done to keep the majority of the data centered on the graph. The same concept can be applied to the abscissa if needed.

### 8.5.5 Histograms and Bar Graphs

Investigators often use histograms and bar graphs to display frequency of data within categories, similar to frequency polygons. In **histograms**, the bars are attached to each other as in Figure 8–7, whereas in **bar graphs**, each bar is detached from one another. The distinction sometimes is based on aesthetic reasons. The histogram shown in Figure 8–7 describes the type of activities in which occupational therapy students participated while completing their level 1 fieldwork experiences. On the abscissa is the type of fieldwork experience; and on the

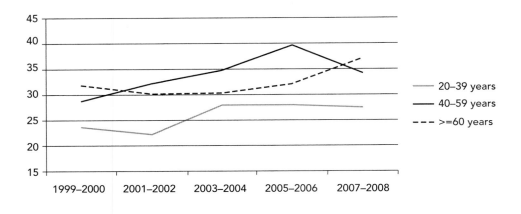

**FIGURE 8-6**  Percentage of U.S. Males Considered Obese (BMI ≥ 30) from 1999 through 2008

Adapted from "Prevalence and Trends in Obesity among US Adults, 1999-2008" by K. M. Flegal, M. D. Carroll, C. L. Ogden, and L. R. Curtin, 2010, *JAMA: The Journal of the American Medical Association*, *303*, 235-241. doi:10.1001/jama.2009.2014

ordinate, the relative frequency or percentage of time spent in a specific activity, such as passive observer, is plotted.

### Constructing a Frequency Polygon, Histogram, or Bar Graph

A frequency polygon, histogram, or bar graph graphically depicts the data provided in a frequency distribution table. The data provided in the *Frequency Distribution of Heart Rate Scores* in Table 8–7 will be used in the following examples.

**Step 1.** *Identify the X axis (abscissa) and the Y axis (ordinate).* This is illustrated in Figure 8–8.

**Step 2.** *Label the abscissa descriptively.* In the example in Table 8–7, the heart rate values range from the lowest score of 47 to the highest of 85. The midpoints of each class interval are located on the abscissa (Figure 8–9). The class intervals are extended on both ends to include zero frequency intervals. The lowest class interval with zero frequency is 44 – 46 with a midpoint of 45. The highest class interval with zero frequency is 86 – 88 with a midpoint of 87. There are now 15 class intervals including the zero frequency intervals.

**Step 3.** *Organize the ordinate into frequency of occurrence.* In the previous example, frequencies of occurrence range from 0 to 7. As a rule of thumb, the number of class intervals for frequency should be between 8 and 15. In this case, there will be 8 class intervals, including 0.

The frequency polygon is depicted in Figure 8–9 with the data from Table 8–7. The histogram is depicted in Figure 8–10 with the same data used in constructing the frequency polygon. Bar graphs are similar to histograms, differing only in that the bars are detached (McCall, 1986).

There are a number of software programs that create any number of graph styles. For example, spreadsheet programs often have a graphing module, as well as a statistical module, that can conveniently facilitate the creation of graphs.

### 8.5.6 Cumulative Frequency Distributive Polygon

A cumulative frequency distribution polygon is a line graph that shows the total number of observations or cases up to the upper real limit of a given class interval. For example, in Section 8.5.2, Step 8, determining

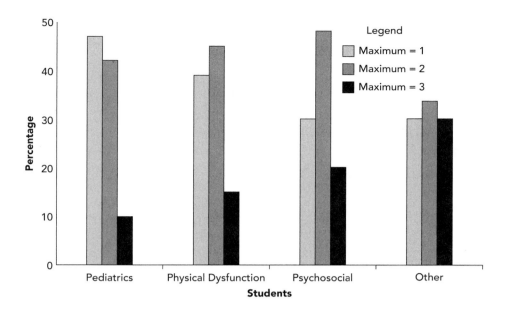

**FIGURE 8-7** Example of a Histogram Depicting the Maximum Number of Level I Fieldwork Students Supervised at One Time in Each Type of Facility

From "The Level I Field Work Process" by L. D. Shalik, 1990, *American Journal of Occupational Therapy, 44,* p. 702. Copyright 1990, *American Journal of Occupational Therapy.* Reprinted with permission.

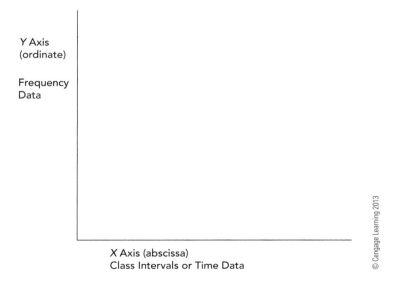

**FIGURE 8-8** Parts of a Frequency Polygon, Histogram, or Bar Graph: The frequency data are plotted along the vertical axis or ordinate (*Y* axis), while the class intervals or time data are plotted along the horizontal axis or abscissa (*X* axis).

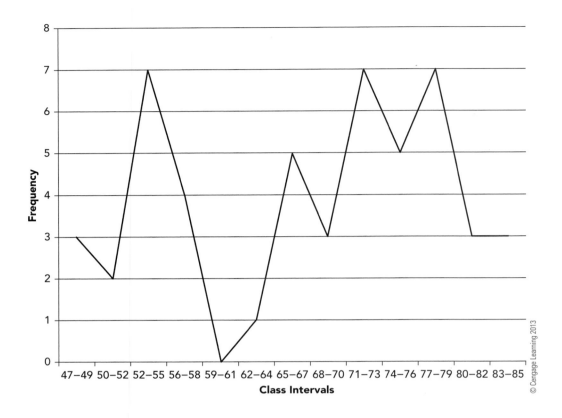

**FIGURE 8-9** Frequency Distribution Polygon Illustrating the Frequencies of Heart Rate Scores for a Hypothetical Population: The data used to plot this polygon are from Table 8–7.

cumulative frequency, the data for the heart rates for 50 subjects are displayed. In Figure 8–11, the cumulative frequency distribution polygon is constructed from the previous table of hypothetical heart rate values (Table 8–7).

Cumulative frequency curves are useful in specifying the individual subject's relative position or standing in a total distribution of scores. For example, someone with a heart rate of 80 in the above distribution is in the 94th percentile or upper 6 percent of the distribution. Cumulative frequency curves often are useful in plotting group test data, such as grip strength, range of motion, blood pressure, and achievement test scores. Individual test data plotted on a cumulative frequency curve can be used to evaluate an individual's function and diagnosis.

In designing a cumulative frequency curve, the ordinate axis is used to display cumulative frequencies, cumulative percentages, or cumulative proportions. The abscissa shows the score values as midpoints or individual scores.

The shape of the cumulative frequency curve reflects the form or shape of the original frequency distribution. As a general rule, the cumulative frequency curve will have the greatest slope or most rapid rate of rise at the point where there is the greatest accumulation of the scores in the original frequency distribution. The cumulative frequency curve levels off and shows the lowest slope for the class intervals when there are fewer scores. Cumulative curves do not describe variations in the data as well as histograms and should not be used

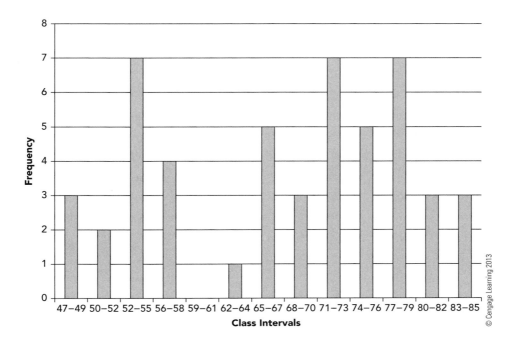

**FIGURE 8-10**  Histogram of Heart Scores in a Hypothetical Population: The data from Table 8–7 and depicted in Figure 8–9 in a frequency polygon are depicted in a histogram here.

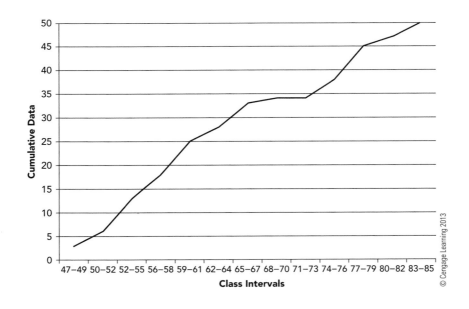

**FIGURE 8-11**  Cumulative Frequency Distribution Polygon Using Data from Table 8–7.

to draw conclusions about the form or shape of the data. The original frequency distribution is best used for this purpose.

### 8.5.7 Statistical Pie

A **statistical pie** is a pictorial representation of the relative percentage of discrete variables or nominal categories, such as health professions, distributions of disease, occupational role functions, types of work injuries, or treatment techniques applied. It is particularly useful to quickly assess the relative percentage of each category. In Figure 8–12, the percentage of placement of students with special needs in each type of educational placement is graphically displayed in a statistical pie.

#### Constructing a Statistical Pie

*Step 1. Make sure the statistical pie is relevant for describing data.* The statistical pie is appropriate when there are between 3 and 10 discrete categories. If there are more than 10 categories, the data will be better presented in a frequency distribution table. The data collected should be categorical and inclusive. For example, data collected regarding the cause of death should include all major causes for a designated population and should add up to 100 percent. Unknown causes should be included in the statistical pie.

*Step 2. First organize data into a frequency distribution table deriving relative percentages for each category.* In the hypothetical example below, specialty areas for female physicians are described. A sample of 250 female physicians was surveyed.

| Medical Specialty | Frequency | Relative Percent |
|---|---|---|
| Pediatrics | 84 | 33.6 |
| Psychiatry and Neurology | 34 | 13.6 |
| Internal Medicine | 25 | 10.0 |
| Anesthesiology | 23 | 9.2 |
| Pathology | 22 | 8.8 |
| General Surgery | 4 | 1.6 |
| Other | 58 | 23.2 |
| **Totals** | **250** | **100** |

*Step 3. Transform relative percent into the degrees of a circle, which is the proportion of 360 degrees.* The relative percent is multiplied by 360 degrees.

*Step 4. To create a pie chart manually, use a protractor and compass to construct the statistical pie.* Divide the statistical pie with a protractor into seven segments running clockwise, starting with the largest category at 12 o'clock, which, in this example, is pediatrics (33.6% or 121°), other (23.2% or 84°), and psychiatry and neurology (13.6% or 49°). Continue with the other specialty areas in completing the 360° circle.

*Step 5. Label each segment category with the relative percent rather than the degrees of arc.* The completed statistical pie is shown in Figure 8–13.

### 8.5.8 Scatter Diagrams

A **scatter diagram** is a graphic representation of the relationship between two variables. In this example, the scatter plot depicts the relationship between age (presumed independent variable) and life expectancy

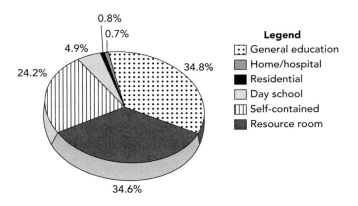

**FIGURE 8-12** An Example of a Statistical Pie Graph that Illustrates the Percentage of Students with Special Needs in Different Types of Educational Placements

Data for this graph are adapted from the *Fifteenth Annual Report to Congress on the Implementation of the Education of the Handicapped Act*, USOE, 1993. The data reflect information collected in 1990.

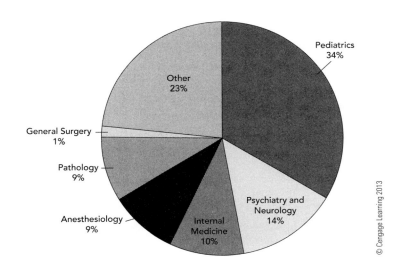

**FIGURE 8-13** Statistical Pie Graph Illustrating Data from the Hypothetical Data of Women Physicians

(presumed dependent variable) in males and females between the age of zero and 100 years (Figure 8–14). The size of the class interval for age ($X$ axis) is 20 years, and the size of the class interval for life expectancy ($Y$ axis) is 10 years. The highest life expectancy is approximately 80 for females and is a few years less for males. This is associated with the youngest age on the $Y$ axis (zero). Visual examination of scatter diagrams often reveals a trend. In Figure 8–14, the trend is that as age increases, the life expectancy (meaning the number of years one is expected to continue to live at a given age) decreases. The points located on the scatter

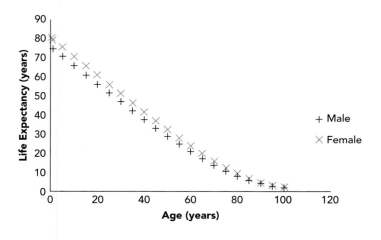

**FIGURE 8-14** Male and Female Life Expectancy in the United States for All Races in 2006

Adapted from "United States Life Tables, 2006" by E. Arias, 2010, *National Vital Statistics Reports, 58*(21). Retrieved from http://www.cdc.gov/nchs/products/life_tables.htm

diagrams are coordinates in which the two variables intersect. For example, in this graph, the expected life expectancy at age 100 is approximately 2 years.

## Constructing a Scatter Diagram

In a hypothetical example a researcher collects the following data, examining the relationship between grip strength as measured by a Jamar dynamometer and Functional Activities of Daily Living (ADL) scores as measured by the *Klein-Bell Test* for patients with muscular dystrophy.

**Step 1.** *Record raw data for hypothetical example of grip strength and ADL scores in patients with muscular dystrophy.*

| Subject | Grip Strength (abscissa) | ADL Score (ordinate) |
|---------|--------------------------|----------------------|
| 01 | 15 | 20 |
| 02 | 40 | 95 |
| 03 | 30 | 50 |
| 04 | 30 | 80 |
| 05 | 10 | 20 |
| 06 | 25 | 15 |
| 07 | 10 | 15 |
| 08 | 20 | 42 |
| 09 | 20 | 15 |
| 10 | 15 | 75 |

| continued | | |
|---|---|---|
| Subject | Grip Strength (abscissa) | ADL Score (ordinate) |
| 11 | 40 | 70 |
| 12 | 30 | 60 |
| 13 | 20 | 45 |
| 14 | 10 | 30 |
| 15 | 40 | 85 |

***Step 2.*** *Determine the range along the abscissa (grip strength) and ordinate (ADL scores).* The range for grip strength is 30 [highest value (40) minus lowest value (10)]. The range for ADL scores is 80 [highest value (95) minus lowest value (15)].

***Step 3.*** *Determine the number of the class intervals for each variable.* Using the convention of 6 to 15 class intervals, we would establish 8 class intervals for grip strength with the size of the interval being 5. The actual score values are 5, 10, 15, 20, 25, 30, 35, 40 (along the abscissa). For ADL scores, the class interval is 20 with a range from 15 to 95. The actual score values plotted along the ordinate are 0, 20, 40, 60, 80, and 100.

***Step 4.*** *Design the scatter diagram (illustrated in Figure 8–15) with the score value on the abscissa (grip strength) and ordinate (ADL scores).* For example, Subject 01 had a grip strength score of 15 and an ADL score of 20. The investigator plots the coordinates for all 15 subjects.

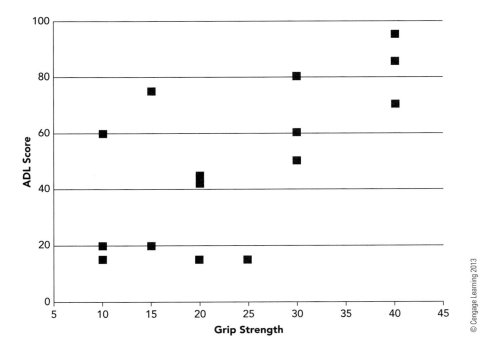

© Cengage Learning 2013

**FIGURE 8-15** Example of a Scattergram: Hypothetical example showing the relationship between grip strength and ADL scores in patients with muscular dystrophy

In the above example, a *positive relationship* is noted because as scores on one variable increase, scores on the other variable increase correspondingly. A negative or inverse relationship is obtained when scores on one variable increase while the corresponding scores on the other variable decrease. The degree of relationship between the two variables of the *correlation coefficient* will be discussed later in this chapter (Section 8.11).

## 8.5.9 Measures of Central Tendency

The first step in organizing data is usually to design a frequency distribution table or graph. The table or graph provides information concerning the form of the data. The properties of a set of data can be further described by calculating a summary statistic, such as a *measure of central tendency*. Measures of central tendency describe "typical" or **average** values in a distribution of data. An index of central tendency provides one value that best captures the distribution as a whole. There are generally three ways to do this:

1. *Mode:* The most frequent score in a distribution
2. *Median:* The point halfway between the top and bottom halves of a distribution (50th percentile)
3. *Mean:* The arithmetic average of all the scores ($\overline{X}$ or $M$)

### Mode

The mode is the easiest measure of central tendency to compute and the simplest to interpret. It may be used to describe any distribution, whether the data are nominal, ordinal, interval, or ratio.

**Definition.** The *mode* is the most frequent score (raw or ungrouped data) or the midpoint of the interval containing the most scores (grouped data). In a frequency distribution graph, the mode is the highest peak in the graph. Figure 8–16 illustrates the mode using the following data on a distribution of scores in which there is only one mode:

| Score (X) | Frequency of Score (f) | |
|---|---|---|
| 3 | 1 | |
| 4 | 2 | |
| 5 | 2 | |
| 6 | 4 | Mode = 6 |
| 7 | 2 | |
| 8 | 3 | |
| 9 | 2 | |

There is no mode in a distribution of scores if all the scores occur with the same frequency (Figure 8–17). For example:

| Score (X) | Frequency of Score (f) |
|---|---|
| 1 | 2 |
| 2 | 2 |
| 3 | 2 |
| 4 | 2 |

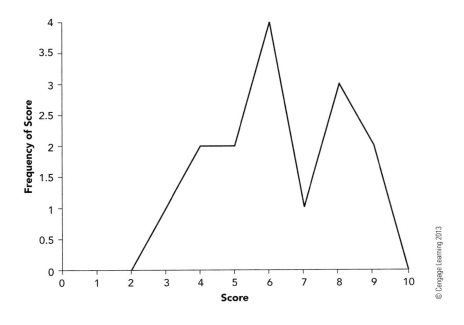

**FIGURE 8-16**  Illustration of a Mode: The highest point is the mode.

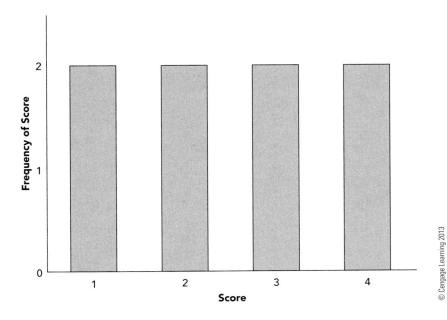

**FIGURE 8-17**  Example of Data Where There Is No Mode: Note that the frequency of each score is the same.

When two adjacent scores have the same frequency and this frequency is higher than any other scores in the distribution, the mode is the average of the two adjacent scores (Figure 8–18). For example:

| Score (X) | Frequency of Score (f) | |
|---|---|---|
| 1 | 1 | |
| 2 | 2 | |
| 3 | 4 | |
| | | Mode = 3.5 |
| 4 | 4 | |
| 5 | 2 | |
| 6 | 1 | |

For grouped data, it is necessary to first calculate the midpoint of each class interval before computing the mode. The mode is then the midpoint of the interval containing the most scores (Figure 8–19).

| Class Interval | Midpoint | Frequency of Scores (f) | |
|---|---|---|---|
| 10 – 12 | 11 | 2 | |
| 13 – 15 | 14 | 2 | |
| 16 – 18 | 17 | 3 | |
| 19 – 21 | 20 | 5 | Mode = 20 |
| 22 – 24 | 23 | 4 | |
| 25 – 27 | 26 | 2 | |
| 28 – 30 | 29 | 1 | |

The mode is the simplest measure of central tendency, but it has two primary limitations:

1. Frequency distributions may have more than one mode, such as a bimodal or even trimodal distribution. In this case, there may be ambiguity about which mode to report, especially if the two (or more) peaks in the distribution are nearly equal. Often one mode is reported as the *primary* or major mode (slightly higher peak), and the other peak is reported as the *secondary* or minor mode (Figure 8–20).
2. When data are grouped, the mode is sensitive to the size and number of class intervals. By changing the class intervals for a distribution, the mode will change—sometimes drastically.

### Median

A second and more sophisticated measure of central tendency is the median. The median is appropriate as a measure of central tendency for ordinal, interval, or ratio data but not for nominal or categorical data from which the mode is the only measure of central tendency that can be calculated.

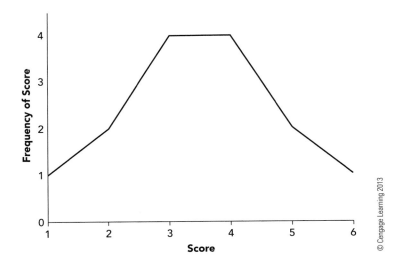

**FIGURE 8-18** Example Illustrating the Mode when the Data Have Two Adjacent Numbers with the Same Frequencies: In this case, the mode is equal to the average of the two adjacent numbers.

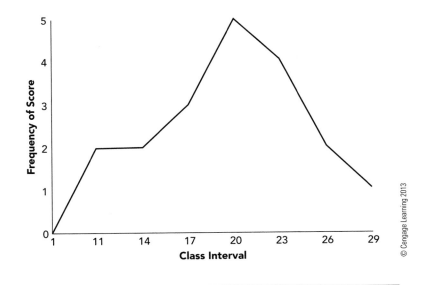

**FIGURE 8-19** Example of a Mode when Grouped Data Are Used

**Definition.** The *median* is the 50th percentile in an ordered group of scores, that is, the point in an array of scores that has 50 percent of the cases below it and 50 percent of the cases above it. The median divides the ranked scores into halves, with one half of the scores below the median and one half of the scores above the median.

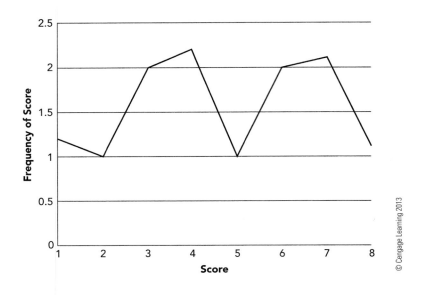

**FIGURE 8-20**   Example of Scores with an Ambiguous Mode: The slightly higher peak is considered the primary or major mode, whereas the next highest peak is considered the secondary or minor mode.

*Calculation.* The calculation of the median is a simple procedure for raw or ungrouped data:

*Step 1. When the number of cases, N, is odd, the median is the score of case (N + 1) / 2 after scores are ranked (either in ascending or descending order).* For example, consider the following array of nine scores:

6, 2, 17, 5, 11, 8, 3, 13, 10

To calculate the median, the nine scores are ranked in order as follows:

| Rank of Score | Score | Frequency | |
|---|---|---|---|
| 1 | 2 | 1 | |
| 2 | 3 | 1 | 4 scores below median |
| 3 | 5 | 1 | |
| 4 | 6 | 1 | |
| 5 | 8 | 1 | Median = 8 |
| 6 | 10 | 1 | |
| 7 | 1 1 | 1 | |
| 8 | 13 | 1 | 4 scores above median |
| 9 | 17 | 1 | |

Median = (score for rank N + 1) / 2
     = (score for rank 9 + 1) / 2
     = score for rank 5

Therefore the median is equal to the score for rank #5, which is equal to the score of 8.

**Step 2.** *When N is even, the median is the score midway between the scores after all scores are ranked.* For example, consider the following scores ($N = 8$):

2, 1, 10, 7, 0, 15, 8, 5

The first step in calculating the median is again to rank order the scores.

| Rank of Score | Score | Frequency | |
|---|---|---|---|
| 1 | 0 | 1 | |
| 2 | I | 1 | 3 scores below median |
| 3 | 2 | 1 | |
| 4 | 5 | 1 | |
| | | | **Median = 6 (midpoint of 5 and 7)** |
| 5 | 7 | 1 | |
| 6 | 8 | 1 | |
| 7 | 10 | 1 | 3 scores above median |
| 8 | 15 | 1 | |

For *grouped data*, the median is the point in a distribution at or below which exactly 50 percent of the cases fall. The median is calculated by constructing a cumulative frequency distribution. The median is then calculated from the cumulative frequency distribution with the following formula:

$$\text{Median} = LL + \left( w_i \left[ \frac{(N/2) - cf}{f_i} \right] \right)$$

Where:

LL = lower real limit of the median interval
$w_i$ = width of class interval
N = number of cases
cf = cumulative frequency up to the median interval
$f_i$ = frequency within the median interval

The first stage in calculating the median is to construct a cumulative frequency distribution beginning with the lowest class interval and proceeding in ascending order to the highest class interval. The next step is to locate the interval that contains the 50th percentile or the median by examining the cumulative frequency column. For example:

| Class Interval | Real Limits | f | Cf | Cumulative Percentile |
|---|---|---|---|---|
| 12 – 14 | 11.5 – 14.5 | 2 | 2 | 10 |
| 15 – 17 | 14.5 – 17.5 | 4 | 6 | 20 |
| 18 – 20 | 17.5 – 20.5 | 3 | 9 | 45 |

*continues*

*continued*

| Class Interval | Real Limits | f | Cf | Cumulative Percentile | |
|---|---|---|---|---|---|
| 21 – 23 | 20.5 – 23.5 | 5 | 14 | 70 | The median is in the class interval in which the 50th percentile rests. |
| 24 – 26 | 23.5 – 26.5 | 3 | 17 | 85 | |
| 27 – 29 | 26.5 – 29.5 | 2 | 19 | 95 | |
| 30 – 32 | 30.5 – 32.5 | 1 | 20 | 100 | |

Inspection of the above cumulative frequency distribution shows that the median or 50th percentile must fall in the class interval of 21–23 because the previous interval of 18–20 has cumulated only 9 of the 20 total cases, that is, 45 percent or 45th percentile.

LL = lower real limit of median interval = 20.5
$w_i$ = width of class interval = 3
N = total number of cases in the frequency distribution = 20
cf = cumulative frequency *up to* median interval = 9 (starting from the lowest to the highest score)
$f_i$ = frequency within median interval = 5
Therefore:

$$\text{Median} = LL + \left( w_i \left[ \frac{[(N/2) - cf]}{f_i} \right] \right)$$

$$= 20.5 + \left( (3) \frac{[(\frac{20}{2}) - 9]}{5} \right)$$

$$= 20.5 + [3 \, (1 \, / \, 5)]$$

$$= 20.5 + 3 \, (.20)$$

$$= 20.5 + .6$$

$$= 21.1$$

The above formula can be used to calculate the median for any grouped frequency distribution, as well as for ungrouped distributions (with or without tied scores).

***Calculation of the Raw Score from the Percentile Rank.*** A modification of the formula allows a generalized method for calculating raw scores corresponding to a given percentile rank (PR).

$$LL + \left[ (w_i) \left( \frac{\{[(PR)(N)/100] - cf\}}{f_i} \right) \right]$$

Where:

LL = lower real limit of the interval containing the given raw score, that is, (PR) (N) / 100
$w_i$ = width of the class interval
PR = percentile rank
N = number of cases in the distribution
cf = cumulative frequency up to the given class interval containing the raw score
$f_i$ = number of cases within the class interval containing the raw score

In the next example, what is the raw score corresponding to the 90th percentile rank?

$$\text{Raw score } (rs) \text{ at 90th percentile rank} = 26.5 + \left[(3)\left(\frac{\{[(90)(N)/100] - cf\}}{f_i}\right)\right]$$

Where:

$LL = 26.5 \qquad cf = 17$
$w_i = 3 \qquad f_i = 2$
$N = 20 \qquad PR = 90$

$$rs = 5 + \left[(3)\left(\frac{\{[(90)(20)/100] - 17\}}{2}\right)\right]$$

$$rs = 26.5 + [(3) * \{[(1800 / 100) - 17] / 2\}]$$

$$rs = 26.5 + \{(3) * [(18 - 17) / 2]\}$$

$$rs = 26.5 + 3 (1 / 2)$$

$$rs = 26.5 + 1.5$$

Therefore, a percentile rank of 90 corresponds to a raw score of 28.

***Calculation of the Percentile Rank (PR) from the Raw Score.*** A researcher may also want to calculate the PR from the raw score. For example, given a raw score of 19 in a group distribution (see above data), what is the PR?

$$PR = \frac{[(f_i)(rs - LL)] + [(W_i)(cf)]}{(N)(w_i)}$$

Where:

$f_i = 3 \qquad rs = 19$
$LL = 17.5 \qquad w_i = 3$
$cf = 6 \qquad N = 20$

$$PR = \frac{[(3)(19 - 17.5)] + [(3)(6)]}{[(20)(3)]}$$

$$= \{[(3)(1.5) - 17.5)] + (18)]\} / 60$$

$$= [(4.5 - 17.5) + 18] / 60$$

$$= 22.5 / 60$$

$$= 37.5$$

Therefore, a raw score of 19 equals a PR of 37.5.

## Mean

The mean is the most widely used and familiar index of central tendency. The *mean* is the arithmetic average of all the scores in a distribution and is calculated by summing all scores and dividing by the total number of scores.

The general formula for the mean ($\overline{X}$) is:

$$\overline{X} = X_1 + X_2 + X_3 \ldots X_n / N$$
$$\overline{X} = \Sigma X / N$$

Where:

$X_1$ = first raw score
$X_2$ = second raw score

$X_3$ = third raw score
$X_n$ = nth raw score
$\Sigma$ = summation or sum of
$N$ = number of subjects in the distribution

The mean may be conceptualized as a "center of gravity" or "balance point" in which the scores or "weights" on one side exactly balance the scores or weights on the other side. Each weight represents a score from a distribution of scores. The arithmetic mean of all the scores or weights is the center of gravity or balance point. The deviation of scores in one direction exactly equals the deviation of scores in the other direction.

***Calculating the Mean with Raw or Ungrouped Data.*** The mean is readily calculated for a distribution of raw scores in which each score occurs only once. The mean is simply the sum of the raw scores divided by the number of scores. For example, consider the following distribution of eight scores:

3, 6, 7, 8, 11, 15, 16, 22

$$\Sigma X = 88$$
$$N = 8$$
$$\overline{X} = \Sigma X / N$$
$$= (3 + 6 + 7 + 8 + 11 + 15 + 16 + 22) / 8$$
$$= 88 / 8$$
$$= 11.0$$

The mean or average value is calculated as 11.0.

For ungrouped data with a small sample of scores, the above procedure may be used to calculate the mean. Alternatively, for grouped data, a frequency distribution should be set up. Then the mean is calculated from the frequency distribution table by multiplying each score by the frequency of occurrence and summing the total across all scores before dividing by the total number of scores.

In the following example, several scores occur more than once:

2, 3, 3, 4, 5, 5, 6, 6, 6, 7, 8, 8, 9, 9, 9

***Step 1.*** *The first stage in computing the mean is to form a frequency distribution table.*

| X | f | fX |
|---|---|---|
| 2 | 1 | 2 |
| 3 | 2 | 6 |
| 4 | 1 | 4 |
| 5 | 2 | 10 |
| 6 | 3 | 18 |
| 7 | 1 | 7 |
| 8 | 2 | 16 |
| 9 | 3 | 27 |
| | | $\Sigma (fX) = 90$ |

The number in the third column is obtained by multiplying each raw score by the frequency of occurrence. The symbol $fX$ represents the product of the scores multiplied by the frequency of scores. This column is then summed and divided by the total number of scores, in this example, 15 scores.

$$\overline{X} = \Sigma fX / N$$

So:

$$\Sigma fX = 90$$
$$N = 15$$
$$= 90 / 15$$
$$= 6.0$$

***Calculating the Mean for Grouped Data.*** When working with grouped data, first find the midpoint of each score interval before calculating the mean.

The general formula to determine the mean for grouped data is:

$$\overline{X} = \Sigma fX / N$$

As an example, consider the following scores grouped into six class intervals:

| Class Interval | Midpoint (X) | f | fX |
|---|---|---|---|
| 3 – 5 | 4 | 2 | 8 |
| 6 – 8 | 7 | 1 | 7 |
| 9 – 11 | 10 | 4 | 40 |
| 12 – 14 | 13 | 6 | 78 |
| 15 – 17 | 16 | 3 | 48 |
| 18 – 20 | 19 | 4 | 76 |
| | | $\Sigma f = 20$ | $\Sigma fX = 257$ |

Therefore:

$$\overline{X} = 257 / 20$$
$$\overline{X} = 12.85$$

In the above example, the midpoint of each class interval ($X$) was multiplied by the frequency in each interval. This product was summed over all the class intervals to give a value equal to 257. This value ($\Sigma fX$) is then divided by the total number of scores or the sum of the frequencies (i.e., $\Sigma f = 20$) to yield the final calculated mean of 12.85.

The mean calculated from a grouped frequency distribution will differ slightly from the mean calculated from raw scores. When scores are grouped, information is lost and a certain amount of inaccuracy introduced. As a general rule, the coarser the grouping of scores, the more the grouped mean will differ from the raw score mean. Nonetheless, for most situations in which 10 to 20 class intervals are typically used, the agreement is close enough between the two calculated means.

### Comparing the Mode, Median, and Mean

1. As a measure of central tendency, the mean takes into account all the scores of distribution and is affected by each single value. One extreme score or **outlier** can influence the mean to a large degree, especially with

small samples. For example, in the following distribution of 10 scores, both the mean and median have a value of 6.0; when an extreme score of 50 is added as the eleventh score, the mean dramatically increases to 10.0, whereas the median changes only to 7.0:

Scores: 2, 3, 4, 4, 5, 7, 8, 8, 9, 10

Mean = 6.0      Median = 6.0

The mean is changed when an extreme score of 50 is added:

Scores: 2, 3, 4, 4, 5, 7, 8, 8, 9, 10, 50

Mean = 10.0      Median = 7.0

1. Therefore, when extreme scores or outliers are present in a frequency distribution of scores, the median may be a more appropriate measure of central tendency than the mean.
2. In distributions that are symmetrical in shape, the mean equals the median, and both are equal to the mode if the distribution is unimodal. This is illustrated in Figure 8–21.
3. In distributions that are symmetrical but not unimodal, it is important to report the mode, mean, and median to provide a clearer picture of the shape and central tendency of the distribution. In Figure 8–22, which depicts a **bimodal** distribution, there are two modes (at 28 and 40) that should be noted: The mean equals the median and both equal 34.
4. In distributions that are skewed to the left or right, the mode, median, and mean will have different values. Note that the mean is pulled either to the right or to the left by the outliers or extreme scores on one end of the **skewed distribution**. The median is the preferred measure of central tendency for skewed distributions, especially when the degree of **skewness** increases. Figures 8–23 and 8–24 illustrate the locations of the three measures of central tendency for right- and left-skewed distributions.

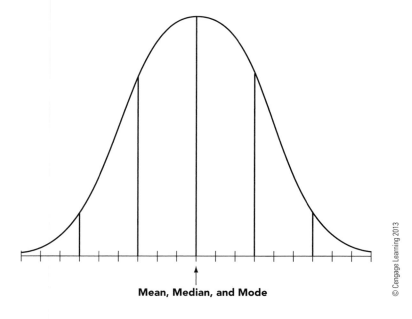

**Mean, Median, and Mode**

© Cengage Learning 2013

**FIGURE 8-21** The Normal Unimodal Curve Depicting the Mean, Median, and Mode: All three fall at the same place on a bell-shaped curve.

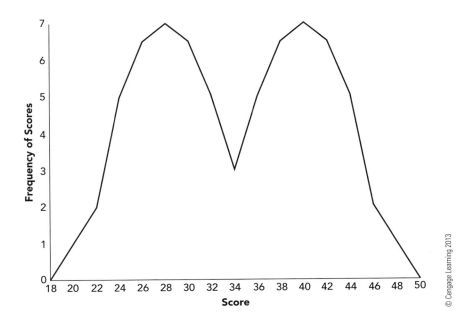

**FIGURE 8-22** Comparison of Mean, Median, and Mode in a Bimodal Distribution: The two modes have the value of 28 and 40. The median and the mean have the same value, 34.

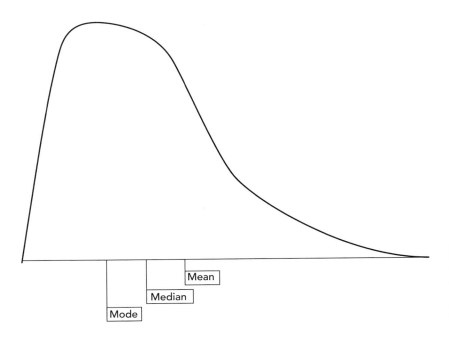

**FIGURE 8-23** A Positively Skewed Distribution: Notice that the figure is pulled to the left, indicating that the scores with the largest frequencies are at the lower end of the distribution.

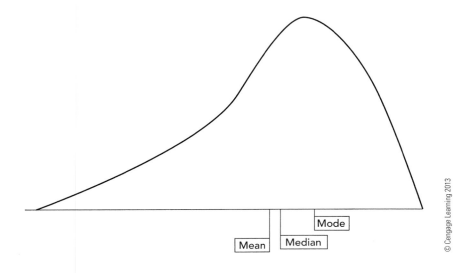

FIGURE 8-24 A Negatively Skewed Distribution: The figure is pulled to the right, indicating that the scores with the largest frequencies are at the upper end of the distribution.

## 8.5.10 Measures of Variability

Measures of variability are descriptive statistics that indicate how scores in a distribution differ from each other and from the mean. For example, in a distribution with the scores 7, 7, 7, 7, the measure of variability is 0 because the scores do not differ from each other and from the mean of 7. The measure of variability increases from zero as the scores vary from each other and from the mean. The *measures of variability* are the range, variance, and standard deviation (*SD*).

### Range

The *range* is the value derived from subtracting the largest score in the distribution from the smallest scores. In the distribution 21, 23, 24, 26, 28, 30, the range is 9. The range is a crude measure of variability because only the highest and the lowest scores of a distribution are used.

### Variance

The *variance* is a measure of the variability of scores in a distribution that takes into account all the scores in that distribution. The computational formula for the variance is:

$$s^2 = [N\Sigma X^2 - (\Sigma X)^2] / N (N - 1)$$

Where:

$N$ = total number of subjects or scores in the distribution
$\Sigma X^2$ = raw scores are squared and then the values are totaled
$(\Sigma X)^2$ = the value which equals the square of the summation of the scores

*Example of Calculating the Variance*

| Subject | Score (X) | X² |
|---|---|---|
| 01 | 2 | 4 |
| 02 | 4 | 16 |
| 03 | 7 | 49 |
| 04 | 9 | 81 |
| 05 | 10 | 100 |
| 06 | 12 | 144 |
| 07 | 14 | 196 |
| N = 7 | ΣX = 58 | ΣX² = 590 |

*Computational Formula for the Variance*

$$s^2 = [N \Sigma X^2 - (\Sigma X)^2] / [N (N - 1)]$$
$$s^2 = [(7) (590) - (58)^2] / [7 (7 - 1)]$$
$$s^2 = [4130 - 3364] / 42$$
$$s^2 = 766 / 42$$
$$s^2 = 18.238$$

### Standard Deviation

The *standard deviation* is the square root of the variance. In the example above, the variance equals 18.238. Therefore, the standard deviation equals 4.27. The standard deviation is an important value that is analogous to the mean. It is used in inferential statistics, such as the *t*-test.

### 8.5.11 Stem and Leaf

Stem and leaf is a method of displaying data developed by Tukey (1977) and is an alternative to the frequency distribution. It derives its name from its display: Any given number is divided into two parts, a stem and a leaf. The first part, the stem, represents a large class into which the number falls, whereas the second number, the leaf, designates the actual placement in the larger class. For example, the number 15 can be divided into 1 (the stem) and 5 (the leaf), whereas the number 216 can be divided into 2 or 21 (the stem) and 16 or 6 (the leaf). When the stem and leaves are displayed in a column, the researcher can easily visualize the organization of the data. The researcher is able to identify the specific scores obtained, as well as the frequency of the class of scores. Once the data have been organized into a **stem and leaf display**, a graph is drawn, allowing the researcher to visualize the structure of the data.

An example of unpublished data helps to explain the concept. Pre- and posttest data were collected to determine the change in understanding of collaboration techniques. The pre- and posttest scores, as well as the ranks for each of the scores, are reproduced in Table 8–8.

TABLE 8-8

**Pretest and Posttest Scores on Collaboration Data**

| Subject | Pretest | | Posttest | |
| | Score | Rank | Score | Rank |
| --- | --- | --- | --- | --- |
| 1 | 118 | 13 | 102 | 11.5 |
| 2 | 59 | 1 | 94 | 8 |
| 3 | 140 | 16 | 114 | 13 |
| 4 | 99 | 9 | 96 | 9 |
| 5 | 96 | 8 | 102 | 11.5 |
| 6 | 63 | 2 | 159 | 16 |
| 7 | 100 | 10 | 71 | 3 |
| 8 | 136 | 15 | 76 | 4 |
| 9 | 152 | 18 | 186 | 18 |
| 10 | 133 | 14 | 198 | 19 |
| 11 | 92 | 6 | 65 | 2 |
| 12 | 62 | 3 | 63 | 1 |
| 13 | 82 | 5 | 148 | 15 |
| 14 | 192 | 19 | 222 | 20 |
| 15 | 106 | 11 | 87 | 7 |
| 16 | 71 | 4 | 82 | 5 |
| 17 | — | — | 101 | 10 |
| 18 | 108 | 12 | 175 | 17 |
| 19 | 151 | 17 | 140 | 14 |
| 20 | 95 | 7 | 84 | 6 |

**Note:** From S. K. Cutler, D. W. Keyes, and M. Urquhart, 1993, unpublished raw data.

The stem and leaf display is as follows:

| Pretest Scores | Pretest Leaf | Stem | Posttest Leaf | Posttest Scores |
| --- | --- | --- | --- | --- |
| 59 | 9 | 5* | | |
| 63, 62 | 3,2 | 6 | 5,3 | 65, 63 |
| 71 | 1 | 7 | 1,6 | 71, 76 |
| 82 | 2 | 8 | 7,2,4 | 87, 82, 84 |

*continued*

| Pretest Scores | Pretest Leaf | Stem | Posttest Leaf | Posttest Scores |
|---|---|---|---|---|
| 99, 96, 92, 95 | 9,6,2,5 | 9 | 4,6 | 94, 96 |
| 106, 108, 118, 136, 133, 140, 100 | 06,08,18,36,33,40,00 | 1 ** | 02,02,01,14,48,40 | 102, 102, 101, 114, 148, 140 |
| 152, 151, 192 | 52,51,92 | 1 | 59,75,86,98 | 159, 175, 186, 198 |
| | | 2 | 22 | 222 |

The asterisks (**) that follow the number in the stem indicate the number of digits that are included in each leaf. For example, 5* means one digit is added to the stem, whereas 1** means two digits are added to the stem. Although commas are not necessary between the leaves, we have chosen to use them. Notice that the number of digits in the leaf can change within a single display. The use of asterisks indicates a change in digits. In this display, the pretest leaves are displayed on the left, and the posttest leaves are displayed on the right. The stem is placed in the center with the leaves on either side. This allows the researcher to compare sets of data easily. For the reader's convenience, the pre- and posttest scores have been listed.

This system has advantages. First, the leaves do not have to be placed sequentially beside the stems; however, when the numbers are ranked later (necessary for the graph), the researcher will want to put them in sequential order. Second, not only is the researcher able to tell the shape of the data, but he or she can also obtain the specific scores. This is not possible in a frequency distribution graph.

When building a stem and leaf display, the number of stems is only limited by the data. The researcher does not want to use so many stems that the data are too spread out or too few lines so that the data are too crowded. Trial and error may be necessary to determine the appropriate number of stems. In general, the last digit of a given number becomes the leaf, and the first digit(s) will be used as the stem. Sometimes, when there are too many leaves on one stem, the stem may be split into parts. By splitting the stem, the leaves may be divided. An example of a split stem can be seen by the repetition of the digit "1."

Once a stem and leaf display has been produced, the researcher needs to make a graph. The graph is called a **box and whisker plot** because of the way in which it is drawn. The graph consists of a box that has lines connected to either side (the whiskers). A box and whisker plot makes use of the ranks of median or middle score, the ranks of the extremes, and the ranks of the hinges. An examination of Table 8–8 shows the median for the pretest to be 100 (rank of 10) and the median of the posttest to be 101.5 (rank of 10.5). The extremes are the ranks of the highest and lowest scores. The pretest extremes are 59 and 192, ranked at 1 and 19. The posttest extremes are 63 and 222, ranked at 1 and 20. The hinges or **quartile** ranks lie halfway between the median and the extremes. They are obtained by the following formula:

Lower hinge = ½ (lower extreme + median)
Upper hinge = ½ (upper extreme + median)

When the rank of a median is not a whole number, drop the decimal (e.g., 10.5 becomes 10). The upper and lower hinges become the upper and lower limits of the box. The whisker is a line that connects the hinges to the extremes. An example of this is seen in Figure 8–25. An examination of the two box plots in this figure reveals that there is little difference between the two scores. Although the upper extreme and the upper hinge is higher on the posttest, the medians, lower extreme, and lower hinge are similar. There is more variability on the posttest.

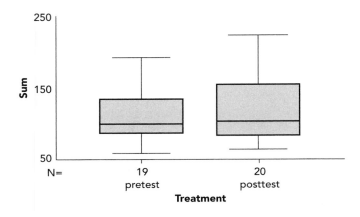

**FIGURE 8-25** An Example of a Box and Whisker Plot Using the Data from Table 8–8. The data are from an unpublished study by Cutler, Keyes, and Urquhart, 1993.

## Construction of a Stem and Leaf Display and Box Plot

**Step 1.** *Make a stem and leaf display.* The following scores have been collected from posttests. Because the scores are between 72 and 97, both the stem and leaf will consist of a single digit. Because of the number of scores that fall between 80 and 89, the stem will be divided into two.

Scores: 88, 82, 75, 93, 96, 81, 83, 82, 97, 96, 87, 88, 72, 75, 95, 82, 80, 87, 89, 88

| Stem | Leaf | Cumulative Rank | Scores Repeated | # of Leaves |
|------|------|-----------------|-----------------|-------------|
| 7* | 525 | 3 | 75, 72, 75 | 3 |
| 8 | 213220 | 9 | 82, 81, 83, 82, 82, 80 | 6 |
| 8 | 878798 | 15 | 88, 87, 88, 87, 89, 88 | 6 |
| 9 | 36765 | 20 | 93, 96, 97, 96, 95 | 5 |

*The asterisk is placed after the 7 to denote that only one digit is used in the leaf.

**Step 2.** *Find the median score.* Because there are 20 scores, the median rank will be 10.5. The score that falls at this rank is 87.

**Step 3.** *Find the extremes.* The extremes are the ranks of the highest and lowest scores or, in this case, those scores with a rank of 1 and 20. The scores for rank 1 and rank 20 are 72 and 97, respectively.

**Step 4.** *Calculate the hinges.* The hinges or quartile ranks lie halfway between the median and the extremes. They are obtained by adding the rank of the extremes to the rank of the median and dividing by 2. When the median rank has a decimal, drop the decimal.

Lower hinge = (1 + 10) / 2 = 11 / 2 = 5.5. The rank for the lower hinge is at 5.5. The score that would fall at this rank is 81.5, obtained by finding the halfway point between the scores that rank at 5 and 6, respectively (e.g., 81, 82).

Upper hinge = (20 + 10) / 2 = 15. The score at this rank is 89.

*Step 5. Draw a box using the lower and upper hinges as the outer limits of the box and connect the extremes to the box with a solid line.* Notice that the box can be drawn horizontally or vertically.

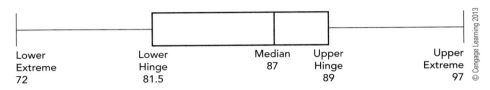

An examination of this box plot suggests that the scores are negatively skewed; that is, more scores are at the upper end of the distribution than at the lower end.

## 8.5.12 z-Scores and the Normal Curve

The **z-scores** are summary values that indicate the distance between a raw score and the mean, using standard deviation units. For example, a z-score of 0 (zero) is equal to the mean. The z-scores are important to describe the relative standing of a raw score. For example, a raw score of 40 is equal to a z-score of +1 in a normal distribution with a mean equal to 30 and one standard deviation equal to 10. Figure 8–26 illustrates the z-score for a raw score of 40.

In this example, a raw score of 40 is equal to a percentile rank of 84, which means that an individual with a z-score of +1 did better than, or is above, 84 percent of the individuals in that distribution.

The formula for calculating z-scores is:

$$z = (\text{raw score} - \text{mean}) / \text{standard deviation or } z = (rs - \overline{X}) / SD$$

In the above example:

$$z = (40 - 30) / 10$$
$$z = 10 / 10$$
$$z = +1$$

The z-scores can be positive or negative, depending on whether the raw score is above or below the mean. These scores are widely used in psychometric testing and are helpful in interpreting raw scores.

## 8.5.13 Normality and the Normal Curve

For the occupational therapist, one of the most difficult decisions is to decide whether a physiological or psychological function is within normal limits. What is normal blood pressure, heart rate, muscle strength, height, visual-perceptual function, or intelligence? Is normality a function of personality or behavior, or is it a statistical value?

When an individual goes in for a physical examination, the physician tests the physiological and neurological functions to determine whether they are within normal limits. The physician uses predetermined values to compare with the patient's results and accepts individual differences within a range of normality to determine whether a function is abnormal. The occupational therapist makes the same judgments in testing range of motion in a specific joint or evaluating muscle strength.

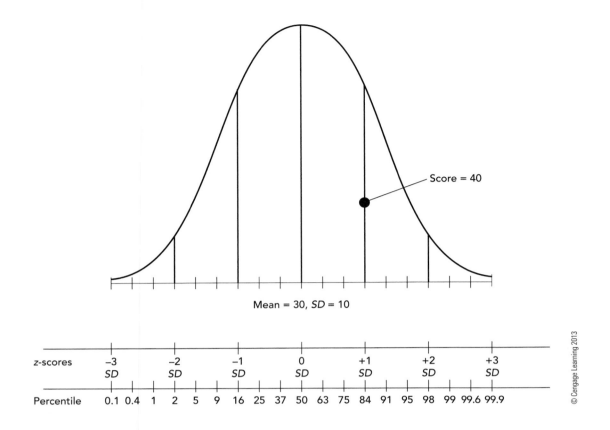

**FIGURE 8-26** Normal Curve Depicting Raw Score of 40, Mean of 30, *SD* of 10: Notice that a raw score of 40 lies one standard deviation above the mean (e.g., z-score of + 1) and at a percentile of 84.

On the other hand, the statistician's definition of "normality" and "abnormality" will depend on the frequency of occurrences within designated class intervals. The statistician interprets **abnormality** as a variance from the mean value, such as 1 or 2 standard deviation units from the mean of a normally distributed variable. In research, scores or values that are abnormal are considered to be outliers or scores that vary widely from expected values. Many times those outliers or abnormal scores are considered at variance with the test of values in a distribution. Consider the scatter diagram in Figure 8–27. Four of the five scores are consistent with a positive relationship with the *X* and *Y* variables. However, one coordinate (50, 5) seems to be an outlier and does not fit into the pattern. The researcher should discuss separately the outlier or abnormal score.

The normal curve (Figure 8–26) is the statistician's guide for examining the relationship between normal values and outliers. In the normal curve, it is expected that 68 percent of the cases will lie within −1 to +1 standard deviation units and 96 percent of the cases will lie within −2 to +2 standard deviations units. If we know that a characteristic is normally distributed, then by calculating the mean and standard deviation of a population, we will be able to determine how many of the cases will be within −2 to +2 standard deviation units from the mean. For example, if we know that the resting heart rate is normally distributed and that the mean value for adults is 72 beats per minute with a standard deviation of 5, then we can determine the percentile ranks (PR) from the raw scores. For example, what is the percentile rank of an individual with a resting heart rate score of 78?

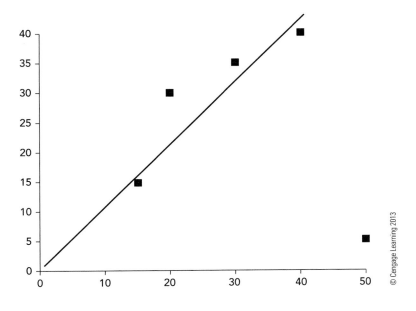

**FIGURE 8-27**  Scattergram Showing an Outlier at the Coordinates of 50, 5: The outlier is the score that appears to be significantly different from the other scores.

The normal curve in Figure 8–28 shows the relationship between the raw score of 78 and the normal values for resting heart rate. We estimate that, based on the diagram, the PR for a raw score of 78 will be slightly above the 84th PR.

### Calculation of PR

First, calculate $z$-scores from raw scores:

$$z = (rs - \overline{X}) / SD$$
$$= (78 - 72) / 5$$
$$= 6 / 5 = 1.2$$
$$z = 1.2$$

Look up the percentile rank from the statistical table (C–2) for the $z$-score of 1.2. Note that in Table C–2 in the appendices, a $z$-score of 1.2 is equal to the percentile rank of .8849.

## 8.5.14 Vital Statistics

The quality of a health care system in a country is usually described by vital statistics such as the infant mortality rate, rates of illnesses and diseases, life expectancy, and mortality rates from specific diseases. In justifying the need for a research study in a clinical area, the researcher first reports the incidence and prevalence rates of a disability or illness to establish the significance of the study. What are some of the most common vital statistics?

### Crude Mortality (Death) or Morbidity (Disease) Rates

The crude mortality or morbidity rate is calculated by dividing the frequency of deaths or illnesses by the total number of individuals in the population. This number is then multiplied by 1,000, 10,000, or 100,000 so it can be used as a comparative figure. For example, if a certain population has a mortality rate of 9.3 per

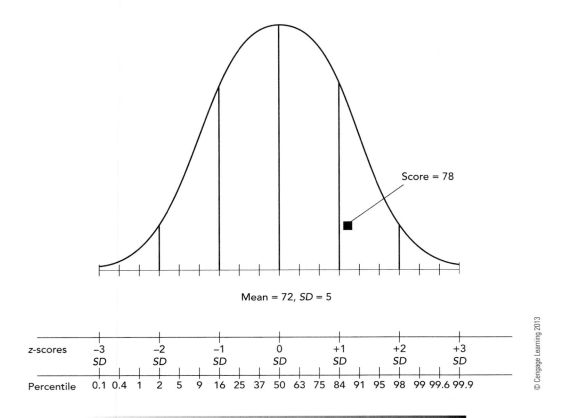

**FIGURE 8-28**  Normal Curve Depicting the Relationship between the Heart Beat Rate of 78 when the Mean Is 72 and the Standard Deviation Is 5: What is the z-score of this heart beat? Is it above or below normal?

1,000 population per year, how does this compare with another population where there are 180,000 deaths in a population of 24,000,000?

### *Calculation of Crude Mortality Rate*

$$\text{Crude death rate} = (180,000 \, / \, 24,000,000) \, (1,000)$$
$$= .0075 \times 1,000$$
$$= 7.5 \text{ per } 1,000 \text{ population}$$

In this hypothetical case, the investigator would conclude that there is a lesser mortality rate in the sample of 180,000 deaths per 24,000,000 population than in the 9.3 per 1,000 population.

### Prevalence and Incidence Rates of Disability or Disease

The terms *prevalence rate* and *incidence rate* are often confused with each other. Prevalence rate refers to the number or proportion of a population who have a given condition. Incidence rate is the number of new cases of a condition within a given time period.

In 2006, the estimated population in the United States was about 299,000,000. In that same year, there were an estimated 1,106,400 people in the United States living with HIV infection (Centers for Disease Control and Prevention, Oct. 2008; http://www.cdc.gov/hiv/topics/surveillance/resources/factsheets/prevalence.htm). In the same year, the estimated incidence rate for new cases of HIV infection was about

56,300 (Centers for Disease Control and Prevention, Sept. 2008; http://www.cdc.gov/hiv/topics/surveillance/incidence.htm).

### Calculation of Prevalence and Incidence Rates

$$\text{Incidence rate} = (56,300 / 299,000,000) (100,000)$$
$$= .000188 (100,000)$$
$$= 18.8 \text{ per } 100,000 \text{ population}$$
$$\text{Prevalence rate} = (1,106,400 / 299,000,000) (100,000)$$
$$= .0037 (100,000)$$
$$= 370 \text{ per } 100,000 \text{ population}$$

### Adjusted Rate

Researchers are also interested in obtaining statistics for specific populations. In these examples, the calculation of rates is adjusted. For example, an investigator is interested in comparing infant mortality rates adjusted for gender. In a hypothetical population, there are 40,000 births of males and 35,000 births of females. In this population, 150 males and 180 females die at birth. What are the adjusted infant mortality rates for females compared with the total crude rates per 1,000 population?

### Calculation of Crude Rate

$$\text{Crude rate} = [(150 + 180) / (40,000 + 35,000)] (1,000)$$
$$= (330 / 75,000) (1,000)$$
$$= (.0044) (1,000)$$
$$= 4.4 \text{ per } 1,000 \text{ (for both males and females)}$$

### Adjusted Rate for Females

$$\text{Adjusted rate} = (180 / 35,000) (1,000)$$
$$= (.0051) (1000)$$
$$= 5.14 \text{ per } 1,000$$

For this hypothetical example, it appears that the infant mortality rate is higher in females compared with the total population.

## 8.6 Inferential Statistics and Testing a Hypothesis

### 8.6.1 Probability and Clinical Research

When an investigator predicts a statistically significant relationship between two variables, it is assumed that the relationship will not exist by chance alone. In other words, the researcher is predicting that $X$ factor is related to $Y$ factor, or that the independent variable, whether manipulated or not, is related to the dependent variable. In clinical research, however, it is difficult to control for all possible factors that could affect the dependent variable.

For example, if a researcher discovers through a thorough search of the literature that arthritis is a psychophysiological disorder, then a set of research investigations would be generated based on this assumption. In a retrospective correlational study, the researcher could select a group of patients with arthritis and investigate personality relationships and the incidence of arthritis. If a statistically significant relationship is found between the incidence of arthritis and personality relationships, it will be beyond a certain probability level, but not necessarily a one-to-one relationship. This means that not all individuals with a certain described characteristic are arthritic. This leads us to the question: Why do we accept a partial relationship rather than a 100 percent probability in clinical research? A number of factors in clinical research impinge on statistically significant results that prevent the perfect 100 percent probability relationships. They are:

- Complex interrelationships among variables in which more than one factor contributes to a disability can affect results in clinical research. For example, in arthritis a multifactorial etiology is assumed. In clinical research, however, we may be able to identify only some portion of the variance associated with the onset of arthritis.
- Diseases in which genetics, age, diet, and numerous other factors influence the course of a disorder can affect research results. There may be individual factors occurring in the individual that are difficult to identify in clinical research during a study.
- The problem of accurately formulating a diagnosis in chronic disabilities such as arthritis, diabetes, multiple sclerosis, cardiovascular disease, schizophrenia, or ulcerative colitis may affect the results in clinical research. Moreover, the sample may not be a homogeneous group, which could contaminate results.
- The **error variance** existing in all clinical research, such as measurement of variables, control of experimental conditions, uniformity of subjects, and data collection procedures, could affect results.

In short, all statistical analysis using hypothesis testing is based on probability. When inferential statistics are applied in a clinical research study, the investigator bases results and conclusions on the probability that any differences between the experimental and control groups are either attributable to chance or are statistically significantly different.

## 8.6.2 Procedure for Statistically Testing a Hypothesis

*Step 1. State the hypothesis.*
A null hypothesis is stated unless the researcher is replicating a previous study or has research evidence to support a directional hypothesis.

1. Null hypothesis is $\mu_1 = \mu_2$ or $r = 0$. *Stated in clinical research study*: There is no statistically significant difference between means or no significantly statistical relationship between variables.
2. Directional hypothesis is $\mu_1 > \mu_2$ or $r$ is statistically significant. This is the reverse of the null hypothesis.

*Step 2. Select a level of significance.*
The researcher usually selects the .05 level of significance in the social sciences. This means that the researcher accepts an error level of 5 percent. The researcher can also state that at $\alpha = .05$, there is a 95 percent confidence level that results are not due to chance.

*Step 3. Apply inferential statistics and select a procedure.*
Selection of a parametric or a nonparametric statistical test will be based on the assumptions underlying the test such as randomness, normal distribution of data, and homogeneity of variance.

*Step 4. Obtain the critical value.*
Refer to the appropriate table for statistical tests based on whether it is one-tailed or two-tailed test, level of statistical significance, and degrees of freedom.

*Step 5. Calculate the value of test statistics.*
This includes *t*-observed, *F*-observed, Chi-square, or correlation coefficient through a mathematical formula.

*Step 6. Accept or reject the research hypothesis (null or directional).*

### 8.6.3 Potential Sources of Research Errors Affecting Statistical Significance

One important aspect of clinical research is to reduce the possible errors in an experiment that could impact on the results. These errors include:

- **Hawthorne effect:** attention given to subjects may increase positive outcome and camouflage the true effects of the independent variable or treatment method. When a Hawthorne effect is present, the subjects' improvement is caused by the attention received from the researcher rather than the direct result of the treatment intervention.
- **Placebo effect:** the suggestion that subjects receiving a treatment, such as medication or a procedure, may produce positive expectations that the treatment will be effective. The subjects may will themselves to improvement. The placebo produces in the subject a desire for improvement. There is some evidence that a psychophysiological effect occurs from the placebo effect.
- **Honeymoon effect:** a short-term effect of a new treatment procedure that subjects hope will impact on a disease. The initial enthusiasm disguises the true effects of the treatment procedure.
- **Researcher bias:** the researcher carrying out a clinical treatment program affects the results through his or her enthusiasm and desire for the treatment to be effective. The researcher's knowledge of the study may affect its outcome.
- **Test administrator bias:** the individual testing the outcome of treatment method is aware of which subjects are in the experimental group and which are in the control group.
- **Sampling errors:** if the researcher's results are based on a sample from a population that is not representative, the results will be skewed or biased to the research sample selected.
- **Systematic variance:** the researcher fails to control for extraneous variables that could possibly affect the results such as age, gender, intelligence, education, socioeconomic status, or degree of disability.
- **Error variance:** the researcher overlooks or minimizes the effects of anxiety, lack of motivation, inattention, distractive environments, and other unexpected problems in the test environment.

### Type I and Type II Errors

All of the above factors and other sources of error in an experiment can potentially affect the results of research. The errors in testing a hypothesis are identified as either a *Type I* or *Type II* error and result from the researcher accepting or rejecting a hypothesis based on the statistical results. The probability of a Type I error in hypothesis testing is typically accepted at the .05 or .01 level. The researcher has confidence that the results are not attributable to chance in 95 or 99 percent of the time. Nonetheless, it is possible that the results are false in 5 out of 100 tries or 1 out of 100 tries purely on the basis of chance errors. Table 8–9 summarizes the relationship between decision errors and hypothesis testing.

The concept in medicine of a false positive or false negative is analogous to describing a Type I or Type II error. A *false positive* in medicine occurs when a disease is falsely detected, whereas a *false negative* exists when a disease is overlooked or not detected. Errors in clinical medicine can occur because of human error because of mistaken judgments in interpreting results, the unreliability of the test equipment or procedure, or unexplained or temporary variables in the patient's condition that can lead to a false diagnosis. Often, clinicians will use more than one test, as well as repeat tests, to confirm or validate a diagnosis. Researchers, on the other hand, try to reduce Type I and Type II errors by replicating experiments with representative samples from different geographical areas.

**In summary:**
- A Type I error is when a researcher rejects a null hypothesis when it should be accepted.
- A Type II error is when a null hypothesis is accepted when it should be rejected.

> **TABLE 8-9**
>
> **Testing the Null Hypothesis, Decision Errors, and Clinical Analogy in Medicine.**
>
> **Null hypothesis $H_0$** predicts that (a) there is no statistically significant difference between means ($\bar{x}_1 = \bar{x}_2$) or (b) there is no statistically significant relationship between variables ($r = 0$).

| Decision by Researcher | True Situation | Analogy in Medicine |
|---|---|---|
| **1. Reject Null Hypothesis:**<br>• $\mu_1 \neq \mu_2 \neq \mu_3 \neq \mu_4 \ldots$<br>• $r \neq 0$ | **Type 1 Error ($\alpha$):** Researcher rejects the null hypothesis when it should be accepted. In reality, there is no significant difference between means or relationship between variables.<br>• $\mu_1 = \mu_2$<br>• $r = 0$<br>*Researcher should accept the null hypothesis* | **False Positive:** Clinician falsely detects the presence of disease or condition when in reality no disease exists. For example, falsely diagnosing breast cancer through mammography screening when in reality breast cancer is not present. |
| **2. Reject Null Hypothesis:**<br>• $\mu_1 \neq \mu_2 \neq \mu_3 \neq \mu_4 \ldots$<br>• $r \neq 0$ | **No Error:** Researcher rejects null hypothesis and concludes that there is a statistically significant difference between the means or that $r$ is greater than zero. | **Correct Diagnosis:** Clinician correctly detects presence of disease and concludes a correct positive diagnosis of a pathological condition. |
| **3. Accept Null Hypothesis:**<br>• $\mu_1 = \mu_2 = \mu_3 = \mu_4 \ldots$<br>• $r = 0$ | **Type II Error ($\beta$):** Researcher accepts null hypothesis when it should be rejected. In reality, there is a significant difference between means or a significant relationship between variables.<br>• $\mu_1 \neq \mu_2$<br>• $r \neq 0$<br>*Researcher should reject null hypothesis.* | **False Negative:** Clinician falsely concludes that based on test results, no disease is present when in reality a disease exists. |
| **4. Accept Null Hypothesis:**<br>• $\mu_1 = \mu_2 = \mu_3 = \mu_4 \ldots$<br>• $r = 0$ | **No Error:** Researcher accepts null hypothesis. | **Correct Diagnosis:** Clinician correctly concludes that no disease is present. |

## 8.6.4 Exploratory Data Analysis

John Tukey (1977) stated, "It is important to understand what you <u>CAN</u> do before you learn to measure how <u>WELL</u> you seem to have done it" (p. v). In clinical research, the question that is usually raised is: How effective is a treatment procedure? For example, are sensory-integration techniques more effective than neurodevelopment treatment? The researcher has to determine at what level of significance the hypothesis would be accepted.

If the researcher is using a standardized test, such as the *Sensory Integration and Praxis Tests* (SIPT; Ayres, 1989), then a definition of "significance" should be decided in advance. Guidelines for the degree of differences between the mean at posttest after intervention should be established. For example, one standard deviation above the mean will show significance. If group 1 had a mean of 100 and group 2 had a mean of 85, on a test in which one standard deviation equaled 15, significance has been demonstrated before a *t*-test or ANOVA was applied to the data. This exploratory data analysis is a method of "eyeballing the data" before applying a statistical test to the results. Exploratory data analysis involves:

a. Calculating group means and standard deviations to determine if the results are clinically significant
b. Screening results by collapsing data in nominal categories and performing a Chi-square test
c. Describing results in scatter diagrams showing the relationship between variables
d. Using stem and leaf displays and box plots to tally the frequency count within designated categories

For a more detailed account of exploratory data analysis, see C. C. Hoaglin, F. Mosteller, and J. N. Tukey, (1991), *Fundamentals of Exploratory Analysis of Variance*. New York: John Wiley and Sons; and J. W. Tukey, (1977), *Exploratory Data Analysis*. Reading, MA: Addison-Wesley Publishing Company.

## 8.6.5 The Concept of Statistical Power and Effect Size

**Statistical power** is the ability of a statistical test to accurately reject the null hypothesis and to detect a difference between groups when one exists. Statistical power is related to the occurrence of a Type II error when the researcher finds that there is no statistically significant difference between the groups when, in reality, there is a significant difference. It is affected by the size of the sample, the probability level of significance such as .05 or .01, and the magnitude of the relationship between the variables measured.

When large samples are used in a clinical study, any statistical analysis will be powerful. For example, a sample of 100 subjects in a clinical study will be more powerful than a sample of 25 subjects. The researcher will have more confidence in rejecting the null hypothesis with a larger number of subjects than with small size samples. However, statistical significance at a .05 level with large numbers of subjects may or may not demonstrate clinical significance. The power of a test, indicating the ability to reject the null hypothesis, also increases when the researcher is willing to accept a higher probability of error (e.g., .05 has more power than.01). What this means is that the researcher is willing to accept more error in interpreting the statistical results. Some researchers recommend a power level of .80 (Ottenbacher & Barrett, 1990).

Nonetheless, a major question for a clinical researcher still remains: Is this treatment method effective? Statistical power should not be manipulated to camouflage clinical results. Clinical research study results should be analyzed to determine if the treatment method is promising, if it is effective with specific patients, and if it can be refined to improve its effectiveness. Statistical confidence should not be compromised to justify the use of treatment methods when they have not demonstrated effectiveness.

Additional concepts associated with determining sample size include the respective means of the dependent variable in each condition, as well as their respective variance. There is a formula that takes all of these concepts into account that is called "Lehr's Equation" (Lehr, 1992). For example:

$$n = \frac{16}{\left(\frac{\mu_0 - \mu_1}{\sigma}\right)^2}$$

Where:

$n$ = number of participants in each condition
$\mu_0$ = the mean of the first condition and
$\mu_1$ = the mean of the second condition
$\sigma$ = the homogenous variance of the means

The number 16 is a constant and is part of Lehr's Equation. This equation assumes $\alpha$ is set at .05 and $\beta$ is set at .2.

In order to use this equation, it is necessary to have access to some data. This can occur through pilot testing where a researcher can obtain some preliminary data, or it could come from other studies that have investigated similar dependent and independent variables. As an example, consider, say, a similar study investigating the efficacy of two types of splints (a hard splint and a soft splint) on the ability to grasp clothespins. Say the mean of the hard splint groups was 11 and the mean of the soft splint group was 17. The homogenized variance between the two means is 8. Lehr's Equation would give the following:

$$n = \frac{16}{\left(\frac{11-17}{8}\right)^2}$$

Therefore:

$$n = 28.44$$

According to this formula, the research would need to recruit 29 participants for each condition, that is, 58 for the entire study.

### Effect Size

In clinical research, researchers present the **effect size** to demonstrate the difference between treatment methods and their impact on improvement. For example, if a researcher is comparing the effectiveness of two types of hand exercise programs to increase grip strength, the researcher should apply an independent $t$-test to evaluate statistical significance. The researcher also may be interested in looking at the clinical impact of the two treatment techniques. Effect size is an important concept that reflects both the variance between the groups and the variance within the groups.

The formula for effect size (ES) is:

$$ES = \mu_0 - \mu_1/s$$

where $s$ is the pooled standard deviation of both groups.

The effect size is zero when the null hypothesis is true (Cohen, 1977). The effect size also serves as an index of the degree of departure from the null hypothesis. For example, a relatively large effect size can be interpreted to mean that the study has high statistical power in accurately rejecting the null hypothesis. Most researchers have defined small, medium, and large effect sizes. Small effect sizes are about .2, medium effect sizes are about .5, and large effect sizes are about .8 (Cohen, 1988).

## 8.7 Model II: One-Sample Problems (One-Sample $t$-Test)

One-sample $t$-tests are applied to research studies in which the investigator is testing whether a sample mean is equal to, less than, or greater than a given value. An example from environmental science is the sampling of air or water to determine if the air or water is polluted. Scientists concerned with the quality of air and water use one-sample $t$-tests to compare samples with parameter values. These parameter values are health standards that have been predetermined by scientific evidence to be at acceptable health levels. At which point is the air considered to be polluted? What are the accepted levels of bacteria for water consumption? These are problems for one-sample $t$-tests. We can also use one-sample $t$-tests for screening populations. For example, is a group sample above or below normal values in height, weight, cholesterol level, blood pressure, heart rate, and hearing acuity? The procedure for applying a one-sample $t$-test is to compare the sample mean with a hypothetical parameter value.

## 8.7.1 Hypothetical Example for Testing for Statistically Significant Differences between Sample Mean and Parameter Mean Values

**Step 1.** *State the research hypothesis.*

1. *Null Hypothesis:* There is no statistically significant difference between the height ($\mu$) of adult Japanese-American men and the standard height ($\mu_0$) of all adult American men.

$$\mu = \mu_0 \text{ (mu, parameter mean value)}$$
$$N = 10{,}000$$

2. *Alternative Hypothesis:* There is a statistically significant difference between the height ($\mu$) of adult Japanese-American men and the height ($\mu_0$) of all adult American men.

$$\mu \neq \mu_0 \text{ (mu, parameter mean value)}$$

**Step 2.** *Select the level of statistical significance:* $\alpha = .05$

**Step 3.** *Select test statistics. Use t-test.*

The formula for a *t*-test is:

$$t = \frac{\overline{X} - \mu_0}{s/\sqrt{N}}$$

(Note: *s* divided by square root of *N*)

**Step 4.** *Identify the* $t_{crit}$ *from the t-distribution table.*

a.  significance level: $\alpha = .05$
b.  two-tailed test of significance
c.  $df = N - 1 = 10{,}000 - 1 = 9{,}999$
$t_{crit} = .196$[1]

**Step 5.** *Calculate the test statistic value.*

From a random sample of 10,000 adult Japanese-American men living in the United States, the following data were collected. An $\overline{X}$ is used, rather than a $\mu$, because only a sample of the total number is used. In this case, the $\overline{X}$ is a value obtained from a representative sample of the population ($\mu$).

$$\overline{X} = 64 \text{ in.}$$
$$\text{standard deviation } (SD) = 1.8 \text{ in.}$$

**Step 6.** *Identify parameter values.*

The parameter values[2] for the average adult American men are:

$$\mu_0 = 69 \text{ in.}$$
$$SD = 1.9 \text{ in.}$$

In this case, $\mu$ is used because the total population is being considered.

**Step 7.** *Graph normal curve for parameter value.*

Because the parameter values are a constant, we can use the normal curve to describe the distribution of parameter values. This is shown in Figure 8–29. For a normal distribution with a mean of 69 and a standard deviation of 1.9, we will expect 68 percent of adult American men to have heights between 67.1 and 70.9 inches.

---

[1]Because *df* = 9,999, which is larger than 120, $t_{crit}$ may be obtained from Table C-2 Normal Curve.
[2]These are hypothetical values set to explain concepts.

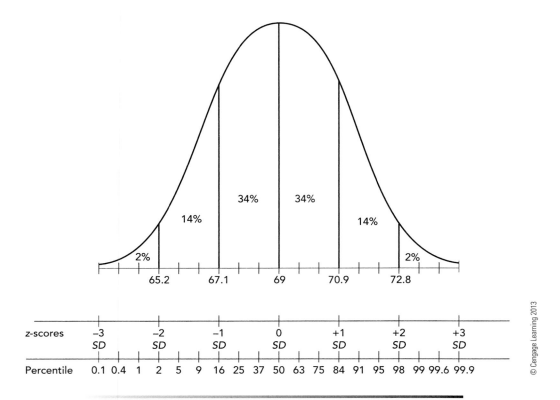

**FIGURE 8-29** Hypothetical Data for Typical Adult American Men (Normal Distribution; Mean Height = 69 inches; Standard Deviation = 1.9): Sixty-eight percent of the adult population should fall between +1 and −1 standard deviations, or heights of 67.1 and 70.9 inches.

**Step 8.** *Graph normal curve for sample.*

This is shown in Figure 8–30. For the sample distribution with a mean of 64 and a standard deviation of 1.8, we will expect 68 percent of the adult Japanese-American men to have heights between 62.2 and 65.8 inches.

**Step 9.** *Calculate the $t_{obs}$ using the formula for t-test.*
(See Step 3.)

$$t = \frac{\overline{X} - \mu_0}{s/\sqrt{N}}$$

Where:

$\overline{X}$ = sample mean equals 64
$s$ = sample standard deviation equals 1.8
$\mu_0$ = parameter mean equals 69
$N$ = sample number of subjects = 10,000

$$t = (64 - 69) / 1.8\sqrt{10,000}$$
$$= (-5) / (1.8 / 100)$$
$$t_{obs} = -5 / .018$$
$$t_{obs} = -277.77$$

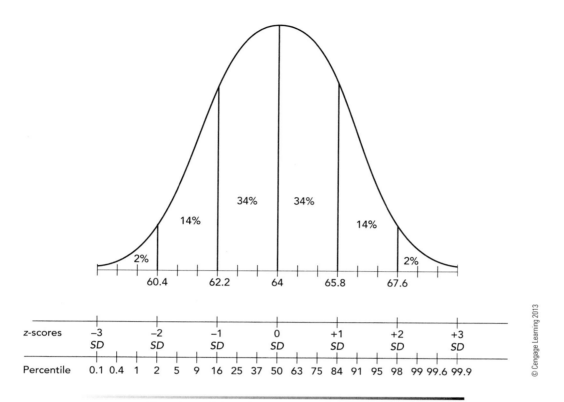

**FIGURE 8-30**  Hypothetical Data for a Sample of 10,000 Adult Japanese and American Men (Normal Distribution; Mean Height = 64 inches; Standard Deviation = 1.8): Sixty-eight percent of the adult population should fall between +1 and −1 standard deviations, or heights of 62.2 and 65.8 inches.

**Step 10.** Compare $t_{obs}$ with $t_{crit}$

$$t_{obs} = -277.77$$
$$t_{crit} = 1.960$$
$$t_{obs} > t_{crit}$$

Thus, the researcher rejects the null hypothesis and concludes that there is a statistically significant difference between the heights of adult Japanese-American men compared with the average height of all adult American men.

## 8.8  Model III: Two Independent Groups

### 8.8.1 Independent *t*-test

The purpose of this statistical model is to test whether there is a statistically significant difference between the means of two independent samples. This frequently is used to test the differences between two clinical techniques applied to an experimental group and a control or comparative group. For example, if a researcher is examining the comparative effectiveness of two treatment techniques in two independent groups, such as

*Progressive Relaxation Exercise* versus *Transcutaneous Electrical Nerve Stimulation* (TENS) in reducing pain, then an independent *t*-test will be applied to the outcome measure for pain (dependent variable).

The *t*-test is also applied when the researcher examines whether there is a statistically significant difference in the characteristic abilities of two groups. In the example below from Liu, Gauthier, and Gauthier (1991), the authors compared performances on 12 perceptual spatial orientation tasks in two independent groups: senile dementia of the Alzheimer type (SDAT) and a comparative control group without dementia. Table 8–10 displays the means for both groups on the perceptual variables and the calculated probability level of significance.

Of the 12 variables tested, only 4 did not reach statistical significance at the *p* < .05 level. The researchers used a two-tailed test for determining the critical level of significance with a total *n* of 30 subjects (15 in each group), at a *df* of *n* − 2. In a two-tailed test with 28 *df*, the critical value of *t* is 2.0484. (See Table C-3 in the appendices.) The observed *t* was above 2.0484 in 8 of the 12 variables tested. The *t*-values reflected the differences between the group means and the comparative homogeneity of the two independent sample standard deviations. In general, a *t*-value is statistically significant when there is a relatively large difference between the group mean and a small difference within the groups.

On the other hand, if the differences within the groups are larger than the differences between the groups, then there will likely not be a statistically significant difference between the groups as reflected in the observed *t*-value. For example, in examining the first variable, figure-ground perception (total), the SDAT group mean was 26.33 and the control group mean was 36.47. The mean difference between the

### TABLE 8-10

**Comparison of Performance on Perceptual Spatial Orientation Tasks**

| Skill | Maximum Score | SDAT Group (n = 15) M (SD) | Control Group (n = 15) M (SD) | p* |
|---|---|---|---|---|
| Figure-ground perception (total) | 48 | 26.33 (6.61) | 36.47 (4.63) | ≤.0001 |
| Figure-ground perception (Part 1) | 24 | 16.00 (3.59) | 20.53 (1.19) | < .0002 |
| Figure-ground perception (Part 2) | 24 | 10.33 (4.15) | 15.93 (3.90) | ≤.001 |
| Shape (visual) | 10 | 9.67 (0.82) | 10.00 (0.00) | ns |
| Shape (tactual) | 10 | 6.13 (2.26) | 8.93 (1.34) | ≤ .0005 |
| Size (visual) | 6 | 6.00 (0.00) | 6.00 (0.00) | ns |
| Size (tactual) | 15 | 14.33 (1.23) | 14.87 (0.35) | ns |
| Position in space (total) | 16 | 11.93 (4.01) | 15.33 (0.82) | ≤.004 |
| Position in space (Part 1 ) | 8 | 7.20 (1.42) | 7.93 (0.26) | ≤.06 |
| Position in space (Part 2) | 8 | 4.73 (2.92) | 7.4 (0.74) | ≤.002 |
| Spatial relations | 15 | 11.47 (2.67) | 14.73 (0.59) | ≤ .0002 |
| Left-right discrimination | 10 | 9.67 (0.72) | 10.00 (0.00) | ns |

**Note:** SDAT = senile dementia of the Alzheimer type; ns = not significant. *Two-tailed *t*-test for independent samples. From "Spatial Disorientation in Persons with Early Senile Dementia of the Alzheimer Type," by L. Liu, L. Gauthier, & S. Gauthier 1991, *The American Journal of Occupational Therapy*, 45, p. 70. Copyright 1991 by American Journal of Occupational Therapy. Reprinted with permission.

groups was 10.14. The standard deviations of 6.61 and 4.63 were comparatively homogeneous. Thus, there was a statically significant difference between the two independent groups. In examining the variable shape (visual), note that the differences between the group means is .33 (10.00 − 9.67), whereas the standard deviation for the SDAT group is .82, thus indicating no statistically significant difference between the two independent group means.

### Operational Procedure for Testing for Statistically Significant Differences between Two Independent Samples

**Step 1.** *State the research hypothesis.*

1. *Null Hypothesis:* There is no statistically significant difference between the mean of group 1 versus the mean of group 2:

$$H_0: \mu_1 = \mu_2$$

2. *Directional Hypothesis:* Mean one is significantly statistically different from mean two in a stated direction:

$$\mu_1 > \mu_2$$

3. *Alternative Hypothesis:* Mean one does not equal mean two, and there is a statistically significant difference between the two means (nondirectional):

$$H_1: \mu_1 \neq \mu_2$$

**Step 2.** *Select the level of statistical significance.* In social sciences research, the .05 level of significance is traditionally selected.

**Step 3.** *Select the statistical test.* Use independent *t*-test.

**Step 4.** *Decide whether to use a one-tailed or two-tailed test for statistical significance.* A two-tailed test is used with a null hypothesis to determine if there are statistically significant differences in either direction of the tail. The model for a two-tailed test is the tails in a normal curve (Figure 8–31). A one-tailed test is used with a directional hypothesis when the researcher predicts that the experimental group mean will be either statistically greater or lesser than a comparison mean.

**Step 5.** *Look up the critical value ($t_{crit}$) from the published statistical table.* The critical value is determined by:

a. the degrees of freedom (*df*)
b. the level of significance ($\alpha < .05$ or $< .01$)
c. the direction of the test (one-tailed or two-tailed)
d. the value of $t_{crit}$ as indicated in the statistical table (See Table C–3 in the appendices.)

**Step 6.** *Calculate the group means and standard deviations.*

**Step 7.** *Do an exploratory data analysis.* This analysis determines if the differences between the two means are clinically significant and that the standard deviations in both groups are approximately equal.

**Step 8.** *Plot a graph.* Use the graph mean and raw scores of group 1 and group 2 to visualize whether there seems to be a statistically significant difference between the group means. (See Figure 8–32.) If there appears to be a difference between the two group means, then go to Step 9 and calculate the values.

**Step 9.** *Calculate the $t_{obs}$ using the formula.* The formula for $t_{obs}$ is:

$$t_{obs} = \frac{\overline{X}_1 - \overline{X}_2}{\sqrt{\{[(n_1 - 1)(s_1^2) + (n_2 - 1)(s_2^2)] / (n_1 + n_2 - 2)\}\,[(1/n_1) + (1/n_2)]}}$$

Where:

$\overline{X}_1$ = mean value of group 1
$\overline{X}_2$ = mean value of group 2

$n_1$ = total number of cases in group 1
$n_2$ = total number of cases in group 2
$s_1^2$ = variance (the standard deviation squared) for group 1
$s_2^2$ = variance for group 2

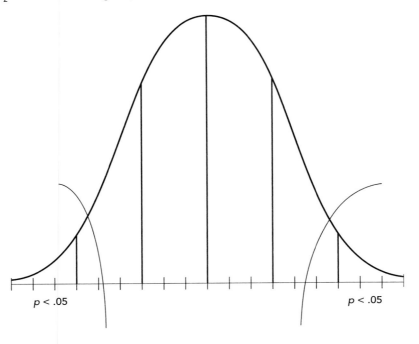

$p < .05$                                                  $p < .05$

© Cengage Learning 2013

**FIGURE 8-31**  Model for a Two-tailed Test: A one-tailed test would use only one of the two marked areas.

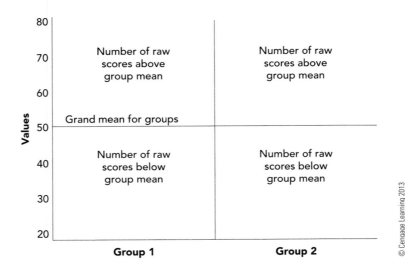

© Cengage Learning 2013

**FIGURE 8-32**  Graph to Visualize Values of Scores: to estimate possible statistical significance between the group means

**Step 10.** *Compare the two values:* $t_{obs}$ *and* $t_{crit}$

a. Accept the null hypothesis if $t_{obs}$ is less than $t_{crit}$
b. Reject the null hypothesis if $t_{obs}$ is equal to or greater than $t_{crit}$
c. Accept the directional hypothesis if $t_{obs}$ is greater than or equal to $t_{crit}$ in the direction that is hypothesized.
d. Reject the directional hypothesis if $t_{obs}$ is less than $t_{crit}$ or if the mean value that is predicted to be greater is less than the mean value of the control or comparative group. For example, a researcher predicts that cognitive training is more effective than behavioral therapy in increasing attention span. The results show a statistically significant difference between the two means, but behavioral therapy demonstrates to be more effective. Because the researcher predicted that cognitive therapy is more effective than behavioral therapy, the directional hypothesis is rejected.

## Two Independent Groups Example

Is there a statistically significant difference between stress management and group psychotherapy in reducing anxiety scores in patients with clinical depression?

| Hypothetical Posttest Scores on the State-Trait Anxiety Inventory[a] | | | | | |
|---|---|---|---|---|---|
| Stress Management Group | | | Psychotherapy Group | | |
| Subject | Score ($X_1$) | $X_1^2$ | Subject | Score ($X_2$) | $X_2^2$ |
| 01 | 35 | 1225 | 01 | 51 | 2601 |
| 02 | 41 | 1681 | 02 | 48 | 2304 |
| 03 | 38 | 1444 | 03 | 52 | 2704 |
| 04 | 42 | 1764 | 04 | 43 | 1849 |
| 05 | 43 | 1849 | 05 | 49 | 2401 |
| 06 | 36 | 1296 | 06 | 54 | 2916 |
| 07 | 32 | 1024 | 07 | 61 | 3721 |
| 08 | 40 | 1600 | 08 | 56 | 3136 |
| 09 | 41 | 1681 | 09 | 54 | 2916 |
| 10 | 43 | 1849 | 10 | 60 | 3600 |
| 11 | 42 | 1764 | 11 | 48 | 2304 |
| 12 | 34 | 1156 | 12 | 46 | 2116 |

$\Sigma X_1 = 467$
$\Sigma X_1^2 = 18333$
$\overline{X}_1 = 38.9$

$\Sigma X_2 = 622$
$\Sigma X_2^2 = 32568$
$\overline{X}_2 = 51.8$

Grand Mean $= (\Sigma X_1 + \Sigma X_2)/24 = (467 + 622)/24 = 45.37$

[a]Smaller score indicates less anxiety.

**Step 1.** *State the research hypothesis.* There is no statistically significant difference between a stress management group and a psychotherapy group in reducing anxiety in a sample of depressed patients. The hypothesis is stated in null form ($\mu_1 = \mu_2$).

**Step 2.** *Select the level of statistical significance.* The $\alpha = .05$ level of statistical significance will be accepted.
**Step 3.** *Decide the test statistic.* This is a nondirectional two-tailed test for statistical significance because a null hypothesis was stated. The independent *t*-test will be used.
**Step 4.** *Determine the critical value for t from published statistical tables.* (See Table C–3 in the appendices.)

a. $df = n_1 + n_2 - 2 = 22$
b. level of significance $\alpha = .05$
c. $t_{crit} = 2.0739$

**Step 5.** *Calculate the mean and standard deviations.*

| Stress Management Group | Psychotherapy Group |
|---|---|
| $\bar{X}_1 = \Sigma X_1 / n = 467 / 12 = 38.9$ | $\bar{X}_2 = \Sigma X_2 / n = 622 / 12 = 51.8$ |
| $\bar{X}_1 = 38.9$ | $\bar{X}_2 = 51.8$ |
| $s_2^2 = 3.80$ | $s_2^2 = 5.45$ |

**Computational Formula for Standard Deviation**

$$s = \sqrt{[n\Sigma X^2 - (\Sigma X)^2] / [n(n - 1)]}$$
$$s_1 = \sqrt{[(12)(18333) - (467)^2] / [12(12 - 1)]}$$
$$s_1 = \sqrt{(219996 - 218089) / [12(12 - 1)]}$$
$$s_1 = \sqrt{1907 / 132}$$
$$s_1 = \sqrt{14.44}$$
$$s_1 = 3.80$$

$$s_2 = \sqrt{[(12)(32568) - (622)^2] / [12(12 - 1)]}$$
$$s_2 = \sqrt{(390816 - 386884) / [12(12 - 1)]}$$
$$s_2 = \sqrt{3932 / 132}$$
$$s_2 = \sqrt{29.78}$$
$$s_2 = 5.45$$

**Step 6.** *Do an exploratory data analysis.*

$$\bar{X}_1 - \bar{X}_2 = 38.9 - 51.8 = 12.9$$
$$s_1 = 3.80$$
$$s_2 = 5.45$$

The mean difference is greater than the standard deviation for group 1 or group 2. Standard deviation difference between the two groups is 1.65. There is a relative homogeneity of variance for the two groups.
**Step 7.** *Do an exploratory graph analysis.* Figure 8–33 shows the graph obtained from the analysis. There appears to be a significant difference between the two groups.
**Step 8.** *Calculate $t_{obs}$.*

$$t_{obs} = \frac{\bar{X}_1 - \bar{X}_2}{\sqrt{\{[(n_1 - 1)(s_1^2) + (n_2 - 1)(s_2^2)] / (n_1 + n_2 - 2)\} [(1/n_1) + (1/n_2)]}}$$

Where:

| Group 1 | Group 2 |
|---|---|
| $\bar{X}_1 = 38.9$ | $\bar{X}_2 = 51.8$ |
| $n_1 = 12$ | $n_2 = 12$ |
| $s_1^2 = (3.80)^2 = 14.44$ | $s_2^2 = (5.45)^2 = 29.70$ |

$$t_{obs} = \frac{38.9 - 51.8}{\sqrt{\{[(12-1)(14.44) + (12-1)(29.78)] / (12 + 12 - 2)\}[(1/12) + (1/12)]}}$$

$$t_{obs} = \frac{-12.9}{\sqrt{[(158.84 + 327.58) / 22][1.667]}}$$

$$t_{obs} = \frac{-12.9}{\sqrt{[(486.12) / 22][1.667]}}$$

$$t_{obs} = -12.9 / \sqrt{3.685}$$

$$t_{obs} = -12.9 / 1.9196$$

$$t_{obs} = -6.72$$

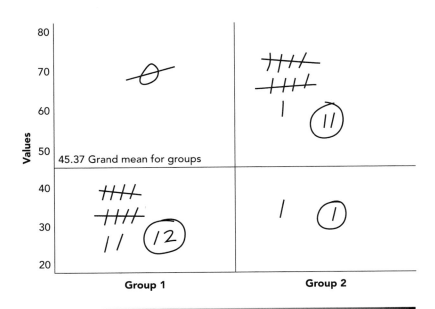

**FIGURE 8-33** Exploratory Graph Analysis for Hypothetical Posttest Scores on the *State-Trait Anxiety Inventory*: The graph shows the difference between scores between two independent groups of patients with clinical depression receiving either stress management training or group psychotherapy. The test being performed is an independent *t*-test.

© Cengage Learning 2013

***Step 9.*** *Compare* $t_{obs}$ *and* $t_{crit}$

$$t_{obs} = -6.72$$
$$t_{crit} = 2.0739$$

The examination shows $|t_{obs}|^3 > t_{crit}$. Reject the null hypothesis. There seems to be a statistically significant difference between the two means, indicating that the stress management group was significantly more effective than the psychotherapy group in the reduction of anxiety in patients with clinical depression.

### 8.8.2 Mann-Whitney *U* Test

#### Rationale

The Mann-Whitney *U* Test, a nonparametric alternative to the independent *t*-test, is used to test whether two independent groups have been drawn from the same population. In practice, the Mann-Whitney *U* test is used with ordinal scale data.

1. The null hypothesis (2-tailed) states that the two independent groups have the same population distribution and there is no significant difference between group means.
2. An alternative, non-directional one-tailed hypothesis states that there is a significant difference between the group means, either an increase or a decrease.

#### Assumptions

1. Random selection of each group.
2. Two mutually independent groups are compared.
3. The measurement scale is at least ordinal.
4. *n* for each group is less than 20.

#### Computation

1. Rank order every raw score combining the two groups (e.g., lowest score is assigned the rank of 1).
2. When two or more raw scores are the same, average the ranks.
3. Add the ranks for one group, obtaining $T_A$ value.

#### Formula for Mann-Whitney U Test

$$U_{obs} = (n_A n_B) + [(n_A)(n_A + 1) / 2] - [T_A]$$

Where:

$n_A$ = number of subjects in 1st group
$n_B$ = number of subjects in 2nd group

#### Example

Language intelligibility scores were compared between an experimental and control group after a 6-month treatment period. There was no significant difference between the groups on the pretest (two-tailed test $\alpha = .05$).

---

$^3 |t_{obs}|$ is an absolute value that disregards the sign. The parallel lines indicate absolute value.

The following data were collected:

| Experimental Group A | | | Control Group P | | |
|---|---|---|---|---|---|
| Subject | Score | Rank | Subject | Score | Rank |
| 101 | 33 | 12 | 201 | 35 | 13 |
| 102 | 30 | 10 | 202 | 32 | 11 |
| 103 | 25 | 8 | 203 | 27 | 9 |
| 104 | 24 | 6.5 | 204 | 24 | 6.5 |
| 105 | 22 | 5 | 205 | 21 | 4 |
| 106 | 19 | 3 | 206 | 18 | 2 |
| | | | 207 | 16 | 1 |
| | $T_A = 44.5$ | | | $T_B = 46.5$ | |
| | $n_A = 6$ | | | $n_B = 7$ | |

$$U_{obs} = [(6)(7)] + [6(6+1)/2] - [44.5]$$
$$U_{obs} = 42 + 21 - 44.5$$
$$U_{obs} = 63 - 44.5$$
$$U_{obs} = 18.5$$

Obtain $U_{crit}$ from table for Mann-Whitney $U$ test. (See Table C–7 in the appendices.)

$$n_A/n_B = 6/7$$
$$U_{crit} = 6/36$$

If $U_{obs}$ is between 6 and 36, do not reject null hypothesis.

### Conclusion

The null hypothesis is not rejected because $U_{obs} = 18.5$, which is between 6 and 36. Thus, the researcher concludes that there is no statistically significant difference in the experimental and control groups in language intelligibility posttest scores.

## 8.9 Model IV: Paired Data Sample

### 8.9.1 Correlated *t*-Test

The correlated *t*-test, often called a *paired t-test*, is applied to data when a researcher compares a group's performance or characteristic on two measures. For example, a researcher compares the difference between pretest and posttest scores of an observed variable. Another example is to compare the difference of two variables in one group, such as intelligence and perceptual motor test scores. The difference between the correlated *t*-test and the independent *t*-test is that the correlated *t*-test is applied with one independent group and two variables, whereas the independent *t*-test is applied to scores for two independent groups.

An example of a correlated *t*-test was found in a study by McFall, Deitz, and Crowe (1993) entitled "Test-Retest Reliability of the Test of Visual Perceptual Skills with Children with Learning Disabilities." In this study, the authors compared the difference in the score on the same test between a 1 to 2 weeks' time period. The following table describes the means, mean differences, and $t_{obs}$.

| | Correlated $t$-tests between Test and Retest Scores | | | |
|---|---|---|---|---|
| **Subtests** | **Pretest Mean** | **Posttest Mean** | **Mean Difference** | **$t$-Value** |
| Visual Discrimination | 11.9 | 13.01 | 1.1 | −1.89 |
| Visual Memory | 9.4 | 10.5 | 1.1 | −2.41* |
| Spatial Relations | 10.4 | 11.1 | .7 | −1.76 |
| Form Consistency | 8.7 | 9.4 | .7 | −1.76 |
| Sequential Memory | 8.4 | 8.4 | 0.0 | 1.76 |
| Figure Ground | 9.2 | 9.3 | .1 | −.11 |
| Visual Closure | 9.5 | 11.4 | .9 | −3.17** |

**Note:** $n = 30$; Critical value for $t_{obs} = 2.0452$; $df = n - 1 = 30 - 1 = 29$; two-tailed test
*$p < .05$
**$p < .01$

There was a statistically significant difference between test and retest means on the variables of visual memory ($|t_{obs}| = -2.41$) and visual closure ($|t_{obs}| = -3.17$). These $t$-values were above the $t_{crit}$ value of 2.0452. The $|t_{obs}|$ in the other tests were all below 2.045. The minus sign is disregarded in a nondirectional test.

On the basis of a significant statistical difference on these two subtests, the researcher will reject the null hypothesis. The null hypothesis is accepted for the other subtests.

### Operational Procedure for Testing for Statistical Significance in a Paired Data Sample

**Step 1.** *State the research hypothesis.*

a. Null Hypothesis: $H_0$: $\mu_1 = \mu_2$
b. Alternative Hypothesis: $\mu_1 \neq \mu_2$
c. Directional Hypothesis: $H_1$: $\mu_1 > \mu_2$

**Step 2.** *Select the level of statistical significance.*

$$\alpha = .05 \text{ or } .01 \text{ level of significance}$$

**Step 3.** *Decide the test statistic and whether to apply a one-tailed or two-tailed test for statistical significance.*
**Step 4.** *Look up the critical value for $t_{crit}$ from statistical table.*

a. determine the degrees of freedom: $df = N - 1$
b. level of significance $\alpha = .05$ or .01
c. one-tailed or two-tailed test
d. $t_{crit}$ derived from table of values (See Table C–3 in the appendices.)

**Step 5.** *Calculate the group means and standard deviations for each variable.*
**Step 6.** *Do an exploratory data analysis.* This analysis determines if the mean differences are greater than the standard deviations for each variable.
**Step 7.** *Plot a graph.* (See Independent $t$-test).
**Step 8.** *Calculate $t_{obs}$ using the formula:*

$$t_{obs} = \frac{\Sigma D_1}{\sqrt{[N\Sigma D_1{}^2 - (\Sigma D_1)^2] / N - 1}}$$

Where:

$\Sigma D_1$ = sum of differences between each subject's score on measured variable
$\Sigma D_1^2$ = sum of the squared differences on each score
$N$ = total number of subjects

**Step 9.** *Accept the null hypothesis if* $t_{obs} < t_{crit}$
**Step 10.** *Reject the null hypothesis if* $t_{obs} \geq t_{crit}$

## Paired Data Sample

Hypothetical example of correlated $t$-test: Is there a statistically significant difference between Performance IQ scores in adults with traumatic brain injury after undergoing an intensive cognitive retraining program?

| | Performance IQ Scores | | | |
|---|---|---|---|---|
| Subject | Baseline (Pretest) | $X_1^2$ | After Treatment (Posttest) | $X_2^2$ |
| 01 | 97 | 9409 | 113 | 12769 |
| 02 | 106 | 11236 | 113 | 12769 |
| 03 | 106 | 11236 | 101 | 10201 |
| 04 | 95 | 9025 | 119 | 14161 |
| 05 | 102 | 10404 | 111 | 12321 |
| 06 | 111 | 12321 | 121 | 14641 |
| 07 | 115 | 13225 | 121 | 14641 |
| 08 | 104 | 10816 | 106 | 11236 |
| 09 | 90 | 8100 | 110 | 12100 |
| 10 | 96 | 9216 | 126 | 15876 |
| | $\Sigma X_1 = 1022$ | $\Sigma X_1^2 = 104988$ | $\Sigma X_2 = 1141$ | $\Sigma X_2^2 = 130715$ |

**Step 1.** *State the research hypothesis.* There is no statistically significant difference between pre- and post-test Performance IQ scores in adults with traumatic brain injury who have undergone an extensive cognitive retraining program. This is a null hypothesis ($H_0$: $\mu_1 = \mu_2$).
**Step 2.** *Select the level of statistical significance.* The level of statistical significance is $\alpha = .05$.
**Step 3.** *Decide whether to use a one-tailed or two-tailed test.* This problem requires a two-tailed test because the hypothesis is stated in null form and the researcher is examining statistical significance without direction.
**Step 4.** *Look up* $t_{crit}$ (See Table C–3 in the appendices.)

a. $df = N - 1 = 9$
b. $\alpha = .05$
c. two-tailed test
d. $t_{crit} = 2.2622$

**Step 5.** *Calculate the group means and standard deviations for the baseline and retest conditions.*

| Group 1 | Group 2 |
|---|---|
| $\overline{X}_1 = \Sigma/N = 1022 / 10 = 102.2$ | $\overline{X}_2 = \Sigma/N = 1141 / 10 = 114.1$ |
| $s_1 = 7.74$ | $s_2 = 7.65$ |

Standard deviation computation formula:

$$s = \sqrt{[N\Sigma X^2 - (\Sigma X)^2] / [N(N - 1)]}$$
$$s_1 = \sqrt{[(10)(104988) - (1022)^2] / [(10)(10 - 1)]}$$
$$s_1 = \sqrt{[1049880 - 1044484] / 90}$$
$$s_1 = \sqrt{5396 / 90}$$
$$s_1 = 7.74$$
$$s_2 = \sqrt{[(10)(130715) - (1141)^2] / [10(10 - 1)]}$$
$$s_2 = \sqrt{[(1307150 - 1301881] / 90}$$
$$s_2 = \sqrt{5269 / 90}$$
$$s_2 = \sqrt{58.54}$$
$$s_2 = 7.65$$

**Step 6.** *Do an exploratory data analysis.*

$$\overline{X}_1 - \overline{X}_2 = 102.2 - 114.1 = 11.9$$
$$s_1 = 7.74$$
$$s_2 = 7.65$$

The mean difference between pre- and posttest scores is greater than the standard deviations for pretest and posttest scores. The difference between the standard deviations is relatively small, indicating a homogeneity of variance for the two groups of scores.

**Step 7.** *Plot an exploratory graph.* This is displayed in Figure 8–34.

From the exploratory data analysis, there appears to be a significant difference between the pretest and posttest scores.

| Subject | Baseline Test | Retest | $D_1$ | $D^2$ |
|---|---|---|---|---|
| 01 | 97 | 113 | −16 | 256 |
| 02 | 106 | 113 | −07 | 49 |
| 03 | 106 | 101 | +05 | 25 |
| 04 | 95 | 119 | −24 | 576 |
| 05 | 102 | 111 | −09 | 81 |
| 06 | 111 | 122 | −11 | 121 |

| Subject | Baseline Test | Retest | $D_1$ | $D^2$ |
|---|---|---|---|---|
| *continued* | | | | |
| 07 | 115 | 121 | −06 | 36 |
| 08 | 104 | 106 | −02 | 4 |
| 09 | 90 | 110 | −20 | 400 |
| 10 | 96 | 126 | −30 | 900 |
| | **1022** | **142** | $\Sigma D_1 = -120$ $(\Sigma D_1)^2 = 14400$ | $\Sigma D^2 = 2448$ |

**Step 8.** *Calculate* $t_{obs}$

$$t_{obs} = \frac{\Sigma D_1}{\sqrt{[N\Sigma D_1{}^2 - (\Sigma D_1)^2 / N - 1}}$$

$$t_{obs} = \frac{-120}{\sqrt{[(10)(2448) - (14400)]/10-1}}$$

$$t_{obs} = \frac{-120}{\sqrt{(24480 - 14400)/9}}$$

$$t_{obs} = \frac{-120}{\sqrt{10080/9}}$$

$$t_{obs} = (-120) / \sqrt{1120}$$

$$t_{obs} = (-120) / 33.460$$

$$t_{obs} = -3.586$$

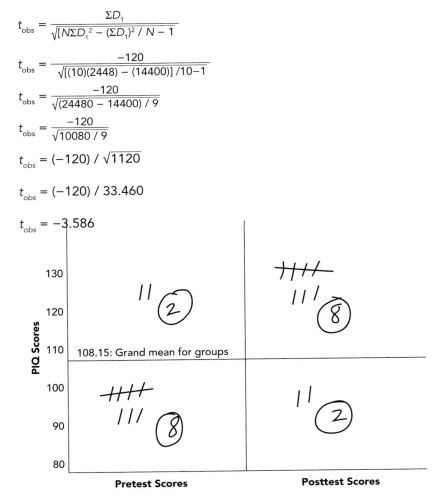

**FIGURE 8-34** Exploratory Graph Analysis Using Hypothetical Data: The graph shows differences between pre- and posttest Performance IQ scores for a group of adults with traumatic brain damage after cognitive retraining. The statistical test being performed is a correlated t-test.

© Cengage Learning 2013

*Step 9. Compare $t_{obs}$ and $t_{crit}$* $t_{obs} = -3.586$. Using Table C–3 in the appendices, we find that $t_{crit} = 2.2622$. The researcher rejects the null hypothesis and concludes that there appears to be a significant difference between the pre- and posttest scores and that cognitive rehabilitation appeared to be effective in raising Performance IQ scores in this sample of individuals with traumatic brain injury.[4]

### 8.9.2 Wilcoxon Signed-Rank Test[5] for Paired Data Samples

The Wilcoxon signed-rank test is a nonparametric alternative to the *t*-test for correlated samples.

#### Assumptions in Applying Wilcoxon signed-rank Test

1. Random selection or random assignment of subjects
2. Measurement scale is at least ordinal

#### Example of Applying Wilcoxon signed-rank Test

An investigator is interested in comparing the pre- and posttest scores for a group of nine subjects. The null hypothesis is stated with $\alpha = .05$. The data for this example are as follows:

| Subject | Pretest Raw Score | Posttest Raw Score | Difference | Rank Difference |
|---------|-------------------|--------------------|------------|-----------------|
| 01 | 10 | 12 | −2 | (−) 4 |
| 02 | 12 | 15 | −3 | (−) 7 |
| 03 | 8 | 6 | 2 | 4 |
| 04 | 6 | 10 | −4 | (−) 8 |
| 05 | 14 | 12 | 2 | 4 |
| 06 | 7 | 6 | 1 | 1 |
| 07 | 10 | 12 | −2 | (−) 4 |
| 08 | 14 | 16 | −2 | (−) 4 |
| 09 | 12 | 18 | −6 | (−) 9 |

#### Stepwise Procedure for Wilcoxon signed-rank Test (Example)

*Step 1. Calculate the difference between the pre- and posttest raw scores.* Subtract the posttest raw scores from the pretest raw scores.

*Step 2. Rank order the differences between raw scores from smallest to largest.* Ignore the negative or positive signs. Notice that in tied ranks, such as with 2 as a difference, the midpoint of the rank is 4 (2, 3, **4**, 5, 6).

*Step 3. Sum the positive rank differences.*

$$
\begin{array}{r}
4 \\
4 \\
+1 \\
\hline
9
\end{array}
$$

---

[4]Note that the negative sign in −3.5 does not affect the value. Both positive and negative values are interpreted equally when compared with the $t_{crit}$ value for the table.

[5]The Wilcoxon signed-rank test is sometimes called the Wilcoxon signed-ranks test.

**Step 4.** *Sum the negative rank differences.*

$$
\begin{array}{r}
-4 \\
-7 \\
-8 \\
-4 \\
-4 \\
(+) \; -9 \\
\hline
-36
\end{array}
$$

**Step 5.** *Determine $T_{obs}$-value. $T_{obs}$ is the absolute value of the smaller sum of the rank differences.*[6]

$$T_{obs} = 9$$

**Step 6.** *Compare the $T_{obs}$ with $T_{crit}$ from the table for critical values to $T$. (See Table C–8 in the appendices.)*

$$N = 9$$
$$\alpha = .05$$
two-tailed test
$$T_{crit} = 5$$

**Step 7.** *If the $T_{obs}$ is equal to or less than $T_{crit}$ then reject the null hypothesis and conclude that there is a statistically significant difference between the pre- and posttest scores.* Because $T_{obs} = 9$ is greater than $T_{crit} = 5$, we accept the null hypothesis and conclude that there are no statistically significant differences between the pre- and posttest scores.

## 8.10 Model V: *k*-independent Samples

### 8.10.1 Analysis of Variance (ANOVA)

ANOVA is a widely used statistical test equivalent to the independent *t*-test when testing for significant differences between two means. ANOVA is applied to statistical data when two or more independent group means are being compared. The statistic for the ANOVA is *F*. (*k* refers to the number of independent groups or conditions in the study.)

$$F = \text{variance between groups} \, / \, \text{variance within groups}$$

The concept of the ANOVA is that if there are large differences between the group means compared with relatively small differences within the variances or scores within the group, then a statistically significant result is evident. ANOVA answers the question: Is there a statistically significant difference between the independent groups being tested? For example, does $\mu_1 = \mu_2 = \mu_3 = \mu_k$? ANOVA is always tested by a null hypothesis. When there is a statistically significant result, the researcher then carries out a post-hoc analysis, such as the Scheffé, Duncan Multiple Range, Neuman-Keuls, and Tukey's procedures. These post-hoc tests are similar to *t*-tests for independent measures, applied to the data after attaining a significant *F*.

---

[6]The "*t*" in *t*-test is not capitalized, whereas the *T* associated with the Wilcoxon is capitalized.

### One-Way ANOVA

A one-way ANOVA simply analyzes the group means for statistically significant differences. The hypothetical table of results that follows is a typical example of a one-way ANOVA for comparing the effectiveness of three handwriting programs among 19 children with handwriting problems.

| ANOVA Summary Table for Comparing Two Treatment Groups | | | | |
|---|---|---|---|---|
| Source of Variance | df | SS | MS | F |
| Between treatment groups | 2 | 16 | 8 | 4.0* |
| Within treatment groups | 16 | 32 | 2 | |
| Total | 18 | | | |

*$p = < .05$, $F_{crit} = 3.63$
Where:
SS = sums of squares
MS = mean squares

$F$ is a derivative value equivalent to $F_{obs}$ that is compared with the $F_{crit}$ derived from a statistical table of values. For example, the $F_{crit}$ for 2 df (treatment groups −1) and 16 df [number of subjects (19) − number of groups (3)] with 2/16, $\alpha = .05$ is 3.63. Degrees of freedom (df) is derived from between treatment groups ($k − 1$) and within treatment groups ($N − k$).

The result in this hypothetical example shows that there is a statistically significant difference between the three treatment methods for handwriting disorders. $F_{obs}$ 4.00 is $> F_{crit}$ 3.63. Thus, the researcher will reject the null hypothesis.

### Example of Two-Factor ANOVA from the Literature

A one-way ANOVA analyzes the group means for statistically significant differences. The two-factor ANOVA looks at the variables from a two-dimensional perspective. It analyzes interactive effects, such as treatment method and therapist personality or treatment method and patient diagnosis. Palmer (1989) studied two methods of bed transfer following back surgery and examined the pain patients experienced preoperative (day 1) and postoperative (day 2). Results are shown in the following table.

| Summary Table of ANOVA on Pain Rating Scores by Transfer Method and Time | | | |
|---|---|---|---|
| Source of Variance | df | F | p Value |
| Time (pre-post operative) | 4 | 17.196 | .000* |
| Method (2 transfer methods) | 1 | 2.435 | .120 |
| Time X method | 4 | 0.911 | .458 |

*$p < .05$ significant

The results show that there was a statistically significant difference between pain ratings during pre- and postoperative time periods. There were no statistically significant differences in the two methods of bed transfer or in the interactional effects of time and method.

### Stepwise Procedures for One-Way ANOVA (Hypothetical Example)

**Step 1.** *State the research hypothesis.* The hypothesis is always stated in the null form when using ANOVA. For example, there is no statistically significant difference between electrical stimulation (ES), acupuncture (A), and proprioceptive neuromuscular facilitation (PNF) in improving upper extremity function in patients with chronic hemiplegia.

$$H_0 = \mu_1 = \mu_2 = \mu_3$$

**Step 2.** *Select the level of statistical significance.*

$$\alpha = .05$$

**Step 3.** *Identify $F_{crit}$ from table.* (See Table C–4 in the appendices.)

a. *df* for the numerator = 2 (three treatment groups −1)
   *df* for the denominator = 15 (number of subjects minus the number of groups = 18 − 3 = 15)
   *df* = 2/15
b. $\alpha = .05$
c. $F_{crit} = 3.68$

**Step 4.** *Calculate means and standard deviations.*[7]

| ES Group | | | A Group | | | PNF Group | | |
|---|---|---|---|---|---|---|---|---|
| Subject | Score (X) | $X_1^2$ | Subject | Score (X) | $X_2^2$ | Subject | Score (X) | $X_3^2$ |
| 01 | 23 | 529 | 01 | 13 | 169 | 01 | 33 | 1089 |
| 02 | 31 | 961 | 02 | 19 | 361 | 02 | 42 | 1764 |
| 03 | 16 | 256 | 03 | 19 | 361 | 03 | 30 | 900 |
| 04 | 27 | 729 | 04 | 25 | 625 | 04 | 38 | 1444 |
| 05 | 32 | 1024 | 05 | 18 | 324 | 05 | 44 | 1936 |
| 06 | 18 | 324 | | | | 06 | 41 | 1681 |
| 07 | 38 | 1444 | | | | | | |
| $\Sigma X_1 = 185$ | | $\Sigma X_1^2 = 5267$ | $\Sigma X_2 = 94$ | | $\Sigma X_2^2 = 1840$ | $\Sigma X_3 = 228$ | | $\Sigma X_3^2 = 8814$ |
| $\bar{X}_1 = 26.4$ | | | $\bar{X}_2 = 18.8$ | | | $\bar{X}_3 = 38.0$ | | |

$$s = \sqrt{N\Sigma X^2 - (\Sigma X)^2 / N(N-1)}$$
$$s_1 = \sqrt{7(5267) - (185)^2 / 7(7-1)}$$
$$s_1 = \sqrt{2644 / 42}$$
$$s_1 = \sqrt{62.95}$$
$$s_1 = 7.93$$

---

[7] The *Fugl-Meyer Poststroke Motor Recovery Test* scores were used for the example. (Range is from 0–60.)

$$s_2 = \sqrt{5(1840) - (94185)^2 / 5(4)}$$
$$s_2 = \sqrt{364 / 20}$$
$$s_2 = \sqrt{18.2}$$
$$s_2 = 4.26$$

$$s_3 = \sqrt{6(8814) - (228)^2 / 6(5)}$$
$$s_3 = \sqrt{(900 / 30)}$$
$$s_3 = \sqrt{30.00}$$
$$s_3 = 5.48$$

**Step 5.** *Do an exploratory data analysis.*

$$\overline{X}_1 = 26 \qquad\qquad s_1 = 7.93$$
$$\overline{X}_2 = 18.8 \qquad\qquad s_2 = 4.26$$
$$\overline{X}_3 = 38.0 \qquad\qquad s_3 = 5.48$$
$$\overline{X}_1 - \overline{X}_2 = 7.6 \qquad\qquad s_1 - s_2 = 3.67$$
$$\overline{X}_1 - \overline{X}_3 = -11.6 \qquad\qquad s_1 - s_3 = 2.45$$
$$\overline{X}_2 - \overline{X}_3 = -19.2 \qquad\qquad s_2 - s_3 = -1.22$$

There appears to be a statistically significant difference between the means and a relatively homogenous variance.

**Step 6.** *Plot an exploratory graph.* This graph is shown in Figure 8–35.

$$\text{Group mean} = (\Sigma\overline{X}_1 + \Sigma\overline{X}_2 + \Sigma\overline{X}_3)/(N_1 + N_2 + N_3)$$
$$= (185 + 94 + 288)/(7 + 5 + 6)$$
$$= 507/18$$
$$= 28.17$$

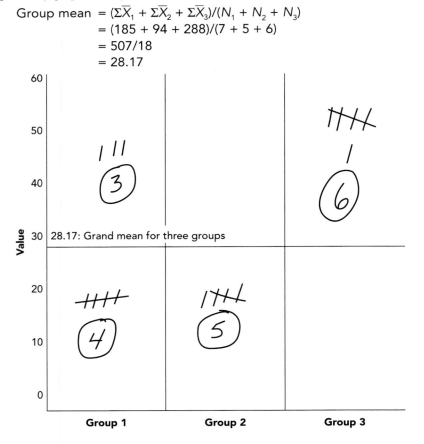

**FIGURE 8-35** Exploratory Graph for ANOVA Using Hypothetical Data: The graph shows differences in scores between three different groups.

There appears to be a statistically significant difference between group 2 and group 3.

**Step 7.** *Calculate F.*

| Summary Table for One-Way ANOVA | | | | |
|---|---|---|---|---|
| **Source of Variance** | *df* | *SS* | *MS* | *F* |
| Between groups (BG) | 2 | 1039.98 | 519.99 | 12.99 |
| Within groups (WG) | 15 | 600.52 | 40.03 | |
| Total | 17 | | | |

### Formulas for ANOVA

a. $F = MS$ between groups / $MS$ within groups

b. $df$ between groups $(df_{bg})$ = Number of groups minus 1 = $(3 - 1)$ = 2

$df$ within groups $(df_{wg})$ = Total number of subjects in all groups minus the number of groups = $18 - 3 = 15$

c. Mean Square between groups = $SS_{bg} / df_{bg}$

Mean Square within groups = $SS_{wg} / df_{wg}$

d. Sum of Squares between groups:

$$SS_{bg} = \Sigma [(\Sigma X_1)^2 / n_1] + [(\Sigma X_2)^2 / n_2] + [(\Sigma X_3)^2 / n_3] - [(\Sigma X_1 + \Sigma X_2 + \Sigma X_3)^2 / \Sigma N]$$

**Group 1**

$(\Sigma X_1)^2 = (185)^2 = 34225$

$n_1 = 7$

$(\Sigma X_1)^2 / n_1 = 4889.29$

**Group 2**

$(\Sigma X_2)^2 = (94)^2 = 8836$

$n_2 = 5$

$(\Sigma X_2)^2 / n_2 = 1767.2$

**Group 3**

$(\Sigma X_3)^2 = (228)^2 = 51984$

$n_3 = 6$

$(\Sigma X_3)^2 / n_3 = 8664.0$

**Total** = $(4889.29 + 1767.2 + 8664.0) = 15320.49$

$(\Sigma X_1 + \Sigma X_2 + \Sigma X_3) / \Sigma N) = 257049 / 18 = 14280.5$

$SS_{bg} = [(4889.29 + 1767.2 + 8664.0)] - [(257049) / 18]$

$SS_{bg} = 15320.49 - 14280.5$

$SS_{bg} = 1039.99$

e. Sums of Squares within Groups

$SS_{wg} = \Sigma (\Sigma X_1^2 + \Sigma X_2^2 + \Sigma X_3^2) - 15320.49$

$SS_{wg} = \Sigma (5267 + 1840 + 8814) - 15320.49$

$SS_{wg} = 15921 - 15320.49$

$SS_{wg} = 600.51$

**Mean Square between groups**

$$SS_{bg} / df_{bg} = 1039.99 / 2 = 519.99$$

**Mean Square within groups**

$$SS_{bg} / df_{wg} = 600.51 / 15 = 40.03$$
$$F = MS_{bg} / MS_{wg} = 519.99 / 40.03 = 12.99$$

***Step 8.*** *Compare* $F_{obs}$ *with* $F_{crit}$.

$$F_{obs} = 12.99 \qquad F_{crit} = 3.68$$

Thus, we reject the null hypothesis and conclude that there is a statistically significant difference between the three groups. This confirms our exploratory data analysis.

***Step 9.*** *Conduct a post-hoc test.* If there is a significant $F$, meaning that the mean values are statistically significant, then the researcher carries out a post-hoc analysis. This analysis is parallel to doing independent $t$-tests and determining which pairs of means have statistically significant differences.

A number of post-hoc tests are available to the researcher, such as:

- Tukey's Honestly Significant Differences (HSD)
- Neuman-Keuls
- Duncan Multiple Range
- Scheffé

### Example of a Post-Hoc Analysis

In the previous example, it was found that $F_{obs}$ is statistically significant when:

$$\overline{X}_1 = 26.4$$
$$\overline{X}_2 = 18.8$$
$$\overline{X}_3 = 38.0.$$

$H_0$: Null hypothesis is rejected and we conclude that all the means are not the same. We can now compare each pair of means, such as:

$$\overline{X}_1 \text{ compared to } \overline{X}_2$$
$$\overline{X}_1 \text{ compared to } \overline{X}_3$$
$$\overline{X}_2 \text{ compared to } \overline{X}_3$$

A significant $F$ means that at least one pair of means are significantly different, that is, the highest and lowest mean. Therefore, $\overline{X}_2$ compared to $\overline{X}_3$ has a statistically significant difference. We do not know whether there is a statistically significant difference between $\overline{X}_1$ and $\overline{X}_2$ and/or $\overline{X}_1$ and $\overline{X}_3$. A post-hoc analysis tests for statistical significant difference in these two situations.

In this example the Tukey ($HSD$), a widely used post-hoc analysis, was selected. The formula for the Tukey is (Gravette & Wellnau, 1985):

$$HSD = q\sqrt{MS_{wg} /n}$$

Where:

$q$ = a derived table value (See Table C–9 in the appendices: The Student Range Statistic.) In this case, $q = 3.67$.

$MS_{wg}$ = the value calculated for mean squares within groups and is taken from the ANOVA table.
In the above example, this value is 40.03.
$n$ = the average of the number of cases in each group.
In the above example, $n_1 = 7$, $n_2 = 5$, and $n_3 = 6$. The average is 6.
$k$ = number of groups $(k) = 3$
df for $MS_{wg} = 15$
$\alpha = .05$

$$HSD = q\sqrt{MS_{wg}/n}$$
$$HSD = 3.67\sqrt{40.03/6}$$
$$HSD = 9.479$$

Therefore, the mean difference between any two group scores must be at least 9.48 to be statistically significant.

a.  $\overline{X}_1 - \overline{X}_2 = 26.4 - 18.8 = 7.6$. Therefore, the null hypothesis is accepted and $\overline{X}_1 = \overline{X}_2$
b.  $\overline{X}_1 - \overline{X}_3 = 26.4 - 38.0 = 11.6$. Therefore, the null hypothesis is rejected and $\overline{X}_1 \neq \overline{X}_3$
c.  $\overline{X}_2 - \overline{X}_3 = 18.8 - 38.0 = 19.2$. Therefore, the null hypothesis is rejected and $\overline{X}_2 \neq \overline{X}_3$

In conclusion, a post-hoc analysis test determines the pairs of means that have statistically significant differences.

## 8.10.2 Kruskal-Wallis Test for *k* Sample

The *Kruskal-Wallis test* is a nonparametric alternative to the one-way ANOVA when comparing three or more independent groups.

### Assumptions

a.  Random selection or random assignment of subjects to each independent group
b.  Ordinal scale measurement
c.  Each group should have at least five subjects

### Example of Applying Kruskal-Wallis

**Step 1.** *The investigator hypothesizes that there is no statistically significant difference between the three groups.*

| Group 1 | | Group 2 | | Group 3 | |
|---|---|---|---|---|---|
| Subj | Raw Score | Subj | Raw Score | Subj | Raw Score |
| 101 | 10 | 201 | 14 | 301 | 12 |
| 102 | 8 | 202 | 12 | 302 | 14 |
| 103 | 6 | 203 | 10 | 303 | 7 |
| 104 | 10 | 204 | 8 | 304 | 6 |
| 105 | 12 | 205 | 9 | 305 | 10 |
| 106 | 14 | | | | |

*Step 2.* *Rank order every raw score, combining all groups (in this example, three groups) with the lowest score assigned a rank of 1. In this example, the raw score of 4 made by Subject 303 is assigned the rank of 1. Note: for tied ranks, take the midpoint of the rank. For example, a raw score of 6 occupies ranks 2 and 3 and becomes rank of 2.5.*

| Subject | Raw Score | Rank | |
|---------|-----------|------|---|
| 101 | 10 | 8.5 | |
| 102 | 8 | 4.5 | |
| 103 | 6 | 2.5 | |
| 104 | 10 | 8.5 | |
| 105 | 12 | 12.0 | |
| 106 | 14 | 15.0 | $\Sigma_{ranks} = 51.0$ |
| 201 | 14 | 15.0 | |
| 202 | 12 | 12.0 | |
| 203 | 10 | 8.5 | |
| 201 | 8 | 4.5 | |
| 205 | 9 | 6.0 | $\Sigma_{ranks} = 46.0$ |
| 301 | 12 | 12.0 | |
| 302 | 14 | 15.0 | |
| 303 | 4 | 1.0 | |
| 304 | 6 | 2.5 | |
| 305 | 10 | 8.5 | $\Sigma_{ranks} = 39.0$ |

**Note:** $n = 16$

*Step 3.* *Sum the ranks for each group.*

| Group 1 | Group 2 | Group 3 |
|---------|---------|---------|
| 8.5 | 15.0 | 12.0 |
| 4.5 | 12.0 | 15.0 |
| 2.5 | 8.5 | 1.0 |
| 8.5 | 4.5 | 2.5 |
| 12.0 | 6.0 | 8.5 |
| 15.0 | | |
| $\Sigma_1 = 51.0$ | $\Sigma_2 = 46.0$ | $\Sigma_3 = 39.0$ |
| $n_1 = 6$ | $n_2 = 5$ | $n_3 = 5$ |

**Step 4.** *Calculate the formula for Kruskal-Wallis ($H_{obs}$).*

$$H_{obs} = 12 / [N(N+1)][(T_1^2 / n_1) + (T_2^2 / n_2) + (T_3^2 / n_3)] - [3(N+1)]$$

Where:

$$N = n_1 + n_2 + n_3 = 16$$
$$T_1^2 = (\Sigma_{1\text{-ranks}})^2 = 51^2 = 2601$$
$$T_2^2 = (\Sigma_{2\text{-ranks}})^2 = 46^2 = 2116$$
$$T_3^2 = (\Sigma_{3\text{-ranks}})^2 = 39^2 = 1521$$
$$\begin{aligned} H_{obs} &= 12 / [16(17)][(2601/6) + (2116/5) + (1521/5)] - [3(17)] \\ &= [12/272][433.5 + 423.2 + 304.2] - [51] \\ &= [.044][1160.9] - [51] \\ &= 51.08 - 51 \\ &= .08 \end{aligned}$$

**Step 5.** *Calculate $H_{crit}$ for $\alpha = .05$, df = number of groups (k) – 1 = 2, $H_{crit}$ = 5.99.* (Use Chi-square, Table C–10, in the appendices to test for statistical significance.)

**Step 6.** *Compare $H_{obs}$ (.08) with $H_{crit}$ (5.991). If $H_{obs}$ is equal to or more than $H_{crit}$, reject the null hypothesis.* In this example, the null hypothesis is accepted and we conclude that there is no statistically significant difference between the three groups tested.

## 8.11 | Model VI: Correlation (Pearson Product-Moment and Spearman Rank Correlation[8])

What is *correlation*? What is the difference between an associational relationship and causality? How do we graph the relationship between variables? What is a *correlation matrix*? What is a *regression line*? What is the difference between the Pearson product-moment correlation and the Spearman rank correlation? Sometimes the word "coefficient" is added to these correlation statistics. Coefficient simply means the actual number that represents the statistic (e.g., $r = .78$). All of these questions relate to the correlational model in statistics.

### 8.11.1 Definition of Correlation

**Correlation** is the reciprocal relationship between two variables. It is a general concept that assumes that variables can be measured and correlated. The index of the degree of relationship between two variables is the correlation coefficient. This index can range from zero, which indicates no relationship, to +1.00 or −1.00, which indicates a perfect correlation between two variables. For example, a correlation coefficient of .30 indicates a low correlation, whereas .90 is a high correlation. The symbol for correlation is $r$. A correlational relationship indicates an association between variables; it does not indicate a causal relationship.

### 8.11.2 Example of a Correlation in the Literature

Table 8–11 displays the relationship between stress and leisure satisfaction among therapeutic recreation personnel examined by an investigator. The table is a **correlation matrix** that measures the degree of associations among five variables. Each variable is correlated with each other. The "Personal Strain Questionnaire" component of the *Occupational Stress Inventory*, as developed by Osipow and Spokane (1987), and the *Leisure Satisfaction Scale* (Beard & Raghab, 1980) was administered to 159 individuals who were members of the National Therapeutic Recreation Society. Data were gathered through a mail questionnaire.

---

[8]In some statistical books, the Spearman rank correlation is called Spearman's Rho.

**TABLE 8-11**

**Correlation Coefficients between Ratings on *Personal Strain Questionnaire* and *Leisure Satisfaction Scale***

|                  | Vocational | Psychological | Interpersonal | Physical | Total |
|------------------|-----------|---------------|---------------|----------|-------|
| Psychological    | .65*      | —             |               |          |       |
| Interpersonal    | .46*      | .57*          | —             |          |       |
| Physical         | .44*      | .61*          | .43*          | —        |       |
| PSQ total        | .75*      | .87*          | .75*          | .81*     | —     |
| Leisure satis.   | −.21      | −.30*         | −.24*         | −.39*    | −.37* |

\* = significant at .05; $N = 85$.
**Note:** From "The Relationship between Stress and Leisure Satisfaction among Therapeutic Recreation Personnel" in P. H. Cunningham and T. Bartuska, 1989, *Therapeutic Recreation Journal, 23*(3), p. 69. Copyright 1989 by *Therapeutic Recreation Journal.*

Fifteen correlation coefficients ($r$) were completed to construct the correlation matrix table. The researchers used $\alpha = .05$ for level of statistical significance. Although statistical significance may be reached at $r — .21$ for 83 $df$ ($N — 2$), ($\alpha = .05$ and a two-tailed test), it is important to note that with correlations, statistical significance is not as important as establishing a clinical level of correlation. For example, in establishing an acceptable reliability for a test, many researchers will accept Pearson product-moment correlation coefficients of $r = .80$ or above as acceptable. In the example in Table 8–11, $r = .60$ is considered by some researchers to be moderate in clinical significance.

In understanding the correlational results, the square of $r$ is the proportion of variance in one variable that is associated with another variable. If $r = .60$, the proportion of variance accounted for is only .36, which means that .64 is that portion of the variance that is not accounted for. Correlation is a measure of predicting the value of one variable $Y$ (unknown) if another variable $X$ is known. If there is a high correlation between the two variables, (e.g., $r = .90$), then the researcher has a high degree of confidence in predicting "if $X$, then $Y$." The degree of confidence in the relationship is more important in clinical research than is the statistical $r$ value.

In the example illustrated in Table 8–11, there are comparatively high correlations between the *Personal Strain Questionnaire* (PSQ) Total and the subscales of the PSQ. Comparatively low-to-moderate correlations exist between the *Leisure Satisfaction Scale* and the subscales of the PSQ. In other words, clinicians could not predict with confidence that persons with higher levels of leisure satisfaction would experience less stress than persons who have low satisfaction with their leisure. On the basis of these results, the researchers should conclude that there is not a strong relationship between stress and leisure satisfaction even though there is a significant statistical relationship at the .05 level.

### 8.11.3 Stepwise Procedure for Correlation

***Step 1.*** *State the research hypothesis.*

For example, there is no statistical significant relationship between variable $X$ and variable $Y$. (Null hypothesis, $r = .00$ or below predetermined level of correlation.)

***Step 2.*** *Determine the degree of relationship that will be acceptable for significance.*

When interpreting correlation coefficients, the following guideline is used (Hinkle, Wiersma, & Jurs 2003):

$r \geq .9$ (Very high)
$r \geq .7$ and $r \leq .9$ (High)

$r \geq .5$ and $r \leq .7$ (Moderate)
$r \geq .3$ and $r \leq .5$ (Low)
$r \geq 0$ and $r \leq .3$ (Very Low to No Correlation)

**Step 3.** *Collect data and arrange raw scores into a table.*

For example:

| Subjects | Variable X Raw Score | Rank | Variable Y Raw Score | Rank | d (difference in ranks between X and Y) | d² (difference squared) |
|---|---|---|---|---|---|---|
| 1 | 31 | 7 | 45 | 5 | 2 | 4 |
| 2 | 22 | 5 | 58 | 8 | –3 | 9 |
| 3 | 19 | 4 | 57 | 7 | –3 | 9 |
| 4 | 16 | 3 | 48 | 6 | –3 | 9 |
| 5 | 78 | 8.5 | 61 | 9 | –0.5 | 0.25 |
| 6 | 3 | 1 | 36 | 4 | –3 | 9 |
| 7 | 93 | 10 | 18 | 3 | 7 | 49 |
| 8 | 78 | 8.5 | 88 | 10 | –1.5 | 2.25 |
| 9 | 23 | 6 | 9 | 1 | 5 | 25 |
| 10 | 15 | 2 | 12 | 2 | 0 | 0 |
| | $\Sigma X = 378$ | | $\Sigma Y = 432$ | | $\Sigma d = 0$ [a] | $\Sigma d^2 = 116.5$ |

**Note:** $d$ = difference in ranks between X and Y; $d^2$ = difference squared.
[a]Note that in computing the differences ($d$), the sum of the rank differences should equal zero when taking into consideration the negative and positive signs.

**Step 4.** *Rank order each raw score, with lowest score being assigned rank of 1.*

Note: for tied ranks, take the midpoint of the rank. For example, a raw score of 78 occupies ranks 8 and 9 and becomes rank of 8.5.

**Step 5.** *Do an exploratory data analysis.*

Note in Figure 8–36 that each point in the scatter diagram is a coordinate value. It appears from the scatter diagram that there is a low correlation between the two variables.

**Step 6.** *Calculate Spearman rank correlation coefficient and estimate degree of relationship between the two variables (X and Y).*

The formula for Spearman $r_s$ is:

$$r_s = 1.00 - [(6)(\Sigma d^2) / (N^3 - N)]$$
$$= 1.00 - [(6)(116.5) / (1{,}000 - 10)]$$
$$= 1.00 - [699 / 990]$$
$$= 1.00 - .71$$
$$r_s = .29$$

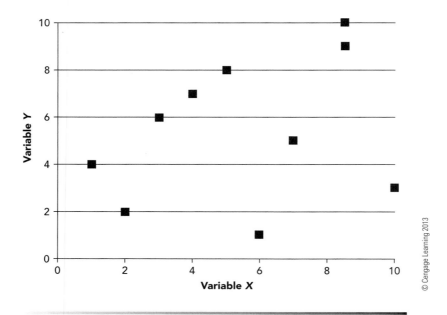

**FIGURE 8-36** Exploratory Data on a Scattergram Using the Ranks of the Scores: Notice that each point is a coordinate value. There appears to be a low correlation between the two variables.

The exploratory data analysis indicates that there is a very low correlation between the $X$ and $Y$ variables.

***Step 7.*** *Calculate the Pearson product-moment correlation coefficient.*

The Spearman (rank order) is a good screening test for the Pearson (product-moment), which is a more accurate test because the Pearson $r$ computes raw scores, whereas the Spearman $r_s$ computes ranks that are transformed scores. The reader will note that the Pearson $r$, which is a parametric test, should be applied to interval or ratio scale data. The Spearman $r_s$ is a nonparametric statistical test that can be used with ordinal scale data. As the reader will note, interval scale data can be transformed to ranks (ordinal scale data).

The formula for the Pearson $r$ product-moment correlation coefficient is:

$$r = [N\Sigma XY - (\Sigma X)(\Sigma Y)] / \sqrt{[N\Sigma X^2 - (\Sigma X)^2][N\Sigma Y^2 - (\Sigma Y)^2]}$$

***Calculation for Pearson Product-Moment Correlation Coefficient***

| Subject | X | X² | Y | Y² | XY |
|---------|-----|------|-----|------|------|
| 01 | 31 | 961 | 45 | 2025 | 1395 |
| 02 | 22 | 484 | 58 | 3364 | 1276 |
| 03 | 19 | 361 | 57 | 3249 | 1083 |
| 04 | 16 | 256 | 48 | 2304 | 768 |
| 05 | 78 | 6084 | 61 | 3721 | 4758 |
| 06 | 3 | 9 | 36 | 1296 | 108 |

*continued*

| Subject | X | X² | Y | Y² | XY |
|---------|-----|-------|-----|-------|-------|
| 07 | 93 | 8649 | 18 | 324 | 1674 |
| 08 | 78 | 6084 | 88 | 7744 | 6864 |
| 09 | 23 | 529 | 9 | 81 | 207 |
| 10 | 15 | 225 | 12 | 144 | 180 |
|  | 378 | 23642 | 432 | 24252 | 18313 |
|  | $\Sigma X = 378$ | $\Sigma X^2 - 23,642$ | $\Sigma Y = 432$ | $\Sigma Y^2 = 24,252$ | $\Sigma XY = 18,313$ |

$$N = 10 \qquad \Sigma X^2 = 23,642$$
$$\Sigma XY = 18,313 \qquad \Sigma Y^2 = 24,252$$
$$\Sigma X = 378 \qquad (\Sigma X)^2 = 142,884$$
$$\Sigma Y = 432 \qquad (\Sigma Y)^2 = 186,624$$

$$r = [(10)(18313) - (378)(432)] / \sqrt{[(10)(23642) - (142884)][(10)(24252) - (186624)]}$$
$$= [183130 - 163296] / \sqrt{(236420 - 142884)(242520 - 186624)}$$
$$= 19834 / \sqrt{(93536)(55896)}$$
$$= 19834 / 72317$$
$$r = .274$$

The Pearson $r$ of .274 is similar to the Spearman $r_s$ of .29. In both computations, the correlation is low and will not be clinically significant because only a small portion of the variance is accounted for.

**Step 8.** *Calculate a regression line.*

A **regression line** describes the relationship between variable $X$ and variable $Y$. The formula for the regression line is:

$$Y = bX + a$$

Where:

$Y$ is a predicted variable from the known $X$ value
$b$ is the slope of the line
$a$ is the $Y$ intercept

The regression line that is calculated assumes that if a perfect correlation 1.00 exists between two variables, then one could predict the $Y$ value if the $X$ value is known. For example, suppose we derive the formula for a specific regression line to be:

$$Y = .3 - X + 1.50$$
$$\text{and } X = .50 -$$
$$Y = .30(.500) + 1.50$$
$$= .15 + 1.5$$
$$Y = 1.65$$

Therefore, if $X = .500$, then $Y = 1.65$ in this example. The calculation of a regression line is useful when there is a high correlation between two variables. On the other hand, a very low correlation of $r = .29$ would not warrant constructing a regression line.

The computational formula for the slope is:

$$b = [N(\Sigma XY) - (\Sigma X)(\Sigma Y)] / [N\Sigma X^2 - (\Sigma X)^2]$$

The formula for the $Y$ intercept is:

$$a = Y - bX$$

**Step 9.** *Identify the critical values for the Spearman rank correlation coefficient.*

a. Determine number of subjects ($N$)
b. Significance level, such as $\alpha = .05, .01$
c. Directional or nondirectional hypothesis

For example, with $N = 10$, $\alpha = .05$, nondirectional test, $r_{s(crit)} = .648$. (See Table C–6 in the appendices.) In the example above, $r_{s(obs)} = .29$. In this result, the researcher will accept the null hypothesis and conclude that there is no statistically significant relationship between the two variables.

**Step 10.** *Identify the critical values for the Pearson product-moment correlation coefficient.*

a. $df = N - 2$
b. Significance level
c. Directional or nondirectional hypothesis

In the example as shown, $df = 8$, $\alpha = .05$, nondirectional test, $r_{crit} = .6319$. (See Table C–5 in the appendices.) Because $r_{obs} = .27$, the null hypothesis is accepted, and the researcher concludes that there is no statistically significant relationship between the two variables.

The reader should note that as the $N$ increases, the $r_{crit}$ decreases. For example, for 100 $df$, $\alpha = .05$ level of significance, $r_{crit} = .1966$, whereas for 20 $df$, $r_{crit} = .4227$.

## 8.12  Model VII: Observed Frequencies (Chi-Square)

When researchers work with nominal data, they frequently are concerned with differences in the number of cases falling into discrete categories such as improved versus not improved or active versus disengaged. The major purpose of this statistical model is to test whether there are statistically significant differences between the observed and the expected frequencies of two independent groups.

For example, this model could be applied if a researcher is interested in determining whether there is a gender difference in the distribution of individuals with multiple sclerosis in a population where there are 51 percent female subjects and 49 percent male subjects. Is there a statistically significant difference between the number of men as compared with women who have a diagnosis of multiple sclerosis? In this hypothetical example, the researcher will compare the observed differences between the number of men and women diagnosed with multiple sclerosis with the expected prevalence, that is, 51 percent for women and 49 percent for men.

### 8.12.1  Example of Chi-Square

In an example from the literature, the investigators examined the factors influencing the successful outcome of tracking individuals with severe psychiatric illnesses in the community compared with those in hospitals. In Table 8–12, the investigators compared the patients treated at home with patients admitted to a hospital in relation to where they were assessed during a psychotic episode.

*Formula for Chi-Square ($\chi^2$)*

$$\chi^2_{obs} = \Sigma \left[ (O - E)^2 \right] / E$$
$$\chi^2_{obs} = [(51 - 42)^2 / 42] + [(3 - 11)^2 / 11] + [(11 - 10)^2 / 10] + [(0 - 2)^2 / 2] + [(13 - 22)^2 / 22] + [(13 - 6)^2 / 6] + [(5 - 5)^2 / 5] + [(3 - 1)^2 / 1]$$
$$\chi^2_{obs} = 1.92 + 5.81 + .09 + 2 + 3.68 + 8.16 + 0 + 4$$

$$\chi^2_{obs} = 25.66$$
$$\chi^2_{crit} = 7.82 \ (3 \ df, \alpha = .05)$$

### Conclusion

The researchers rejected the null hypothesis and concluded that there is a statistically significant difference where patients are assessed if they are treated at home or admitted to a hospital. From the results, the researchers concluded that if patients are assessed at home, they will have significant less probability of hospitalization for a psychiatric illness. The results of the study reinforced their hypothesis that home treatment is a feasible alternative to hospital treatment for many individuals with psychiatric illness. The application of Chi-square is an appropriate statistical test when comparing nominal categories of data. It is a simple but powerful statistic that can be applied to outcome studies of clinical populations.

## 8.12.2 Operational Procedure of Observed Versus Expected Frequencies (Chi-Square)

**Step 1.** *State the research hypothesis.*

The null hypothesis is: There is no statistically significant difference between the observed versus expected frequencies in normal groups ($\chi^2_{obs} < \chi^2_{crit}$). The **alternative hypothesis** is: There is a statistically significant difference between the observed versus expected frequencies in nominal groups ($\chi^2_{obs} \geq \chi^2_{crit}$).

**Step 2.** *Select the level of statistical significance.*

This is usually $a = .05$.

**Step 3.** *Determine the degrees of freedom (df) for the contingency table.*

$$df = (r - 1)(c - 1)$$
$$r = \text{number of rows in the table}$$
$$c = \text{number of columns in the table}$$

For example, in a $2 \times 2$ contingency table, the degree of freedom is 1. In a $3 \times 6$ contingency table, $df = 10$.

### TABLE 8-12

**Location of Assessment during a Psychiatric Episode**

| Location of Assessment | Patients Treated at Home | | Patients Admitted to Hospital | | Total Patients |
|---|---|---|---|---|---|
| | Observed | Expected | Observed | Expected | |
| Home | 51 | 42 | 13 | 22 | 65 |
| Hospitals | 3 | 11 | 13 | 6 | 16 |
| Outpatient Clinic | 11 | 10 | 5 | 5 | 16 |
| Police Station | 0 | 2 | 3 | 1 | 3 |
| | 65 | 65 | 34 | 34 | 99 |

**Note:** Reproduced from "Home Treatment for Acute Psychiatric Illness," by C. Dean and E. M. Gadd, 1990, *British Medical Journal, 201,* p. 1023 with permission from BMJ Publishing Group Ltd.

**Step 4.** *Identify $\chi^2_{crit}$ (Chi-square critical) from the statistical table of values.*

The critical value is determined by:

a. Level of significance
b. *df*

For example, $\chi^2_{crit} = 18.307$ for $\alpha = .05$, nondirectional test, with *df* = 10. (See Table C–10 in the appendices.)

**Step 5.** *Identify the discrete nominal categories being compared.*

For example, diagnostic groups, gender, and health care settings.

**Step 6.** *Determine the number of columns and rows in the Chi-square contingency table.*

Chi-square **contingency tables** are based on the number of columns and rows being compared. Contingency tables range from two rows and columns ($2 \times 2$ contingency table) to larger number of rows and columns, such as ($2 \times 3$), ($3 \times 5$), ($6 \times 8$).

**Step 7.** *Tabulate the observed number of frequencies within each discrete category or group.*

| | Nonsmokers | | Smokers | | Total Observed |
| --- | --- | --- | --- | --- | --- |
| | Observed | Expected | Observed | Expected | |
| Lung Cancer | 500 | 1,000 | 1,500 | 1,000 | 2,000 |
| No Lung Cancer | 4,500 | 4,000 | 3,500 | 4,000 | 8,000 |
| | 5,000 | | 5,000 | | 10,000 |

The researcher counts the number of individuals with lung cancer who were smokers or nonsmokers in a population.

**Step 8.** *Calculate the expected frequencies based on the probability of chance.*

The expected frequencies in a cell are computed by multiplying the total frequencies of a row that contains the cell by the total frequencies of the column that contains the cell and dividing this product by the total number of cases in the population. In the example above, the expected frequencies for nonsmokers with lung cancer is equal to:

$$(2000)(5000) / 10,000 = 1,000$$

**Step 9.** *Calculate Chi-square ($\chi^2_{obs}$).*

The formula for Chi-square is:

$$\chi^2_{obs} = \Sigma[(O - E)^2 / E]$$

Where:

$\Sigma$ = grand sum of all the cells
$O$ = observed frequency in each cell
$E$ = expected frequency in each cell

**Step 10.** *Compare the two values: $\chi^2_{obs}$ and $\chi^2_{crit}$.*

(See Table C–10 in the appendices for critical score.)

a. Accept the null hypothesis if $\chi^2_{obs}$ is less than $\chi^2_{crit}$
b. Reject the null hypothesis if $\chi^2_{obs}$ is equal to or more than $\chi^2_{crit}$

### Observed Frequencies, Chi-square Example

**Research Problem.** Is cognitive-behavioral treatment as effective as antidepressant medication in treating individuals with clinical depression?

**Step 1.** *State the research hypothesis.* Null hypothesis: There is no statistically significant difference between the number of individuals with depression who improve with medication (Med) compared to those who receive cognitive-behavioral treatment (CBT).

**Step 2.** *Determine the level of significance:* $\alpha = .05$.

**Step 3.** *Determine the df from the contingency table.*

$$df = (r - l)\,(c - l)$$
$$df = (2 - 1)\,(3 - 1) = 2$$

**Step 4.** *Identify $\chi^2_{crit}$ from the statistical table of values.*

a. $\alpha = .05$
b. $df = 2$
c. $\chi^2_{crit} = 5.99$. (See Table C–10 in the appendices.)

**Step 5.** *Identify the nominal categories.* In this example, the nominal categories are:

a. Those individuals treated with CBT who regressed,
b. Those individuals treated with CBT who showed no improvement,
c. Those individuals treated with CBT who improved,
d. Those treated with medication who showed no improvement, and
e. Those treated with medication who improved.

**Step 6.** *There are two rows and three columns: (2 × 3 contingency table).*

**Step 7.** *Enumerate the observed number of frequencies within each nominal category and place in 2 × 3 contingency table.*

| Treatment | Regressed O | Regressed E | No Improvement O | No Improvement E | Improvement O | Improvement E | Total Observed |
|---|---|---|---|---|---|---|---|
| Cognitive-Behavioral | 20 | 24.70 | 40 | 57.64 | 150 | 127.64 | 210 |
| Medication | 40 | 35.29 | 100 | 82.35 | 160 | 182.35 | 300 |
| Totals | 60 | | 140 | | 310 | | 510 |

In this example, 210 individuals received CBT and 300 individuals received medication. A total of 510 individuals with depression were included in the study. Out of 310 individuals who improved, 160 received medication while the remaining 150 received CBT. The rest of the group (200 individuals) showed either no improvement (remained the same) or regressed.

**Step 8.** *Calculate the expected frequencies for each nominal category or cell based on the formula.*

To complete the expected frequency of any cell, multiply the marginal total for the row that contains the cell by the marginal total for the column that contains the cell, and divide this product by the total number of cases in the table. (McCall, 1986, p. 321)

CBT (Regressed) = (210) (60) / 510 = 24.70
CBT (No Improvement) = (210) (140) / 510 = 57.64
CBT (Improved) = (210) (310) / 510 = 127.64
Med (Regressed) = (300) (60) / 510 = 35.29
Med (No Improvement) = (300) (140) / 510 = 82.35
Med (Improved) = (300) (60) / 510 = 182.35

**Step 9.** *Calculate Chi-square* $(\chi^2_{obs})$.

$$\chi^2_{obs} = \Sigma [ (O - E)^2 / E]$$
$$\chi^2_{obs} = [(20 - 24.70)^2 / 24.70] + [(40 - 57.64)^2 / 57.64] + [(150 - 127.64)^2 / 127.64] +$$
$$[(40 - 35.29)^2 / 35.29] + [(100 - 82.35)^2 / 82.35] + [(160 - 182.35)^2 / 182.35]$$
$$\chi^2_{obs} = .89 + 5.39 + 3.91 + .62 + 3.78 + 2.73$$
$$\chi^2_{obs} = 17.32$$

**Step 10.** *Compare* $\chi^2_{obs}$ *with* $\chi^2_{crit}$.

$$\chi^2_{obs} = 17.32$$
$$\chi^2_{crit} = 5.991$$

Reject the null hypothesis. There is a statistically significant difference between CBT and medications in the treatment of depression. It appears that CBT is more effective than medication in the improvement of depression in this hypothetical example. Of the 210 individuals, 150 (or 71 percent) of the CBT group improved, while 160 out of the 300 individuals (or 53 percent) of the medication group improved.

### 8.12.3 Kappa

#### Purpose

Kappa's purpose is to determine the degree of agreement between two or more judges independently ranking a variable. The **Kappa test (k)** can be used to measure **interrater reliability**. Kappa can range from +1.00 to −1.00

#### Assumptions

a. The units are independent, that is, completed by independent observations.
b. The categories are nominal scale measurements, are fully mutually exclusive, and exhaustive.
c. The judges operate independently.
d. There are no criteria for correctness, choices, clinical judgment, or client attitudes.
e. Judges have equal competence, education, or ability to make ratings.
f. There are no restrictions placed on ranking or rating the variable.

#### Formula for Kappa

$$Kappa = P_0 - P_c / 1 - P_c$$

Where:

$P_0$ = the observed proportion of agreement
$P_c$ = the proportion of agreement expected by chance alone

#### Example

In a hypothetical observation, two independent observers rate the level of depression indicated by a behavioral scale. One individual is observed by two independent raters during 10 sessions to evaluate the level of depression (i.e., low depression [LD], medium depression [MD], and severe depression [SD]). Each category of depression is operationally defined, and each rater has been trained previously using a standardized rating scale. They independently observe a patient on a ward applying a behavior rating scale. Is there a high interrater relationship between the two observers using a standardized rating scale? The data from the observations follow:

| Sessions | Observer 1 | Observer 2 | Agreement |
|---|---|---|---|
| 1 | LD | MD | no |
| 2 | MD | MD | yes |
| 3 | LD | LD | yes |
| 4 | MD | MD | yes |
| 5 | LD | LD | yes |
| 6 | LD | LD | yes |
| 7 | MD | MD | yes |
| 8 | LD | MD | no |
| 9 | MD | MD | yes |
| 10 | LD | LD | yes |
| Totals | 6 LD, 4 MD, 0 SD | 4 LD, 6 MD, 0 SD | Agreements: 8/10 = 80% |

### Stepwise Procedure for Kappa

**Step 1.** *Place data into a 3 × 3 contingency table to display agreements.* Use three categories of depression, MD, LD, and SD.

| | LD | MD | SD | Marginal Totals |
|---|---|---|---|---|
| LD | 4 | 2 | 0 | 6 |
| MD | 0 | 4 | 0 | 4 |
| SD | 0 | 0 | 0 | 0 |
| Marginal Totals | 4 | 6 | 0 | (10) |

Notice that there were four instances of both observers agreeing on low depression and four instances of both observers agreeing on moderate depression. There were no observations of severe depression. The agreements will always be the numbers in the diagonal cells when there are 2 observers and 1 subject. Also note that when adding frequencies in cells that observer one usually is on the $Y$ axis and observer two is on the $X$ axis of the table. In this example, the discrepancy between the two raters occurred in the cell containing 2. This is where observer 1 rated the subject twice as LD and observer 2 rated the same subject for sessions 1 and 8 as MD.

**Step 2.** *Calculate for Kappa applying the formula.*

$$Kappa = P_0 - P_c / 1 - P_c$$

$P_0$ is obtained by adding all the frequencies in the cells that both observers agree.

|  | | Observer 2 | |
|---|---|---|---|
|  | 11 | 12 | 13 |
| Observer 1 | 21 | 22 | 23 |
|  | 31 | 32 | 33 |

Each cell is numbered to represent the rating of each observer. For example, cells 11, 22, and 33 represent agreements of observers 1 and 2. On the other hand, cell 21 represents discrepancy between observers 1 and 2.

$P_0$ = the frequency of agreement over the total number of observations ($N$).

The formula is:

$$P_0 = (n_{11} + n_{22} + n_{33} + n_{ii}...) / \text{Sum of Marginal Cells}$$

Where:

$n_{ii}$ = and other cells
The marginal total is the sum of each row or column.

$$n_{11} = 4$$
$$n_{22} = 4$$
$$n_{33} = 0$$
$$P_0 = 8 / 10 = .80$$

$P_c$ = marginal totals of observer 1 times marginal totals of observer 2, divided by the total number of observation periods of sessions squared.

$$P_c = \{[ (6)(4) ] + [ (4)(6) ] + [ (0)(0) ]\} / 10^2$$
$$P_c = [ (24) + (24) + (0)] / 100$$
$$P_c = 48 / 100$$
$$P_c = .48$$

$$Kappa = P_0 - P_c / 1 - P_c$$
$$Kappa = (.80 - .48) /(1 - .48)$$
$$Kappa = 32 / 52$$
$$Kappa = .61$$

A Kappa of .70 is considered to indicate an acceptable level of agreement (Sattler, 1988). The results indicate a slightly lower interrater agreement than what statisticians consider acceptable interrater reliability. Note that the percentage of agreement, that is, 80 percent, is uncorrected for chance. From a pragmatic perspective, Kappa should always be interpreted in terms of its value to the clinician. In this example, the clinical researcher would interpret a Kappa of .61 as acceptable.

For further information see:

Cohen, J. (1960). A coefficient of agreement for nominal scales. *Educational and Psychological Measurement, 20,* 37-46.

Sattler, J. M. (1988). *Assessment of children* (3rd ed.). San Diego, CA: Sattler.

Simon, S. (2005). *What is a Kappa coefficient?* (*Cohen's kappa*). Retrieved from http://www.childrens-mercy.org/stats/definitions/kappa.htm

### 8.12.4 Rasch Analysis

**Rasch analysis** is a statistical method that calculates the likelihood of something being true based on the probabilities of how strong effects are while considering the probabilities of the effectiveness of "control" variables (http://www.rasch-analysis.com). Rasch analysis is particularly suited for evaluating psychometric concepts such as attitudes, abilities, and personality traits. This statistical method has been used frequently for testing the validity and reliability of psychometric scales and assessments (Velozo, Kielhofner, & Lai, 1999).

A good example in occupational therapy that uses the Rasch method is the *Assessment of Motor and Process Skills* (AMPS; AMPS Project International, 2010; Fisher, 1994). In this instance, the Rasch model predicts the probability of how well an individual performs a task based on many different factors, including but not limited to the person's ability to perform the task, the skill required to complete the task, how simple the task is, and the leniency associated with the examiner. The Rasch model is able to take into account all of these (and more) factors and predict the probability of how well a person performs a certain task.

Another example using Rasch analysis is from a study by Lehman, Sindhu, Shectman, Romero, and Velozo (2010) comparing the effectiveness of two separate upper extremity assessments to measure change. Based on the results from the Rasch analysis, these researchers determined that there was no clear advantage of using the *Disabilities of Arm, Shoulder, and Hand over Upper Extremity Functional Index* to measure clinical change.

For further information, see Rasch Analysis http://www.rasch-analysis.com/ and Velozo, C.A., Kielhofner, G., & Lai, J. (1999). The use of Rasch analysis to produce scale-free measurement of functional ability. *American Journal of Occupational Therapy*, 53, 83-90.

## 8.13  Statistical Software Packages

Although the authors have used hand calculations to solve the examples presented in this book, in actuality, many statistical problems can be solved through one of a number of statistical packages available for computers. Three widely used computer programs designed for the health and social sciences are detailed below.

### 8.13.1 Statistical Package for the Social Sciences (SPSS©)

This company, now owned by IBM, produces a data analysis package for research scientists. It has been widely used within the social science fields, as well as other disciplines. SPSS© includes the capabilities to perform basic analyses (e.g., frequencies, correlations) and more advanced analyses (e.g., regression, ANOVA, general linear models, contingency tables, factor and discriminant analysis, nonparametric statistics, and time series). A Graduate Pack, containing the full version of SPSS©, is available at a reduced price for students working on an advanced degree (http://www.spss.com/gradpack/).

The following information was obtained from the SPSS© website (http://www.spss.com/vertical_markets/healthcare/).

**Manage Resources to Ensure Quality of Care**

Healthcare organizations today face numerous challenges, including concern about their ability to deliver the quality of care people expect—and the increasing cost of such care.

There is a growing awareness that information technology can play a critical role in meeting some of these challenges. SPSS© solutions help researchers, healthcare providers, and "payer" organizations-both private health insurers and public sector programs like Medicare—manage existing resources more efficiently, combat waste and fraud, and achieve their goals.

SPSS© solutions enable healthcare organizations to:

- Support medical research: Analyze large, complex datasets easily and efficiently
- Improve disease management: Identify the most effective treatments and therapies for your patients or for the public
- Monitor the quality of patient care: Compare your organization's practices with regional and national benchmarks and identify areas needing improvement
- Improve operational efficiency: Monitor key performance indicators and strengthen your bottom line
- Maintain accreditation: Support your internal processes for meeting accreditation requirements
- Combat healthcare fraud: Detect changing patterns in fraud, waste, and abuse so you can minimize their impact on your ability to deliver needed care
- Protect public health: Speed the discovery of patterns in disease and facilitate the communication of results through open, interoperable predictive analytics solutions
- For more than 38 years, SPSS© has helped organizations involved in healthcare collect and analyze data and gain insight. SPSS© solutions for healthcare can be found at:
    - Five of the seven largest healthcare provider organizations in the U.S.
    - 14 of the 16 hospitals on U.S. News & World Report magazine's 2005 "honor roll"
    - More than 300 hospitals in the U.K. NHS Trust system
    - The top five private payers in the U.S., who insure more than 150 million consumers
    - AXA and BUPA, two of the leading insurers in the U.K.
    - Many county, state, and national healthcare agencies, including those serving densely populated areas
    - Medical researchers at numerous universities and public health agencies, including those conducting research on genomics and other groundbreaking therapies
    - Leading medical associations and not-for-profit foundations

(SPSS©, Inc., 2010, para. 1-4)

### SPSS© Example

Statistical software packages such as SPSS© make it possible to obtain statistical results with relative ease. The following is an example of an SPSS© printout of an ANOVA, first discussed in an earlier section: 8.10 Model V: $k$-independent Samples. The data comes from the hypothetical *Fugl-Meyer Poststroke Motor Recovery Test Scores* listed in Section 8.10.1. SPS Statistics version 17.0.1 was used (IBM-SPSS©, http://www-01.ibm.com/). In this experiment, a comparison was being made between the performance of subjects on the Fugl-Meyer test based on their random assignment to the electrical stimulation (ES), acupuncture (A), or the proprioceptive neuromuscular facilitation (PNF) groups.

In order to have the software calculate various statistical procedures, data need to be arranged in a specific manner, depending on the type of statistical procedure. Generally, for SPSS©, data can be arranged by columns or by rows, depending on the data collected. In this example, the data representing the dependent variable are listed in a column format, labeled as "SCORE," and the independent variable is organized by rows. For example, the factor labeled "GROUP" represents the independent variable and is listed as being either "ES," "A," or "PNF," depending on the row. If this example had contained two dependent variables, there would have been two columns representing the dependent variables.

| Subject | Group* | Score |
|---------|--------|-------|
| 1 | ES | 23 |
| 2 | ES | 31 |
| 3 | ES | 161 |
| 4 | ES | 27 |
| 5 | ES | 32 |
| 6 | ES | 18 |
| 7 | ES | 38 |
| 8 | A | 13 |
| 9 | A | 19 |
| 10 | A | 19 |
| 11 | A | 25 |
| 12 | A | 18 |
| 13 | PNF | 33 |
| 14 | PNF | 42 |
| 15 | PNF | 30 |
| 16 | PNF | 38 |
| 17 | PNF | 44 |
| 18 | PNF | 41 |

*ES = electrical stimulation; A = acupuncture;
PNF = proprioceptive neuromuscular facilitation

A typical manner in which to enter this type of data into an SPSS© spreadsheet (i.e., SPSS© Statistics Data Editor) would look like the following:

Note that all of the subjects are labeled from 1 – 18. Once the data are entered, it is important to make sure the column labeled "score" is categorized as "NUMERICAL." This can be done using the "VARIABLE VIEW" within the SPSS© Statistics Data Editor. Next, it is good practice to make sure the data have a bell-shaped distribution, also referred to as being "normally distributed." If data are not normally distributed, they may be skewed. If the skewness measure is greater than 1 or less than −1, the data are skewed. However, if the skewness measure is between −1 and +1, then the data are considered to be not skewed. If the data are skewed, apply a nonparametric statistic such as Kruskal-Wallis (See Section 8.10.2).

***Calculating the Skewness.***    This can be done in the SPSS© Statistics Data Editor.

1. Under the "ANALYZE" pull-down menu, select "DESCRIPTIVE STATISTICS."
2. Choose "EXPLORE."
3. Once the "EXPLORE" window opens, identify the "DEPENDENT LIST" (i.e., score) and the "FACTOR LIST" (i.e., Group).
4. Click "OK." This action will open the SPSS© Statistics Viewer and, among other things, a "DESCRIP-TIVES" table that lists various descriptive statistics. See the following descriptive table for this set of data:

| Descriptives | | | | |
|---|---|---|---|---|
| Group | | Statistic | Score | Std.Error |
| A | Mean | | 18.800 | 1.908 |
| | 95% Confidence Interval for Mean | Lower Bound | 13.500 | |
| | | Upper Bound | 24.100 | |
| | 5% Trimmed Mean | | 18.780 | |
| | Median | | 19.000 | |
| | Variance | | 18.200 | |
| | Std. Deviation | | 4.266 | |
| | Minimum | | 13.000 | |
| | Maximum | | 25.000 | |
| | Range | | 12.000 | |
| | Interquartile Range | | 7.000 | |
| | Skewness | | 0.229 | 0.913 |
| | Kurtosis | | 1.848 | 2.000 |
| ES | Mean | | 26.430 | 2.999 |
| | 95% Confidence Interval for Mean | Lower Bound | 19.090 | |
| | | Upper Bound | 33.770 | |
| | 5% Trimmed Mean | | 26.370 | |
| | Median | | 27.000 | |
| | Variance | | 69.952 | |
| | Std. Deviation | | 7.934 | |
| | Minimum | | 16.000 | |
| | Maximum | | 38.000 | |
| | Range | | 22.000 | |
| | Interquartile Range | | 14.000 | |
| | Skewness | | 0.021 | 0.794 |
| | Kurtosis | | −1.121 | 1.587 |
| PNF | Mean | | 38.000 | 2.236 |
| | 95% Confidence Interval for Mean | Lower Bound | 32.250 | |
| | | Upper Bound | 43.750 | |
| | 5% Trimmed Mean | | 38.110 | |
| | Median | | 39.500 | |
| | Variance | | 30.000 | |
| | Std. Deviation | | 5.477 | |
| | Minimum | | 30.000 | |

*continued*

| Descriptives | | | |
|---|---|---|---|
| Group | Statistic | Score | Std.Error |
| | Maximum | 44.000 | |
| | Range | 14.000 | |
| | Interquartile Range | 10.000 | |
| | Skewness | −0.602 | 0.845 |
| | Kurtosis | −1.308 | 1.741 |

5. Examine the skewness. The skewness for Group A is .229; for Group ES, .021; and for PNF, −.602. Because all skewness values are $> -1$ and $< 1$, it is safe to assume that these data are appropriate for an ANOVA with regard to skewness.

### Calculating the ANOVA.

1. Go back to the SPSS© Statistics Data Editor, select the "ANALYZE" menu pull-down and select "GENERAL LINEAR MODEL."
2. Select "UNIVARIATE."
3. Move the "SCORE" variable to the "DEPENDENT VARIABLE" box and the "GROUP" variable to the "FIXED FACTOR" box using the little arrow buttons.
4. Click "OK." The SPSS© Statistics Viewer will reopen and display several tables including one labeled, "Tests of Between-Subjects Effects."

| Tests of Between-Subjects Effects | | | | | |
|---|---|---|---|---|---|

Dependent Variable: Score

| Source | Type III Sum of Squares | df | Mean Square | F | Sig |
|---|---|---|---|---|---|
| Corrected Model | 1039.986[a] | 2 | 519.993 | 12.989 | .001 |
| Intercept | 13595.037 | 1 | 13595.037 | 339.585 | .000 |
| Group | 1039.986 | 2 | 519.993 | 12.989 | .001 |
| Error | 600.514 | 15 | 40.034 | | |
| Total | 15921.000 | 18 | | | |
| Corrected Total | 1640.500 | 17 | | | |

[a] R Squared = .634 (Adjusted R Squared = .585)

*Discussion of Specific Results from SPSS© Analysis.* Notice that some of the same information in this table is identical to that shown in the Summary Table for One-Way ANOVA in Section 8.10.1. As a part of interpreting the results, it is important to consider whether the observed F-value is larger than the critical F-value. SPSS© does not automatically provide a table of critical F-values, but more conveniently produces the associated p-value which is labeled in the table as "SIG," meaning significance. In this comparison, the important items to consider are the F- and p-values associated with the variable labeled "Group," which, in our case, is labeled as 12.989 and .001, respectively.

Because the *p*-value is $< .05$, it can be assumed that there is a statistically significant difference between the three groups. However, this test does not say which groups are actually significantly different from each other. In order to determine which groups are significant from each other, a post-hoc comparison is necessary.

If the original research hypothesis was not to just determine whether there would be a significant difference between the three groups, but rather to determine which individual groups are significantly different from the other individual groups, then this should be stated in the original statistical plan. Proper protocol stresses that it is only appropriate to execute a post-hoc comparison if statistical significance exists between the three groups. In our hypothetical example, this is indeed the case because of having a *p*-value $< .05$.

### Post-Hoc Tests of ANOVA.

1. In order to run a post-hoc comparison, go back to the SPSS© Statistics Viewer or the SPSS© Statistics Data Editor and select the "ANALYZE" pull-down menu, then select the "GENERAL LINEAR MODEL," then select "UNIVARIATE." If this is done after completing the previous steps, the "DEPENDENT VARIABLE" and "FIXED FACTOR(s)" will not need to be redefined again.
2. In the UNIVARIATE window, select the "POST HOC" button.
3. At the top of the "UNIVARIATE: POST HOC MULTIPLE COMPARISONS FOR OBSERVED MEANS" window select the "GROUP" factor and move it to the "POST HOC TESTS FOR:" window using the little arrow button.
4. Once this occurs, you will notice that all of the post-hoc options are no longer grayed out. You will notice that there are nearly 20 different options from which to choose. Each option is unique in its own right and should be chosen depending on specific statistical assumptions and strategies. Common options include the Bonferroni, the Tukey, SchefFÈ, and Dunnett comparisons.
5. For this example, the Bonferroni option was chosen before clicking the "CONTINUE" button. This will bring you back to the "UNIVARIATE" window where the arrangement of the dependent variable and the fixed factors should be the same as you recently left them.
6. Click the "OK" button to run the new analysis. The SPSS© Statistics Viewer will generate an ANOVA table identical to the one without the post-hoc analysis. The bottom of the ANOVA table should be a section labeled as "Post Hoc Tests." You should see a "Multiple Comparisons" table that also identifies "Bonferroni" at the top. The "Multiple Comparison" table for this set of data is shown here.

| **Multiple Comparisons** | | | | | | |
|---|---|---|---|---|---|---|
| Score: Bonferroni | | | | | | |
| (I) Group | (J) Group | Mean Difference (I-J) | Std. Error | Sig. | 95% Confidence Interval | |
| | | | | | Lower Bound | Upper Bound |
| A | ES | −7.63 | 3.705 | .172 | −17.61 | 2.35 |
| | PNF | −19.20* | 3.831 | .000 | −29.52 | −8.88 |
| ES | A | 7.63 | 3.705 | .172 | −2.35 | 17.61 |
| | PNF | −11.57* | 3.520 | .015 | −21.05 | −2.09 |
| PNF | A | 19.20* | 3.831 | .000 | 8.88 | 29.52 |
| | ES | 11.57* | 3.520 | .015 | 2.09 | 21.05 |

Based on observed means.
The error term is Mean Square (Error) = 40.034.
*The mean difference is significant at the 0.05 level.

This table individually compares each intervention group with the other intervention groups. There is some redundancy within the table. The left columns are labeled (I) Group and (J) Group. The (I) group is compared with the other groups (J). In the first row, the "A" group is being compared to the "ES" and the "PNF" groups. The third column is the mean difference between the "I" and "J" groups, and the fourth column is the associated standard error. The fifth column is labeled as "Sig" (significance) which is how SPSS© labels the $p$-value.

In the first row, there is no significant difference between the A and the ES group because the $p$-value is $> .05$, and indeed is .172. However, there is a statistically significant difference between the A group and the PNF group because the $p$-value is .000. In this table, the $p$-values have 3 decimal places. It would not be accurate to report the $p$-value, in this case as being $= .000$. In actuality, the $p$-value, while being very small, still is actually $> 0$; it is just that it would require more than 3 decimal points to give the exact value. Therefore, the proper way to report this would be "$< .001$." The 95 percent confidence intervals (both the lower and upper bounds) for the comparisons are listed in the two most right columns.

When examining the remainder of the Multiple Comparisons table, we learn that there are statistically significant differences between the A and the PNF groups, and the ES and the PNF groups, but not the A and the ES groups. This knowledge, considered along with the means of the respective groups, allows one to interpret with confidence (within the bounds of being at least 95 percent certain) that the proprioceptive neuromuscular facilitation (PNF) group and the electrical stimulation (ES) groups outperformed, at a statistically significant level, the acupuncture (A) group on the Fugl-Meyer Poststroke Motor Recovery Test.

## 8.13.2 Statistical Analysis Software (SAS)

This statistical package is an integrated system of data access, management, analysis, and presentation, which is not limited to a particular computer system. The software is available for mainframes and PCs. Basic and advanced statistics are available, and the analysis can be integrated into a presentation for any type of reporting needs. Training and support are available. Further information regarding SAS can be obtained through the Internet at (http://www.sas.com).

Information obtained on the SAS website (http://www.sas.com/industry/healthcare/provider/) indicates that it is useful for healthcare statistics:

Rapid change is a way of life in the health care industry, and even the most agile provider organization can find it difficult to keep pace. Take, for example, the sheer volume of clinical and operational data being generated on a daily basis. How do you harness all of that data and turn it into evidence-based knowledge that you can act on?

The SAS Health Care Provider Practice is committed to helping you keep pace with change by delivering software solutions and strategic services designed to spark innovation and drive improvement based on best evidence. More than 500 US hospitals use SAS software to improve their quality of care, productivity and patient/staff relations…to enable better and more informed decisions…and to drive their organizations forward.

Only SAS addresses the entire process of translating raw data into useful, trusted and timely information for evidence-based decisions. Only SAS gives you THE POWER TO KNOW® how to improve:

*Patient Safety and Quality of Care*
- Identify best practices by measuring performance against benchmarks.
- Drive evidence-based practice by sharing information at the point of service.
- Optimize outcomes by understanding the cause-and-effect relationships between performance metrics.

*Financial/Operational Performance*

- Control rising costs, respond to increasing regulatory and consumer scrutiny, and implement initiatives such as pay-for-performance.
- Adapt easily to new business models.
- Identify strategies to address revenue cycle and performance management issues.
- Maximize allocation of scarce resources, and eliminate waste and duplication of effort by analyzing operational data.
- Enhance communication and collaboration across the delivery system.

(SAS Institute Inc., n.d., para. 1–5)

### 8.13.3 SYSTAT

This statistical package is available through the website at http://www.systat.com/. A menu-driven data analysis tool enables data to be analyzed in basic statistics (e.g., descriptive, *t*-test, correlation) and more advanced statistics (e.g., ANOVA, multiple regression, and factor analysis). As with most packages, graphics are available.

### 8.13.4 UNISTAT

This statistical program for Windows® was first made available in 1984. It is described by the company as a "fully fledged spreadsheet for data handling, a wide range of statistics and powerful 2D and 3D presentation quality graphics" (http://www.unistat.com). It can be used alone, or combined with Excel®.

## 8.14 Summary

In this chapter, the authors have presented the basic statistical concepts and tests that are applied in clinical research. Statistics is both an art and a science. The art of statistics is the decision making involving the selection of the appropriate statistical test for a research study. There are a number of possibilities in this decision, based on the level of measurement, the probability level for statistical significance, and the number of subjects in the study. The science of statistics is based on mathematical reasoning and use of statistical tables. Mastery of statistics means approaching the subject with an objective attitude and open mind. Statistics should not be applied mechanically such as "throwing data in a computer." The researcher should use statistics in a reflective manner while interpreting and analyzing the results. In this way, statistical analysis is integrated into the research study.

## CHAPTER 9

# Selecting a Test Instrument

*For all such areas of research—and for many others—the precise measurement of individual differences made possible by well-constructed tests is an essential prerequisite.*

—A. Anastasi, 1988, *Psychological Testing* (p. 4)

## Operational Learning Objectives

By the end of the chapter, the learner will:
- Define key concepts in testing.
- Discuss the early history in the development of testing.
- Identify the major purposes of testing.
- Know where to look for bibliographies of tests in books, test catalogues, and online.
- Know how to select a test for a specific function and target population.
- Know how to evaluate reliability and validity of tests.
- Know how to incorporate tests into a research study.
- Determine the skills necessary in:
  - Administering tests;
  - Scoring tests; and
  - Interpreting results of tests.
- Develop an objective attitude in selecting a test instrument and evaluating its effectiveness.
- Identify the potential sources of error in testing.

## 9.1 Key Concepts in Testing

To understand testing and evaluation, one should be able to define the key concepts. How is a test defined? How does the evaluator determine what is normal behavior and what is atypical behavior? Why are tests used? What are potential sources of error in testing? What is the difference between norm-referenced and criterion-referenced tests? These key concepts, listed in Table 9–1, are elaborated upon in this chapter.

## 9.2 Early History of Test Development

Tests have been used for generations for problem solving and decision making. For example, in the twelfth century, the Chinese used civil service examinations to make hiring decisions (Têng, 1943). The ancient Greeks administered physical and intellectual tests as part of the educational process. In Europe, from the time of the Middle Ages, universities gave tests as part of the process of awarding

---

### TABLE 9-1

**Key Concepts in Tests and Measurements**

- **Assessment** refers to the "specific tools or instruments that are used during the evaluation process" (AOTA, 2005, p. 663).

- **Evaluation** refers to "the process of obtaining and interpreting data necessary for intervention. This includes planning for and documenting the evaluation process and results" (AOTA, 2005, p. 663).

- **Measurement** is "a process of assigning quantitative values to objects or events according to certain rules" (Sattler, 2008, p. 92).

- A **measurement scale** is a system of assigning scores to a trait or characteristic.

- A **test** is essentially an objective and standardized measure of a sample of behavior (Anastasi & Urbina, 1997).

- A **major purpose** of a test is to predict future performance based on a current sample of behaviors.

- An **extremely important quality** of a test is to accurately detect change in an individual's behavior (e.g., improvement).

- The **value** of a test depends on its purposes, ability to predict outcome, and the degree of consistency and precision in defining a variable.

- The **degree of accuracy** of a test is based on its ability to be consistent (reliability) and to test what it claims to measure (validity).

- The **sources of error in measurement** are derived, for example, from the unreliability of the instrument, bias of the test administrator, behavior from the client, and adverse test environment.

- **Distributions of data** from heterogeneous populations tend to be normally distributed, whereas data from homogeneous populations tend to be skewed.

- A **norm-referenced test** is a standardized sampling of behavior that uses data from a heterogeneous group of individuals in interpreting results.

- A **criterion-referenced test** is a standardized sampling of behavior that bases performance on accepted standards of competency.

**Note:** Adapted from *Psychological Testing* (7th ed.) by A. Anastasi and S. Urbina, 1997, and *Assessment of Children: Cognitive Foundations* (5th ed.) by J. M. Sattler, 2008.

professional degrees and bestowing honors. In the United States, procedures for testing applicants to the U. S. Civil Service were introduced in 1883. Not until the nineteenth century, however, when an interest in providing humane treatment to individuals with intellectual disabilities and mental illness arose, were tests developed that could identify and distinguish between intellectual disability and emotional disturbance (Anastasi & Urbina, 1997; Sattler, 2008; see Table 9–2 for a summary of major events in test development during the nineteenth and twentieth centuries).

### TABLE 9-2

**Early History of the Test Movement**

| Theorist | Occupation | Contribution to Testing |
|---|---|---|
| Jean-Étienne Dominique Esquirol (1838) | Physician | Classified individuals with intellectual disabilities into various levels of disability; believed that language provided the best measure of intelligence |
| Paul Broca (1864) | Surgeon | Proposed a relationship between the volume of the brain and intelligence |
| Sir Francis Galton (1883) | Biologist | Theorized that physical traits (visual and hearing acuity, muscular strength) and reaction speed could serve as a measure of gauging intellectual abilities |
| James McKeen Cattell (1890) | Psychologist | Developed norms in sensory, motor, and simple perceptual processes for comparing individuals, helping to create the concept of mental measurement |
| Emil Kraepelin (1895) | Psychiatrist | Developed assessment of daily living skills based on perception, memory, attention, and motor functioning; interested in the clinical examinations of patients with psychiatric disorders; designed tests of critical functions to measure practice effects in memory and susceptibility to fatigue and to distraction |
| Charles E. Spearman (1904) | Psychologist | Proposed that intelligence was comprised of a primary factor (g) and specific factors (s) |
| Alfred Binet (1905) | Psychologist | Along with Simon, developed a test that identified children who could not benefit from formal education; this instrument consisted of short tests measuring perception, judgment, comprehension, and reasoning |
| Lewis M. Terman (1916) | Psychologist | Popularized and revised Binet's scale by including tasks to identify superior adult intelligence and by assigning age equivalents to items |
| H. H. Goddard (1919) | Educator | Introduced Binet's scale in America, adding categories of intellectual ability and identifying "morons" and "idiots" |
| Robert M. Yerkes (1921) | Psychologist | Instrumental in developing the Army Alpha, a verbal test, and the Army Beta, a visual test, for group testing; also espoused the idea of point-scales rather than age scales |
| Louis L. Thurstone (1938) | Psychologist | Proposed that intelligence was comprised of several different factors, which he called primary mental abilities, all of which could be considered equally important |
| David Wechsler (1939) | Psychologist | Developed the Wechsler-Bellevue, the precursor to the Wechsler Scales; this test had a verbal scale and a performance scale |

*continues*

| TABLE 9-2 | | |
|---|---|---|

**Early History of the Test Movement** *continued*

| Theorist | Occupation | Contribution to Testing |
|---|---|---|
| Raymond B. Cattell (1979) | Psychologist | Along with John Horn, proposed that intelligence was comprised of fluid (nonverbal, novel, and relatively culture-free) and crystallized reasoning (acquired skills strongly dependent on culture) |
| Jagannath Das (1963) | Psychologist | Used an information-processing model to describe cognitive functioning; information obtained through two distinct methods: simultaneously and sequentially |
| J. P. Guilford (1967) | Psychologist | Attempted to link theory to test development by proposing a three-dimensional Structure of Intellect with 120 factors that led to a test that measured each factor |
| Howard Gardner (1983) | Psychologist | Proposed that there are several autonomous intellectual competencies or multiple intelligences, which are manifested differently in different individuals |
| Robert Sternberg (1985) | Psychologist | Developed 3-part theory of intelligence (*Triarchic Theory of Intelligence*) based on cognitive theory and composed of meta-components, performance components, and knowledge-acquisition components |

© Cengage Learning 2013

Traditionally, test theorists have taken the viewpoint that human characteristics and abilities are normally distributed. Thus, researchers involved in early test development sought to demonstrate what was normal in an effort to identify those individuals who differed significantly from the typical population. Sir Francis Galton (1822–1911; Galton, 1865; 1883/1907/1973), advocating the importance of individual differences, postulated that differences in physical characteristics such as vision, hearing, reaction time, and physical strength could be used to determine mental capabilities. He tried to validate his beliefs through the use of statistical methods developed by Karl Pearson (1857–1936; Pearson, 1911). Although Galton was unsuccessful in showing that mental abilities were related to physical characteristics, our use of a normative sample is a direct result of his hypothesis (Swanson & Watson, 1989). James McKeen Cattell (1860–1944; Cattell, 1890), an assistant to Galton, supported Galton's views that "mental tests" measuring sensory and physical abilities differentiated individuals.

Although he found no relationship between these abilities and school achievement, Cattell contributed to the understanding of tests and measurement by demonstrating that mental ability could be examined empirically (Sattler, 2008).

Eduardo Séquin (1812–1880; Séquin, 1846/1997) also believed that individuals could be differentiated by sensory and motor-control abilities. Galton had believed that the differences were inherent and unchangeable; however, Séquin believed that training in these areas could improve one's intellectual potential. Currently his materials, such as the form board (a task in which individuals place wooden or plastic shapes into puzzle frames) are used as a part of a test battery for young children (Swanson & Watson, 1989).

One of the first attempts to classify individuals with intellectual disabilities was made by Jean-Étienne Dominique Esquirol (1772–1840; de Esquirol, 1838). He recognized that individuals with intellectual disabilities had diverse abilities and concluded that language development was the most important characteristic for distinguishing between degrees of intellectual capacity. His appreciation for the importance of language in the development of intellectual capacity influenced the development of intelligence tests (Anastasi & Urbina, 1997).

While researchers in the United States tried to measure intellectual development through performance on sensory and motor tasks, clinicians in Germany turned toward more complex and abstract tasks as a means of measuring aptitude. Emil Kraepelin (1855–1926; Kraepelin, 1919), recognizing the importance of measuring skills needed for daily living, developed a battery that measured such skills as perception, memory, motor functioning, and attention. H. Ebbinghaus (1850–1909; Ebbinghaus, 1885/1913), after teachers in Germany requested that he develop an aptitude test, produced a timed completion task consisting of reading passages from which words had been left out. This test was a forerunner of group intelligence tests. He also produced tests that assessed arithmetic and memory skills. Carl Wernicke (1849–1905; Wernicke 1875/1994), noted for his work on aphasia and brain localization, investigated individual differences in verbal conceptual thinking and generalization.

### 9.2.1 Influence of Binet on IQ Testing

In 1905, the French government commissioned Alfred Binet (1857–1911; Binet & Simon, 1905/1916), a French psychologist, and a colleague, Theodore Simon (1873–1961), to develop a test that would identify those children who could not benefit from formal education. The content of Binet's test came from educational research and through a deductive analysis of the factors that underlie academic achievement. The Binet–Simon test was developed pragmatically, without a theory of intelligence to guide its contents. Nonetheless, the influence of individuals such as Esquirol and Séquin was apparent in that Binet included items measuring sensory perception, motor control, and language. In addition, the Binet–Simon intelligence test:

> had several unique characteristics: (1) questions were arranged in a hierarchy of difficulty, (2) levels were established for different ages (establishment of mental age), (3) a quantitative scoring system was applied, and (4) specific instructions for administration were built into the test. (Swanson & Watson, 1989, p. 9)

The initial test consisted of 30 items related to following simple directions, defining words, constructing sentences, and answering judgmental questions of a psychological nature.

Binet's test was translated into English by H. H. Goddard (1866–1957; Goddard, 1920) in 1910, while Lewis Terman (1877–1956) revised the Binet–Simon Intelligence test in 1916 for use in the United States (Sattler, 2008; Swanson & Watson, 1989; Terman & Merrill, 1973). Although Binet had perceived his instrument as a way to identify those students who needed to be instructed through alternative methods, Goddard, in the early nineteenth century, linked intelligence test scores to occupation and social status (Gould, 1996). Terman extended Binet's test by adding additional items suitable for testing adults and by adding the concept of "mental quotient" to that of mental age. Terman's revision became known as the Stanford–Binet, so named because he was a professor at Stanford University in California.

### 9.2.2 Alternative Tests to the Binet

Binet's test and the revisions by Terman were developed on the premise that one's ability to successfully complete a particular task was related to developmental level. Thus, in a heterogeneous set of items arranged in a developmental sequence, age-scores could be assigned based on the ability of a majority of children at a given age level to do a particular task. Mental ability was determined by obtaining a ratio between the obtained age-score and one's chronological age. Tests that use this format to find mental abilities are said to have an **age-scale**.

Discontent with age-scores led individuals such as Robert M. Yerkes (1876–1966; Yerkes, 1921; 1930) and David Wechsler (1896–1981; Wechsler, 1939) to develop tests with a radically different scoring format. Rather than using age-score, similar items were put together and points were assigned to each item. Then the raw score, determined by the number of points received, was converted into standard scores, and subsequently into an overall score. Scales with this type of scoring are known as a **point-scale**. The IQ scores derived in this manner are called "**Deviation IQs**." At this time, most tests developed for school-age children, adolescents, and adults use the point-scale, whereas developmental scales, developed for infants, toddlers, and preschoolers, use an age-scale.

Another concern regarding intelligence testing was the emphasis on verbal reasoning seen on the Stanford–Binet. Tests such as the *Leiter International Performance Scale* (LIPS; Leiter, 1948), the Arthur adaptation of the *Leiter International Performance Scale* (Arthur, 1949), the *Kohs Block Design Tests* (Kohs, 1923), and the *Culture-Fair Intelligence Scale* (Cattell, 1950) were developed to counterbalance the highly verbal influence of the *Stanford–Binet*. The Wechsler–Bellevue, developed in 1939 by Wechsler, consisted of a verbal and a performance scale. This test, based on Wechsler's conception that intelligence was global, included tasks from various sources (e.g., *Kohs Block Design Test*, *Army Alpha*, and *Army Beta*). Although the items have changed over time, many of the same types of items are included in the present-day Wechsler scales (Sattler, 2008).

### 9.2.3 Factor Analytical Theories of Intelligence

With the development of computers and more advanced statistical methods (e.g., factor analysis), the concept of intelligence has changed drastically. Although both Binet and Wechsler believed that intelligence was composed of many different abilities, neither one had proposed a theory that identified the components of intelligence. Binet had used items that he believed would assess skills necessary to succeed in an academic setting. Wechsler, on the other hand, had borrowed from a number of available tests, all of which he believed were factors in the construct of intelligence (Sattler, 2008). It fell

to theorists like Charles E. Spearman (1863–1936; 1927), Edward L. Thorndike (1874–1949; 1927), and Louis L. Thurstone (1887–1955; 1938) to suggest the components contained in the construct of intelligence. In general, there were three viewpoints regarding the structure of intelligence:

1. Intelligence was composed of a primary factor called *g* made up of complex mental tasks, such as reasoning and problem solving, and specific factors called *s* that required less complex processes, such as speed of processing, visual-motor, and rote learning (Spearman, 1927).
2. Intelligence was multifactorial and similar abilities clustered to form more complex skills (Thorndike, 1927).
3. Intelligence was comprised of primary factors (e.g., verbal, perceptual speed, inductive reasoning, work fluency, and space or visualization) rather than a single unitary factor (Thurstone, 1938).

More recently, others (e.g., Gardner, 1983; Guilford, 1967; Sternberg, 1985) have proposed alternative theories to account for the nature of intelligence. J. P. Guilford (1897–1987), in an effort to link theory to intelligence tests, proposed in *The Nature of Human Intelligence* (1967) that human intellect could be understood by a three-dimensional model, which he called the Structure of Intellect. This structure contained (a) five operations, which defined the way we process information (e.g., divergent or convergent), (b) four contents, which defined the manner in which the material is presented (e.g., visual or verbal); and (c) six products, which defined the outcome of the mental process (e.g., units or classes). By using combinations of one attribute from each dimension, 120 factors of intelligence can be identified (5 operations × 4 contents × 6 products). Theoretically, if one were to assess a student in each of these 120 factors, one would have a better understanding of how the student learned and could provide an appropriate educational program for that student. Unfortunately, Guilford's model has not been widely accepted, nor has it been used in many research studies.

Raymond B. Cattell (1963) and John L. Horn (1968) agreed with Guilford (1967) that intelligence was not a unitary concept but disagreed in the specific components comprising intelligence. They suggested, instead, that intelligence is made up of two constructs, fluid (*Gf*) and crystallized (*Gc*). Tasks considered to be fluid intelligence include unlearned, culture-free, novel experiences in which adaptation or generalization of previously learned tasks is required (e.g., nonverbal analogies, block building, speed of processing, and problem solving). Crystallized intelligence, on the other hand, is defined as acquired knowledge, such as what is learned in school or in cultural experiences. Examples of tasks measuring crystallized intelligence include vocabulary tests, verbal analogies, rote learning, and rule learning. Two tests that were developed using the concept of crystallized and fluid intelligence are the *Stanford-Binet Intelligence Scale–Fifth Edition* (SB5; Roid, 2003) and the *Kaufman Adolescent and Adult Intelligence Test* (KAIT; Kaufman & Kaufman, 1993). The most recent revisions of the Wechsler scales have also incorporated this theory.

In 1993, John Carroll at Cambridge, England, proposed that intelligence "could be understood best via three strata that differed in breadth and generality" (Miller, 2010, p. 104).

> Each stratum represents a different level of abstraction. Stratum I includes approximately 70 narrow abilities derived from more than 400 data sets; Stratum II represents Carroll's groupings of differentiated broad abilities that are similar to the *Gf-Gc* factors recognized by Horn and others; Stratum III represents the construct of general intellectual ability (*g*). (Schrank, Miller, Wendling, & Woodcock, 2010, p. 2)

The integration of Cattell-Horn and Carroll's work has resulted in the Cattell-Horn-Carroll (CHC) theory. As a result of continued research by McGrew (McGrew, 2005) and Flanagan (McGrew, Flanagan, Keith, & Vanderwood, 1997), the theory has become the framework for the development of the Woodcock-Johnson (Woodcock, McGrew, & Mather, 2001) assessment family (e.g., *WJ–III Tests of Cognition, WJ–III Tests of Achievement*). These assessments are widely used in education to determine eligibility for special education services.

## 9.2.4 Alternative Theories of Intelligence

Although factor analysis theories of intelligence are still the most widely accepted, two additional approaches to intelligence should be mentioned. One approach, information processing, involves the understanding of the ways in which individuals take in and transform the information so that it can be used. While information processing is frequently linked with memory processes, the concept has been extended by individuals such as Das (Das, Kirby, & Jarman, 1975) and Campione and Brown (1978). Das conceptualized intelligence as having two processes: (a) simultaneous, in which information is processed in a spatial, gestalt manner, and (b) sequential, in which material is sequenced in temporal order. Campione and Brown theorized that intelligence consisted of structures that enabled learning (e.g., memory and efficiency) and an executive system that controlled and managed the components involved in problem solving (e.g., knowledge, metacognition, and use of learning strategies). The latter theory has led special educators to emphasize the use of strategies in the learning process as a means of improving problem solving and learning. Continued research is needed to identify ways to teach learning strategies so that learners can benefit from the process.

A second approach to intelligence other than factor analysis is that proposed by Howard Gardner. In *Frames of Mind: The Theory of Multiple Intelligences*, Gardner (1983) proposed that there are several autonomous competencies, each of which can be thought of as separate intelligences. Although he only identified seven of these separate intelligences (linguistic, musical, logical-mathematical, spatial, bodily-kinesthetic, interpersonal, and intrapersonal), he suggested that there may be others. More recently Gardner has added naturalist to his list and has considered spiritual, existential, and moral intelligences (Gardner, 1999). Gardner's theory has taken hold in many educational circles, and curriculums have been developed to encourage development of each of these.

Another important influence has been emotional intelligence (EI), defined as the ability or capacity to identify, assess, and control one's emotions (Mayer, Salovey, & Caruso, 2008). Although E. L. Thorndike (1920; 1927) first introduced the idea as social intelligence, the concept has been expanded in the 20 years by Salovey and Mayer (1990) and Goleman (1995). Proponents of emotional intelligence suggest that EI may be more important than IQ in predicting success in the corporate field:

> IQ washes out when it comes to predicting who, among a talented pool of candidates *within* an intellectually demanding profession will become the strongest leader. In part this is because of the floor effect: everyone at the top echelons of a given profession, or at the top levels of a large organization, has already been sifted for intellect and expertise. At those lofty levels a high IQ becomes a threshold ability, one needed just to get into and stay in the game. (Goleman, 1995, xiv–xv)

More information about emotional intelligence can be found at Daniel Goleman's website, danielgoleman, which can be found at http://danielgoleman.info/topics/emotional-intelligence/ (Daniel Goleman, 2011).

### 9.2.5 Group Aptitude and Achievement Tests

Although the early IQ tests were administered individually, the advent of World War I resulted in a need for group aptitude (mental ability) testing. In 1917, the American Psychological Association appointed Yerkes, an American psychologist and professor at Yale, to develop group mental tests that could effectively evaluate military recruits. Working with Goddard and Terman, Yerkes developed the *Army Alpha*, a verbal test, and the *Army Beta*, a perceptual/nonverbal test, to be administered to recruits who failed the *Army Alpha*. Although the army made little use of their tests, the major result was the obtaining of normative data on 1.75 million

men and the recognition that levels of "intelligence" could be obtained through group testing.

What transpired after that was the massive development and the multiplication of group testing for all groups in society. Students and job applicants were routinely administered tests to determine aptitude and achievement. Two factors led to this phenomenon of mass testing: (a) individuals could be tested simultaneously in less time and with fewer personnel needed to administer the tests, and (b) simplified instructions enabled individuals without professional training in testing to administer the tests. As a result, many professionals working with groups (e.g., teachers, therapists, counselors, personnel directors) are able to administer group tests (Anastasi & Urbina, 1997; Gould, 1996).

Although group testing developed because of the need to determine intellectual ability, issues regarding academic achievement soon became a concern of the nation. Group written examinations were first introduced in the Boston schools in 1845 as a substitute for individual oral examinations. The Stanford Achievement Test, developed in 1923, was the first achievement test to be standardized by using statistical principles of measurement (Sattler, 1988). The practice of mass educational testing continues today at the national level, where students enrolled in public schools are administered a group achievement test during the spring semester (NCLB, 2002). Entrance into postsecondary schools is partially based on the results of the *American College Test* (ACT) and the *Scholastic Aptitude Test* (SAT) tests. Entrance into a profession is routinely accompanied by a test (e.g., *Graduate Record Exam* [GRE], *Graduate Management Admissions Test* [GMAT], *Law School Admissions Test* [LSAT]) developed specifically to evaluate proficiency and knowledge of the profession.

### 9.3 Outline of Overall Evaluative Process of Testing

The steps in the overall evaluative process of testing are listed in Table 9–3 and are elaborated upon in the following section.

**TABLE 9-3**

**Steps in the Evaluation Process**

1. Identify the function to be measured.

2. Identify a published instrument to measure condition, or develop a new standardized procedure for evaluation of function.

3. Identify the skill level necessary to use a test instrument.

4. Identify the possible factors in the environment, tester, subject, or test instrument that can potentially distort the test results.

5. Identify the target population for whom the test is intended and for whom norms have been established.

6. Strictly follow the directions and procedures for administering and scoring the test or for modifying the test procedure to enable the client with disabilities to perform at a maximum level.

7. Interpret the results based on:

   a. Norm-referenced data based on the general population, or

   b. Criterion-referenced data for client performance or competence.

The first step in the process of testing is to determine what will be measured and to operationally define the variable. The researcher must be precise and state clearly what is to be discovered. For example, a clinical researcher is interested in evaluating visual perception. Visual perception consists of a number of different skills, such as discrimination, spatial orientation, form-constancy, memory, figure ground, closure, and visual-motor integration. Although it is possible to evaluate visual perception as a whole, effective treatment necessitates an understanding of the individual's ability in each of the various components.

Once the researcher has identified the function to be measured, he or she selects an instrument to measure that function. Often a published instrument is available. Sometimes published instruments may be better because of the known psychometric properties; however, it may be that there is no instrument, and the researcher has to develop one. This is frequently true when designing an interview or survey questionnaire (see methodological research in Chapter 3).

If the clinical researcher chooses to use a published instrument, then it will be necessary to determine what qualifications are needed to administer the test. Qualification levels are set by the APA Standards for Educational and Psychological Testing (AERA, APA, & NCME, 1999), and most test publishers adhere to this policy.

- *Level A:* There are no special qualifications to purchase these products.
- *Level B:* Tests can be purchased by individuals with (a) certification by or full active membership in a professional organization (ASHA, AOTA, APA, AERA, ACA, AMA, NASP, NAN, INS) that requires training and experience in a relevant area of assessment; or (b) a master's degree in psychology, education, occupational therapy, speech-language pathology, social work, or in a field closely related to the intended use of the assessment, and formal training in the ethical administration, scoring, and interpretation of clinical assessments.
- *Level C:* Tests with a C qualification require a high level of expertise in test interpretation, and can be purchased by individuals with (a) licensure or certification to practice in your state in a field related to the purchase; or (b) a doctorate degree in psychology, education, or closely related field with formal training in the ethical

administration, scoring, and interpretation of clinical assessments related to the intended use of the assessment.

- *Level Q*: Tests can be purchased by individuals with one of the following backgrounds as determined by the particular purchase, along with formal training in the ethical use, administration, and interpretation of standardized assessment tools and psychometrics: (a) Q1: a degree or license to practice in the health care or allied health care field; or (b) Q2: formal supervised mental health, speech/language, and/or educational training specific to working with parents

and assessing children, or formal supervised training in infant and child development. (Pearson Assessments, 2010, para. 4–6)

The fourth step in the process involves identifying the possible factors in the environment, tester, subject, or test instrument that can potentially distort the test results. These factors are outlined in Figure 9–1. The researcher will want to eliminate as many of these factors as possible.

Once the researcher has identified the variable to be measured, the tests to be used, and the potential error factors that need to be eliminated or reduced, he

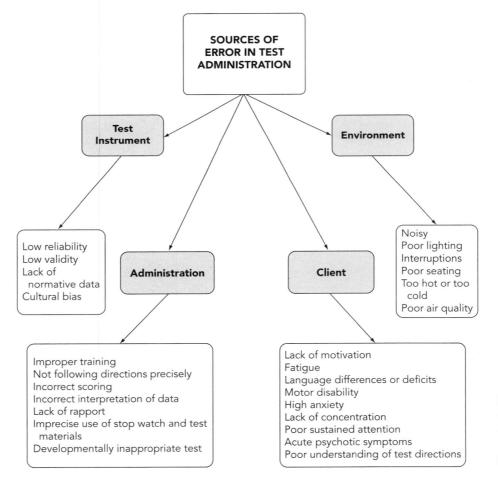

**FIGURE 9-1**  Potential Sources of Error in Test Administration: Errors come from four main areas: the instrument itself, the administration of the test, the client or subject, and the environment.

or she must identify the target population for whom the test is intended and for whom norms have been established. Sometimes this will seem unclear. For example, a clinical researcher may want to examine the psychological effect and impact or behavior that a child with disabilities has on a parent. The target population may, at first, appear to be the parent; however, the question being asked is how the child with disabilities impacts the parent. Although a questionnaire will be given to the parents, items on the instrument will relate to the child with disabilities. Therefore, the target population is, in reality, the child.

Whether the clinical researcher is administering a standardized test or one that he or she developed, the instrument must be administered the same way every time. An alteration in the test directions or administration will confound the results and make them unreliable. When the directions or procedures are altered or modified, this must be stated in the final report. Keep in mind that the alteration or modification of administering a test will make the norms invalid.

The final step is to interpret the results based on either the typical performance as determined by the norms from a general population or a standard set prior to administration of the test. For example, a researcher wants to see the effect of treatment on reduction of anxiety. The researcher has a choice of measurements: (a) a standardized test that measures the level of anxiety (e.g., *State-Trait Anxiety Inventory* by Spielberger, 1983) and compares the results with the expected level based on the norms for the general population, or (b) a custom-designed self-evaluation administered before and after treatment.

## 9.4 Characteristics of a Good Test in Clinical Research

The accuracy and precision in evaluating a client's performance or improvement in a clinical research study depend on the quality of the test instrument. What are the characteristics of a good test instrument? What are some essential questions in evaluating the purposes and "goodness" of a test?

- What is the population for whom the test is targeted (e.g., children with learning difficulties,

individuals with schizophrenia, persons with muscular dystrophy)?
- What are the specific purposes of the test (e.g., planning treatment goals, determining prognosis, establishing baseline data, or documenting progress)?
- What are the areas of function identified in the test (e.g., social development, pre-vocational, personality, leisure interests, perceptual-motor abilities, ADL skills, independent living, cognitive level)?
- What are the methods used to evaluate a client? Primary sources for evaluating a client include:

  - *Medical records:* demographics, previous treatment, and outcomes
  - *Educational records:* educational attainment, achievement scores
  - *Clinical observation of performance:* therapists and teacher observations
  - *Interviews:* formal or unstructured individual interviews
  - *Objective tests:* objectively scored paper-and-pencil tests, performance scales, and verbal tests
  - *Survey questionnaires:* group tests, **forced choice test items** or **open-ended questions**
  - *Self-reports:* evaluation of treatment effectiveness through client's perspective
  - *Reports from peers, teacher/therapist, or family:* informal reports or observations
  - *Biomechanical or physiological measurement of human factors:* machine monitoring, test procedures

- Is there a standardized procedure or manual of instructions in administering the test and interpreting results? Are there tables of normative data?
- Are there special skills or certifications that are necessary to administer, score, and interpret results of the test?
- Is the scale of measurement used in collecting data identifiable (i.e., continuous, such as interval or ratio, or discrete, such as nominal or ordinal)?
- Are error factors controlled that can potentially interfere with obtaining reliable test results?
- Are research data reported (such as those derived from previous studies, including reliability, validity, and normative scores)?

## 9.5 Assumptions in Clinical Evaluation

What are some of the assumptions in clinical evaluation that guide a clinician in assessment? The major assumptions are outlined below:

- Evaluation is an essential factor in the treatment process. It is used to determine the client's abilities, interests, potentials, and work traits.
- Evaluation is used to establish baseline data so as to compare with outcome results.
- Evaluation is based on reliable and valid instrumentation. The degree of accuracy in measurement depends on the degree of reliability (consistency) and validity (accuracy).
- Error is always present to a degree in evaluation, owing to anomalies in the examiner's presentation of test materials, degree of anxiety or fatigue, client's motivation, less-than-perfect reliability of the test, and a less-than-ideal testing environment. Test scores obtained are a sample of the client's performance and represent an approximation of abilities within a given time frame.
- The reliability of the test score is increased by eliminating potential error factors that could endanger or distort the test results.
- Evaluation can provide data for documentation and the basis for establishing clinical efficacy and quality assurance. Evaluation is an excellent method for objectively determining client progress.

## 9.6 Major Purposes of Testing in Clinical Research

The major purposes of testing are as follows:

- Establish baseline data (experimental research, pretest).
- Evaluate outcome or effectiveness of treatment procedure (experimental research, posttest).
- Assess the degree of relationship between two variables (correlational research).
- Evaluate quality of health care or education progress for accreditation (evaluative research).
- Assess developmental landmarks (developmental research).
- Assess individual values, interests, or attitudes (survey research).
- Evaluate differences between groups (correlational, experimental research).
- Evaluate functional assessment (screening target population).

## 9.7 Conceptual Model for Selecting a Test Instrument for Clinical Research

The decision whether to select a test from a published source or to construct a new test to measure a defined variable is a frequent dilemma. The measuring instrument is an essential part of a research study and represents the operational definition of a variable. Figure 9–2 shows this process.

The conceptual definition of a variable should lead the investigator to a specific test that is the most appropriate for operationally defining a variable. In clinical research, it is crucial that the investigator selects a measuring instrument that has a high reliability and is a valid measurement of outcome. Measuring improvement in such areas as personality, physical capacity, cognitive functions, independent living skills, vocational skills, and perceptual-motor abilities depends directly on the adequacy and sensitivity of the instrument to measure changes. A crude measuring device that does not have the capacity to record subtle changes in an individual's functioning or behavior is of either limited or no value to the researcher.

When deciding on the instrument to use for the outcome measure, the researcher must ask the following questions:

- *What is the target population?* Examples include:
  - Typical children, adolescents, adults, older adults
  - Intellectual deficiencies
  - Psychiatric diagnosis
  - People with physical challenges (specify diagnosis)

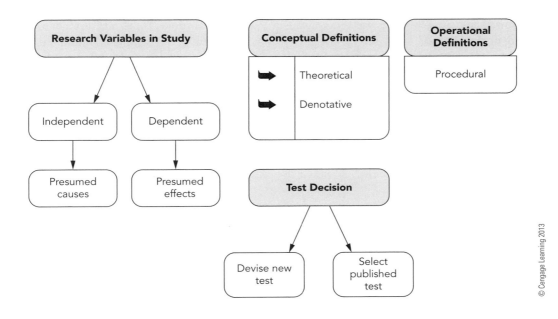

© Cengage Learning 2013

**FIGURE 9-2**    Critical Steps in Determining an Appropriate Test Instrument

    – Social, economic variables
    – Demographic variables

● *What are the specific areas of function to be measured?* Examples of these areas include:

    – Manual dexterity
    – Intellectual aptitude
    – Vocational interests
    – Independent living
    – Personality
    – Job readiness
    – Attitudes toward work
    – Work experiences
    – Work tolerance
    – Social skills
    – Self-care
    – Communication
    – Mobility and transportation
    – Educational level

● *Where will the client be assessed?* Some places for assessment include:

    – Home
    – Sheltered workshop

    – Clinical environment
    – School
    – Office
    – Hospital

● *What are the methods for evaluating function, and how will the individual be assessed?* Some methods include:

    – Observation of performance
    – Paper-and-pencil test
    – Interview
    – Self-report and self-evaluation
    – Direct measure of function through standardized test instrument
    – Evaluation by teacher, therapist, or parent
    – Work samples
    – Parent, therapist, or teacher report
    – Computerized test

● *Is the test reliable and valid?*

    – Are there standardized directions for administration?
    – Are norm scores available for comparison purposes?

– How many subjects were used in collecting norm values?

– How was reliability of the test established (e.g., test-retest, split half, equivalent forms)?

– How was the validity of the test established (e.g., concurrent, construct, predictive)?

● *Are the test results easily interpreted?*

● *What is the scale of measurement (i.e., ordinal, nominal, interval, or ratio)?*

● *How will the individual be tested?*

– In a single session? (summative evaluation) or over several sessions? (formative evaluation)

– In a large group, small group, or individually?

## 9.8 Bibliographic Sources

Another consideration for testing involves asking the following question: Where can I find the most appropriate test instrument? Examples and names of test instruments can be found in a number of sources, as listed in the following sections.

### 9.8.1 Books on Psychological Testing

The researcher has available several books on psychological testing, such as the following:

Anastasi, A., & Urbina, S. (1997). *Psychological testing* (7th ed.). Saddle River, NJ: Prentice Hall.

Asher, I. E. (Ed.) (2007). *Occupational therapy assessment tools: An annotated index* (3rd ed.; with CD-ROM). Rockville, MD: American Occupational Therapy Association.

Bowling, A. (2005). *Measuring health: A review of quality of life measurement scales* (3rd ed.). Buckingham, Great Britain: Open University Press/McGraw Hill.

Dittmar, S. S., & Gresham, G. E. (2005). *Functional assessment and outcome measures for the rehabilitation health professional.* Austin, TX: Pro-Ed.

Finch, E., Brooks, D., Stratford, P., & Mayo, N. (2002). *Physical rehabilitation outcome measures* (2nd ed.; PROM-II with CD-ROM). Hamilton, ON: BC Decker Inc.

Fischer, J., & Corcoran, K. (2007). *Measures for clinical practice: A sourcebook. Volume 1: Couples, family and children* (4th ed.). New York: Oxford University Press.

Hemphill-Pearson, B. J. (Ed.). (2008). *Assessments in occupational therapy mental health: An integrative approach* (2nd ed.). Thorofare, NJ: SLACK.

Lewis, C. B., & McNerney, T. (1994). *The functional tool box: Clinical measures of functional outcomes.* Washington, DC: Learn.

Lezak, M. D., Howieson, D. B., & Loring, D. W. (2004). *Neuropsychological assessment* (4th ed.). New York: Oxford University Press.

*Mental measurements yearbook (MMY), Mental measurements supplement, or Tests in print.* Published by The University of Nebraska Press. In 1989, the MMY began an alternate-year publication schedule with the *Supplement to the Mental Measurements Yearbook or MMY-S.* The 18th edition was published in September, 2010 (http://www.unl.edu/buros/).

Neistadt, N. E., (2000). Occupational therapy evaluation for adults: *A pocket guide.* Baltimore: Lippincott.

Paul, S., & Orchanian, D. (2003). *Pocketguide to assessment in occupational therapy* (1st ed.). Clifton Park, NY: Delmar, Cengage Learning.

Power, P. (2006). *A guide to vocational assessment* (4th ed.). Austin, TX: Pro-Ed.

Sattler, J. M. (2008). *Assessment of children: Cognitive foundations* (5th ed.). San Diego: Sattler.

Stein, F., & Cutler, S. K. (2002). *Psychosocial occupational therapy: A holistic approach* (2nd ed.). Clifton Park, NY: Delmar, Cengage Learning.

Van Deusen, J., & Brunk, D. (1997). *Assessment in occupational therapy and physical therapy.* Philadelphia: Saunders.

## 9.8.2 Internet Sources

Several Internet sites containing databases of assessment tools are available. Here is a list of some of them:

- *meta-OT: Tools and Discussion of Occupational Therapy* (Meta-OT/Occupation-Matters, 2009). Contains a comprehensive database of assessment tools titled *OT Assessments and Outcome Measures*. Readers have the option of adding tools or providing information about outdated assessments. http://metaot.com/ot-assessments-outcome-measures

- *Spinal Cord Injury Rehabilitation Evidence (SCIRE; 2010).* This Internet site, maintained by the SCIRE Project, provides the reader with information about outcome measures, as well as references for further reading. http://www.scireproject.com/outcome-measures

- *Patient Reported Outcome and Quality of Life Instruments Databases* (ProQoild; Mapi Research Institute, 2001–2011). Contains over 700 descriptions of instruments (711) and almost 200 review copies of user manuals, as well as original instruments, translations of instruments, and descriptions of other databases. http://www.proqolid.org/

- *The Internet Stroke Center* (1997–2011). Valuable resource maintained by the Stroke Center at Barnes-Jewish Hospital and Washington University School of Medicine in St. Louis, MO, that contains information about tools that are used in assessing individuals with stroke (*Stroke Scales and Clinical Assessment Tools*): http://www.strokecenter.org/trials/scales/scales-overview.htm#l

- Pain Intensity Scales, used by the National Institutes of Health Pain Consortium (2007). The Internet site contains six pain scales, some of which can be used with children or infants. http://painconsortium.nih.gov/pain_scales/

- Pain inventories and assessments, maintained by Pain Treatment Topics (2005–2011). http://pain-topics.org/

## 9.9  Test Instruments

Testing instruments and procedures can be found for almost every functional area that health professionals might want to assess. Figure 9–3 diagrams the major categories of tests used in occupational therapy, and the following paragraphs and sections describe the major tests. We have tried to select tests that are commonly used or are important for specific reasons (e.g., they have normative data for populations of individuals with special needs; they are used more frequently by occupational therapists; they have high validity and reliability). We recognize that not all tests are listed. For a more complete list, the reader should refer to one of the books on assessment and testing listed in the previous section or to a publisher's catalog (listed at the end of the chapter in Section 9.12). As a caution, tests are developed or revised yearly, and even the most up-to-date book may not have a description of the test. In case of doubt, it is wise to contact the publisher directly.

### 9.9.1 Psychosocial Tests

Assessment of psychosocial functioning occurs in several different ways. Observation of a client may occur in a hospital or residential setting. Professionals and paraprofessionals may complete checklists or rating scales as part of the evaluation. Self-report scales used for assessment of self-concept, role identity, stress management, and leisure activities are valuable in the assessment of a client's perceptions. Some of the more widely used psychosocial scales are described in Table 9–4 (Checklists and Self-Report Scales), Table 9–5 (Cognitive and General Assessments), Table 9–6 (Independent Living Skills), Table 9–7 (Stress Management), and Table 9–8 (Leisure Interests). Additional tests are described in the following paragraphs. Other examples can be found in the publishers' catalogs.

#### Behavior Rating Scales

Therapists, teachers, and clinicians use behavior rating scales to obtain information about a client's behavior. Usually, the rating scales are paper-pencil instruments filled out by the client's parents

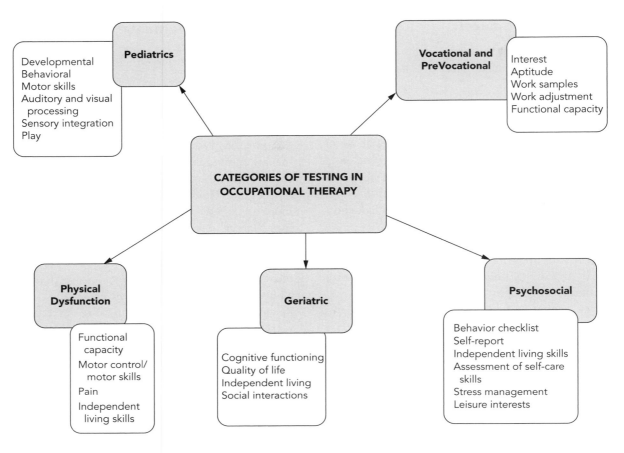

**FIGURE 9-3** Categories of Tests Used in Occupational Therapy Assessment

or family. Occasionally, rating scales may be completed by a member of the peer group (e.g., another student in the classroom) or as a self-report measuring.

Although rating scales are widely used, there are some disadvantages and cautions to be considered when using them. Because the rating scale is a subjective measurement, response bias is possible. For example, the responder may rate the individual either too harshly or too positively (e.g., halo effect) than is realistic, or the respondent may restrict the scores to the central range of the scale, leaving the impression that the individual being rated has few strengths or weaknesses. Second, results from rating scales obtained from different settings (e.g., individual therapy and large classroom settings) may show very different scores. This is frequently attributable to the client's varied behavior in different settings. Finally, differences obtained on the scales may occur because of the day on which the rating scale was completed (Martin, Hooper, & Snow, 1986), thereby reflecting the behavioral variability of either the respondent or the client. For these reasons, more than one informant should be used to complete the rating scale. If possible, each informant should complete a couple of rating scales over a short period of time.

### Objective Personality Tests

Measurement of personality variables through paper-and-pencil tests are widely used in research studies of treatment outcome in psychiatry.

continues

### TABLE 9-4

#### Psychosocial Assessment in Occupational Therapy: Checklists and Self-Reports

| Test | Target Population | Purpose | Variables Assessed | Publisher/Source |
|---|---|---|---|---|
| *Behavior Assessment System for Children* (2nd ed; BASC-2; Reynolds & Kamphaus, 2004) | Children/Adolescents ages 2 through 21 | Teacher, parent, and self-rating scales designed to examine maladaptive and adaptive behavior | Three maladaptive scales (externalizing, internalizing, school problems), Behavioral Symptoms Index, Atypicality, Withdrawal; 1 adaptive scale (adaptability). Content scales further define behaviors. | Pearson Assessment/Psych Corp Attn: Customer Service 19500 Bulverde Road San Antonio, TX 78259-3701 Phone: (800) 627-7271 Fax: (800) 232-1223 http://psychcorp.pearsonassessments.com/pai/ca/cahome.htm/ |
| *Devereaux Scales of Mental Disorders* (DSMD; Naglieri, LeBuffe, & Pfeiffer, 1994), and *Behavior Rating Scales–School Form* (Naglieri, LeBuffe, & Pfeiffer 1992) | Children ages 3 through 18 | Allow teachers and other professionals to evaluate and identify behavior in individuals perceived as having an emotional dysfunction | Behaviors associated with psychopathology, including conduct, attention, anxiety, depression, autism, and acute problems | Pearson Assessment/Psych Corp Attn: Customer Service 19500 Bulverde Road San Antonio, TX 78259-3701 Phone: (800) 627-7271 Fax: (800) 232-1223 http://psychcorp.pearsonassessments.com/pai/ca/cahome.htm |
| *Hamilton Depression Inventory* (HDI; Reynolds & Kobak, 1995) | Adults | Self-report measure designed to screen for symptoms of depression | Symptoms of depression as defined by the DSM-IV. An overall score defines the level of depression. | Psychological Publications, Inc. P.O. Box 3577 Thousand Oaks, CA 91359-0577 Phone: (800) 345–TEST (8378) http://www.tjta.com/products/TST_020.htm |
| *Health Status Questionnaire 2.0* (HSQ® 2.0) (Health Outcomes Institute; 1995) | Ages 14–Adults | Designed as a general outcomes measure to be used in all settings that provide primary or mental health care services, it captures aspects of both physical and emotional health. | Overall health attributes, health status change, and risk for the presence of a depressive disorder. This instrument is designed to be easily administered via self-report, personal interview, or telephone interview. | Pearson Assessment/Psych Corp Attn: Customer Service 19500 Bulverde Road San Antonio, TX 78259-3701 Phone: (800) 627-7271 Fax: (800) 232-1223 http://psychcorp.pearsonassessments.com/pai/ca/cahome.htm |

## TABLE 9-4

**Psychosocial Assessment in Occupational Therapy: Checklists and Self-Reports** *continued*

| Test | Target Population | Purpose | Variables Assessed | Publisher/Source |
|------|-------------------|---------|--------------------|------------------|
| MOHO, the Model of Human Occupation, developed by Gary Kielhofner at the University of Illinois in Chicago. These assessment tools can be accessed through http://www.moho.uic.edu/intro.htmlhttp://www.moho.uic.edu/intro.html (Kramer, J., Kielhofner, G., Forsyth, K., 2008). | Children, adolescents, adults | Self-inventory of daily activities and volitional issues for those activities | Activity patterns, classification of activities and ranking of activities according to value, interest, and personal causation | Available from: UIC COLLEGE OF APPLIED HEALTH SCIENCES 1919 West Taylor Street Room 560 AHSB MC 528 Chicago, IL 60612–7249 or http://www.moho.uic.edu/assessments See also B. J. Hemphill-Pearson (2008), *Assessments in occupational therapy mental health: An integrative approach* (2nd ed., pp. 159–184) |
| Occupational Therapy Trait Rating Scale (Clark, Koch, & Nichols, 1965) | Adults with psychosocial dysfunction who are inpatients | Rating scale used by mental health workers; assesses an individual's personality traits | Dominance-manipulativeness; energy or enthusiasm; social isolation; orderliness | *American Journal of Occupational Therapy*, (1965), 19, 14–18. |
| State-Trait Anxiety Inventory (STAI; Spielberger, 1983) and State-Trait Anxiety Inventory for Children (STAIC; Spielberger, in collaboration with Edwards, Lushene, Montuori, & Platzek, 1973) | High school students, adults, children | Assess how anxious an individual feels at a given moment (state) or in general (trait) | State of anxiety (i.e., feeling at a given moment) and trait of anxiety (i.e., how a person generally feels) | Multi-Health Systems Inc. (MHS Inc.) P.O. Box 950 North Tonawanda, NY 14120-0950 Phone: (800).456–3003 http://www.mhs.com/default.aspx |
| State-Trait Anger Expression Inventory: Adolescents/Child (STAXI-2™ C/A, Brunner & Spielberger, 2009) | Children and adolescents, age 9–18 | Assess both state and trait anger, along with anger expression and control | State anger (feelings, expression); trait anger (temperament, reactions), anger expression (out), anger expression (in), anger control | SIGMA Assessment Systems, Inc. P.O. Box 610757 Port Huron, MI 48061-0757 Phone: (800) 265–1285 http://www.sigmaassessmentsystems.com/ |

### TABLE 9-5

**Psychosocial Assessment in Occupational Therapy: Cognitive and General Assessment**

| Test | Target Population | Purpose | Variables Assessed | Publisher |
|---|---|---|---|---|
| *Adolescent Role Assessment* (Black, 1976; Huebner, Emery, & Shordike, 2002) | Adolescents with psychosocial dysfunction | To assess past history and present role development in home, school, and community | Six areas, including childhood play, adolescent socialization, school performance, occupational choice, and work | *American Journal of Occupational Therapy* (1976), 30, 73–79. |
| *Allen Cognitive Levels (ACL;* Allen, 1985; Allen, Earhart, & Blue, 1992; Allen et al., 2007; Earhart & Allen, 1988) http://www.allen-cognitive-network.org/ | Clients with psychiatric or cognitive impairment | Screening tool to classify people into one of six cognitive levels based on Allen's theory | Six cognitive levels: • automatic actions • postural actions • manual actions • goal-directed actions • exploratory actions • planned actions | Available from: S & S Arts 75 Mill St. Colchester, CT 06415 (800) 288–9941 http://www.ssww.com/therapy-and-rehab/allen-diagnostic-module/ |
| *B. H. Battery* (Hemphill-Pearson, 1999b) | Children and adolescents | Structured instrument to assess the psychological area of human function | Cognitive and psychosocial factors, including problem solving and abstraction, frustration tolerance, organization and internal structure, and self-awareness | In B. J. Hemphill-Pearson (1999a), Assessments in occupational therapy mental health: An integrative approach (pp. 139–152) |
| *Build A City: A Projective Task Concept* (Clark, 1999) | Adults with psychosocial dysfunction who are in group therapy | Group task or activity that evaluates interactions within a standardized situation and utilizes the constructive, doing process valued in occupational therapy | Communication and work skills within a group; positive and negative interactions between group members | In B. J. Hemphill-Pearson (1999a), Assessments in occupational therapy mental health: An integrative approach (pp. 155–170) |
| *Canadian Occupational Performance Measure* (COPM; Bowman & Llewellyn, 2002; Law et al., 1991; 1994) | Individuals age 7 through adults; individuals with disabilities | Outcome measured designed to detect changes in client's perception of occupational performance; based on the Model of Occupational Performance | Three subareas are measured (self-care, productivity, and leisure) with total scores obtained for performance and satisfaction; based on the Canadian Model of Occupational Performance | Canadian Association of Occupational Therapists CTTC Bldg 3400-1125 Colonel By Drive Ottawa, ON K1S 5R1 Canada |

*continues*

## TABLE 9-5

### Psychosocial Assessment in Occupational Therapy: Cognitive and General Assessment continued

| Test | Target Population | Purpose | Variables Assessed | Publisher |
|---|---|---|---|---|
| Cognitive Adaptive Skills Evaluation (CASE; Masagatani, 1994; 1999) | Clients with psychosocial dysfunction; can be used with adults and adolescents with developmental delays or cognitive dysfunction | Survey functional skills to examine individual's cognitive skills while performing a task and responding to interview questions | Performance summary using defined behavioral criteria based on analysis of task completion and responses to interview questions | In B. J. Hemphill-Pearson (1999a), Assessments in occupational therapy mental health: An integrative approach (pp. 279–284) |
| Functional Life Scale (FLS; Dittmar & Gresham, 1997; Sarno, Sarno, & Levita, 1973; Sapountzi-Krepiaet et al., 1998) | Adults in the community | Assessment of an individual's ability to participate in activities of daily living performed by most people | · Forty-four items in five categories:<br>• cognition<br>• activities of daily living<br>• activities in the home<br>• outside activities<br>• social interaction | In Archives of Physical Medicine and Rehabilitation (1973), 54, 214–220 |
| Goal Attainment Scaling (GAS; Cot & Finch, 1991; Ottenbacher & Cusick, 1990; Rockwood, Joyce, & Stolee, 1997; Stolee, Rockwood, Fox, & Streiner, 1992) | Adolescents through adults | Assess changes in performance self-care goals | Range of change from expected change (0) to below average (−2, −1) and above average (+2, +1) | In:<br>American Journal of Occupational Therapy (1990), 44, 519–525<br>Journal of the American Geriatrics Society (1992), 4, 575–578<br>Physiotherapy Canada (1991), 43, 19–22 |
| Independent Living Behavior Checklist (ILBC; Walls, Zane, & Thveldt, 1979) | Adults with intellectual disabilities or psychosocial disorder | Assess the ability for adults with disabilities to function in society | • mobility skills<br>• self-care skills<br>• home maintenance and safety skills<br>• food skills<br>• social and communication skills<br>• functional academic skills. | West Virginia Research and Training Center One Dunbar Plaza, Suite E, Dunbar, WV 25064 Or: http://www.eric.ed.gov/ PDFS/ED193848.pdf |

### TABLE 9-6

## Psychosocial Assessment of Independent Living Skills

| Test | Target Population | Purpose | Variables Assessed | Publisher |
|---|---|---|---|---|
| *Bay Area Functional Performance Evaluation* (BaFPE; 2nd ed.; Klyczek, 1999; Klyczek & Stanton, 2008; Williams & Bloomer, 1987) | Adults with psychosocial dysfunction | Two components: Task Oriented Assessment (TOA), which assesses goal-directed abilities, as well as cognitive, performance, and affective areas of function; Social Interaction Scale (SIS), which assesses social behaviors observed in 5 different settings | 12 functional parameters (e.g., memory, organization, attention, abstraction, task completion, affective and behavioral impression) and 7 categories of verbal and nonverbal social interaction | Available from: Allegro 1833 West Main Street, Suite 131 Mesa, AZ 85201 http://www.allegromedical.com/patient-care-c530/bafpe-bay-area-functional-performance-evaluation-p192719.html |
| *Canadian Occupational Performance Measure* (COPM, 4th ed.; Baptiste & Rochon, 1999; Law et al., 1991; 1994; 2004) | Clients with disabilities; can be used with children as young as age 7 | Outcome measured designed to detect changes in client's perception of occupational performance | Self-care, productivity, leisure, performance and satisfaction; based on the Canadian Model of Occupational Performance | Canadian Association of Occupational Therapists CTTC Bldg 3400–1125 Colonel By Drive Ottawa, ON K1S 5R1 Canada Phone: (613) 523–CAOT (2268) |
| *Comprehensive Occupational Therapy Evaluation* (COTE; Brayman, 2008; Brayman, Kirby, Meisenheimer, & Short, 1976; Kunz & Brayman, 1999) | Adults with acute psychosocial dysfunction who are hospitalized | Provides standard, objective means of rating behaviors of hospitalized patients on a frequent basis | General behavior, interpersonal behavior, task behaviors | In B. J. Hemphill-Pearson (2008), *Assessments in occupational therapy mental health: An integrative approach* (2nd. ed; pp. 113–124; 405–412) |
| *FIM™* Formerly known as Functional Independent Measure (Granger, Sherwood, Greer, 1977; Keith, Granger, Hamilton, & Sherwin, 1987; Granger et al., 2010); http://www.scireproject.com/outcome-measures/functional-independence-measure-fim | Adults | Developed as part of the Uniform Data System for Medical Rehabilitation to assess independent performance in self-care, toileting, transfers, locomotion, communication, and social cognition | 18 activities, 13 with motor emphasis related to self-care; 5 with a cognitive emphasis involving communication | Available from: Uniform Data System for Medical Rehabilitation 270 Northpointe Parkway, Suite 300 Amherst, New York 14228 Phone: (716) 817–7800 FAX: (716) 568–0037 http://www.udsmr.org/ |

*continues*

## TABLE 9-6

**Psychosocial Assessment of Independent Living Skills** *continued*

| Test | Target Population | Purpose | Variables Assessed | Publisher |
|---|---|---|---|---|
| *Independent Living Skills Evaluation* (ILSE; Johnson, Vinnicombe, & Merrill, 1981) | Adults (age 18 and above) with chronic psychosocial dysfunction who are living in independent living arrangements or living independently | Assess levels of living skills in areas necessary for independent community living | Ten major categories of independent living in home, community, and personal areas | Community Living Experiences, Inc. The Independent Living Project 291 North Tenth Street San Jose, CA 95112 Or: http://www.informaworld.com/smpp/content-db=all~content=a904375711 |
| *Kohlman Evaluation of Living Skills* (KELS; 3rd ed.; McGourty, 1988; Pickens et al., 2007; Thomson, 1992; 1999) | Clients with acute psychiatric disorders, older patients in acute care hospitals; adolescent through older must be used cautiously with individuals hospitalized for more than 1 month | Quick assessment to provide information about a person's ability in everyday functioning in daily living skills, independent living, and work/leisure | Seventeen living skills in areas of self-care, safety/health, money management, transportation/telephone, work/leisure | American Occupational Therapy Association 4720 Montgomery Lane P.O. Box 31220 Bethesda, MD 20824-1220 Phone: (301) 652-2682 |
| *Milwaukee Evaluation of Daily Living Skills* (MEDLS; Haertlein, 1999; Leonardelli, 1988) | Adults with chronic mental illness who are inpatients or outpatients in a community mental health clinic (CMHC) | Assessment of behavior and skills needed for adequate functioning in the client's living situation | Twenty subtests measuring basic living skills, safety, communication, and transportation | In B. J. Hemphill-Pearson (1999a), *Assessments in occupational therapy mental health: An integrative approach* (pp. 245–257) |
| *Performance Assessment of Self-Care Skill: Version 3.1* (PASS; Holm & Rogers, 2008) | Adults | Assess the types of assistance needed to stay in or remain in the community | MOB, ADL, and IADL from perspectives of independence, safety, and task outcome | In B. J. Hemphill-Pearson (2008), *Assessments in occupational therapy mental health: An integrative approach* (2nd ed.; pp. 101–110) |
| *Street Survival Skills Questionnaire* (SSSQ; Linkenhoker & McCarron, 1979; 1993) | Adolescents and adults with developmental disabilities, including psychosocial dysfunction | Assessment of specific aspects of adaptive behavior needed for independent living | Nine areas of adaptive behavior, including functional signs, tools, health and safety, time, and money | McCarron-Dial Systems, Inc. P.O. Box 35285 Dallas, TX 75235-0285 Phone: (214) 634-2863 Fax: (214) 634-9970 http://www.mccarrondial.com/index.html#anchor556866 |

## TABLE 9-7

**Psychosocial Assessment of Stress**

| Test | Target Population | Purpose | Variables Assessed | Publisher |
|------|------------------|---------|--------------------|-----------|
| Occupational Stress Inventory–Revised (OSI-R; Osipow & Spokane, 1987) | Employed adults (age 18 to 70) | Generic occupational stress inventory that applies across different occupations, built on a theoretical model | Occupational adjustment, stress, psychological strain, and coping resources | SIGMA Assessment Systems, Inc. P.O. Box 610757 Port Huron, MI 48061-0757 Phone: (800) 265–1285 http://sigmaassessmentsystems.com/ |
| Stress Audit Questionnaire (Miller & Smith, 1983; Miller, Smith, & Mehler, 1988) | Adults | Operationalization of biobehavioral model of stress into a self-report questionnaire | Situational stress, symptoms and vulnerability factors | Biobehavioral Institute 13309 Beacon Street Suite 202 Brookline, MA 02146 |
| Stress Management Questionnaire (SMQ; Stein, 1987; Stein, Bentley, & Natz, 1999; Stein & Cutler, 2002; Stein, Grueschow, Hoffman, Taylor, & Tronback, 2003) | Typical adults and adults (18 and above) with disabilities | Assess symptoms precipitated by stress, stressors that cause a stress response, and coping activities used to manage stress | Symptoms of stress, stressors, and copers | In B. J. Hemphill-Pearson (2008), Assessments in occupational therapy mental health: An integrative approach (2nd ed.; pp. 293–307) Or: Cengage Learning, Inc. P.O. Box 6904, Florence, KY 41022-6904 Phone: (800) 354–9706 http://www.cengage.com/search/productOverview.do?N=+14&Ntk=P_Isbn13&Ntt=9780766842588 |
| Survey of Recent Life Experiences (SLRE: de Jong, Timmerman, & Emmelkamp, 1996; Kohn & McDonald, 1992) | Adults | Measure of daily hassles in the lives of adults over the past month | Social and cultural difficulties; work; time pressure; finances; social acceptability; and social victimization | Journal of Behavioral Medicine (1992), 15, 221–236 |

**TABLE 9-8**

## Psychosocial Assessment of Leisure Skills

| Test | Target Population | Purpose | Variables Assessed | Publisher |
|------|-------------------|---------|--------------------|-----------|
| *Leisure Activities Finder* (LAF; Holmberg, Rosen, & Holland, 1999) Part of the Self-Directed Search products | Adults | Identify leisure time activities | Identification of leisure time activities using the self-directed search summary codes | Psychological Publications, Inc. P.O. Box 3577 Thousand Oaks, CA 91359-0577 Phone: (800) 345–TEST (8378) http://www.tjta.com/products/TST_038.htm |
| *Occupational Performance History Interview* (OPH-II; Kielhofner et al., 2004) | Adolescents and adults who are capable of responding to a life-history questionnaire. | Gather history of work, play, and self-care performance in order to determine the impact of disability and future goals | Five content areas of occupational performance, based on the Model of Human Occupation | Available from: UIC COLLEGE OF APPLIED HEALTH SCIENCES 1919 West Taylor Street Room 560 AHSB MC 528 Chicago, IL 60612–7249 Or: http://www.moho.uic.edu/assess/ophi%202.1.html |
| *Role Activity Performance Scale* (RAPS; Good-Ellis, 1999; Good-Ellis, Fine, Spencer, & Divittis, 1987) | Adults with acute or chronic psychiatric disorders | Measure range of past and present role functioning as basis for treatment planning | Twelve role domains in home, community, or interpersonal relationships up to an 18-month period | In B.J. Hemphill-Pearson (1999a), Assessments in occupational therapy mental health: An integrative approach, (pp. 205–226) |

## TABLE 9-8

### Psychosocial Assessment of Leisure Skills

| Test | Target Population | Purpose | Variables Assessed | Publisher |
|------|-------------------|---------|--------------------|-----------|
| Role Checklist (Dickerson, 2008; Oakley, 1988; Oakley, Kielhofner, Barris, & Reichler 1986) | Adults, adolescents, and older people with psychosocial or physical dysfunction | Assess individual's perception of and identification with roles | Continuous, disrupted changes in past, present, and future roles, and the degree of value for each role | In B. J. Hemphill-Pearson (2008), Assessments in occupational therapy mental health: An integrative approach (2nd ed., pp. 251–258, 440-440) Also available from: http://www.moho.uic.edu/images/assessments/Accessible%20Role%20Checklist.pdf |
| Volitional Questionnaire–Version 4.1. (VQ; Chern, Kielhofner, de las Heras, & Magalhaes, 1996; de las Heras, Geist, Kielhofner, & Li, 2007; Li & Kielhofner, 2004) | Adolescents and adults | Provide insight into an individual's inner motives and how the environment affects volition | Level of volition in achievement, competency, and exploration | American Journal of Occupational Therapy (1996), 50, 516–525 Available from: MOHO Clearing House at: http://www.moho.uic.edu/assess/vq.html |

The *Minnesota Multiphasic Personality Inventory* (MMPI), first published in 1942, is the most extensively used test for diagnosing psychological maladjustment. The researcher using objective personality tests should use caution in interpreting results. The methods of administering the tests and the subject's attitude toward the tests potentially can affect the results. Factors such as noise distractions, unmotivated and uncooperative subjects, and subject faking (sometimes referred to as *malingering)* are some of the problems encountered in personality testing. The ethical consideration in personality testing is another major consideration. The researcher should make efforts to ensure the subject's anonymity and confidentiality. Most of the tests can only be given by evaluators trained in personality assessment. Some of the more common tests are described in the following paragraphs.

- *Minnesota Multiphasic Personality Inventory-2* (MMPI-2; Hathaway & McKinley, 1970; PsychCorp/Pearson Assessments) consists of 550 true-false items used for measuring adjustment on 10 psychiatric diagnostic scales. The test takes from 2–3 hours and is given to adults.
- *Million Adolescent Personality Inventory* (MAPI; Million, Green, & Meagher, 1982; PsychCorp/Pearson Assessments) is a personality test for adolescents ages 13 and up. The test is written in language understood by adolescents and is based on a model of personality development rather than clinical pathology. The paper-and-pencil test must be scored by computer through the National Computer Systems.
- *Personality Inventory for Children-2* (PIC–2; Lachar & Gruber, 2001; Western Psychological Services) is a questionnaire containing true-false items completed by an informant (usually the parent). The scale consists of three broad scales covering categories such as behaviors at home and school, family interactions, educational achievement, and possible diagnoses. Results can be compared with 12 clinical types for use in differential diagnosis. The scale can be used with children ages 3 through 16.

- *Children's Depression Inventory* (CDI-2; Kovacs, 2011; Pearson Assessment), consists of self-rating items in which the client must choose between one of three sentences that best describes his or her experience in the past two weeks. The test is sensitive to changes in mood and provides a valid severity level of depression. The test is designed for ages 7 to 17 and takes about 15 minutes to complete.
- *Sixteen Personality Factor Questionnaire* (5th ed.; 16PF; Cattell, Cattell, & Cattell, 1993; PsychCorp/Pearson Assessments) is a forced choice test used for measuring 16 independent factors of personality. It is designed for high school students and college and adult subjects and takes about an hour to administer.

### 9.9.2 Physical Dysfunction, Motor Control, Pain, and Independent Living

Tests of functional capacity, vocational aptitude, pain, and independent living assess the degree to which an individual can live and work independently in the community. They assess an individual's ability to perform physical movements as they relate to work, vocational activities, and activities of daily living. These measures are extremely important to rehabilitation research in determining whether an individual can return to work or live in independent housing.

**Functional capacity evaluations (FCEs)** are comprehensive and systematic approaches that measure the client's overall physical ability such as muscle strength, endurance, joint range of motion, ambulation, sitting, standing, and lifting. According to the American Physical Therapy Association (APTA, 2008) guidelines for evaluating functional capacity:

A Functional Capacity Evaluation (FCE) is a comprehensive battery of performance based tests that is used commonly to determine ability for work, activities of daily living, or leisure activities. ... The Functional Capacity Evaluation today quantifies safe functional abilities, and is a pivotal resource for

   1.1 Return-to-work and job-placement decisions

   1.2 Disability evaluation

   1.3 Determination of how non-work-related illness and injuries impact work performance

   1.4 Determination of functioning in non-occupational setting

   1.5 Intervention and treatment planning

   1.6 Case management and case closure (p.1)

Additional information about FCEs, including the relationship of function to job requirements, can be found in APTA guidelines, located at http://www.apta.org/AM/Template.cfm?Section=Home&Template=/CM/ContentDisplay.cfm&ContentID=68532

**Work samples** are well-defined activities that are similar to actual jobs. They can be used to assess an individual's vocational aptitudes, worker characteristics, and vocational interests. **Independent living evaluations** test the degree to which an individual can perform the activities of daily living. They include self-care, communication, leisure, shopping, mobility, and related areas. Table 9–9 summarizes information about each of these areas and gives examples of evaluation instruments.

### Outcome Measures and Functional Assessment

There is a rising trend in health care to demonstrate effectiveness and client satisfaction. **Outcome measures** have been designed to evaluate the overall functional status of clients who have received treatment and rehabilitation services in hospitals, outpatient clinics, rehabilitation centers, and home environments. These outcome measures (Keith, 1984) are usually designed for specific populations such as individuals with stroke, brain injury, spinal cord injury, low back pain, psychological diagnoses, and developmental disabilities. The outcome measures evaluate the client's ability to perform functional activities of daily living, the degree of

pain intensity, ability to work, to engage in leisure activities, to have restful sleep, to drive, to be mobile in the community, to communicate, to ambulate, to academically achieve, and to perform other activities related to functional abilities. Following is a list of some commonly used outcome measures for rehabilitation (also see Applegate, Blass, & Williams, 1990).

- *Levels of Rehabilitation Scale* (LORS-II; Carey & Posavac, 1980; 1982), designed to obtain functional ratings from individuals who are in hospital-based rehabilitation programs.
- *Katz Index of Independence in ADL* (Katz, Ford, Moskowitz, Jackson, & Jaffe, 1963), developed for use with rehabilitation in patients.
- *Functional Assessment Screening Questionnaire* (Granger & Wright, 1993), an instrument used with patients who have undergone rehabilitation.
- *Global Assessment of Functioning* (American Psychiatric Association, 2000), used with individuals with psychosocial diagnoses.
- *The Multilevel Assessment Instrument* (Lawton, Moss, Fulcomer, & Kleban, 1982), designed for older individuals.
- *Unified ADL Evaluation Form* (Donaldson, Wagner, & Gresham, 1973).
- *Functional Life Scale* (Sarno, Sarno, & Levita, 1973).
- *Community Integration Questionnaire* (Willer, Ottenbacher, & Coad, 1994), used with individuals with traumatic brain injury.
- *Barthel Index* (Mahoney & Barthel, 1965), designed to evaluate the degree of assistance required by an individual on 10 items of self-care and mobility.
- *Health Status Questionnaire* 2.0 (HSQ® 2.0; Pearson Assessments), used to assess the functional status of adults with chronic illnesses.
- The *Sickness Impact Profile* (Bergner, Bobbitt, Carter, & Gilson, 1981; Gilson et al., 1975), used to assess a patient's function in such areas as sleep and rest, work, social interactions, leisure, and emotional behavior.

## TABLE 9-9

### Functional Assessment of Physical Dysfunction

| | Functional Capacity Evaluations | Motor Control/Motor Skills | Pain | Independent Living Skills |
|---|---|---|---|---|
| **Purpose** | To evaluate a person's functional physical abilities as they relate to work performance (Lechner, Page, & Sheffield, 2008; Lechner, Roth, & Straaton, 1991) | To evaluate a person's functional motor activities | To evaluate a client's pain to determine effectiveness of treatment (Ross & LaStayo, 1997) | To assess activities of daily living skills needed to function successfully in the community (Power, 2006) |
| **Sample of Variables Assessed** | • range of motion<br>• muscle strength<br>• coordination<br>• manual dexterity<br>• muscle endurance<br>• position tolerance | • muscle tone<br>• postural control<br>• gross mobility<br>• somatosensory function<br>• functional hand skills<br>• ambulation<br>• balance | • pain intensity<br>• pain tolerance<br>• pain location<br><br>See:<br><br>http://www.painedu.org/Downloads/NIPC/Pain%20Assessment%20Scales.pdf and http://painconsortium.nih.gov/pain_scales/ | • social skills<br>• self-care<br>• safety and health<br>• communication<br>• transportation<br>• money management<br>• home making<br>• leisure activities |
| **Examples of Widely Used Instruments** | BTE Technologies (formerly Baltimore Therapeutic Equipment; 2010) http://www.btetech.com/eval_rehab_systems.htm<br><br>Grip Dynamometers (Bohannon, Peolsson, Massy-Westropp, Desrosiers, & Bear-Lehman, 2006; Gilliam & Barstow, 1997) Available from: Rehabilitation outlet (http://www.rehaboutlet.com/grip_hand_dynamometer.htm) or Sammons Preston (http://www.pattersonmedical.com/app.aspx?cmd=get_subsections&id=100565) | Assessment of Motor and Process Skills (AMPS; Fisher, 1994) http://www.ampsintl.com/AMPS/index.php<br><br>Bruininks-Oseretsky Test of Motor Proficiency, Second Edition (BOT-2; Bruinicks, 1978; Bruininks & Bruininks, 2005) | Descriptor Differential Scale (DDS; Gracely & Kwilosz, 1988) Available from: http://www.painedu.org/Downloads/NIPC/Pain%20Assessment%20Scales.pdf<br><br>McGill Pain Questionnaire (MPQ; Melzack, 1975) Available from: https://www.cebp.nl/vault_public/filesystem/?ID=1400 | Barthel Index (Collin, Wade, Davies, & Horne, 1988; Mahoney & Barthel, 1965; Sainsbury, Seebass, Bansal, & Young, 2005) http://www.strokecenter.org/trials/scales/barthel.pdf<br><br>Functional Autonomy Measurement System (SMAF; Hébert, Carrier, & Bilodeau, 1988) |

## TABLE 9-9

**Functional Assessment of Physical Dysfunction**

| Functional Capacity Evaluations | Motor Control/Motor Skills | Pain | Independent Living Skills |
|---|---|---|---|
| Goniometric Range of Motion (Gilliam & Barstow, 1997) Available from: Rehab Outlet (http://www.rehaboutlet.com/goniometers.htm) or Sammons Preston (http://www.pattersonmedical.com/app.aspx?cmd=get_subsections&id=100571) | Carr and Shepherd's Motor Assessment Scale for Stroke Patients (Carr, Shepherd, Nordholm, & Lynne, 1985; Poole & Whitney, 1988) | Medical Rehabilitation Follow Along™ (MRFA; Baker, Granger, & Fiedler, 1997) | FIM™ Formerly known as Functional Independent Measure (Granger, Sherwood, Greer, 1977; Keith, Granger, Hamilton, & Sherwin, 1987) http://www.scireproject.com/outcome-measures/functional-independence-measure-fim |
| Isointertal Back Testing (Simmonds, 1997; Vissing et al., 2008) | Functional Test for the Hemiparetic Upper Extremity (Okkema & Culler, 1988; Wilson, Baker, & Craddock, 1984) | Numerical Pain Rating Scale (Childs, Piva, & Fritz, 2005; Jensen, Karoly, & Braver, 1986) | Functional Status Index (FSI; Jette, 1980; 1987) |
| Jebsen Hand Function Test (Jebsen, Taylor, Trieschmann, Trotter, & Howard, 1969; SCIRE, 2010) | Fugl-Meyer Assessment (Fugl-Meyer, Jääskö, Leyman, Olsson, & Steglind, 1975; Gladstone, Danells, & Black, 2002) | Oswestry Disability Index (Fairbank & Pynsent, 2000a; 2000b) Available from: http://http://www.spineguys.com/images/pdfs/ROQ.pdf | Katz Index of Activities of Daily Living (KATZ-ADL; Katz, Down, Cash, & Grotz, 1970; Katz, Ford, Moskowitz, Jackson, & Jaffe, 1963; Staff of the Benjamin Rose Hospital, 1959; Wallace & Shelkey, 2006) |
| KEYMethod (Key, 1996; Key Functional Methods, 2010) Available from: Key Functional Assessments, Inc. 300 Carlsbad Village Drive Suite 108A,# 99 Carlsbad, CA 92008 Phone: 800–333–3KEY (3539) or 760–729-2732 http://www.keymethod.com/key_system/ | Rivermead Mobility Index (Collen, Wade, Robb, Bradshaw, 1991; Wade, Collen, Robb, Warlow, 1992) http://www.scireproject.com/outcome-measures/rivermead-mobility-index-rmi Available from: http://www.medicaleducation.co.uk/resources/Rivmob.pdf | Pain Discomfort Scale (PDS; Jensen, Karoly, & Harris, 1991) | Kenny Self-Care Evaluation (Schoening et al., 1965; Schoening & Iversen, 1968) |

continues

## TABLE 9-9

### Functional Assessment of Physical Dysfunction *continued*

| Functional Capacity Evaluations | Motor Control/Motor Skills | Pain | Independent Living Skills |
|---|---|---|---|
| Manual muscle tests (MMTs; Daniels & Worthingham, 1986; Hislop & Montgomery, 2002; Kendall, McCreary, & Provance, 1993) | | Pain Drawing (Margolis, Chibnall, & Tait, 1988; Margolis, Tait, & Krause, 1986; Ransford, Cairns, & Mooney, 1976; Schwartz & DeGood, 1984) Available from: http://www.aapmr.org/zdocs/condtreat/paindrawing.pdf | Klein-Bell Activities of Daily Living Scale (Klein-Bell ADL Scale; Dahlgren Karlsson, Lundgren Nilsson, Fridén, & Claesson, 2007; Klein & Bell, 1982; 1993) |
| Medical Rehabilitation Follow Along™ (MRFA; Baker, Granger, & Fiedler, 1997) | | Short-Form McGill Pain Questionnaire –2 (SFMPQ–2; Dworkin et al., 2009; Melzack, R. 1987) Originally published, 1984; revised 2009 | Level of Rehabilitation Scale (LORS-II; Carey & Posavac, 1980; 1982) |
| Pinch meters and gauges: Available from: Sammons Preston (http://www.pattersonmedical.com/app.aspx?cmd=get_subsections&id=100566) Abledata (http://www.abledata.com/abledata.cfm?pageid=19327&ksectionid=19327&top=13607) | | Standardized Evaluation of Pain (StEP; Scholtz et al., 2009) http://www.plosmedicine.org/article/info%3Adoi%2F10.1371%2Fjournal.pmed.1000047 | Patient Evaluations Conference System (PECS®; Harvey & Jellinek, 1981) Available from: Hollis M. Jellinek, Dept of Rehabilitation Medicine, E3/350 Clinical Science Center, 600 Highland Ave, Madison WI 53792, USA. Dr. R. F. Harvey MD, Vice President and Chief of Medical Staff, Marianjoy Hospital, Roosevelt Road, PO Box 795, Wheaton, Illinois USA 60189. |

## TABLE 9-9

### Functional Assessment of Physical Dysfunction

| Functional Capacity Evaluations | Motor Control/Motor Skills | Pain | Independent Living Skills |
|---|---|---|---|
| Work Capacity Evaluation (Matheson, 1988; Matheson & Ogden, 1987) Available from: Matheson (http://www.roymatheson.com/products/all-products) | | Verbal Rating Scale (VSR; Cork et al., 2004; Gracely, McGrath, & Dubner, 1978) | PULSES Profile (Granger, 1976; Marshall, Heisel, & Grinnell, 1999; Moskowitz & McCann, 1957) Available from: https://www.cebp.nl/vault_public/filesystem/?ID=1471 |
| | | Visual Analog Scale (VAS; Carlsson, 1983; Cork et al., 2004) | Safety Assessment of Function and the Environment for Rehabilitation (SAFER; Chiu, Oliver, Marshall, & Letts, 2001; Oliver, Blathwayt, Brackley, & Tamaki, 1993) SAVER-HOME (Chui & Oliver, 2006; Oliver, Chiu, Marshall, & Goldsilver, 2003) |
| | | | Structured Assessment of Independent Living Skills (SAILS; Mahurin, DeBettingnies, & Pirozzolo, 1991) |

- *FIM-TM (previously called Functional Independence Measure*; Keith, Granger, Hamilton, & Sherwin, 1987), designed as a tool to evaluate the patient's ability to complete activities of daily living.
- *Rehabilitation Best Practices* standards, published by the Vancouver Health Authority Rehabilitation Services, found at http://www.viha.ca/NR/rdonlyres/B9279155-0172-40E7-86F4-80D026B68855/0/iadl1_stnd_13_doc.pdf

### 9.9.3 Vocational and Prevocational

In assessing an individual's prevocational ability, an evaluator seeks information on basic ability levels required for specific occupations. Most prevocational tests involve some aspect of motor coordination. Such tests as the *Bennett Mechanical Comprehension Test* (2nd ed. Bennett, 1994), *Crawford Small Parts Dexterity Test* (Crawford & Crawford, 1985), *Strömberg Dexterity Test*, and *O'Conner Tweezer Dexterity Test* (see Table 9–10) require the subject to perform tasks using small tools in an assembly operation. Work samples are used to assess an individual's vocational aptitudes, worker characteristics, and vocational interests (Nadolsky, 1974) in areas of vocational potential in various fields, gross and fine manual dexterity, visual and tactile discrimination, and work habits. The tests purport to measure skill proficiencies related to industrial work. Tests have been devised, such as the *McCarron-Dial Systems* (MDS, n.d.; McCarron & Dial, 1973) to evaluate work behavior at a sheltered workshop as indicative of vocational aptitude. Other work sampling tests include the *Micro Tower System of Vocational Evaluation* (ICD Rehabilitation and Research Center, NY, 1977) and the *VITAS: Vocational Interest, Temperament and Aptitude System* (Abrams, 1979; Vocational Research Institute, 1980). More elaborate methods for assessing vocational aptitude in various industrial occupations are available through the Valpar International Corporation (http://www.valpar int.com) and Stout University.

There are many self-devised, unpublished, prevocational tests that are used in sheltered workshops, occupational therapy clinics, and special schools. Some of the more common prevocational tests are listed in Table 9–10, and Table 9–11 provides examples of the more common work sample systems and their addresses.

#### Vocational Interest Tests

Most investigators constructing **vocational interest tests** assume that:

- Vocational interests are stable characteristics.
- Vocational interests can be measured by paper-and-pencil tests.
- Vocational interests are grouped around clusters of interest.
- Individuals in occupations share common interests and characteristics.
- There is a positive relationship between vocational interests and choice of occupation.
- Job satisfaction is related to vocational interest and aptitude.

The *Strong Vocational Interest Test* (SCII; Strong, Campbell, & Hansen, 1985) is the test most widely used by clinical psychologists and social researchers. Table 9–12 lists other widely used tests available for measuring vocational interest.

### 9.9.4 Geriatrics

A number of tests have been developed specifically for the geriatric population. Many of these tests can be administered in a hospital, nursing home, or home setting. Table 9–13 describes some of the most commonly used tests administered by occupational therapists.

### 9.9.5 Pediatrics

The basic assumption underlying all child development scales is that development is vertical, sequential, and hierarchical. Arnold Gesell and associates in the Children's Development Laboratories at Yale University during the 1920s and 1930s used observational analysis of children's behavior to develop norms. Gesell provided the earliest data correlating age with task attainment in such areas as perceptual-motor, language, and personal-social.

Since Gesell, other developmental researchers have provided data demonstrating that the growth of human abilities are linked to a biological clock

## TABLE 9-10

### Vocational and Prevocational Tests

| Test | Target Population | Purpose | Variables Assessed | Publisher |
|------|-------------------|---------|--------------------|-----------|
| *Bennett Hand Tool Dexterity Test* (Bennett, 1946) | Adolescents through adults | Assesses basic skills necessary for any job requiring hand tools | • fine motor coordination<br>• manual dexterity | Pearson Assessment/Psych Corp<br>Attn: Customer Service<br>19500 Bulverde Road<br>San Antonio, TX 78259-3701<br>Phone: (800) 627–7271<br>Fax: (800) 232–1223<br>http://psychcorp.<br>pearsonassessments.com/<br>pai/ca/cahome.htm |
| *Bennett Mechanical Comprehension Test* (Bennett, 1994) | Adolescents through adults | Paper-pencil test that measures the understanding of mechanical principles or general physical concepts in practical situations | • mechanical comprehension | Pearson Assessment/Psych Corp<br>Attn: Customer Service<br>19500 Bulverde Road<br>San Antonio, TX 78259-3701<br>Phone: (800) 627–7271<br>Fax: (800) 232–1223<br>http://psychcorp.<br>pearsonassessments.com/<br>pai/ca/cahome.htm |
| *Complete Minnesota Dexterity Test* (n.d.; also known as Minnesota Rate of Manipulation Test) | Adolescents through adults | Measures simple hand-eye coordination and gross motor skills | • placing<br>• turning<br>• displacing<br>• one-hand turning and placing<br>• two-hand turning and placing | Lafayette Instrument Company<br>P.O. Box 5729<br>Lafayette, IN 47903-5729<br>Phone: (765) 423–1505<br>Fax: (765) 423–4111<br>Toll Free: (800) 428–7545 (US Only)<br>http://www.<br>lafayetteevaluation.<br>com/product_detail.<br>asp?ItemID=165 |

*continues*

## TABLE 9-10

**Vocational and Prevocational Tests** *continued*

| Test | Target Population | Purpose | Variables Assessed | Publisher |
|------|-------------------|---------|--------------------|-----------|
| *Crawford Small Parts Dexterity Test* (Crawford & Crawford, 1985) | Adolescents through adults | Measure fine eye-hand coordination for vocational skills | • fine-motor coordination<br>• manual dexterity | Pearson Assessment/Psych Corp<br>Attn: Customer Service<br>19500 Bulverde Road<br>San Antonio, TX 78259-3701<br>Phone: (800) 627-7271<br>Fax: (800) 232-1223<br>http://psychcorp.<br>pearsonassessments.com/<br>pai/ca/cahome.htm |
| *O'Connor Finger Dexterity Test* (O'Connor, circa 1920a) | Adolescents through adults | Assess rapid manipulation of small objects | • finger dexterity<br>• speed | Lafayette Instrument Company<br>P.O. Box 5729<br>Lafayette, IN 47903-5729<br>http://www.lafayetteevaluation.com/product_detail.asp?ItemID=161 |
| *O'Connor Tweezer Dexterity Test* (O'Connor, circa 1920b) | Adolescents through adults | Assess aptitude for work involving precision with small tool usage | • fine-motor coordination<br>• speed | Lafayette Instrument Company<br>P.O. Box 5729<br>Lafayette, IN 47903-5729<br>http://www.lafayetteevaluation.com/product_detail.asp?ItemID=162 |

## Vocational and Prevocational Tests

| Test | Target Population | Purpose | Variables Assessed | Publisher |
|------|-------------------|---------|--------------------|-----------|
| *Purdue Pegboard* (Tiffin, 1948) | Adults | Assess fine-motor dexterity | • gross movements of hands, fingers, and arms<br>• fingertip dexterity necessary for assembly tasks | Lafayette Instrument Company<br>P.O. Box 5729<br>Lafayette, IN 47903–5729<br>Phone: (765) 423–1505<br>Fax: (765) 423–4111<br>Toll Free: (800) 428–7545 (US Only)<br>http://www.lafayetteevaluation.com/product_detail.asp?ItemID=159 |
| *Roeder Manipulative Aptitude Test* (Roeder, 1970) | Adults | Assess fine-motor dexterity | • speed and accuracy for eye-hand coordination<br>• finger dexterity | Lafayette Instrument Company<br>P.O. Box 5729,<br>Lafayette, IN 47903–5729<br>Phone: (765) 423–1505<br>Fax: (765) 423–4111<br>Toll Free: (800) 428–7545 (US Only)<br>http://www.lafayetteevaluation.com/product_detail.asp?ItemID=169 |

## TABLE 9-11

**Examples of Work Sample Systems**

- *McCarron-Dial Systems, Inc.*
  http://www.mccarrondial.com/
     McCarron-Dial Systems, Inc., P.O. Box 35285, Dallas, TX 75235–0285
     Telephone: (214) 634–2863    Fax: (214) 634–9970
     E-mail: mds@mccarrondial.com

  An assessment system that assesses strengths and weaknesses in verbal-cognitive-language, sensory, motor; emotional, and integration-coping. Information from these factors "may be used to estimate the appropriate program level for serving individuals in a preschool, transitional planning, prevocational or vocational setting" (McCarron-Dial, n.d., p. 1 ). Used with individuals aged 4 through adult.

- *Micro-Tower System of Vocational Education*
  http://www.icdnyc.org/content/view/16/39/
     International Center for Disability ICD, 340 East 24th Street, New York, NY 10010
     Phone: (212) 585–6000    FAX: (212) 585–6262

  Work sample tests used to measure aptitudes (e.g., motor clerical skill, spatial perception, verbal, and numerical) required for semiskilled and unskilled jobs. Appropriate for adolescents through adults.

- *Mobile Vocational Evaluation* (MVE; Hester, 1994)
  http://www.lafayetteevaluation.com/product_detail.asp?ItemID=239
     Lafayette Instrument Company, P.O. Box 5729, Lafayette, IN 47903
     Telephone: (765) 423–1505    Fax: (765) 423–4111
     Toll Free: (800) 428–7545 (US Only)
     E-mail: info@lafayetteinstrument.com

  Normed on more than 1,500 individuals and linked to the Dictionary of Occupational Titles, this system is composed of a number of tests used in vocational assessment (e.g., *Minnesota Manual Dexterity Test, Lafayette Pegboard Test, Hester Reaction Time Test*) and designed to assist any individual with a disability to obtain a suitable vocation. For use with adolescents and adults in secondary and postsecondary schools, rehabilitation agencies, hospitals, and clinics. A Windows compatible computer-assisted testing system is used to analyze the data and present a listing of specific vocations based on client interests and abilities.

- *Physical Work Capacity Fitness Evaluation System*
  (PWC-FES; http://www.lafayetteevaluation.com/product_detail.asp?ItemID=223)
     Lafayette Instrument Company, P.O. Box 5729, Lafayette, IN 47903
     Telephone: (765) 423–1505    Fax: (765) 423–4111
     Toll Free: (800) 428–7545 (US Only)
     E-mail: info@lafayetteinstrument.com

  Well-researched and comprehensive evaluation using the *Physical Work Capacity* (PWC) and *Functional Capacity* (FC), which allows objective worker baseline physical information for physically demanding jobs. Evaluation provides data to develop treatment protocols for clients in rehabilitation. Application software is required for scoring and analyzing the results. The report can be used to make decisions about clients returning to work or new employees.

- *Talent Assessment Programs* (TAP; Nighswonger, 1981)
  http://www.talentassessment.com/programs_tap.php#test1
     Talent Assessment Inc., P.O. Box 5087, Jacksonville, FL 32247
     Toll Free Call: (800) 634–1472

  Comprehensive assessment program measuring visualization and retention, discrimination, and dexterity through 10 manual tests related to production level capacities and vocational aptitudes of individuals in areas applicable for occupations in trade, industrial, technical, and professional. A computer program is used to analyze the results and link abilities to occupations listed in the *Dictionary of Occupational Titles* (DOR) and occupational data from the Department of Labor. The test is appropriately used with adolescents through adults.

- *Valpar Component Work Samples* (Valpar, 1973)
  http://www.valparint.com/
     Valpar International Corporation, P. O. Box 5767, Tucson, AZ 85703
     Sales Office: (800) 633–3321      Fax: (262) 797–8488
     E-mail: sales@valparint.com

  A comprehensive work evaluation system designed to assess vocational abilities through 23 different work samples. The original samples were developed in 1973, but have been updated as needed. Tasks include mechanical, size, discrimination, range of motion and physical capacity, clerical abilities, assembly, coordination and motor dexterity, drafting skill, and electronic skills. Scores are obtained through computer-based programs, with the criterion-referenced scores linked to the *Revised Handbook for Analyzing Jobs* (RHAJ) and the *Dictionary of Occupational Titles* (DOT).

Additional information about work sample assessment and systems can be found in *A Guide to Vocational Assessment* (4th ed.) by P. W. Power, 2006, published by Pro-Ed in Austin, TX (http://www.proedinc.com/customer/default.aspx), or by contacting the Stout Vocational Rehabilitation Institute at the University of Wisconsin-Stout (http://www3.uwstout.edu/svri/index.cfm)

that determines when behavior unfolds at certain critical periods along an age continuum. Differences among child development tests are based on the factors identified and the methods used for assessment. These tests also vary in the time involved in administering a test and in the requirements needed to validly interpret results. For example, the *Denver Developmental Screening Test* (Frankenburg, Dodds, Archer, Shapiro, & Bresnick, 1990) takes about 15 minutes to administer by nonprofessional health aides, whereas the *Gesell Developmental Scale* requires at least 2 hours to administer by a professionally trained psychometrician. Examples of the most widely used child development scales are described in Table 9–14.

### 9.9.6 Special Populations

In addition to general tests in psychosocial function and physical disabilities, assessments have been developed for specific populations such as individuals with arthritis or stroke. These tests have been standardized for these specific populations and should not be used with typical individuals. Table 9–15 provides information about many of these tests.

### 9.9.7 Neuropsychological Batteries

Clinical neuropsychology is a relatively new field that attempts to relate behavior to brain functioning. Clinicians, therapists, and educators request neuropsychological testing in special cases. For example, neuropsychological testing is usually requested when a client has sustained a traumatic or acquired

brain injury. Neuropsychological testing may also be requested when a more specific understanding of an individual's strengths and weaknesses is desired. Although individual neuropsychological tests can be given, frequently neuropsychologists use a specific battery of tests generated by their particular philosophical stance.

The *Halsted-Reitan Neuropsychological Test Battery* (HRNTB; Reitan & Wolfson, 1985; 1993), used with adults, consists of up to 37 individual tests, each of which must be administered to obtain a complete profile of an individual's brain functioning. Diagnosis is dependent on (a) comparing the client's score with a comparison group, (b) comparing scores between individual tests, and (c) comparing differences between scores performed on the right or left side of the body. Based on the profile of scores, treatments for deficits are suggested. Although the original *Halsted-Reitan* has not been renormed, many of the individual tests have been renormed and incorporated into the *Dean-Woodcock Sensory-Motor Battery* (DWSMB; Dean & Woodcock, 2003).

Luria (1980) developed a second approach to neuropsychological testing by developing specific test items that would allow the clinician to identify the way in which a person approached a task. The *Luria-Nebraska Neuropsychological Battery* (LNNB; Golden, Purisch, & Hammeke, 1985) is an outgrowth of Luria's work. Although this battery is not frequently used, it does provide information for the clinician regarding brain-behavior relationships.

## TABLE 9-12

### Vocational Interest Tests

| Test | Target Population | Purpose | Variables Assessed | Publisher |
|------|-------------------|---------|--------------------|-----------|
| COPSystem (Knapp & Knapp, 1982; Knapp & Knapp-Lee, 1995; Knapp-Lee, Knapp, & Knapp, 1982) | Adolescents through adults | Identify occupational choices based on 14 occupational clusters through interests (COPS), abilities (CAPS), and values (COPES) | Self-administered inventory measures interests and values and paper-and-pencil tests assess abilities in 8 dimensions; results of all assessments are linked to 14 COPSystem Career Clusters | Educational & Industrial Testing Service, (EdITS) P.O. Box 7234 San Diego, CA 92126 Phone: (800) 416-1666 FAX: (619) 226-1666 http://www.edits.net/ |
| Geist Picture Interest Inventory-Revised (Geist, 1988) | Grade 8 through adult | Identify vocational and avocational interests using a minimum of language | Picture selection test measures occupational interest; Spanish and deaf forms available | Western Psychological Services 12031 Wilshire Blvd. Los Angeles, CA 90025-1251 Phone: (800) 648-8857 FAX: (310) 478-7838 http://portal.wpspublish.com/portal/page?_pageid=53,267719&_dad=portal&_schema=PORTAL |
| Kuder Career Search with Person Match (KCS; Zytowski, n.d.). Takes the place of the Kuder Occupational Interest Survey (Kuder, 1979; Kuder & Zytowski, 1991) | Middle school students, high school students, adults; not recommended for career choice at middle school level | Forced choice interest inventory using triads in which individual marks "most," "next most," and "least preferred"; use of the Kuder Skills Assessment (Zytowski & Luzzo, 2002) and Super'sWork Values (Zytowski, 2001) provides comprehensive career assessment | Pattern of interests similar to groups of people in six career clusters: <br>• Outdoor/Mechanical <br>• Science/Technical <br>• Arts/Communication <br>• Social/Personal Services <br>• Sales/Management | Kuder® Inc., 302 Visions Parkway Adel, IA 50003 Phone (800) 314-8972 http://www.kuder.com/solutions/kuder-assessments.html#kuder_career_search |

## TABLE 9-12

### Vocational Interest Tests

| Test | Target Population | Purpose | Variables Assessed | Publisher |
|---|---|---|---|---|
| *Reading-Free Vocational Interest Inventory* (Becker, 1981; 2000) | Adolescence and older people who are learning disabled, intellectually disabled, and disadvantaged | Measure vocational interests with special populations | Picture format measuring occupational interests; specifically designed for individuals who cannot read | PRO-ED, Inc. 8700 Shoal Creek Blvd. Austin, TX 78757–6897 Phone: (800) 897–3202 Fax: (800) 397–7633 http://www.proedinc.com/Customer/default.aspx |
| *Self-Directed Search® Form R* (4th ed.; SDS-R; Holland, 1994) and *Self-Directed Search ® Form E* (4th ed., SDS-E; Holland, 1994) | Form R: Ages 11 to 72 Form E: Ages 15 to 72 | Assess career interests using Holland's RIASEC theory. Form E is for those with poor reading skills; Form R, for typical individuals | Yields 3-letter summary code related to one's personality, using these factors: Realistic, Investigative, Artistic, Social, Enterprising, and Conventional | PAR, Inc. 16204 N. Florida Ave, Lutz, FL 33549 Phone: (800) 331–8378 http://www4.parinc.com/Products/Product.aspx?ProductID=SDS_R |
| *Strong Interest Inventory and Skills Confidence Inventory* (SCII; Betz, Borgen, & Harmon, 2004; Strong, Campbell, & Hansen, 1985) | Adolescents through adults | Assess occupational and leisure interests for individuals oriented toward college graduation and professional occupations | General Occupational Themes (GOTs), Basic Interest Scales (BISs), Personal Style Scales (PSSs), and Occupational Scales (OSs); scoring available online or mail-in | CPP, Inc. 1055 Joaquin Road, 2nd Floor Mountain View, CA 94043 Tel: (800) 624–1765 https://www.cpp.com/products/strong/index.aspx |
| *Wide Range Interest and Occupation Test—Second Edition* (WRIOT—2; 2003; Glutting & Wilkinson, 2003) | Junior high school through adult | Assess occupational interests | Picture format measuring occupational interest; adaptations for individuals who are blind; computer format available, to take in two sessions | Pearson Assessment/Psych Corp Attn: Customer Service 19500 Bulverde Road San Antonio, TX 78259-3701 Phone: (800) 627–7271 Fax: (800) 232–1223 http://psychcorp.pearsonassessments.com/pai/ca/cahome.htm |

## TABLE 9-13

### Geriatric Scales

| Test | Purpose | Variables Assessed | Format | Publisher |
|------|---------|--------------------|--------|-----------|
| **Cognitive Function** | | | | |
| Mini-Mental® State Examination, 2nd Edition™ (MMSE®-2™; Folstein & Folstein, 2010); User's Manual by Folstein, Folstein, White, & Messer, 2010) | Obtain a quantitative measure of cognitive performance for older adults with neurological dysfunction quickly Standard version (MMSE-2:SV) and Expanded version (MMSE-2:EV) available | Five areas of cognition:<br>• orientation<br>• memory<br>• attention and calculation<br>• recall<br>• following oral and written instructions | Oral questionnaire administered by examiner | *Journal of Psychiatric Research* (1975), 12, 189–198<br>PAR, Inc.<br>16204 N. Florida Ave, Lutz, FL 33549<br>Phone: (800) 331–8378<br>http://www4.parinc.com/Products/Product.aspx?ProductID=MMSE-2 |
| *Rivermead Behavioral Memory Test 3* (RBMT3; 3rd ed.; Wilson, Baddley, Cockburn, & Hiorns, n.d.; Wilson, Cockburn, & Baddley, 1991; Wilson et al., 2008) | Assess problems in memory and provide means for monitoring treatment outcomes | • immediate memory<br>• short-delay<br>• long-term memory<br>• overall memory function | Visual or verbal presentation of questions with verbal response | Pearson Assessment/Psych Corp<br>Attn: Customer Service<br>19500 Bulverde Road<br>San Antonio, TX 78259-3701<br>Phone: (800) 627–7271<br>Fax: (800) 232–1223<br>http://psychcorp.pearsonassessments.com/pai/ca/cahome.htm |
| *Short Portable Mental Status Questionnaire* (SPMSQ; Pfeiffer; 1975) | Quick assessment of the degree of intellectual impairment in older patients in the home or in a clinical setting | Level of intellectual functioning, taking into account educational level | Question and answer using pencil-and-paper | *Journal of the American Geriatrics Society* (1975), 23, 433–441<br>Available from http://www.npcrc.org/usr_doc/adhoc/psychosocial/SPMSQ.pdf |
| **Independent Living** | | | | |
| *Assessment of Living Skills and Resources-Revised 2* (ALSAR-R2; Clemson, Bundy Unsworth, & Fiatarone Singh, 2008; Williams et al., 1991) | Assess the living skills and resources in a community-dwelling of older residents to determine treatment protocol and assist in problem-solving | Assesses areas of IADL including:<br>• use of community resources<br>• leisure time<br>• medication<br>• finances<br>• home management | Rating scale, with scores combined to determine risk | Available from:<br>http://sydney.edu.au/health_sciences/ageing_work_health/docs/Clemson_ALSAR.pdf |

## TABLE 9-13

### Geriatric Scales

| Test | Purpose | Independent Living | | |
| | | Variables Assessed | Format | Publisher |
| --- | --- | --- | --- | --- |
| *Functional Assessment Scale* (FAS; Breines, 1988; 1996) | Scale designed to rate self-care function in patients who are in nursing homes or hospitals | Provides a single level of function, ranging from 1 "total care" to 10 "prepared to live independently" | Checklist-type rating scale | Geri-Rehab, Inc. 15 Hibbler Road Lebanon, NJ 08833 |
| *Instrumental Activities of Daily Living* (IADL Scale; Graf, 2007; Lawton & Brody, 1969) | Assess skills needed by older individuals to live independently | Eight categories of IADL (e.g., housekeeping, food preparation, finances) rated according to level of independence | Rating scale, with higher scores indicating need for more assistance | *Gerontologist* (1969), 9, 179–186 Available from: http://www.abramsoncenter. org/pri/documents/iadl.pdf |
| *Klein-Bell Activities of Daily Living Scale* (K-B Scale; Klein & Bell, 1982; 1993) | Developed to measure ADL independence in both adults and children and determine present status, changes in status, and activities for rehabilitation | Subdimensions:<br>• mobility<br>• emergency communication<br>• dressing<br>• elimination<br>• bathing/hygiene<br>• eating | Performance tasks in which individual is given a rating of "able to perform," "unable to perform," or "not applicable" | *Archives of Physical Medicine and Rehabilitation* (1982), 63, 335–338 Available from Health Sciences Center for Educational Resources, University of Washington, T–281 Health Sciences Building, Box 357161, Seattle, WA or from www.youngseo.ac.kr/ dep_info/homepage/dep_ home33/dep4/do... |
| *Maguire's Trilevel ADL Assessment* (Maguire, 1995) | Assess ADL abilities in older clients in personal areas, home, or sheltered environment | • communication<br>• food needs<br>• dressing<br>• hygiene<br>• organization<br>• mobility | Observation | In C. Lewis (1995), *Aging: The health care challenge: An interdisciplinary approach to assessment and rehabilitative management of the elderly* (pp. 61–71) |

*continues*

## TABLE 9-13

**Geriatric Scales** *continued*

| Test | Purpose | Independent Living | | Publisher |
|------|---------|-------------------|---|-----------|
| | | **Variables Assessed** | **Format** | |
| *Older Adults Resources and Services* (OARS; Duke University Center for the Study of Aging and Human Development, 1978; updated electronically, 2005) | Multidimensional instrument to obtain information in basic and instrumental activities of daily living for older clients living in the community | • social resources<br>• economic resources<br>• mental health<br>• physical health<br>• activities of daily living | Structured interview, now available online exclusively | Available from:<br>OARS<br>Center for the Study of Aging and Human Development<br>Box 3003<br>Duke University Medical Center<br>Durham, NC 27710, USA<br>http://www.geri.duke.edu/service/oars.htm |
| *Paracek Geriatric Rating Scale* (3rd ed.; Paracek & King, 1986) | Screening tool to assist mental health workers in treatment planning for older patients | • level of physical capabilities<br>• self-care skills<br>• social interaction skills | Likert scale, rated by mental health workers or clinicians | Center for Neurodevelopmental Studies<br>5340 West Glenn Drive<br>Glendale, AZ 85301<br>(623) 915–0345<br>In D. J. Mangen and W. A. Peterson (1992), *Research instruments in social gerontology* (Vol. 3, pp. 29–30, 79–81) |
| *Rapid Disability Rating Scale-2* (RDRS-2; Linn, 1967; Linn & Linn, 1982) | Assessment of functional disabilities in older clients | 16 items grouped into:<br>• activities of daily life<br>• sensory and communication<br>• mental/cognition | Rating scale | *Journal of the American Geriatrics Society* (1982), *30*, 378–382 |
| *Geriatric Hopelessness Scale* (Fry, 1984; Heisel, & Flett, 2005) | Assess attitudes of pessimism and futility in older clients toward themselves and their future | Attitudes toward:<br>• physical and cognitive abilities<br>• personal and interpersonal worth<br>• spiritual faith<br>• nurturance and respect | Rating scale | *Journal of Counseling Psychology* (1984), *31*, 322–331 |

## TABLE 9-13

**Geriatric Scales**

### Quality of Life

| Test | Purpose | Variables Assessed | Format | Publisher |
|------|---------|--------------------|--------|-----------|
| *Life Satisfaction Index* (LSI-K; Barrett & Murk, 2006; Koyano & Shibata, 1994; Neugarten, Havighurst & Tobin, 1961) | Quick measure of one's self-perception of well-being in older clients<br>Several different versions; originally conceived of by Neugarten, Havighurst, & Tobin (1961) | • cognitive/short-term<br>• cognitive/long-term<br>• emotional/short-term well-being | Self-administered paper-pencil test | The measurement of life satisfaction, in *Journal of Gerontology* (1961), 16, 134–143<br>Facts and Research in Gerontology (1994), Suppl. 2, 181–187<br>Barrett & Murk, 2006, http://hdl.handle.net/1805/1160 |

### Social Interaction

| Test | Purpose | Variables Assessed | Format | Publisher |
|------|---------|--------------------|--------|-----------|
| *Geriatric Depression Scale* (Sheikh & Yesavage 1986; Sheikh et al., 1991; Yesavage et al., 1983) | Easily administered survey used as screening instrument to evaluate depression | Level of depression:<br>• normal<br>• mild<br>• severe | Paper-and-pencil survey test, completed by client or clinician<br>Electronic version (short edition) also available at: http://www.stanford.edu/~yesavage/Testing.htm | *Journal of Psychiatric Research* (1983), 17, 37–49 |
| *Geriatric Rating Scale* (GRS; Plutchik et al., 1970) | Assessment of readiness of older patients to leave a hospital setting | • physical disability<br>• apathy<br>• communication failure<br>• socially irritating behavior | Observational based behavioral rating scale | *Journal of the Geriatric Society* (1970), 18, 491–500 |

## TABLE 9-14

**Pediatric Assessments**

| Developmental | Behavior | Motor and Sensory Integration | Visual, Auditory, and Motor Processing | Play |
|---|---|---|---|---|
| Assessment of Preterm Infants' Behavior (ABIP; Als, 1984; Als, Butler, Kosta, & McAnulty, 2005; Als, Duffy, & McAnulty, 1988a; 1988b) | Achenbach System of Empirically Based Assessment (ASEBA, Achenbach, 1991; Achenbach & Rescorla 2001; 2007; 2010) http://www.aseba.org/ | Alberta Infant Motor Scales (AIMS; Piper & Darrah, 1994; Piper, Pinnell, Darrah, Macguire, & Byrne, 1992) | Bender Visual-Motor Gestalt II (Bender, 1938; Koppitz, 1963; 1975; revised by Brannigan & Decker, 2003) http://psychcorp.pearsonassessments.com/pai/ca/cahome.htm Koppitz-II (Koppitz Developmental Screening; Reynolds, 2007) http://www.proedinc.com/Customer/default.aspx | Knox Preschool Play Scale–Revised Edition (Knox, 1974; 1997) |
| Bayley Scales of Infant and Toddler Development®, Third Edition (Bayley-III®; Pearson Assessments, 2005) http://psychcorp.pearsonassessments.com/pai/ca/cahome.htm | Attention Deficit Disorders Evaluation Scale (3rd ed.; ADDES-3; McCarney & Arthuad, 2004) http://www.hawthorne-ed.com/pages/adhd/ad2.html | DeGangi-Berk Test of Sensory Integration (DeGangi & Berk, 1983) http://portal.wpspublish.com/portal/page?_pageid=53,69337&_dad=portal&_schema=PORTAL | Brunicks-Osteresky Motor Proficiency (2nd ed; BOT-2; Bruinicks & Bruinicks, 2005) http://psychcorp.pearsonassessments.com/pai/ca/cahome.htm | Play History (Takata, 1969; 1974) |
| Denver Developmental Screening Test–II (DDST-II; Frankenburg, Dodds, Archer, Shapiro, & Bresnick, 1992) http://www.denverii.com/DenverII.html | Behavioral Assessment Scale of Oral Functions in Feeding (Stratton, 1981) | Erhardt Developmental Prehension Assessment (3rd ed.; Erhardt, 1994) http://www.erhardtproducts.com/edpa.html | Beery-Buktenica Developmental Test of Visual-Motor Integration, (6th ed.; BEERY™ VMI; Berry, Buktenica, & Berry, 2010) http://psychcorp.pearsonassessments.com/pai/ca/cahome.htm | Play Observation (Kalverboer, 1977) |

## TABLE 9-14

**Pediatric Assessments**

| Developmental | Behavior | Motor and Sensory Integration | Visual, Auditory, and Motor Processing | Play |
|---|---|---|---|---|
| Developmental Profile–3 (DP3; Alpern, 2007) http://portal.wpspublish.com/portal/page?_pageid=53,186601&_dad=portal&_schema=PORTAL | Behavior Assessment System for Children–2 (BASC–2; 2nd ed.; Reynolds & Kamphaus, 2004) http://psychcorp.pearsonassessments.com/pai/ca/cahome.htm | Miller Assessment for Preschoolers (MAP; Miller, 1988) http://portal.wpspublish.com/portal/page?_pageid=53,69640&_dad=portal&_schema=PORTAL | Motor-Free Visual Perception Test–3 (MVPT-3; 3rd ed.; Colarusso & Hammill, 2002) http://portal.wpspublish.com/portal/page?_pageid=53,69183&_dad=portal&_schema=PORTAL | Transdisciplinary Play-Based Assessment -2 (TPBA2; Linder, 2008) http://www.brookespublishing.com/store/books/linder-tpbai2/index.htm |
| Mullen Scales of Early Learning (Mullen, 1995) http://psychcorp.pearsonassessments.com/pai/ca/cahome.htm | Burks' Behavior Rating Scales, Second Edition (BBRS-2; Burks & Gruber, 2006) http://portal.wpspublish.com/portal/page?_pageid=53,267719&_dad=portal&_schema=PORTAL | QUEST: Quality of Upper Extremity Skills Test (QUEST; DeMatteo, Law, Russell, Pollock, Rosenbaum, & Walter, 1992; 1993). http://www.canchild.ca/en/measures/resources/1992_quest_manual.pdf | Peabody Developmental Motor Scales–2 (PDMS-2, 2nd ed.; Folio & Fewell, 2000) http://www.proedinc.com/customer/productView.aspx?ID=1783 | Westby Symbolic Play Scale (Westby, 1991; 2000) |
| Pediatric Evaluation of Disability Inventory (PEDI; Haley, Coster, Ludlow, Haltiwanger, & Andrellos, 1992) http://psychcorp.pearsonassessments.com/pai/ca/cahome.htm | Children's Depression Inventory–2™ (CDI-2; Kovacs, 2011) http://www.mhs.com/product.aspx?gr=edu&prod=cdi2&id=overview | Sensory Integration and Praxis Tests (SIPT; Ayres, 1989) http://portal.wpspublish.com/portal/page?_pageid=53,267719&_dad=portal&_schema=PORTAL | Test of Visual-Perceptual Skills (nonmotor)–3 (TVPS–3; Martin, 2006) http://portal.wpspublish.com/portal/page?_pageid=53,267719&_dad=portal&_schema=PORTAL | |
| | Conners 3 (3rd ed.; Conners, 2008) http://www.mhs.com/default.aspx | Sensory Processing Measure (SPM; Kuhaneck, Henry, & Glennon, 2007) http://portal.wpspublish.com/portal/page?_pageid=53,267719&_dad=portal&_schema=PORTAL | Test of Visual-Motor Skills–3 (TVMS–3; Martin, 2006) http://portal.wpspublish.com/portal/page?_pageid=53,267719&_dad=portal&_schema=PORTAL | |

continues

TABLE 9-14

**Pediatric Assessments** *continued*

| Developmental | Behavior | Motor and Sensory Integration | Visual, Auditory, and Motor Processing | Play |
|---|---|---|---|---|
| | *Devereaux Scales of Mental Disorders* (DSMD; Naglieri, LeBuffe, & Pfeiffer, 1994), *and Behavior Rating Scales–School Form* (Naglieri, LeBuffe, & Pfeiffer 1992)<br><br>http://psychcorp. pearsonassessments.com/ pai/ca/cahome.htm | *Toddler and Infant Motor Evaluation* (TIME; Miller & Roid, 1994)<br><br>http://psychcorp. pearsonassessments.com/ pai/ca/cahome.htm | | |
| | *Personality Inventory for Children-2* (PIC-2; Lachar & Gruber, 2001)<br><br>http://portal.wpspublish. com/portal/page?_ pageid=53,267719&_ dad=portal&_ schema=PORTAL | *Touch Inventory for Elementary School* (TIE; Royeen, 1987a; Royeen & Fortune, 1990)<br><br>and<br><br>*Touch Inventory for Preschoolers* (TIP; Royeen, 1987b) | | |

TABLE 9-15

## Assessments for Special Populations

| Arthritis | ***Arthritis Impact Measurement Scales*** |
|---|---|

**Arthritis**

***Arthritis Impact Measurement Scales***
(https://www.rheumatology.org/practice/clinical/clinicianresearchers/outcomes-instrumentation/AIMS.asp and http://www.proqolid.org/instruments/arthritis_impact_measurement_scales_aims2)

*Purpose:* To measure changes in pain, mobility, social function, and global health in patients with arthritis

*Versions:* An original version (AIMS), an expanded version (AIMS2; Meenan, Mason, Anderson, Guccione, & Kazis, 1992), a short-form of the AIMS2 (AIMS2-SF; Ren, Kazis, & Meenan (1999); Haavardsholm, Kvien, Uhlig, Smedstad, & Guillemin, 2000), a children's version, and a version for older adults (Geri-AIMS).

*Available:*
- Robert F. Meenan, M. D., Boston University School of Public Health, 715 Albany Street, Talbot Building, Boston, MA 02118, USA.
  Phone: (617) 638–4644 Fax: (617) 638–5299
- A free edition of the AIMS2 questionnaire is available at http://www.proqolid.org/

***Edinburgh Rehabilitation Status Scale*** (ERSS; Affleck, Aitken, Hunter; McGuire, & Roy, 1988)

*Purpose:* To measure levels of performance and changes during rehabilitation in independence, activity, social integration, and effects of symptoms on lifestyles areas

*Available from*: Rehabilitation Studies Unit, Princess Margaret Rose Hospital, Edinburgh, Scotland EH 10 7ED

***Functional Status Index*** (FSI; Jette, 1980; 1987)

*Purpose*: To assess adult patients with arthritis living in the community

*References:*
- *Jette, A. M. (1980).* Functional Status Index: Reliability of a chronic disease evaluation instrument. *Archives of Physical Medicine and Rehabilitation, 61,* 395–401.
- Jette, A. M. (1987). The Functional Status Index: Reliability and validity of a self–report functional disability measure. *Journal of Rheumatology (1987), 14*(Supplement 15), 15–19.

***Standardized Test of Patient Mobility*** (Jebsen et al., 1970; Mikulic, Griffith, & Jebsen, 1976)

*Purpose*: To assess patient mobility in categories of bed mobility, wheelchair activities, transfers, and ambulation

*References:*
- Jebsen, R. H., Trieschmann, R. B., Mikulic, M. A., Hartley, R. B., McMillan, J. A., & Snook, M.E. (1970). Measurement of time in a standardized test of patient mobility *Archives of Physical Medicine and Rehabilitation, 51,* 170–175.

**Low back pain**

***Oswestry Low Back Pain Disability Questionnaire*** (Fairbank, Couper, Davies, & O'Brien, 1980)

*Purpose:* Self-rating questionnaire used to assess patients with low back pain by determining its impact on the activities of daily living

*Limitations:* Because this is a self-rating questionnaire, the response may be subjective and items may be left out.

*Versions*: Several versions are available on the internet, including an electronic form.

*Available:*
- http://www.orthopaedicscore.com/scorepages/oswestry_low_back_pain.html
- http://etd.library.pitt.edu/ETD/available/etd-08222003-013408/unrestricted/Childsl.pdf
- http://www.dallaspaincontrol.com/pdfs/pci-back-form.pdf

*continues*

| TABLE 9-15 |
| --- |

### Assessments for Special Populations *continued*

| | |
| --- | --- |
| **Low back pain** | *Sickness Impact Profile™* (SIP; Gilson et al., 1975; Bergnen, Bobbitt, Carter, & Gilson,1981); http://ajph.aphapublications.org/cgi/reprint/65/12/1304.pdf |
| | *Purpose:* To provide a descriptive profile of changes in a person's behavior as a result of sickness |
| | *Available from*: Johns Hopkins University, School of Public Health, Department of Health Policy and Management, 624 N. Broadway, Room 647, Baltimore, MD 21205-1901. (http://www.techtransfer.jhu.edu/bin/m/d/C01822.pdf) |
| | **Research Study:** Pain measurement in elders with chronic low back pain: Traditional and alternative approaches, by D. Weiner, C. Pieper, E. McConnell, S. Martinez, and F. Keefe (1996), *Pain, 67,* 461–467 |
| **Osteoarthritis** | **Research Study:** Measuring functioning in patients with hand osteoarthritis—content comparison of questionnaires based on the *International Classification of Functioning, Disability and Health* (ICF), by T. Stamm, S. Geyh, A. Cieza, K. Machold, B. Kollerits, M. Kloppenburg, M. … G. Stucki, (2006), *Rheumatology, 45, 1534–1541. Full text available:* http://rheumatology.oxfordjournals.org/content/45/12/1534.full.pdf+html?sid=1c5f5fb4-52d6-4f0c-bbcb-13871810d105 |
| | *Purpose:* To analyze and compare the content of questionnaires that have been used to assess functioning in patients with hand osteoarthritis (OA) based on the *International Classification of Functioning, Disability and Health* (ICF). Authors concluded that a "comprehensive measurements of functioning in hand OA, … [should] include both one instrument with a low diversity ratio (for disease-specific aspects) and another instrument with a high diversity ratio (for broader aspects of functioning including some aspects of participation)" (Stamm et al., p. 1540). |
| **Spinal cord injury** | *Quadriplegic Index of Function* (**QIF;** http://www.scireproject.com/outcome-measures/quadriplegia-index-of-function-qif-short-form |
| | *Purpose*: To provide a sensitive functional assessment that could document the small but clinically significant gains in functional patient recovery made by quadriplegics throughout in-patient rehabilitation |
| | *Versions:* Long form (Gresham et al., 1986) and short form (Marino & Goin, 1999). Short form was designed for spinal cord injuries. |
| | *References:*<br>• Gresham, G. E., Labi, M. L., Dittmar, S. S., Hicks, J. T., Joyce, S. Z., & Phillips-Stehlik, M. A. (1986), The Quadriplegia Index of Function (QIF): Sensitivity and reliability demonstrated in a study of thirty quadriplegic patients, *Paraplegia. 24,* 38–44.<br>• Marino, R. J., & Goin, J. E. (1999). Development of a short form Quadriplegia Index of Function scale. *Spinal Cord, 37,* 289–296. |
| **Stroke** | *Frenchay Activities Index* (FAI; Holbrook & Skilbeck, 1983; https://www.cebp.nl/vault_public/filesystem/?ID=1327) |
| | *Purpose:* To assess the frequency of doing Instrumental Activities of Daily Living (IADL) through a survey or interview format |
| | *References:*<br>• Holbrook, M, & Skilbeck, C. E. (1983). An activities index for use with stroke patients. *Age and Ageing, 12,* 166–170.<br>• Schuling, J., deHaan, R., Limburg, M., & Groenier, K. (1993). The Frenchay Activities Index: Assessment of functional status in stroke patients. *Stroke, 13,* 1173, 1177. |

| | |
|---|---|
| **Stroke** | **Fugl-Meyer Assessment** (Fugl-Meyer, Jääskö, Leyman, Olsson, & Steglind, 1975; Gladstone, Danells, & Black, 2002) |

*Purpose*: To assess motor functioning, balance, sensation and joint functioning in patients with post-stroke hemiplegia

*Available*: Contact: Institute of Rehabilitation Medicine, University of Goteberg, Goteberg, Sweden. A version of the measure is given in Fugl-Meyer et al. (1975) and Dittmar, S. S., & Gresham, G. E., (1997).

**Time Care Profile** (Halstead & Hartley, 1975)

*Purpose*: to describe the use of a diary method to record the amount of time the patient receives assistance during the course of a normal day as an index of dependency in ADL

*References*:
- Halstead, L., & Hartley, R. B. (1975). Time care profile: An evaluation of a new method of assessing ADL dependence. *Archives of Physical Medicine and Rehabilitation, 56,*110–115.

**Traumatic brain injury**    **Agitated Behavior Scale** (ABS; Corrigan, 1989; http://www.ohiovalley.org/agitation/agbe.html)

*Purpose*: To assess the nature and extent of agitation during the acute phase of recovery from acquired brain injury

*References*: A list of references describing the use of the ABS can be found at http://www.ohiovalley.org/agitation/ref.html

*Available*:
- http://www.ohiovalley.org/agitation/agbe.html (includes a description, rating forms, directions for scoring, and references)
- http://www.tbims.org/combi/abs/abs.pdf

**Community Integration Questionnaire** (CIQ; Corrigan & Deming, 1995; Willer, Ottenbacher, & Coad, 1994)

*Purpose*: To provide an objective measure for community integration after traumatic brain injury by measuring frequency of performance of activities in home integration, social integration, and productive activities

*Available*:
- http://tbims.org/combi/ciq/index.html (including description, rating forms, directions for scoring, references and a forum for discussion).

**Disability Rating Scale** (Rappaport, 2005; Rappaport, Hall, Hopkins, Belleza, & Cope, 1982)

*Purpose*: Intended to measure accurately general functional changes over the course of recovery

*Available*:
- http://www.tbims.org/combi/drs/index.html (including description, rating forms, directions for scoring, references and a forum for discussion).
- http://www.neuroskills.com/tbi/drs.shtml

**Rabideau Kitchen Evaluation-Revised: An Assessment of Meal Preparation Skill** (RKE-R; Neistadt, 1992; 1993; 1994; 2000)

*Purpose*: Used to evaluate functional sequencing abilities of individuals with traumatic or anoxic brain trauma by the use of a meal preparation treatment protocol

*References*:
- Neistadt, M. E. (1992). The Rabideau kitchen evaluation, revised: An assessment of meal preparation skill. *Occupational Therapy Journal of Research, 12,* 242–255.
- Neistadt, M. E. (1993).The relationship between constructional and meal preparation skills. *Archives of Physical Medicine and Rehabilitation, 74,*144–148.

*continues*

| TABLE 9-15 |
| --- |

**Assessments for Special Populations** *continued*

| | |
| --- | --- |
| **Traumatic brain injury** | • Neistadt, M. E. (1994). A meal preparation treatment protocol for adults with brain injury. *American Journal of Occupational Therapy, 48,* 431–438.<br>• Neistadt, M. E. (2000). Rabideau Kitchen Evaluation-Revised: An assessment of meal preparation skill. In M. E. Neistadt, *Occupational therapy evaluation for adults: A pocket guide* (pp. 136–137). Baltimore: Lippincott. |

*Available:* University of New Hampshire, Department of Occupational Therapy, School of Health and Human Services, Durham, NH

***Rivermead Perceptual Assessment Battery*** (RPAB; Whiting, Lincoln, Bhavnani & Cockburn, 1985)

*Purpose:* To provide a detailed picture of a client's visual perceptual ability before treatment, following head injury, or a stroke

*Available:* GL Assessment, The Chiswick Centre, 414 Chiswick High Road, London, W4 5TF | T +44 (0) 20 8996 3333 | F +44 (0)20 8742 8767 http://shop.gl-assessment.co.uk/home.php?cat=359

Edith Kaplan, using the philosophy and work of Luria, has proposed a third approach to neuropsychological testing: an evaluation should result in an understanding of the way in which a person approaches a task, regardless of which tests are used. This method, called the Boston Process Approach (Milberg, Hebben, & Kaplan, 1996), relies less on specific instruments and more on observation of behavior during the evaluation. All neurological functioning (e.g., cognitive, perceptual, memory, language, organization, and personality) is evaluated in this approach. The *Wechsler Adult Intelligence Scale-IV* (WAIS-IV; Wechsler, 2008) and the *Wechsler Intelligence Scale for Children–Fourth Edition, Integrated* (WISC-IV–Integrated, 2004), are examples of instruments that incorporate the Boston process approach.

In addition to these test batteries, several new assessment instruments have been developed for use with children and adults. The *Test of Memory and Learning–II* (TOMAL–II; Reynolds & Voress, 2007), *Wide-Range Assessment of Memory and Learning–II* (WRAML-II; Sheslow & Adams, 2003), *NEPSY-II* (Korkman, Kirk, & Kemp, 2007), *Delis–Kaplan Executive Functioning System* (K–DEFs; Delis, Kaplan, & Kramer, 2001), and the *Dean-Woodcock Sensory-Motor Battery* (DWSMB; Dean & Woodcock, 2003)

are examples of these assessments. With the exception of the *NEPSY-II*, which is appropriate for ages 3 through 16, these assessment instruments are appropriate for children, adolescents, and adults.

Clinical researchers may not, at first, be involved in neuropsychological testing as part of their research. Nonetheless, information obtained from these tests, as well as use of pre- and posttest data can be useful as outcome measures in examining the relationship between changes in behavior and interventions.

## 9.10 Reviewing and Evaluating Tests

For the researcher, the selection of a valid and reliable instrument is critical. Knowledge in assessing the adequacy of a measuring instrument is extremely important in view of the literally thousands of instruments that test corporations publish. Before choosing a test to use in research, the clinical researcher must determine the purpose for the test. Does the researcher need to screen participants for normal intelligence or average achievement? Is adaptive behavior a concern? If the purpose of the

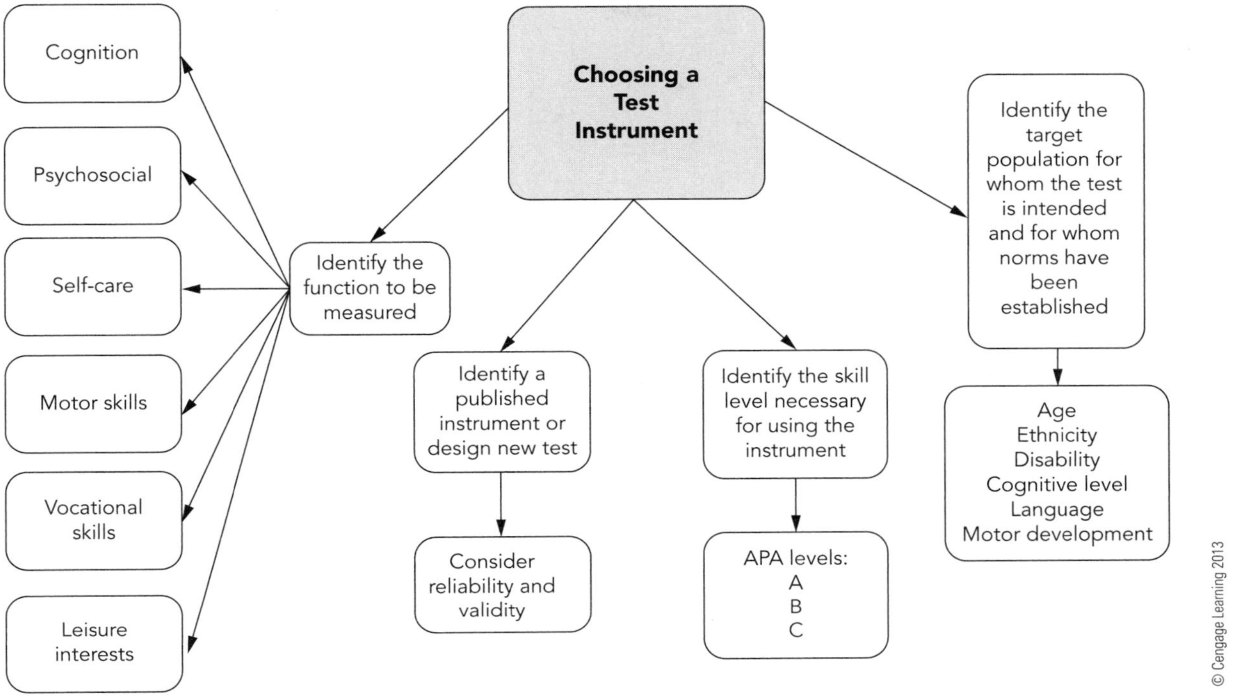

**FIGURE 9-4**    Factors in Choosing a Test Instrument

investigation is to evaluate the effect of a treatment on reducing low back pain, the researcher will want to make sure that all subjects have clinically significant low back pain (see Figure 9–4).

The next step in determining which test to use is to review the appropriate tests that are available, taking into account the psychometric properties, including the reliability, validity, and measurement scales of each test. If there are special qualifications in administering the test, the researcher must know who is able to administer the test and how long the test will take to administer. The following outline and examples of reviews of tests will illustrate the manner in which tests are analyzed (Stein, 1988).

### 9.10.1 Outline for Reviewing Tests

1. **Title**
2. **Date published, date revised**
3. **Authors**
4. **Publisher:** Distributor of test or where test is available
5. **Target Population:** What was the original sample from which data were collected in terms of age, diagnostic group, and geographical location? Is there a specific target population for whom the test is appropriate?
6. **Variables Assessed:** What are the specific areas of function, behavior, or personality that are being assessed? What are the major stated purposes of the test?
7. **Measurement Scales:** What is the level of measurement in the test?

   A. Qualitative (subjective judgment)

      i. Nominal scale of measurement refers to evaluating variables using independent categories such as *can* or *cannot perform a specific task.*

ii. Ordinal scale of measurement refers to evaluating variables using magnitude and ranking such as *completely dependent in task*, *needs assistance*, or *independent functioning*. Variables can also be rated on a numerical scale from 1 to 5, for example, where 1 indicates *no self-care* and 5 indicates *cares for self independently*.

**B.** Quantitative (objective evaluation)

i. Interval scale of measurement refers to scoring variables on a continuous scale with equal distances between score values. Pulse rate, blood pressure, height, and weight are usually measured on interval scales using tests that produce mathematical data.

ii. Ratio scale of measurement incorporates the concept of an absolute zero.

8. **Examiner's Manual:** Is there an examiner's manual? Does the manual identify the theoretical framework used to develop the test? Are references available for further study of the framework? Is there a chapter on psychometric properties, including reliability and validity? Are the directions for administering the test clear? Does the manual discuss adaptations which can be used with special populations (e.g., blind, physically impaired)? Are there tables of norms? Does the manual identify the way in which the norms were obtained? Is there a chapter on interpretation? If so, does the chapter adequately discuss ways in which the information can be applied to treatment?

9. **Administration of Instrument:** Who administers the test and when is it administered? How long does the test take to administer? Is there special training to administer the test? Are special materials or environments required?

10. **Scoring and Interpretation of Results:** Are there overall scores or subtest scores derived from the test results? Are there norms available to interpret raw scores? How are the results used in treatment planning, documentation of progress, and discharge recommendations?

11. **Test Reliability and Validity:** Are the types of reliability and validity identified? Are reliability and validity co-efficients present? Was the test correlated with any other test? What was the correlation? Is the reliability above .8?

12. **Other Comments:** Included in this section are miscellaneous comments such as the theoretical orientation or conceptual framework of the test and its appropriateness for the clinical researcher.

13. **References:** Includes books, journals, test manuals, and other sources where the test has been published or critically evaluated.

## 9.10.2 Example of Test Review

1. *Kohlman Evaluation of Living Skills* (KELS; Thomson, 1992)
2. Originally published in 1978, revised in 1992
3. Linda Kohlman Thomson, MOT, OTR, OT(C), FAOTA
4. American Occupational Therapy Association, 4720 Montgomery Lane, P.O. Box 31220, Bethesda, MD 20824–1220
5. Clients with acute psychiatric disorders, older patients in acute care hospitals; adolescent through older must be used cautiously with individuals hospitalized for more than 1 month.
6. Seventeen living skills categorized into five main domains: self-care, safety and health, money management, transportation and telephone, and work and leisure are measured.
7. Measurement Scales: Nominal and ordinal scales.
8. Manual is well written and easy to follow.
9. The test can be given by an occupational therapist or occupational therapist assistant when supervised by the occupational therapist.

10. Each of the 17 living skills are scored for either "independent" or "needs assistance" with a score of 1 (½ point for the work and leisure category) given if the client needs assistance. Items scored as independent are given a score of 0. Individuals obtaining an overall score of 5 ½ or less are considered able to live independently; scores equal to or above 6 indicate the client needs assistance to live in the community.

11. Interrater reliability ranges from $r$ = .84 to 1.00. Concurrent validity has been measured at $r$ = .78 to .89 with Global Assessment Scale; −.84 with BaFPE. The test has successfully predicted which older patients could live independently.

12. The test provides a quick assessment to provide information about a person's ability in everyday functioning in daily living skills, independent living, and work/leisure.

13. McGourty, L. K. (1988). Kohlman Evaluation of Living Skills (KELS). In B. J. Hemphill, *Mental health assessment in occupational therapy: A integrative approach to the evaluative process* (pp. 131–146). Thorofare, NJ: SLACK.

Burnett, J., Dyer, C. M., & Naik, A. D. (2009). Convergent validation of the Kohlman Evaluation of Living Skills as a screening tool of older adults' ability to live safely and independently in the community. *Archives of Physical Medicine and Rehabilitation, 90,* 1948–1952.

Pickens, S. Naik, A. D., Burnett, J., Kelly, P.A., Gleason, M., & Dyer, C. B. (2007). The utility of the KELS test in substantiated cases of elder self-neglect. *Journal of the American Academy of Nurse Practitioners, 19,* 137–142. doi: 10.1111/j.1745-7599.2007.00205.x

Thomson, L. K. (1992). *The Kohlman Evaluation of Living Skills* (KELS, 3rd ed.). Rockville, MD: American Occupational Therapy Association.

Thomson, L. K. (1999). The Kohlman Evaluation of Living Skills. In B. J. Hemphill-Pearson, *Assessment in occupational therapy mental health: An integrative approach* (pp. 231–242). Thorofare, NJ: SLACK.

## 9.11  Criterion-Referenced Tests and Norm-Referenced Tests

Until recently, most tests were **norm-referenced tests**, or NRTs. These tests, described previously, were developed to classify individuals into levels of instructional groups. The scores obtained by the normative sample on a norm-referenced test are distributed along a normal curve. Raw scores obtained by individuals taking a norm-referenced test are compared with the normative sample and can be converted into standard scores and percentiles.

There are several advantages to NRTs. Individuals taking the test are compared with the general population; thus, the performance of a student or patient can be judged to be typical or atypical. Because NRTs are usually commercially published, psychometric characteristics such as reliability and item analysis are carefully considered in the development. Additionally, standardization of an NRT includes administering the test to large samples of individuals stratified across many socioeconomic groups, ages, ethnic backgrounds, and educational levels. In this way, raw scores obtained from a given individual can be compared to the raw score obtained by most of the population having the same characteristics.

At the same time, there are disadvantages to an NRT. First, because the tests are broad measures of a subject and contain a limited number of items from many areas within that subject, they are often referred to as "survey tests." It is not uncommon for an NRT designed to be used in grades 1 through 12 to include only 100 sight words. Second, because there is no national or state curriculum, the content found on the test may not match the curriculum of a particular school or community. Finally, because the number of items in each area is limited, the test results cannot be used to measure small gains in progress. Likewise, there is limited value for using the results of an NRT in determining an instructional or therapeutic program.

The purposes of NRTs are (a) to compare an individual's achievement or performance with other individuals of the same age, educational level, and socioeconomic status and (b) to obtain information regarding the normal population. When these tests are used with atypical populations, there may be a bias, which results in systematic error. In spite of these disadvantages, NRTs are useful in clinical research.

In testing circles during the last 40 years, there has been a growing interest in devising criterion-referenced tests in lieu of norm-referenced tests (Deno, 1985). **Criterion-referenced tests** (CRTs), first proposed by Glaser (1963), use content or curricular domains to set the standard of performance. They compare the performance of an individual with a specified level of mastery or achievement rather than with a normative population. Because the performance is compared with a criterion, performance on these tests allows the therapist or teacher to suggest specific classroom goals and objectives to use in program planning. Progress can be monitored more effectively and more discretely.

CRTs are based on a comprehensive theory that generates ideas for a specific content domain. In CRTs, items are selected systematically to represent the content domain. For example, if an investigator is interested in determining the visual perceptual skills of individuals, the first task would be to determine the dimensions of visual perception from the theoretical and experiential perspectives. The investigator would use the theoretical framework to guide the writing of test items, making sure that each aspect of the framework is covered by test items in the CRT. Operational performance standards, obtained by surveying a representational sample of the general population, are used in writing test items. For example, a survey of 10-year-olds would reveal that most of them have no difficulty with activities involving visual closure or visual figure ground. The operational performance standard, therefore, might be set at a criterion level of 90 percent accuracy for recognition of figures in tasks involving visual figure ground or visual closure.

One example of criterion-referenced testing occurs when measuring an individual's independent living skills. For instance, in the criteria of dressing completely, we might include the act of putting on all clothes right-side out and frontwards, tying shoes, and fastening all fasteners. The individual's ability to perform this activity is measured by a given standard. Until the individual has mastered the expected standard, the individual is not considered to have reached competency. Social skills and self-help skills are often evaluated by CRTs.

CRTs are sometimes referred to as "curriculum-based measures" (CBMs) or "curriculum-based assessments" (CBAs). CBAs and CBMs establish a student's instructional needs in relationship to the requirements of the actual curriculum being used. Just as with CRTs, the CBAs and CBMs assess mastery of learning by providing an operational performance criterion as a necessary standard for passing. Although commercial CRTs are available, teachers and occupational therapists frequently develop the measurement instrument based on their own criteria.

In summary, a CRT is constructed to obtain measurements that can be interpreted in terms of specific criteria or performance standards. Scores obtained on NRTs, however, are interpreted in terms of comparison to a population. The choice of which test to use depends on the outcome desired. If a researcher is interested in the progress of a particular student over time, a CRT is more appropriate; however, if the researcher is interested in the differences between two groups of subjects, then an NRT may be more appropriate.

A summary of the differences between criterion- and norm-referenced tests is given in Table 9–16. This summary may help in deciding which type of test to use.

## 9.11.1 Applying Criterion-Referenced Concepts to Research

The major content areas for clinical researchers in evaluation include basic living skills, interests, work behavior, and skill attainment. If one uses a

© Cengage Learning 2013

**TABLE 9-16**

**Comparison of Criterion-Referenced Tests and Norm-Referenced Tests**

| Criterion-Referenced Tests | Norm-Referenced Tests |
| --- | --- |
| Absolute standards of competence or mastery are established based on theory. | Relative standards are based on normal standards. |
| Scores are derived from standards or behaviors or competency. | Scores are compared to established norms. |
| Scores are interpreted based on what the student can or cannot do and then used diagnostically. | Scores are interpreted by percentile ranks, standard scores, and organized along a normal curve. |
| Content or items are comprehensive of domain. | Content of items are a sample of domain. |
| Cut-off score for passing is based on minimal standards of competency. | Cut-off score for passing is based on pre-established percentile rank. |
| Theoretically all can pass or all can fail. | The number of failures is predicted before test is administered. |

criterion-referenced approach to these areas, one should look for the following factors:

- The theory underlying these concepts is identified.
- Research evidence supporting any assumptions of the test is stated.
- The content domain of the test that considers a comprehensive view of skills, interests, and behavior is discussed.
- The specific target population is operationally defined in terms of age, intelligence, education, and degree of disability.
- The test items are generated by selecting representative samples of behavior.
- Performance standards in the test are based on systematically collected data from representative samples of the target population.
- Test items are pilot-tested for clarity and ease of administration.
- Scoring methods are devised that are operationally defined.
- Reliability and validity data are documented.
- A test manual for administering, scoring, and interpreting data is provided.
- The degree of competency in the administration of the test is included in test descriptions.

## 9.12 Test Publishers

The development of new tests and measuring instruments is a relatively recent event in the occupational therapy professions. The clinical nature of these fields and the service-oriented process of treatment have led to the emphasis in the past on developing new treatment techniques rather than on measuring outcome variables. However, as the need for accountability and validation for treatment continue on federal and state governmental levels (e.g., through laws such as Individuals with Disabilities Improvement Education Act [IDEIA-2004] and Americans with Disabilities Act [ADA]), the use of tests and measuring instruments to justify therapeutic and educational intervention has become more important. Many tests have been developed for use by occupational therapists in the past 20 years. In addition to publishing their own tests, most test corporations distribute the most widely used tests. Thus, in general, a researcher is not limited to one corporation to obtain a specific test.

The following list includes test publishers that occupational therapists and other clinicians frequently use.

American Occupational Therapy Association (AOTA): http:// www.aota.org/
CPP, Inc.: https://www.cpp.com/en/index.aspx
Curriculum Associates, Inc.: http://www.curriculumassociates.com
Educational Testing Service: http://www.ets.org
Educational and Industrial Testing Service (EdITS): http://www.edits.net
Flaghouse Rehabilitation http: http://www.flaghouse.com
Institute for Personality and Ability Testing (IPAT): http://www.ipat.com/pages/home.aspx
Lafayette Instrument: http://www.lafayetteinstrument.com/
McGraw-Hill: http: //www.mcgraw-hill.com/
Multi-Health Systems (MHS): http://www.mhs.com/
PAR, Inc.: http://www4.parinc.com/
Pearson Assessments (also PsychCorp): http://www.pearsonassessments.com/pai/
Pro-Ed, Inc.: http://www.proedinc.com/Customer/default.aspx
Psychological Publications, Inc.: https://www.tjta.com/asp/index.asp
Riverside Publishing: http://www.riversidepublishing.com/
Western Psychological Services (WPS): http://portal.wpspublish.com/portal/page?_pageid=53,53086&_
    dad=portal&_schema=PORTAL
Stoelting Publishing: https://www.stoeltingco.com/stoelting/templates/99/Default
Stout Vocational Rehabilitation Institute: http://www3.uwstout.edu/scri/index.cfm
Trace Research and Development Center: http://trace.wisc.edu/
Valpar International Corporation: http://www.valparint.com/

## 9.13 Ethical Considerations in Testing

"Competence in test use is a combination of knowledge of psychometric principles, knowledge of the problem situation in which the testing is to be done, technical skill and some wisdom" (Davis, 1974, p. 6). This quote is from the Standards for Educational and Psychological Tests published by the American Psychological Association. To protect psychological tests from abuse, standards fall into three areas: guidelines for devising a new psychological test, qualifications for administering tests, and guidelines for interpreting results. The following guidelines should be adhered to in using tests:

1. The researcher publishing a new test should provide reliability, validity, normative data, scoring procedure, and qualifications for using the test in an accompanying manual.
2. A standardized test procedure should be carefully followed by the tester.
3. Results should be reported that can be compared to specified populations.
4. The researcher using psychological tests should obtain informed consent for the subject and assure the subject's confidentiality.

## 9.14 Summary

In the last 30 years, literally hundreds of tests have been developed for use with individuals with disabilities. In this chapter, the authors have presented descriptions of tests that are the most commonly used in clinical practice. These tests are available to use by occupational therapists knowledgeable in the administration, scoring, and interpretation of test results. These tests can be used as outcome or descriptive measures in clinical research. The use of a specific test is a key component in the research process and could affect the results if the test selected is not sensitive to changes in individuals or is not reliable or valid; therefore, the researcher should have knowledge of reliability and validity of the test before using it. When using a test in research, the researcher must be aware of the level of qualification needed to administer it.

Because new tests are developed frequently, the researcher should keep informed of newly published tests. Annual catalogs obtained from the test publishers listed in Section 9.12 are helpful in locating new tests. Online listings of tests are also available. Before developing a new test, occupational therapists should search the literature, references in testing, textbooks, publishers' catalogs, and websites for locating new tests.

## CHAPTER 10

# Scientific Writing and Thesis Preparation

*Vigorous writing is concise. A sentence should contain no unnecessary words, a paragraph no unnecessary sentences, for the same reason that a drawing should have no unnecessary lines and a machine no unnecessary parts. This requires not that the writer make all his sentences short, or that he avoid all detail and treat his subjects only in outline, but that every word tell.*

—W. Strunk Jr. and E. B. White, 1979,
*The Elements of Style*, p. 23

## Operational Learning Objectives

By the end of this chapter, the learner will:

- State ways to prepare for writing a research paper.
- Name the important divisions of a research paper.
- Identify and correct sexist and racist language in the research paper.
- Use *People First language*.
- Recognize reasons for revising the original draft.

- Write a bibliography using American Psychological Association (APA) format.
- Proof for errors in language mechanics and style.
- Critically evaluate one's own writing.
- Identify the major parts of the final format.
- Design a research proposal.
- Communicate results of research study.

## 10.1 Preparation for Writing

It is as important to prepare oneself for writing as it is to complete the review of literature and collect the data for the research project. Prior to writing the research paper, the researcher should take into consideration the many processes that facilitate writing.

One hindrance to the completion of the writing task is the failure to actually sit down and write, but allowing frequent interruptions during the actual writing period is equally problematic. The first task in the preparation for writing is to get oneself into the proper frame of mind. This includes taking care of as many "settling activities" that might lead to interruptions. This can be likened to an animal preparing to go to sleep: The animal roughs up the bed, circles the bed a number of times, grooms, and finally settles down. Similarly, settling activities for writers include planning a large block of time, getting one's coffee or drink, assembling all the materials needed, finding a quiet and comfortable place (preferably away from a phone), arranging for child care, putting the dog or cat outside, and taking care of any needed personal toiletries. Once one has completed those tasks and is settled, writing is made easier.

Effective writing is a skill that becomes more refined as it is practiced. Clear and simple language is the hallmark of good scientific writing, and its most important quality is objective self-criticism. For some individuals, a major block to the task of writing is the initial step of organizing their ideas on paper. The desire to write as if whatever one first put on paper is chipped forever in granite sometimes prevents the flow of ideas.

The place and time in which one writes are important initial considerations. Some individuals do their best writing during the morning in a quiet, sunny room with a large table where they can spread out reference books, scrap paper, and notes filed in manila folders. Others work better in the late evening. Some individuals can work 12–14 hours for several days, followed by several days of complete rest. Some students do their best work in a college library or cafeteria, despite visual and auditory distractions. Some can write using paper and pencil, whereas others prefer writing on a computer or word processor or dictating by using speech recognition software such as Dragon NaturallySpeaking® (http://www.nuance.com/talk/). Whatever the method and place, one must be aware of the environment that best facilitates creative writing.

Another consideration for writers is a time schedule. Some writers report that they compose in spurts of creative inspiration, whereas others work daily whether or not they feel inspired. Setting aside enough time is important, however, so that the writer does not feel rushed or under time constraints, allowing the writer to feel that something can be accomplished. Writing a research paper or article is unlike casual writing in which an individual can use spare minutes throughout the day to complete the task. Scientific writing takes mental energy and therefore requires concentrated effort.

A third consideration consists of assembling the materials to be used before beginning any writing task. Writing materials (e.g., pens, paper, computer), note cards prepared during the literature review, statistical analyses, and other references should be available and at hand. Just as one would not consider doing therapy without having all the tools and equipment available, one cannot expect to write adequately without having the proper tools and materials.

Writing a book, journal article, or thesis requires self-discipline. In a way, the individual should prepare for writing much as an athlete trains for a sporting event. A period of "conditioning" and mental rigor prior to writing is important. Some individuals take long walks, ride bicycles for miles, climb mountains, or take part in physical sports in preparation for writing. Others prepare mentally by playing chess, doing crossword puzzles, solving arithmetic problems, reading prolifically, or doing intricate manual work. Sleeping on an idea or letting it brew beneath the surface for a while also may be helpful. After the first draft, there will be ample time for revision, which in most cases will involve excision. For the author or research investigator, the completed document is analogous to giving birth. Writing is a continuous process with much editing and revision, but one should be careful not to abandon the initial efforts prematurely.

In Chapter 5, we talked about choosing a research topic. We stated that although the research topic must be meaningful to the researcher, the implications of the findings should lead to changes in the way the disability is viewed. These implications may affect evaluation or treatment of the disability or result in changes in administrative or educational practices. The purpose of the research paper includes an explanation of why the question was formulated and how the research methodology serves to answer the question. In the final project, that is, the research paper, the writer summarizes the literature, discusses the findings, and makes specific recommendations based on these findings. In this way, the final scientific paper becomes a part of the body of literature, placing the research findings within the context of previous works (Locke, Spirduso, & Silverman, 1997).

A well-conceived research paper requires active contemplation by the writer. The conceptual relationships between previous research and present findings must be considered. The hypothesis or guiding question(s) proposed by the researcher must be concisely and clearly stated and should cover all the points covered in the paper (Slade, Campbell, & Ballou, 1997). The summary and arguments used in the paper to advance one's theory must be compared with viewpoints held by established researchers. On the other hand, a researcher may present findings that are contradictory to accepted beliefs in the scientific community. Under attack, the researcher must be able to defend the validity of the research findings. For example, in spite of common belief that dyslexia is a result of visual-perceptual deficits, such as seeing and writing letters backwards, researchers such as Liberman (1973), Shaywitz and Shaywitz (2008), and Kamhi and Catts (1998) have espoused the underlying deficit in dyslexia to be language related.

Another essential component for writing a research paper is to understand the literature encompassing the topic as fully as possible. This is accomplished by completing an exhaustive literature review as described in Chapter 6. The researcher will discover quickly, however, that much more literature has been reviewed than will be discussed in the paper. This fact does not minimize the need for an extensive literature review; rather, it emphasizes the need for the researcher to understand and master the relationship of a specific literature within the context of a body of knowledge. For example, a cogent understanding of the methods used to teach students with dyslexia to read requires an examination of landmark studies directly related to the identification and diagnosis of this disability. It is not uncommon to revise the initial hypothesis or guiding question several times as one's knowledge base increases through reading and reviewing the literature.

Writing and reviewing literature is like an organic process that helps researchers to modify their thinking while extending their knowledge base. It is a creative process that allows one to be objective and self-critical. This process is sometimes referred to as "cognitive dissonance" (the state in which there is conflict between one's attitudes and one's behavior, generally resulting in changing one's thinking so that there is equilibrium between the two), "reflective decision making" (the process of making decisions by critically examining all sides of the issue), or the "Socratic method of learning." All these methods rely on the individual's ability to question and rethink a body of knowledge.

## 10.2   Outlining the Research Study

The overall organization of the research study, outlined in Table 10–1, is dictated by tradition. Each of the major sections within the research paper contains specific issues and topics.

### 10.2.1   Introduction to the Research Paper

The first part of the research paper contains a brief introduction to the present study, including the purpose, the research or guiding question(s), and the significance when examined beside findings from landmark studies (Best & Kahn, 2005). Epidemiological data should be cited to reinforce the significance of the study. A pivotal part of this portion of the research paper, article, or manuscript

**TABLE 10-1**

**Major Parts of a Research Paper**

   **I.** Introduction to the Research Paper
      **A.** Statement of the Research Problem or Guiding Question
      **B.** Significance of the Research Problem
      **C.** Purposes of the Study
      **D.** Specific Definitions or Terms
      **E.** Assumptions

  **II.** Review of the Literature
      **A.** Major Studies
      **B.** Critical Analysis of Key Studies

 **III.** Method
      **A.** Research Design
         **1.** Subjects (number; demographic data; inclusion and exclusion criteria)
         **2.** Procedures (tests, collection of data)
         **3.** Statistical Analyses

 **IV.** Results
      **A.** Presentation and Analysis of Data
      **B.** Relevant Tables and Figures

  **V.** Discussion, Summary, Conclusions, and Implications of the Findings
      **A.** Limitations of the Study
      **B.** Significance of Study Related to Prior Research
      **C.** Clinical Implications of Study
      **D.** Future Research

 **VI.** Reference List and Appendices

**VII.** Abstract (Placed after the Title Page)

© Cengage Learning 2013

is a clear statement of the hypotheses or guiding questions such that they are (a) well understood, (b) lead the reader to anticipate the major sections of the paper, and (c) indicate the direction or argument in which the paper will be written (Winkler & McCuen, 1998). Finally, this part of the research paper should include definitions for any terminology that are uncommon or might not be understood by the reader (Best & Kahn, 2005).

### 10.2.2 Review of the Literature

The second part of the research paper, which contains the literature review, is to some extent a measure of what the student knows about the subject (Best & Kahn, 2005; Krathwohl, 1988). In some papers, this section and the previous section are written as a single part. In a thesis or dissertation, this section is traditionally identified as Chapter 2 or, if written with the introduction, as Chapter 1.

The purpose of this section is to introduce further the reason for the study by reviewing previous research in the same area and by building a background for the study. Although it is not necessary to cite or review every article or book in the subject, as the researcher must presume that the reader has some knowledge in this area, the major studies must be discussed (American Psychological Association, 2010). For example, a student is interested in learning more about the relationship between cerebral damage and spasticity. In a preliminary literature review, the student will have read or identified many articles on the etiology and prognosis of a motor dysfunction plus some clinical descriptions of cerebral damage. A more in-depth review will yield studies regarding the relationship between specific types of cerebral damage as it relates to a motor dysfunction. A final review will examine those articles related to cerebral damage and spasticity. Although all these articles may be important, only the articles related directly to the research question will be discussed at length.

One way to outline this portion of the research paper is to organize the articles reviewed (described in Chapter 6). If the researcher used note cards, organization becomes a logical task of putting the note cards in the order in which they will be discussed. The selection of appropriate articles will be based both on the findings and on the relationship of the article to the research question. Some note cards will be put aside, because the articles will not be linked directly to the research question. Others will be mentioned only briefly as a means of presenting a background underlying the rationale behind the research question. Some articles will be especially important to build a strong argument for the research design, and a critical analysis of these articles will be an integral part of the literature review. Research literature and theory need to be reviewed and discussed objectively, citing both positive and negative research findings that relate to the present research question. In this way, one can avoid researcher bias, as shown in the following example from literature on treating depression.

A student is interested in the relationship between depression and use of cognitive-behavioral therapy. A review of literature identifies the following categories of studies involving the use of cognitive-behavioral therapy to treat individuals with depression: (a) those in whom there was no improvement (e.g., Jacobson et al., 1996; Twisk & Maes, 2009), (b) those in whom there was improvement (e.g., Clarke, Rohde, Lewinsohn, Hops, & Seeley, 1999; Pinninti, Rissmiller, & Steer, 2010), and (c) those in whom there was mixed success (e.g., McIntosh, Carter, Bulik, Frampton, & Joyce, 2010). Each of these articles should be critically analyzed and critiqued, with special attention

given to the methodology used in the studies and the relationship of the findings to the present research question. The student should present studies in which both favorable and unfavorable results were found. In doing this, the student demonstrates objectivity in reviewing the literature and avoids research bias.

Once the note cards have been placed in a logical order, a formal outline should be written. There are many ways to write an outline. Some people prefer to use phrases or single words, whereas others prefer to use sentences for each level. Occasionally, a student may find it easier to jot down a paragraph describing and expanding on the topic. This paragraph becomes the outer edifice of the particular section. Regardless of the method that one chooses when organizing the topics, the outline facilitates the organization of the literature review.

An effective way to organize the outline and make it functional is to use parallel or grammatical structure. For example, a list written as:

a. planning a therapy session
b. obtaining materials
c. positioning the student

is easier to comprehend than one written as:

a. plan the therapy session
b. obtaining materials
c. to position the student

Use of parallel or grammatical structures in an outline is effective in clarifying one's writing. (Refer to the Section 10.6, Format of a Paper, for further discussion regarding parallel construction.)

### 10.2.3 Method

The third section of the research paper includes a discussion of the methodology used in the study. This portion of the research paper should be written in a concise and succinct manner, with enough information available so that others can replicate the study.

Traditionally, there are three subdivisions in the methods section: (a) subjects, (b) the apparatus or tests, and (c) the procedures used for data collection and analysis. Demographic information, such as the number of subjects, ages, gender, and ethnicity, is critical. Other additional demographic information that may be essential for the study might include education level, socioeconomic level, handedness, disabilities, prior testing, and previous need for therapies, especially occupational therapy. If a control group is used, the demographics of the control group must be contrasted with the experimental group. The manner in which subjects were chosen (e.g., stratified random sample, voluntary response to a newspaper ad) is also described in this section.

A description of the tests or apparatus includes the names of the tests or surveys used, any laboratory equipment needed, and any specific directions or adaptations to the test or procedure that might not be found in a test manual. For example, if only part of a perceptual motor test is used, one must name the subtests chosen and justify the modification. When a standardized test is used, the reliability and validity of the test (or test portions) used must be indicated. If a survey or questionnaire has been developed for the study, a copy is put into the appendix following the major divisions of the paper.

Finally, the researcher describes the methods of data collection and the statistical procedures used to analyze it (Best & Kahn, 2005). For example, did the researcher collect data alone, in person, or by telephone? Were others trained to collect the data? If a questionnaire was used, was it mailed or left in a public place for people to fill out as desired? Was a second letter sent as a follow-up? How long did data collection occur? Was it collected in one or two sessions? Was it collected by outcome measures (pre- and posttesting)? What types of statistical procedures were used to analyze the data?

## 10.2.4 Results

The fourth section of the research paper presents the results and statistical findings from the study without attempting to interpret them. Each hypothesis is discussed separately, with statistical interactions and main effects reported. Tables and figures depicting significant relationships between variables often

make the text more understandable; however, they should be self-explanatory and add to the information in the text rather than add new information.

## 10.2.5 Summary, Discussion, and Implications of the Findings

In the final section, the writer summarizes the findings and attempts to interpret them in the context of previous studies in the same field. Conclusions regarding acceptance or rejection of hypotheses are stated in this section. Although statements of generalization can be made here, one must be careful not to overgeneralize or overstate the significance of the findings. The writer should be aware of the limitations of the study and state them, expressing any cautions regarding generalization to populations not included in the sample. Implications for further research, present practice, or policy changes are advanced, along with the arguments for these changes. The internal and external validity of the study should be discussed.

According to Best and Kahn (2005), the discussion section of the research paper is the most difficult part to write. Inexperienced authors tend to over- or undergeneralize, thinking their results less or more important than the data would support (Winkler & McCuen, 1998). The discussion section should be a critical and analytical summary of the findings, rather than a superficial overview of the results. Because this part of the research paper is the most frequently read (Best & Kahn, 2005), it is crucial that the researchers summarize the results and critically review these findings in the context of prior studies. The usefulness of the research paper, despite the findings, can be determined by the way in which the discussion section is written.

## 10.2.6 Reference List and Appendices

In the last section of the research paper, the writer needs to list all of the cited references. The writer must be careful not to leave out any reference, to include all information in the citation, and to check for accuracy and correct spelling of information. There is nothing more frustrating than an incomplete or inaccurate citation when one wishes to obtain further information from the original article. (Refer to Section 10.5, Quotations, Referenced Material, and Bibliographic Citations, for further information.)

Sometimes a writer wishes to place a bibliography and a reference list into the research paper. A bibliography contains any article, book, or chapter that might be helpful in understanding the topic. A reference list, on the other hand, includes journal articles, books, or other sources used in the research and preparation of the paper and cited within the article (American Psychological Association, 2010). Any tables or figures used in the research paper are placed after the reference list. Any additional information (e.g., copy of the survey or test protocol, drawing of specific apparatus) can be placed in an appendix at the very end.

### 10.2.7 Abstract

The abstract of a research study, which is written last and then placed at the beginning of the study, contains summary statements of each independent unit or section (i.e., the problem, literature review, research design, methods, results, discussion, and conclusions). The abstract should contain enough information so that the reader will know the purposes of the study, the specific variables or groups investigated, the number of subjects, the measuring instruments used, the results, and the conclusions presented. An abstract of a research study is usually limited to between 150 and 300 words.

When preparing an abstract, it is useful to extract key sentences from each part of the study and then integrate the sentences through transitional phrases. Abstracts are extremely important to investigators reviewing literature; therefore, it is vital to present as complete a summary of the total study as possible within the number of words permitted. Abstracts are not merely a summary or discussion of the results as perceived by some investigators. An abstract should be a complete statement representative of the total study. Whenever possible, key words or phrases should be identified by the author and placed below the abstract. These key words are used in data retrieval systems (see Chapter 6).

## 10.3 Writing the First Draft

Writers begin the first draft after completing the outline. As stated above, the outline aids in organizing the literature review, but the outline is not set in stone. After the first draft has been written, the organization may need to be revised. Nonetheless, having an outline allows the writer to have a sense of the direction in which the paper is going.

Perhaps the hardest part of writing is putting initial thoughts on paper. Writers should compose these initial thoughts with the expectation of revising them later. There will be plenty of time for revision after the first draft has been written, and writers should expect to revise their first work a number of times.

A difficult skill for inexperienced writers is the ability to use notes effectively. There is a tendency to quote extensively rather than to paraphrase the author's words. Frequently, this is caused by a lack of understanding about what the author meant. If this is the case, researchers must do additional reading and studying until they completely understand the material. Although quotes from the original source can be an effective means of relating information, too many quotations make the research paper difficult to read and leave "the impression that students have done [no more than] 'cut and paste' from books and articles they have read" (Winkler & McCuen, 1979, p. 114). It is better to use quotations sparingly, intermixing the quotations with summaries and paraphrases of the original sources. When quoting or paraphrasing, one must document the source (see section on quotations).

The literary and scientific styles used for citations often are determined by a particular discipline. The four most commonly used systems are *The Chicago Manual of Style* (University of Chicago Press, 2010), the *Modern Language Association* (MLA, 2009), the *American Medical Association Manual of Style* (Iverson, 2007), and the *Publication Manual of the American Psychological Association* (APA, 2010). The latter style is used most frequently in psychology, education, and social and health sciences and will be discussed in this text.

The essential reference book for APA style is the sixth edition of the *Publication Manual of the American Psychological Association* (APA, 2010), generally available in university or college bookstores. If the university or local technical bookstore does not have one, it can be obtained from the American Psychological Association in Washington, DC. Because of the extensiveness of the APA style, one will need to refer to this manual frequently. It is wise to get into the habit of referring to the APA Manual whenever there is a question about style, language mechanics, or format of the paper. Major highlights of the APA Manual will be discussed in the following sections of this chapter;

however, because of space limitations, not all topics will be covered in detail.

## 10.4 Making Revisions

Once the research paper has been written, revisions will be necessary. Revising the research paper five or six times is not uncommon. Each time the writer reviews the research paper for accuracy and cohesiveness, he or she may discover additional ways for revision or clarity.

The function of revision is to make sure that specific editing requirements have been followed. These editing requirements are summarized in Table 10–2.

---

### TABLE 10-2

**Checklist for Proofing One's Article**

**1. Gender and Ethnic Bias**
- Is the article free of language that might be ambiguous or stereotypical?

**2. *People First***
- Is the manuscript written with the individual emphasized rather than the disability?
- Have all references to a disability been written in the form "individual with …"?

**3. Grammar**
- Are there run-on sentences or sentence fragments?
- Are there split infinitives, dangling modifiers, or errors in verb-subject agreement?
- Is the writing in parallel structure?
- Are relative pronouns used appropriately?
- Has a grammar program been used to check the language?
- Has past tense been used rather than presence tense (e.g., the author *said*)

**4. Spelling/Punctuation**
- Has a spell check been used to check spelling?
- Has the article been reviewed for commas, quotation marks, hyphens, and apostrophes?

**5. Abbreviations**
- Is the abbreviation placed in parentheses following the full term the first time it is used?
- Are the Latin abbreviations used correctly and according to APA style?
- Are abbreviations invented by the author kept to a minimum?

**6. Transitional Words, Phrases, and Sentences**
- Are there transitional statements or words between ideas?
- Is there a sense of unity and integration in the paper?
- Do words such as "however," "although," or "nevertheless" need to be added?

### 7. Clarity

- Is the language clear and simple?
- Do any unusual terms need to be explained or defined?
- Would a figure or table help explain the information?
- Has the material been reviewed by a second reader?

### 8. Organization

- Do the hypotheses or guiding question(s) drive the content of the research paper?
- Is there consistency between sections?
- Are unnecessary repetitions removed?
- Is the sequence of the research paper logical and coherent?

## 10.4.1  Bias

*First*, the writer will want to make sure that no type of bias (gender, sexual orientation, racial or ethnic, disability, age, or historical and interpretive inaccuracies) has been introduced into the paper or into the study. Several guidelines have been established by the APA for avoiding bias in one's writing. "Part of writing without bias is recognizing that differences should be mentioned only when relevant. Marital status, sexual orientation, racial and ethnic identity, or the fact that a person has a disability, should not be mentioned gratuitously" (APA, 2010, p. 71).

"Gender" refers to role (APA, 2010, p. 73), whereas "sex" is biological (APA, 2010, p. 71). Both gender and sexual bias can be avoided by specifically describing participants, rather than using a general term to describe the population. For example, bias occurs when the writer uses the term *man* to mean the human race rather than using a less ambiguous term such as *person, people,* or *individual*. Additionally, use of specific gender words (e.g., *his, her*) or using terms that end in *man* or *men* (e.g., *postman, chairman, policemen* must be avoided. Stereotyping (e.g., *the psychologist … he; mothering*) can be avoided by using specific language (e.g., *boys enjoyed playing with Legos while girls enjoyed reading*), by using parallel language (e.g., *men and women* rather than *men and girls*), or by changing the term to a plural (e.g., *their* instead of *his* or *her*). Compounds, such as *his/her,* or *(s)he* should be avoided (American Psychological Association, 2010). The term *sexual orientation* is preferred over *sexual preference*.

Bias involving disabilities occurs when the writer attributes to a specific group something that has no supporting data (American Psychological Association, 2010). An example of this stereotyping occurs when someone writes, "In general, all individuals with traumatic brain injury tend to have psychosocial difficulties."

Ethnic or racial bias can be avoided by using commonly accepted designations, such as the census categories, while being sensitive to the preferred designations. For example, persons of Hispanic background in New Mexico prefer to be called Hispanic or Spanish, whereas persons of Hispanic background in southern California or southern Texas consider themselves Mexicans. Avoid terms that are either dated or derogatory. Finally, terms used to refer to racial or ethnic groups are proper nouns, and therefore should be capitalized. By asking the participants their preference, ethnic or racial bias can be avoided. APA suggests that an informal test can be completed by substituting another group (e.g., your own) for the group being discussed. If the writer perceives offense in the revised statement, then bias is probably present.

When referring to individuals by age, specific ranges should be used. APA suggests that individuals under 12 should be referred to as *girls* or *boys*, whereas *young men* or *young women* is used for individuals between 13 and 18. Individuals older than 18 are referred to as *women* or *men*. Terms such as *elderly* or *senior* are generally not acceptable, as some participants will find these terms perjorative. The acceptable term is *older adults*. Other guidelines can be found in the APA Manual.

### 10.4.2 *People First* Language

A *second reason* for revision is to make sure that the writing is in **People First** language. Because of the Individuals with Disabilities Education Act (1990), all references to disabilities must be written with the individual placed first. Thus, *child with autism* is correct, whereas the *autistic child* is incorrect. This convention emphasizes the value of the human being and delegates the disability to secondary importance.

The writer must distinguish also between the terms *handicap* and *disability*. A handicap can be thought of as a disadvantage imposed on an individual by the environment or by another person, whereas a disability is something that an individual is unable to do, a lack of a body part, or physical or psychosocial impairment. For example, an individual with a spinal cord injury may not be able to walk; the inability to walk is a disability. However, this disability becomes a handicap if there is no wheelchair access, or if the individual refuses to use a wheelchair. The presence of a disability does not make an individual handicapped.

### 10.4.3 Mechanics of Writing

Clear writing requires use of a formal writing style and using grammatically correct language. A *third reason* to revise the manuscript is to make sure that there are no grammatical errors. Errors such as subject-verb agreement (e.g., using *data is* rather than *data are*), punctuation and capitalization, run-on sentences, and sentence fragments are common for inexperienced writers. Run-on sentences and sentence fragments are an indication that either the writer is careless and has not proofread the research paper or that the writer needs help with writing skills.

Other common errors include (a) failing to use parallel structure for grammatical units (e.g., using different parts of speech in a series or in connecting phrases), (b) having dangling modifiers (e.g., sentences in which the modifier is misplaced, such as "It is however believed," rather than "However, it is believed"), (c) splitting infinitives (e.g., "to swiftly complete the task" rather than "to complete the task swiftly"), (d) improperly using relative pronouns (e.g., "an individual must keep their head" rather than "an individual must keep his or her head"), (e) using the passive tense rather than the active tense (e.g., "There were seven subjects" instead of "Seven subjects"), and (f) placing prepositions at the end of sentences ("ethical and legal obligations that occupational therapists are faced with" rather than "ethical and legal obligations that occupational therapists face"). If one is unsure about the proper grammatical structure, a basic grammar book is indispensable. Additional examples of these errors, as well as the correct usages, are illustrated in Figure 10–1.

Many excellent sources are available to help writers avoid grammatical errors and improve their writing. The following list provides major references and online programs:

- Strunk, W., & White, E. B. (1999). The *elements of style* (4th ed.). Boston: Allyn & Bacon.
  A classic containing a gold mine of writing ideas, including rules of usage, principles of composition form, and writing style. The epitome of concise, effective writing.
- American Psychological Association (2010). *Publication manual of the American Psychological Association* (6th ed.). Washington, DC: Author.
  An exhaustive guide to organizing a journal article for publication. Includes content areas such as headings, quotations, references, tables, figures and graphs, and other matters of style that can keep a writer up all night.
- University of Chicago Staff (Ed.). (2010). *The Chicago manual of style: The essential guide for writers, editors, and publishers.* (16th ed.). Chicago: University of Chicago Press.
  If the APA Manual is confusing on a question of style, the CMS is the final word.
- Slade, C., & Perrin, R. (2007). *Form and style: Research papers, reports, theses* (13th ed.). Florence, KY: Cengage Learning/Watsworth.
  A classic guide for writing research papers. Focuses on the processes of writing and gives detailed coverage of *The Chicago Manual of Style*, Modern Language Association, American Psychological Association, and Columbia Guide to Online Style (CGOS). Many examples are given in the text.

| TYPE | RULES | INCORRECT EXAMPLE | CORRECT EXAMPLE |
|---|---|---|---|
| **Dangling or Misplaced Modifier or Participles** | Modifiers and participles should be put as close as possible to the word they are to modify to prevent ambiguity or missing referents. | ... would first determine | ... would determine first... |
| | | ... local issues in that particular clinic that affect job satisfaction | ... local issues that affect job satisfaction in that particular clinic |
| | Place *only* next to the word it modifies. | The participants were screened only ... | The participants only were screened ... |
| **Split Infinitives** | Place adverbs that modify the verb after the phrase "to ... " rather than between the "to" and the verb. | Occupational therapists need to carefully observe behaviors ... | Occupational therapists need to observe carefully behaviors ... |
| **Parallel Structure** | Expressions similar in function or content should be in the same grammatical construction. | (a) Identification of.... (b) clarifying ... (c) assessing to ... and (d) determine whether ... | (a) Identification of ... (b) clarification of ... . (c) assessment of ... and (d) determination of ... |
| | With coordinating conjunctions (i.e., and, but, or, nor), make sure to use all elements of the parallel structure. | The children wanted both to run and play. Neither the directions or the examples were ... | The children wanted both to run and to play. Neither the directions nor the examples were ... |
| **Relative Pronoun** | Use *that* with a restrictive clause (i.e., one that is essential to the passage). | | The chimps that participated in the study were all kept unrestrained in an open testing area. |
| | Use *which* with an unrestrictive clause surrounded by commas (adds information, but is not essential to the sentence). | | The glasses, which were on top of the container, belonged to the patient. |
| | Use *who* in unrestrictive clauses in reference to people. | | The students, who all had ADHD, won ribbons at the races. |

**FIGURE 10-1**   Common Errors of Writing Style

| TYPE | RULES | INCORRECT EXAMPLE | CORRECT EXAMPLE |
|---|---|---|---|
| **Voice (Active/Passive)** | Use *since* when you mean "after that," and *while* when you mean "during." | | Since the development of the WISC-IV, ... <br><br> While the music was playing, the participants ... |
| | Use the active voice whenever possible. | The information examined by the authors ... | The authors examined ... |
| **Tense** | Use past tense to report something that occurred in the past, such as discussion of another author's results or reporting your results. | Jones and Smith (2005) state ... | Jones and Smith (2005) stated ... |
| **Possessives** | Place an apostrophe after the noun or pronoun to show possession. **Exception:** Do not use an apostrophe after the word "it" when showing possession. | The subjects score ... <br><br> It's major strengths are ... | The subject's score was ... <br><br> The Wechsler has 12 subtests. Its first score is ... <br><br> **But:** It's cold (it is cold). |
| **Seriation** | Place elements in a series in parallel form. <br><br> (See Figure 10–2 for correct punctuation.) | ... asked to read the directions, fill out the information, and then to turn in the form. | ... asked to read the directions, fill out the information, and turn in the form. |
| | When the series of items is written in one sentence, use letters in parentheses to separate each item. Use commas to separate the items, unless there are internal commas. Use semicolons to separate items of major categories. | The subjects were administered four tests: clinical observations, *Stress Management Questionnaire*, *Crawford Small Parts Dexterity Test*, and *Strong Vocational Interest Test* | The subjects were administered four tests: (a) clinical observations, (b) *Stress Management Questionnaire*, (c) *Crawford Small Parts Dexterity Test*, and (d) *Strong Vocational Interest Test*. |

**FIGURE 10-1**  *(continued)*

| TYPE | RULES | INCORRECT EXAMPLE | CORRECT EXAMPLE |
|---|---|---|---|
| | When each item in the series is placed into separate sentences or separate paragraphs, use numbers to separate the items. | | The subjects were administered three outcome measures:<br>1. *Stress Management Questionnaire* to examine coping skills,<br>2. *Crawford Small Parts Dexterity Test* to assess dexterity, and<br>3. *Strong Vocational Interest Test* to determine interests. |
| Pronouns | Make sure that the reference for the pronoun is clear. | This was completed. | This self-report scale was completed. |
| | | Those were put over there. | Those books were put over there, on the bottom shelf. |
| | Make sure that the pronoun agrees in number with the noun it replaces and/or modifies. | His chart was placed in their folder. | His chart was placed in his folder. |
| | | The group took their packages. | The group took its packages .... |
| Subject-Verb Agreement | Verbs must agree with the subject, regardless of intervening phrases and/or use of pronouns. | Data is... | Data are ... ["Data" is plural] |
| | | Phenomena is... | Phenomena are ... [Phenomenon is the singular form] |
| | | The articles that were taken from a single journal was ... | The articles that were taken from a single journal were [articles ...were] |
| Misplaced Prepositions | Avoid placing prepositions at the end of sentences. | ... the next area the clinicians were questioned in ... | ...the next area in which the clinicians were questioned ... |

**FIGURE 10-1**   (*continued*)

- Kipfer, B. A., (2010). *Roget's international thesaurus* (7th ed.), New York: Collins Ref.
  An invaluable guide to the writer for selecting the most appropriate word. It is helpful both in locating a specific word and in varying one's language. There are many different versions of this reference, as well as many formats. It is also available online at http://education.yahoo.com/reference/thesaurus/ and on Kindle®.
- Venes, D. (Ed.). (2009). *Taber's cyclopedic medical dictionary* (21st ed.). Philadelphia: F. A. Davis.
  An essential guide for those researchers needing medical terms defined and clarified. Taber's also has an online version at http://www.tabers.com/tabersonline/ub
- *Merriam-Webster's Collegiate Dictionary* (11th ed.). (2003). Springfield, MA: Merriam-Webster.
  Having a dictionary is a must, both for finding meanings of words and for using correct spelling. This is also available online at http://www.merriam-webster.com/ and available on Kindle®.
- Purdue Online Writing Lab (or OWLS), available at http://owl.english.purdue.edu/
  This online resource provides over 200 resources for writing, including format and style guides for MLA and APA, help with writing and grammar, English as a Second Language, and ways to avoid plagiarism.

A *fourth reason* for revision is to check for spelling and punctuation errors. It is critical to check one's spelling with a spell checker (available with most word-processing programs) to ensure that there are no errors. One must be careful, however, to read the article and proof for errors, rather than relying on the computerized speller to find all the errors. It cannot find errors when the words are spelled correctly but misused. For example, if the words *to* and *too* are used incorrectly, the speller will not identify the errors.

Punctuation errors must be found and corrected. Figure 10–2, adapted from the APA Manual (2010), summarizes common punctuation rules. Reading the paper aloud is one method to revise the paper and find errors in punctuation and grammar.

In scientific articles, it is common practice to abbreviate terms used repeatedly (e.g., proprioceptive facilitation as [PF], neurodevelopmental therapy as [NDT], learning disability as [LD or SLD], perceptual-motor training as [PMT], and quality food index as [QFI]). Abbreviations invented by the writer should be kept to a minimum and used only for terms that are long and frequently repeated. Tables of statistical data containing abbreviations should contain a footnote defining the abbreviations.

Latin abbreviations are useful for shortening sentences. The following are the most commonly used abbreviations in scientific articles. Notice that they are not italicized.

- ca. (circa): about a certain time, e.g., ca. BC 130
- e.g. (exempli grata): for example.
- et al. (et alii): and others
- et seq. (et sequens): and the following
- ibid, (ibidem): in the same place
- i.e. (id est): that is to say.
- viz. (videlicet): namely, used to introduce lists

Be sure to refer to the APA Manual for the proper way to use abbreviations. For example, many abbreviations, (including i.e. and e.g.) must be used only within parentheses.

### 10.4.4 Transitional Words, Phrases, and Sentences

A *fifth reason* for revision is to make sure that transitional statements are present so that the flow of ideas is smooth. Writing a well-organized, integrated manuscript requires the use of words and phrases that connect ideas and summarize a section of a paper. In reviewing scientific literature, it is important to integrate the studies under topical areas and to develop a logical sequence. Writing should be coherent. The use of transitional words such as *however, although,* or *nevertheless,* can be used to make the transition smoother and the paper unified. (Note that many style guides frown on beginning a sentence with *however.*) In addition, sentences can be used to permit the smooth transition from one idea to another.

| TYPE | | RULE | EXAMPLE |
|---|---|---|---|
| Spacing | With all punctuation marks | In final copies, use one space in most instances after all punctuation marks. Do not put a space in abbreviations. In a draft copy, double spacing makes it easier to read. | The research was completed by 10 a.m. By 11 a.m., ... Mathews, R. J. ... for the participants. Results ... |
| Comma | Seriation | Use a comma after each word in a series of three or more items. | ... equipment, apparatus, and tools ... |
| | Parenthetical expression | Use a comma before and after a phrase that adds information but is not essential. | Collaboration can be an informal process, where two individuals meet to discuss a problem, or ... |
| | Independent clause | Use a comma to separate independent clauses, but do not use a comma to separate the two parts of a compound predicate. | Five of the participants were Black, and seven of the subjects were Anglo. (But notice: Six students were in seventh grade and were taking history.) |
| | Essential or restrictive clauses | Do not use a comma when the modifying phrase is used to identify, limit, or define a word and is essential to the meaning. | The subjects who were used for the control group included seven occupational therapists. |
| | Dependent clauses | Use a comma rather than a semicolon to separate a dependent and independent phrase. | Although the participants with developmental disabilities were separated from the rest of the participants, all the subjects were placed into a single group for evaluation. |
| Semicolon | Independent clauses | Use a semicolon when the independent clauses are not separated by a coordinating conjunction or when the clauses are separated by a conjunctive adverb. | The apparatus was put on the shelves; the writing materials were put into the desk. The client was interviewed ...; however ... |
| | Seriation | Use a semicolon when there is a comma contained in any part of the seriation. | ...: (a) red box, which contained 3 balls; (b) blue box, which contained 2 balls; and (c) yellow box, which contained 6 balls. |
| Colon | References | Use a colon after the place of publication and before the publisher. | Boston: Pearson/Allyn & Bacon. |
| | | Use a colon before a phrase or example of explanatory material with an introductory phrase. If the example is a complete sentence, start it with a capital letter. | The recorded scores were in the following order: 37, 50, 24, 70. The material was made up of the following parts: two blue boxes, each containing four toys. |

**FIGURE 10-2** Common Errors of Punctuation

| TYPE | | RULE | EXAMPLE |
|---|---|---|---|
| **Quotation Marks** | **Direct quote (fewer than 40 words)** | Put quotations marks around any direct quote of 40 words or fewer. | Lock, Spirduso, and Silverman (1987) cautioned that "[t]he problem in writing a proposal is essentially the same as in writing the final report" (p. 19).<br><br>"The problem in writing a proposal is essentially the same as in writing the final report" (Locke, Spirduso, & Silverman, 1987, p. 19). |
| | **Direct quote (more than 40 words)** | If the direct quote is more than 40 words, offset it in a paragraph and indent on both right and left margins. Do not use quotation marks. End the quotation with a period. Cite the reference with the author, date, and page, or just the page (if the author and date have been previously identified), in parentheses following the quote. Do not put a period at the end of the parenthesis. | |
| | **With other punctuation** | Period and commas should be placed inside closing single or double quotation marks, whereas other punctuation marks are placed outside of the quotations, unless they are part of the quote. | Smith stated, "General educators look at the forest, while special educators look at the trees." |
| | **Titles** | Put quotation marks around any title of a chapter or article cited in the text. Do not put around any title in the reference list. | John's review discussed Chapter 2, "The Scientific Method." |
| | **Terms** | Use quotation marks when introducing a word or phrase used as slang, irony, or invented term. Use italics to introduce a technical or key term. Do not use quotation marks or italics when the word or phrase is used a second time. Do not use quotations (or italics) with commonly used foreign terms. | Ninja coined the term "normalization" …<br><br>Removing a previously given reinforcement is called cost response.<br><br>But:<br><br>per se<br><br>vis-á-vis |

**FIGURE 10-2** *(continued)*

Adapted from the *Publication Manual of the American Psychological Association* (2010).

| TYPE | | RULE | EXAMPLE |
|---|---|---|---|
| **Parentheses** | **Parenthetical information** | Use parentheses to set off material that is independent of the rest of the information. Put punctuation marks inside the parentheses if the material is a sentence and outside the parentheses if the material is a phrase. | The subjects (15 boys and 2 girls) were ...<br><br>(The subjects consisted of 15 boys and 2 girls.) |
| | **References** | Enclose reference citations in text with parentheses. | (Jones & Smith, 1994)<br><br>Jones and Smith (1994) |
| | **Abbreviations** | Abbreviations should be put in parentheses the first time the full term is used. Thereafter, the abbreviation can be used instead of the full term. | Sensory therapy ... (SI)... SI ... |
| | **Seriation** | Enclose the letters used in seriation within a sentence or paragraph in parentheses.<br><br>Use periods if each item in the series is placed in a different paragraph. | (a) ..., (b) ..., and (c) ...<br><br>1. ...<br>2. ...<br>3. ... |
| **Brackets** | **Parenthetical material** | Enclose parenthetical material that is within parentheses in brackets unless the use of the commas will not confuse the reader. | (*Miller Assessment for Preschoolers* [MAP, 1988])<br><br>(Johns, 1998; Smith, 2009). |
| | **References** | Enclose material inserted into a quotation with brackets. | " ... [the participants in the study] were asked to come ... "<br><br>"[T]he study showed ..." |

**FIGURE 10-2**   *(continued)*

The reader should have no difficulty following the train of thought or the arguments used to build a case. Additionally, reading the research paper as a whole will uncover any inconsistencies or repetitions between sections (Slade & Perrin, 2007). Often, having someone unacquainted with the topic read the work serves to ensure clarity, understanding, and consistency.

### 10.4.5 Clarity of Thought

The scientific writer should try to communicate ideas simply and rigorously. Some of the most profound ideas can be expressed in clear, direct language. It is not a sign of intellectual prowess to present ideas so that they are difficult to understand. Therefore, a *sixth reason* for revision is to ensure that the paper is written clearly. Scientific writing is particularly prone to abstruseness and ambiguity, especially in clinical areas where language is used loosely without precise operational definitions. One method of ensuring clarity is to include a conceptual or operational definition for unusual terms or for terms specific to a certain discipline. Even if the writer chooses not to create a glossary, uncommon terms must be defined operationally. Use of well-thought-out charts, tables, or figures can facilitate the clarity of the research paper. It is not unusual for readers to look at charts, tables, or figures before reading the text, especially when these visual aids provide an overall summary of the principle finding.

### 10.4.6 Organization

*Finally*, the author should examine whether the background information is represented accurately, whether ideas unrelated to the topic have been introduced, and whether the hypothesis or guiding statement(s) have directed the writing (Slade & Perrin, 2007). Each statement of results should be supported by data. Differences or contradictions in findings compared with previous studies need to be discussed and, when possible, explained. The whole research paper should be reviewed for sequence of ideas. Eventually, even though additional changes are possible, the writer must accept the paper as it is.

[T]he secret of good writing is to strip every sentence to its cleanest components. Every word that serves no function, every long word that could be a short word, every adverb which carries the same meaning that is already in the verb, every passive construction that leaves the reader unsure of who is doing what—these are the thousand and one adulterants that weaken the strength of a sentence. (Zinsser, 1990, pp. 7–8)

## 10.5 Quotations, Referenced Material, and Bibliographic Citations

Whenever one uses material written by another person, whether the material is directly quoted or only paraphrased, one must make reference to the original author(s). Failure to do so is **plagiarism**. Some authors (Winkler & McCuen, 1998) have suggested that plagiarism is common in everyday language. One might use in speech an example stated in a lecture by a professor and fail to give that professor the credit, for example. In another case, one may use a proverb such as "A stitch in time saves nine" and fail to give Benjamin Franklin the credit. Although these examples are not routinely considered plagiarism and are generally acceptable in everyday speech, plagiarism is not accepted in a research or scholarly paper.

Plagiarism occurs when a researcher deliberately takes another person's ideas and incorporates them into his or her own writing without giving any credit to the original author. Examples of plagiarism include the following: (a) taking another's research ideas and submitting them as one's own, (b) paraphrasing an article without giving credit to the author, or (c) directly copying part of an article without citing the authors. Any copyright material used without giving credit to the original author is considered plagiarism (Winkler & McCuen, 1998).

If the material used is a direct quote from another author or authors, the writer must cite the author(s), year of publication, and page number of the quotation in the text. There must be no change in spelling, phrasing, capitalization, or punctuation from the original. The exception to this rule is when the first word of a quotation needs to be capitalized or placed in lower case to make the statement grammatically correct. When it is necessary to make changes (e.g., when a pronoun must be clarified or a word added to make the content more understandable), the change must be put in square brackets ([ ]). When a word is misspelled or the grammar is incorrect in the original, *[sic]* follows the misspelling or grammatical error to show that the quotation is reproduced exactly. For example, "The article was written by an england *[sic]* author."

A quote can be introduced as part of a grammatical sentence, or it may stand alone as a sentence. When material is omitted from the quotation, then an ellipsis (…) replaces the material that is left out. When the quote is more than 40 words, it should stand alone as a separate paragraph. In this case, the quoted material is punctuated, and the reference for the quoted material is placed after the paragraph and in parenthesis with no punctuation. Examine the following:

> Slang, hackneyed or flippant phrases, and folksy style should be avoided. Since objectivity is the primary goal, there should be no element of exhortation or persuasion. The research report should describe and explain, rather than try to convince or move to action. In this respect, the research report differs from the essay or the feature article. (Best, 1977, p. 317)

When the material has fewer than 40 words, it is placed within the paragraph. The reference is placed in parentheses at the end of the quote. For example: According to Best (1977), "The research report should be presented in a style that is creative, clear, and concise" (p. 317).

When the writer wishes to paraphrase another author's material, then the writer must cite the author(s) and date of publication. Examine the following two examples:

> 1. Best & Kahn (2005) suggested that when writing a research article, one must be careful to write concisely and clearly.
> 2. When writing a research article, one must be careful to write concisely and clearly (Best & Kahn, 2005; Winkler & McCuen, 1998).

Notice that no page numbers are used in either reference and that the authors' names are put within parentheses at the end of the sentence if it has not been used as part of the sentence structure. Additional information regarding common citations of authors in the text is summarized in Figure 10–3.

Whether the writer has quoted the source directly or paraphrased the material, a complete reference must be placed in the reference list at the end of the research paper. Figure 10–4 summarizes the different styles for common reference citations, and Table 10–3 shows some examples of these citations. Further information regarding the appropriate style for dissertations, secondary sources, movies, or films can be found in the APA Manual. Regardless of the type of publication, all citations must include enough information so that the reader can locate the original source.

## 10.6 Format of a Paper

The format of the research paper is dictated by the style of writing used. For journal publications using the APA style, the size of the margins, line spacing, and size of print are specified. Individual professors and non-APA style journals may have different requirements. In a thesis or dissertation, additional sections are required. A typical organization of the sequence for a thesis or dissertation is listed below:

1. Title page (see Figure 10–5)
2. Approval page indicating names and titles of thesis readers (required for a thesis or dissertation only)
3. Acknowledgments, including individuals who aided in the study and any grant support accepted

| | FIRST CITATION | ADDITIONAL CITATIONS IN THE TEXT |
|---|---|---|
| **One Author, Citation with Page Numbers** | Last name, year, page (when applicable):<br><br>Sanchez (2010) … (p. 94); (Sanchez, 2010, p. 94)<br><br>Page number is used only when there is a direct quote. No page numbers are used when the material is paraphrased. | Same as the first citation. |
| **One Author, Citation with No Page Numbers** | Last name, year, paragraph (when applicable):<br><br>Miller (2009) … (para. 4.)<br><br>When there are short headings in the article use the heading and paragraph following the heading:<br><br>Miller (2010) … (Results, para. 1).<br><br>If the heading is too long, shorten the title and put it in quotation marks:<br><br>Miller (2010) … ("Covering Schools with no AYP," para. 2). [The original heading was Covering Urban Schools which Have Not Received AYP.]<br><br>Paragraph number is used only when there is a direct quote. No paragraph number is used when the material is paraphrased. | Same as the first citation. |
| **Two Authors** | Last names; use "and" or "&":<br><br>Smith and Miller (2011); (Smith & Miller, 2011) | Same as the first citation. |
| **Three to Five Authors** | Last name of all authors; "and" or "&" placed before the last author:<br><br>Rasmussen, Miller, Sanchez, Rogers, and Thomas (2011) …<br><br>(Rasmussen, Miller, Sanchez, Rogers, & Thomas, 2011) …<br><br>**But** if two or more references would shorten to the same citation, cite as many authors as necessary to distinguish between the two citations and follow with (comma) et al.:<br><br>DeWitt, Sherer, Johnson, and Smith (2011) versus De Witt, Sherer, Jones, Johnson, and Dennis, (2011) | List the first author and replace the rest of the authors with et al.<br><br>Rasmussen et al., (2011); (Rasmussen et al., 2011)<br><br><br><br>Shorten to DeWitt, Sherer, Johnson, et al., 2011) and (De Witt, Sherer, Jones, et al., 2011) |
| **Six or More Authors** | Last name of first author followed by et al., year:<br>Steinberg et al. (2009)<br><br>When two or more references would shorten to the same citation, cite as many authors as necessary to distinguish between citations, followed by (comma) et al. (See Three to Five authors). | Same as the first citation. |
| **Two or More Citations** | List citations alphabetically by first author's name, followed by a semicolon:<br><br>(James, Smith, & Johnson, 2009; Marley & Barnett, 2008). | Same as the first citation. |

**FIGURE 10-3** Using Citations in Text using APA Style: The sequence of authors is determined by the sequence in the article. When the citation is used a second time in the same paragraph, leave out the date unless there are two citations by the same author, or the citation can be confused with another citation.

| | BOOK | JOURNAL | CHAPTER FROM A BOOK | INTERNET ARTICLE |
|---|---|---|---|---|
| Author(s)— Seven or Fewer | Last name(s), initials ... & last name, initials; no additional punctuation at the end.<br><br>**Jones, M. J., Smith, J. C., & Merrill, M. M.** | Same as book.<br><br>**Jones, M. J., Smith, J. C., Merrill, M. M., Simon, J., Bills, S., & Jones, C. C.** | Same as book.<br><br>**Jones, M. J., Smith, J. C., Merrill, M. M., & Simon, J.** | If the article has an author, same as the others. If not, the title of the page becomes the author. The title of the page is found above the URL in the browser.<br><br>**Schoolneuropsychology.com: Home page.** |
| Author(s)— Seven or more | Last name(s), initials of first six authors, comma, ellipsis (...) last name, initials of last author. No ampersand is used; no additional punctuation at the end.<br><br>**Johnson, A. B., Martin, B. C., Jones, M. J., Smith, J. C., Merrill, M. M., Smith, D. K., ... Brown, D. A.** | Same as book.<br><br>**Johnson, A. B., Martin, B. C., Jones, M. J., Smith, J. C., Merrill, M. M., Smith, D. K., ... Brown, D. A.** | Same as book.<br><br>**Johnson, A. B., Martin, B. C., Jones, M. J., Smith, J. C., Merrill, M. M., Smith, D. K., ... Brown, D. A.** | Same as book.<br><br>**Johnson, A. B., Martin, B. C., Jones, M. J., Smith, J. C., Merrill, M. M., Smith, D. K., ... Brown, D. A.** |
| Editor | Place the terms (Ed.) or (Eds.) before the date. Place a period after the parentheses.<br><br>**James, J. B., & Jones, J. J. (Eds). (2010). *Evaluation procedures.*** | | Same as book.<br><br>**James, J. B., & Jones, J. J. (Eds). (2010). *Evaluation procedures.*** | |

**FIGURE 10-4** Common Bibliographic References: Additional information regarding the appropriate style of dissertations, secondary sources, movies or films, or other sources can be found in the APA Manual.

| | BOOK | JOURNAL | CHAPTER FROM A BOOK | INTERNET ARTICLE |
|---|---|---|---|---|
| **Year** | Place the year in parentheses and put a period after the parentheses.<br><br>**(2010).** | Same as book, except:<br><br>For weekly issues or magazines, put the year, month (and day if it is weekly) in parentheses. If there is no date, put n.d. (i.e., no date)<br><br>**(2010).**<br><br>**(n.d.)**<br><br>**(2010, Oct 17).** | Same as book.<br><br>**(2010).** | Same as journal. The date is often found at the bottom of the page as the copyright.<br><br>**(2010).**<br><br>**(2010, November).**<br><br>**(n.d.).** |
| **Title of Book, Article, Chapter** | Capitalize the first word of the book and first word after a colon or ending punctuation. End with a period, unless there is an edition number. Underline the title of book or put in italics.<br><br>*Evaluation in therapeutic settings.* | Capitalize first word of the journal and first word after a colon or ending punctuation. End with a period. DO NOT underline the title of article or put in italics.<br><br>**Evaluation of therapeutic progress: Part 1.** | Capitalize first word of the chapter from a book and first word after a colon or ending punctuation. End with a period. DO NOT use italics or underline.<br><br>**The role of the COTA in evaluating therapeutic progress.** | Capitalize first word of the title of the article and first word after a colon or ending punctuation. End with a period. Underline or italicize the title.<br><br>***Thank you for visiting the*** *www.schoolneuropsychology.com* ***website.*** |
| **Edition** | Put the edition number of the book in parentheses following the title of the book. Place a period at the end. Do not italicize.<br><br>*Evaluation of therapeutic progress (2nd ed.).* | | Same as journal. The edition goes after the title of the book, not the title of the chapter.<br><br>In *Evaluation of therapeutic progress (2nd ed.; pp. 199–255)* by J. W. Smith and M. C. Thompson. | |
| **Title of Journal** | | Capitalize important words in the journal title and underline it or put in italics. Put a comma after the title.<br><br>*Journal of Aging,* | | |

**FIGURE 10-4** *(continued)*

| | BOOK | JOURNAL | CHAPTER FROM A BOOK | INTERNET ARTICLE |
|---|---|---|---|---|
| **Volume** | | Place after the title of the journal. Underline (or italicize) the volume and comma. *Journal of Aging, 35,* | | Include the issue if present with the title of journal and volume. *Journal of Aging, 35(3).* |
| **Issue** | | Do not include an issue number, unless each issue begins with page 1. If needed, place in parentheses following the volume, with no space in between. Do not italicize. Follow with a comma. *Journal of Aging, 35(3),* | | |
| **Page or Paragraph** | | Place the page number after the volume (or issue) number. Put a period after the page number. Don't use p. or pp. *Journal of Aging, 35, 179–195.* | | If the electronic article has page numbers, follow the rule of a journal. |
| **Place of publication** | City, State: Publisher. Do not use state for major cities. Use the 2-letter abbreviation for state, when needed. Boston: Allyn & Bacon. Thorofare, NJ: SLACK. | | Same as book. | Provide the URL where the electronic source was retrieved. DO NOT put a period after the URL. Retrieved from http://www.ninds.nih.gov/disorders/cerebral_palsy/cerebral_palsy.htm#What_is |

**FIGURE 10-4**   *(continued)*

Adapted from the *Publication Manual of the American Psychological Association* (2010), Slade & Perrin (2007)), and the Purdue Online Writing Lab at http://owl.english.purdue.edu/owl/section/2/10/

| | |
|---|---|
| **TABLE 10-3** | |

**Examples of Bibliographic References using APA Style**

| | |
|---|---|
| *Book* | Locke, L. F., Spirduso, W. W, & Silverman, S. J. (1997). *Proposals that work* (3rd ed.). Newbury Park: Sage. |
| *Journal Article* | Smith, J. G., & Jones, J. M. ( 1993). Reconstructing the facial features. *Journal of Paleontology, 17,* 339–431. |
| *Chapter in a Book* | Rutter, M., Chadwick, O., & Shaffer, D. (1983). Head injury. In M. Rutter (Ed.), *Developmental neuropsychiatry* (pp. 83–111). New York: Guilford. |
| *Electronic Sources: Online Journal* | Badge, J., Johnson, S., Moseley, A., & Cann, A. (2010, March). Observing emerging student networks on a microblogging service. *Journal of Online Teaching and Learning, 7*(1). Retrieved from http://jolt.merlot.org/vol7no1/cann_0311.htm |
| *Online Article with Assigned DOI* | Gallardo, G., Guardia, J., Villasenor, T., & McNeil, M. R. (2011). Psychometric data for the revised Token Test in normally developing Mexican children ages 4-12 years. *Archives of Clinical Neuropsychology, 26,* 225–234. First published online March 25, 2011 doi:10.1093/arclin/acr018 |
| *Online Books* | Mowrer, R. R., & Klein, S. B. (Eds.) (2001). *Contemporary learning theories.* Mahwah, NJ: Lawrence Erlbaum. Available at http://www.questia.com/PM.qst?a=o&d=58896999 |

**Note:** Additional information regarding the appropriate style for other electronic sources, including dissertations, secondary sources, movies, films, or podcasts can be found in the APA Manual.

Adapted from the *Publication Manual of the American Psychological Association, 6th edition,* (2010); Slade & Perrin (2007); and the Purdue Online Writing Lab at http://owl.english.purdue.edu/owl/section/2/10/

4. Table of contents, including chapter and section headings, appendix, and bibliography
5. List of statistical tables
6. List of illustrations, photographs, and figures
7. Abstract
8. The content of the text

   a. Introduction
   b. Review of the literature
   c. Method
   d. Results
   e. Discussion, including clinical implications of findings and limitations of study
   f. Conclusions and further research

9. References
10. Acknowledgements
11. Tables
12. Figures
13. Appendix
14. Vita, listing professional education, work history, and previous publications

A running title, consisting of no more than 50 words, is placed in capital letters in the upper left hand corner of each page. One inch margins are used for the top, bottom, and both sides. APA style dictates the position of page numbers (usually below the running title), the use of Roman and Arabic numbers, the type of paper, the levels of headings, spacing, and use of quotations.

### 10.6.1 Outline of a Research Proposal

1. Title of study
2. Investigator
3. Date

Boston University: Sargent College

College of Health and Rehabilitation Sciences

The Effect of Sensory Integration

on a 10-Year-Old Child with Learning Disabilities

By

Barbara Stein, B. S.

Submitted in partial fulfillment

of the requirements for the degree of

Master of Occupational Therapy (MOT)

September, 2012

© Cengage Learning 2013

**FIGURE 10-5**    Example of a Title Page for a Research Paper, Thesis, or Dissertation

4. The research problem

   a. Statement of problem in question form
   b. Justification and need for the study
   c. Implications of anticipated results in relation to clinical treatment, professional, education, or administrative problems

5. The literature review

   a. Outline of major areas to be reviewed
   b. Plan for search of related literature
   c. Annotated bibliographical notation organized under major areas reviewed

6. Research design

   a. Research model, (e.g., experimental, correlational, or methodological)
   b. Operational definitions of variables

   c. Statement of hypotheses or guiding questions
   d. Identification of presumed independent or dependent variables
   e. Theoretical explanation underlying study

7. Method

   a. Procedure for selecting sample and screening criteria for subject inclusion
   b. Setting for study and procedure for collecting data
   c. Tests, questionnaires, or instruments applied to study
   d. Methodological studies to include evaluation of

      i. reliability
      ii. validity

e. Tentative time schedule for study

    i. time period for literature review
    ii. collection of data: number of hours required
    iii. date for completion of research

f. Projected costs for study

    i. clerical
    ii. instrumentation
    iii. other

## 10.7 Sample Proposal of a Graduate Research Project

An example of a graduate research project is listed at the end of this chapter. The project has been reprinted by permission of the author.

## 10.8 Preparation for Presentation

### 10.8.1 Poster Session

A **poster display** is an opportunity for researchers to present their research in a discussion-like format. At many conferences, a portion of the conference area is set aside for poster displays. Usually the researcher stays with the poster and discusses the data analysis and procedures with the conference participants. This is an opportunity for the participants to ask questions related to the research.

The poster should be presented in a clear and comprehensive manner. Components of the poster itself include (a) an abstract written in 25–50 words; (b) the purpose or aim of the study; (c) the methodology including subject selection, measurements, procedures, or treatment techniques; (d) results presented in graphic form; and (e) a summary of the conclusions. In addition to the poster, a handout is usually available that may include all the components, plus a summary of literature review and a means of contacting the researchers.

Use of a graphic program, such as the SmartArt in WORD, will make the presentation look more professional. Graphs should be completed with a graphics program, such as Microsoft Excel.

### Key Points in Preparing a Poster

- **Size of print:** The print size should be large enough for participants to read it at a distance of 4 feet, generally a font size of 18–24 points.
- **Layout:** The layout is determined by the space provided at the conference and directions from the conference committee. Try different layout designs. The material should be arranged to facilitate understanding of the material, generally top to bottom in a left-to-right sequence (see Figure 10–6).
- **Amount of information:** Information should be written in bullets (three-to-four word phrases) rather than in sentences. Include essential information about the design, procedure, and results. Figures, charts, and photographs are helpful in displaying results. Additional information can be included in the handout.
- **Color:** Use color in highlighting the results and conclusions. A light color (e.g., yellow) printed on a dark paper is frequently easier to read.
- **Background:** Use of contrasting color or border behind the individual components will make the poster visually attractive.

### 10.8.2 Conference Paper

Researchers are encouraged to present the results of their findings at local, state, national, and international conferences. A call for papers is issued in *OT Practice*. When presenting a paper, it is important to recognize that those in attendance are adult learners with a heterogeneous knowledge base.

### Key Points of Presenting a Paper

- Rehearse the presentation, considering time available for the presentation.
- Consider the number of people and the size of the room when preparing the paper. If a presenter has only 10–15 minutes, discussing one or two major points is more feasible than if the presentation is a 90-minute workshop.
- Consider who will be in the audience (e.g., parents, professionals, new graduates, experienced clinicians) and plan your presentation accordingly.

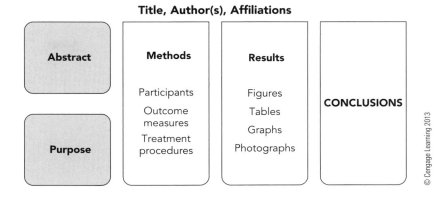

**FIGURE 10-6**  Sample Layout of a Poster Session

- If the paper must be read verbatim, use conversational expression and eye contact with members of the audience.
- When presentations are more than 15 minutes long, prepare a visual presentation, such as a PowerPoint presentation that can be used to discuss the paper rather than reading it verbatim.
- Use 3 × 5 cards to organize and remember the key points to present.
- Allow 5–10 minutes for questions from the audience.
- Speak loudly enough for everyone in the audience to hear.
- Prepare the visual presentation so that people in the last row can see them. If possible, provide handouts of the overheads (in smaller fonts).
- When preparing PowerPoint presentations, be sure that the print is large (fonts of 36 points or above) and that students have handouts of the presentations. A light print with a dark background (dark blue background with yellow print) is easier to read. A sans serif font (e.g., Arial) is also preferable. Although adding animations can be entertaining, they may distract from the presentation.
- Be sure that equipment works prior to the presentation. Go to the room at least 10 minutes before the presentation and try out the equipment.

- Include a beginning, middle, and ending in your presentation. The beginning should establish rapport and set the purpose of the presentation with the audience. The ending should summarize the presentation. Make your conclusion memorable.
- Generally, the audience will be adult learners. Adult learners are pragmatic, eager to apply what they learn, have a variety of experiences, and often challenge the presenter.
- Include a one-page handout with references, in addition to the handouts from the PPT presentation.

### Audiovisual Aids

- **PowerPoint:** This is a useful tool for the organization of material. Individual points can be displayed as they are discussed, rather than all at once, as they would be on a transparency or slide. Sequencing and timing are easier than when using slides or overheads. Handouts should be used to help the audience follow the program. In addition, speaker notes can be scripted to remind the speaker of specific points. Because PowerPoint is updated frequently, the speaker should verify that the software and hardware are compatible.
- **Overhead transparencies:** Overhead transparencies are used less frequently than in the

past. In general, prepare these with a word-processing program rather than free-hand print. Use color transparencies if possible. Pictures can be scanned into a document and printed. The print should be large enough for those in the back to see (36 point or larger). Graphics should be clear without distracting material.

- **Slides:** Arrange slides in a carousel and test prior to presentation. Use a dark background with highly contrasted and large lettering.
- **Flip charts:** Use dark-colored markers, write in large lettering, and place the easel on a platform above the audience so those in the back can see the chart.

## 10.8.3 Publication

Numerous opportunities exist for students and clinicians to publish their research in occupational therapy journals. The following outline lists the steps in selecting a journal and preparing the research study for publication. In addition, based on the first author's experience as an editor, questions used to evaluate a submitted manuscript to a referred journal have been included.

### Selecting the Appropriate Journal

An extensive list of all occupational therapy journals is found in Chapter 6. The researcher should obtain the instructions for submission before submitting the paper. The style (e.g., APA, CMS), margins, page length, manuscript length, number of copies, and the arrangement of the manuscript are specific to each journal. Most journals require work to be submitted electronically, either through e-mail or on a CD or DVD.

### Classifying the Manuscript

- Research paper, presenting original data (quantitative and qualitative)
- The position paper, (e.g., advocating change in health care system)
- Review article (integration of research studies)
- Description of clinical program
- Description of clinical device
- Book review
- Letter to the editor

### Components of Manuscript

- **Title:** include variables, subjects, settings
- **Author(s):** include degrees, affiliation, e-mail address, and correspondence address
- **Abstract:** 100–175 word summary of article
- **Key words:** 4–5 descriptive words
- **Literature review and introduction**
- **Method**
- **Results**
- **Discussion**
- **Conclusions**
- **Recommendations for further research and limitations of study**
- **Acknowledgments**
- **References**
- **Tables and figures**

### Process of Getting into Print

- Rewriting and multiple drafts are necessary.
- Keep in mind that 30 percent of manuscripts are rejected.
- The lag between submitting an article and seeing it in print is often up to 1 year.
- Refereed journals: The types of decisions made include (a) accept with minor revisions, (b) accept with major revisions, (c) resubmit for additional review, and (d) reject.

### The Journal Review Process (Questions Posed for the Reviewer)

- Is the title representative of the article?
- Is the abstract a summary of the main points of the study?
- Does the author justify the need and significance of research?
- Is the literature review comprehensive and up to date?
- Is the research design rigorous? (Internal validity)
- Is generalization to target population valid? (External validity)
- Does the investigator use the appropriate statistical tests?
- Are results consistent with statistical findings?
- Are the conclusions justified?

- Are the references up to date and from a variety of sources?
- Does the author recommend further research and state limitations of study?
- Are the figures and graphs labeled correctly?
- Do the figures and graphs add to the information presented?

## 10.9 Summary

One of the important purposes of this text is to help the student and practitioner generate clinical research studies that validate practice. The authors have presented the research process in a systematic method. The research process presented incorporates both qualitative and quantitative research models. For the clinical researcher, these models can be used to validate practice. Research does not exist in a vacuum. There is a strong historical background for research that has led to the progress in medicine, rehabilitation, and habilitation. Occupational therapists are part of the behavioral medicine tradition that applies nonsurgical and nonpharmaceutical methods. Occupational therapists employing behavioral techniques and assistive technology, such as sensory-integration therapy, neurodevelopmental theory, creative arts, relaxation therapy, splinting, and prescriptive exercise can use the clinical research methods described to establish evidence-based practice for the twenty-first century. It is the authors' intention that the development of treatment protocols can be useful in the establishment of a scientific foundation for occupational therapy.

# KR and Learning to Tell Time in Persons with Cognitive Developmental Disabilities

*Samantha Applegate*
*The University of Toledo*
*June, 2006*

## TABLE OF CONTENTS

# 1.0 THE RESEARCH PROBLEM

## 1.1    Statement of Research Problem in Question Form

- What is a developmental disability?
- What is the cause of developmental disabilities?
- How is mental retardation *[sic]* /developmental disabilities categorized?
- How do people with developmental disabilities acquire skill?
- What are effective strategies for teaching people with developmental disabilities new skills?
- What type of services do people with developmental disabilities typically receive?
- What is occupational therapy's typical focus when treating a person with developmental disabilities?
- What is Knowledge of Results?
- What are effective strategies employed using Knowledge of Results?
- Is the use of Knowledge of Results effective in teaching people with developmental disabilities?

## 1.2    Justification and Need for Study

The American Association on Mental Retardation (Mental Retardation, 1993) defines developmental disabilities (DD) as a substantial limitation in present functioning that is characterized by significantly subaverage intellectual functioning, along with related limitations in two of ten areas, including communication, self-care, home living, social skills, and safety. The American Psychiatric Association also states that the age of onset must occur before age 18 years (1994). Developmental disabilities can occur prenatal, perinatal or in early childhood (Merrill & Mulligan, 2003).

There is no cure for DD, but those who have DD can learn to do many things. It may just take them more time and effort than others, depending on the severity of involvement. One way of categorizing DD is in four distinct levels. These levels have been established based upon intelligence quotient scores (IQ); however these levels are not universally used. The highest level of DD, mild DD, is associated with the highest IQ range. For instance individuals over the age of 21 years of age with IQs ranging from 52–68, are considered to have mild DD. These individuals usually have achieved enough social and vocational skills for self support; however, they do need support under social or economical stress (dealing with relationship or financial needs). The moderate level of DD involves an IQ range of 36–51. Individuals in this range may achieve self support by performing in assisted conditions and needs support in mildly stressful social and economic situations. The third level of DD, referred to as severe, involves an IQ range of 20–35. Individuals in this category need complete supervision but are able to contribute partially to their own self care. Profound is the lowest level of DD. The IQ range for a person who is profoundly mentally retarded is 19 or below. As an adult, a person in this category may achieve very little independent self care and usually requires nursing assistance (Merck, 2003). One way to understand the levels of classification are to associate how the level of IQ relates to the abilities of the individual with DD. The relationship is proportional in that the higher the IQ, the greater the ability. Conversely needing support or complete supervision is often associated with a reduced ability to meet self-care, household, community interaction, social interaction, leisure time, and vocational needs and goals.

The care and treatment of those with DD has changed greatly as societal attitudes have evolved through the past century and beyond. Most recently, the shift has involved deinstitutionalization resulting in placing those with DD into family or group homes. Some individuals with DD are even living independently while requiring minimal assistance. There are several advantages for community based group homes compared to institutional life. One advantage to those who move to group settings is that they have increased contact with their families and are provided more time in a wider variety of activities outside the house (Firth, 1987). They also provide opportunities for clients to learn both basic and advanced living skills. This is important for two reasons. First, it is a "real life" living situation. For instance, household chores need to be done or more self care is done by the individual with DD due to the fact that there is less staff available to them. They also learn skills in real life situations that might be hard to simulate in institutions, like going grocery shopping or taking care of a dog (Neistadt, 1987). Secondly, the social structure of the group home provides a ready-made peer support network. Peer support can increase their social skills. They will also learn to offer emotional and physical assistance as needed (Neistadt, 1987). It has been shown that individuals living in institutions are also less active, mobile, social, and independent compared to a nondisabled reference group (O'Neill, Brown, Gordon, & Schonhorn, 1985). Individuals placed in communities also have a greater level of cognitive and social skills than those not placed in community living (Eastwood & Fisher, 1988). However, adults with developmental disabilities residing in group homes generally have not yet reached the peak of their functional abilities in spite of being placed in a more naturalistic community setting (Neistadt, 1987). Occupational therapy has the opportunity to help those with DD fulfill some of those cognitive and psychosocial abilities given the right interventions.

Although there is great variability among individuals with DD, many higher functioning individuals may want to enter the work environment or socialize outside the group home. A basic skill that is essential for being able to hold a job or engage in social events in the community is the skill of telling time. This is a very important Instrumental Activities of Daily Living (IADL) because telling time is an essential precursor for knowing when to leave for a job or social gathering, how long they have to get to their destination, and when they need to leave to return home. Therefore the purpose of the present study is to see if there is an effect on learning to telling time when KR is present in a population with DD who is residing in a group home. Telling time is an important IADL that can lead to increased independence in the home and work settings. This is an important skill to any subpopulation of DD, but it is especially important to those interested in prevocational opportunities.

## 2.0 THE LITERATURE REVIEW

### 2.1   How the Literature Was Searched

- PubMed
- MEDLINE
- CINAHL

- Google Scholar
- Internet Resources
- AOTA
- AOTF

### 2.2   Underlying Theoretical Assumptions

- There is variability in the cognitive abilities of people with cognitive developmental disabilities (Merck, 2003).
- Learning activities of daily living and instrumental activities of daily living is possible in people with cognitive developmental disabilities (Merck, 2003).
- Providing a reduced frequency of Knowledge of Results is an effective strategy for teaching motor skills (Schmidt & Lee, 2005).
- People with cognitive developmental disabilities can learn a skill through using reduced frequency of Knowledge of Results (Rice & Hernandez, 2006).

### 2.3   Target Population

The target population is adult-aged people with cognitive developmental disabilities

### 2.4   Literature Review Summary

Occupational therapists work with a broad range of clientele, helping them develop useful life skills that will permit them to be more independent, successful, and to improve their quality of life. One population occupational therapists work directly with is the mentally retarded/developmentally disabled population. As many as 3 out of every 100 people in the country have developmental disabilities (The Arc, 2004). As occupational therapists, we have the responsibility to ensure the most appropriate and efficacious intervention programs are provided to all populations. Evidence based practice is needed in occupational therapy to establish important strategies for assessment and treatment. By giving those with developmental disabilities the best possible treatment, the occupational therapist can help these individuals reach their maximum potential in life. This population has a wide array of characteristics and abilities.

There are many different causes of developmental disabilities (DD). Some are genetic, where DD results from the abnormality of genes inherited from parents during conception. The use of drugs and alcohol by the mother while pregnant can also cause DD. Malnutrition, rubella, granular disorders and diabetes, cytomegalovirus, human immunodeficiency virus (HIV), and many other illnesses of the mother during pregnancy can also cause DD. An unusual amount of stress during birth can also injure the baby's brain, as can insufficient oxygen, and extreme premature birth. Other causes of DD include childhood diseases such as whooping cough, chicken pox, measles, and haemophilus influenzae type B disease which may lead to meningitis and encephalitis, all of which can damage the brain. Accidents that affect the brain similar to a blow to the head or a near drowning accident can also cause DD. Toxic substances such as mercury or lead can cause permanent damage to the brain and nervous system. Children in deprived families may become mentally retarded because of malnutrition or inadequate medical care. Overall, damage to the brain occurs resulting in cognitive mental retardation (*The Merck Manual of Diagnosis and Therapy,* 1992; The Arc, California Edition, 1977).

A study done by Eastwood and Fisher (1988) compared skill acquisition among those institutionalized to those who had been moved from an institution to a community setting. They found that clients who were in the community setting had a significantly greater level of cognitive and social skills after placement than did a matched group of control clients who were still residing in institutions. The community group scored higher than the institution group on seven of eight skill areas including reading/writing, quantitative, independent living, community orientation, recreation/leisure time, vocational, and social interaction.

O'Neill et al. (1985) evaluated the change in activity pattern and skills of severely and profoundly DD individuals *[sic]* after they moved from an institution to community living. They found that when compared to a nondisabled reference group the individuals with DD become much more similar to the reference group in their activity patterns after being deinstitutionalized. They also improved in 4 of 16 skill areas within three months of leaving the institutions. The skill areas they improved in were expressive communication, eating, serving meals/washing dishes, and meal preparation, all of which are occupations of daily living (ODL).

Poole et al. (1991) stated, "The overall goal of occupational therapy for the person with cognitive impairments is to enhance performance in daily living" (Poole, Dunn, Schell, Tiernan, & Barnhart, 1991). Occupational therapists also focus on improving instrumental activities of daily living (IADL) skills with their clients. An IADL is a complex occupation or task that a person does to maintain independence in the home and community (Law, 2002). This could include meal planning, taking care of pets, cleaning the house, or telling time. Increasing these skills in an individual with DD can drastically improve his/her quality of life, independence level, and social functioning.

One of the main objectives of occupational therapy is to enhance the learning process (Flinn & Radomski, 2002). Unfortunately group homes can also make it very difficult for clients to learn, due to the high turnover rate of staff and the stresses that are associated with the turnover rates (Neistadt, 1987). The hope is that occupational therapists facilitate learning processes in ways that enhance the probability that their clients will remember the learned information.

A strategy that has been shown to be effective in motor learning uses a certain type of augmented feedback known as *Knowledge of Results.* Knowledge of Results (KR) is extrinsic, or external, information presented after the task is completed (Flinn & Radomski, 2002). It is a type of feedback given to the client so that he/she can change responses or behaviors on subsequent trials to increase the likelihood of reaching a desired goal. Knowledge of Results is not feedback about the movement itself ("Your wrist was locked.") but it is about movement outcome in terms of an environmental goal ("You missed your target.") (Schmidt & Lee, 2005). This type of feedback has shown to increase the chances of learning fine and gross motor skills in "normal" populations. Knowledge of Results has typically been used with motor learning tasks. Motor learning, as defined by Schmidt and Lee (2005), is a process of how movements are produced and learned as a direct result of practice and experience by the individual.

A large number of recent studies using "normal" participants investigated whether KR works better at 100% or at a reduced frequency. Giving 100% KR involves providing feedback after every trial, giving KR at 50% or 75%, involves providing feedback after every other or after every three trials, respectively. Overall these studies found that when given 100% KR individuals perform better in the acquisition phase and those given KR at a reduced frequency performed better in the retention phase. One reason behind this thought as explained by Sidaway, Fairweather, Powell, and Hall (1992) is that KR functions to guide performance rather than enhance the learning process. Another suggestion is that the individual becomes reliant on the KR and does not use environmental and task cues to encode the skills to long term memory (Schmidt, Lange, & Young 1990). Shea and Wulf (2005) stated that when compared with constant practice (trial-to-trial practice), variable practice generally resulted in more effective retention and transfer. Little is known about the applicability of using KR strategies with individuals with DD. The few studies that have been completed with participants with DD focused more on whether 100% KR was more effective than when KR is given less than 100% of the time.

Gillespie (2003) recruited 32 individuals with mild intellectual disabilities and found that participants in the 100% KR performed better in the acquisition phase than those with 50% KR. Conversely participants with 50% KR performed better in the retention phase than the 100% KR group did. The task involved in this study was putting a golf ball [sic]. They performed 50 acquisition trials, 25 one-day trials retention trials, and 25 one week retention trials.

In a more recent study, Rice and Hernandez (2006) investigated the effect of 100% KR versus 50% KR in a group of individuals with developmental disabilities and a group of age-matched average individuals. The task involved matching a yellow bar to a blue target bar on a computer screen by moving the access device (i.e., a knob). Participants received KR in the form of a green bar that indicated the level of success in matching the blue bar to the position of the yellow bar on the computer screen. There were 30 trials in the first phase where KR was provided (acquisition) and five in the second phase (retention) where KR was not provided. Knowledge of Results was provided directly after each trial. The results show that participants with developmental disabilities who were assigned to the 100% KR group performed better during the acquisition phase than the participants assigned to the 50% KR group. Similar to the results in the Gillespie (2003) study, the 50% KR group performed better than the 100% KR group in the retention phase. This was the case for both the individuals with developmental disabilities and the age matched individuals without developmental disabilities.

Presently, a large number of individuals with DD reside in group homes, which some might say is a more conductive environment for learning. It appears that KR may facilitate the individual's ability to perform a motor task; unfortunately the tasks involved in these KR studies did not indicate any type of ADL or IADL training. Consequently no research has been done to investigate this strategy using a task where the individual learns an ADL or an IADL. Learning ADLs or IADLs can help any individual reach his/her full potential.

One of the advantages to working in a group home is that the client gets more individualized attention from all health care providers, due to the fact that the ratio of healthcare providers to residents is higher. Leaning an IADL is very specific to every individual. How one individual learns to tell time may be completely different than how another individual learns that same skill. Single case research studies, are focused on providing individualized treatment to a certain individual, producing changes that are specifically designed and appropriate for that individual (AOTA, 1985). One advantage of single case research studies is that the researcher does not need to obtain a group that is homogenous, especially within the special population where there is often great variability person to person. It is often difficult to attain a homogenous group for a study when certain conditions vary extensively depending on the individual and the deficits and needs (Payton, 1988). A second reason single case research designs are important is that they focus on the individual's abilities and what treatments are particularly effective for him/her (Payton, 1988). Single case research designs let the therapist focus directly on the individual and allow the therapist to tailor the intervention to the individual's needs and situation (Ottenbacher & York, 1984). Another reason single case research designs are useful is that they can be used as a precursor to investigating a phenomenon using a large number of individuals. For instance, a case study using a few individuals can be used as a pilot study to see if the phenomenon exists. Therefore, a single case study involving participants with DD, who will be learning an IADL (telling time), is particularly suited and needed at this point in time. Single case research designs show the difference between one treatment (A) and another type of treatment (B) (Payton, 1988). In most situations, treatment A is a non-treatment control (Payton, 1988). The A phase is also called a baseline or no treatment condition (Ottenbacher & York, 1984). B phase is called the treatment condition (Payton, 1988). It is during this phase that acquisition of the task should take place. Some single case studies will repeat the A phase after the treatment is withdrawn to strengthen the findings and to see if the patient was able to obtain the information learned (Ottenbacher & York, 1984). This phase can also be termed as the retention phase.

Knowledge of Results may provide, and hopefully improve task performance for a long term result. It may however only elicit short term or temporary results. Some studies report that participants were more interested and put more effort into the task when KR was present (Arps, 1920; Crawley, 1926; Elwell & Grindley, 1938). Salmoni, Schmidt, and Walter (1984) noted this as a temporary phenomenon, which can dissipate with a brief rest or alter in condition from the original task. Similar to that, KR can also provide a strong guidance function for future performance. It may provide the participant with the information needed to change his/her performance before the next performance occurs. This too could be a temporary effect in which performance deteriorates quickly (Salmoni et al., 1984).

# 3.0 RESEARCH DESIGN

This study will use an ABAB single case experimental design. The A phases will represent no treatment and the B phases will represent when treatment is present. Each phase will consist of six trials per time period given. The times given on the clock will be six on the hour and six on the half hour. The task will last approximately 20 minutes each day for four consecutive weeks.

## 3.1   Research Design Questions

- How will persons with developmental disabilities be found?
- Where will data be collected?
- How will the independent variable be administered?

- How can compliance be ensured during the data collection process?
- How will the data be collected?
- How will the data be analyzed?

### 3.2    Guiding Question

We first hypothesize that performance during intervention phases (B1 and B2) will be significantly better than during the baseline performance (A1 and A2). We also hypothesize that performance during post phases (A2 and B2) will be significantly better than during the initial phases (A1 and B1 respectively).

### 3.3    Diagrammatical Relationship between Variables

*Target Population:*    Adults with cognitive developmental disabilities

*Representative Sample:*    Adults with cognitive developmental disabilities located in NW Ohio

*Method:*    ABAB single subject research design.

*Guiding Question:*    We first hypothesize that performance during intervention phases (B1 and B2) will be significantly better than during the baseline performance (A1 and A2). We also hypothesize that performance during post phases (A2 and B2) will be significantly better than during the initial phases (A1 and B1 respectively).

*Statistical Test:*    Visual observation of 'celebration lines and Wilcoxon Signed-Rank test

### 3.4    Possible Limitations of the Study

There will be several possible limitations to the study. As this is a single subject research design, which by design employs a small sample size, the ability to generalize the study's results to a larger population is limited. Another potential limitation will be the lack of control over participant compliance during the data collection process. Lastly, the researcher is aware of the hypothesis and could therefore influence the study by introducing bias.

## 4.0 METHODS

### 4.1    Target Population

Participants will consist of four to eight individuals with DD. Participants will be selected from a large group of individuals with DD who reside in community based housing. Each participant will be classified as an individual with mild to moderate DD. Inclusion criteria includes that [sic] individuals have mild to moderate DD, be over 18 years of age, and currently have not demonstrated the ability to consistently tell time accurately. Participant's age, gender, diagnosis, and years of schooling will be recorded. The identities of the participants will be kept confidential.

### 4.2   Apparatus

A Pentium IV laptop computer with custom software will be used to deliver the independent variable.

### 4.3   Data Collection Procedure

Prior to any data collection, informed consent will be obtained. To ensure participant's understanding of his or her rights and the study's procedures, the participants will state back their understanding of their rights and the study's procedures. Each participant will complete the task independently of each other. Participants will be given the directions of the task and will be given a chance to become familiar with all of the equipment. Each participant will be given 3 practice trials each day to ensure he/she understands the task and how to use the equipment. These practice trials will not be used in the results.

During the explanation of the task, the participants will each be shown the face clock on the computer screen and will be told that they are to match the correct digital time with what is being shown on the face clock. Demonstration will be provided to show the participants how to select their desired digital time using the computer mouse.

During the treatment trials (B1 and B2), it will then be explained to the participant, that if he or she chooses the correct digital time, balloons will be shown on the screen and "Great Job" will be heard along with the time that the participant chose. If the participant chooses the wrong digital time, one that does not match what was shown on the face clock, the phrase "Sorry" will be heard along with the time that was chosen and the desired time. A new face clock will also appear on the computer screen displaying the correct time and the time chosen by the participant. The hands of the clock will be in red to show the difference between the two times. Each time will be repeated six times to increase the chance that learning will occur in the individual. This will give the participant verbal and visual feedback on the performance. The feedback will be provided directly after each trial.

During the "A" phases, the same procedure will be followed as in the "B" phases, only no feedback of any kind will be given. That is, after the participant selects a time, the next trial will appear.

### 4.4   Projected Time Schedule for Completing Study

Selection of Topic . . . . . . . . . . . . . . . . . . . . . . . . . . . . . . . . . . . . . . . . . . . . . . . . . . . . . . 3 hours
Literature Review . . . . . . . . . . . . . . . . . . . . . . . . . . . . . . . . . . . . . . . . . . . . . . . . . . . . . 50 hours
Research Proposal . . . . . . . . . . . . . . . . . . . . . . . . . . . . . . . . . . . . . . . . . . . . . . . . . . . . 45 hours
Recruitment Activity . . . . . . . . . . . . . . . . . . . . . . . . . . . . . . . . . . . . . . . . . . . . . . . . . . 10 hours
Software development and testing . . . . . . . . . . . . . . . . . . . . . . . . . . . . . . . . . . . . . . . . 80 hours
Travel . . . . . . . . . . . . . . . . . . . . . . . . . . . . . . . . . . . . . . . . . . . . . . . . . . . . . . . . . . . . . . . 20 hours
Data Analysis . . . . . . . . . . . . . . . . . . . . . . . . . . . . . . . . . . . . . . . . . . . . . . . . . . . . . . . . 30 hours
Write Discussion . . . . . . . . . . . . . . . . . . . . . . . . . . . . . . . . . . . . . . . . . . . . . . . . . . . . . 10 hours
Complete Research . . . . . . . . . . . . . . . . . . . . . . . . . . . . . . . . . . . . . . . . . . . . . . . . . . . 10 hours
Total Time to Complete Study . . . . . . . . . . . . . . . . . . . . . . . . . . . . . . Approximately 12 months

### 4.5    Research and Statistical Design

This study will use an A1B1A2B2 single case experimental design. The A phases will represent no treatment and the B phases will represent when treatment is present. Each phase will consist of six trials per time period given. The times given will be six on the hour and six on the half hour, lasting approximately 20 minutes each day for four weeks straight.

Visual observation through a 'celeration line will be used to see if the slopes differed over the four phases. Observation of the slopes will also include an analysis to test if the slopes are different from zero during each phase. If the slopes differ from zero in each phase then all phases will be combined to see if slope made any differences across all phases. A positive slope for number of correct responses indicates an improvement in the participant's performance. When analyzing time differences, if a negative slope is observed, that also indicates improvement in the participant's performance. A Wilcoxon Signed-Rank Test will compare the performance between each subject for each block of time, and distinguish any significant differences between the blocks of time, particularly between phases B1 and B2, and between A1 and A2. Finally the B phases will be compared to the A phases for both correct responses and time.

### 4.6    Projected Costs of Study

Travel . . . . . . . . . . . . . . . . . . . . . . . . . . . . . . . . . . . . . . . . . . . . . . . . . . . . . . . . . . . . $100
Photo Copies . . . . . . . . . . . . . . . . . . . . . . . . . . . . . . . . . . . . . . . . . . . . . . . . . . . . . . $20
Computer Thumb Drive . . . . . . . . . . . . . . . . . . . . . . . . . . . . . . . . . . . . . . . . . . . . . . $20
Binder for Study . . . . . . . . . . . . . . . . . . . . . . . . . . . . . . . . . . . . . . . . . . . . . . . . . . . . . $5
Total cost of Study . . . . . . . . . . . . . . . . . . . . . . . . . . . . . . . . . . . . . . Approximately $145

### 4.7    Definition of Terms

***Mental Retardation:*** A generalized term referring to an impairment in adaptive functioning and cognition that occurs prior to the age of 18 years and has an intelligent quotient score of 70.

***Developmental Disabilities:*** A term to describe a chronic condition of either physical or cognitive impairments lasting throughout one's life and whose manifestation of symptoms occurs prior to the age of 18 years.

***Cognitive Impairment:*** Lack of cognitive development and adaptive behavior often manifesting itself during the developmental years. Persons with cognitive impairment are diagnosed with a psychiatric disorder, organic impairment, or a developmental disorder where cognitive abilities including judgment and reasoning are diminished.

***Motor Learning:*** "a set of [internal] processes associated with practice or experience leading to relatively permanent changes in the capability for responding" (Schmidt, 1988, p. 346).

***Knowledge of Results:*** a type of extrinsic feedback provided after a task is completed that gives information regarding how accurate the performance was based upon a desired goal.

***Instrumental Activities of Daily Living (IADLs):*** Personal tasks beyond fundamental tasks associated with activities of daily living. IADLs involve those tasks often associated with maintaining one's independence and can include activities such as, but not limited to time management, money management, and grocery shopping.

***Activities of Daily Living:*** Fundamental and personal tasks required on a daily basis to maintain personal hygiene, adaptive functioning and cognitive, physical and emotional health.

***Single Subject Research Design:*** A general term for research that involves a small sample size and is not intended for external validity, rather it is intended for comparing behavior on an individual basis.

***Intelligence Quotient:*** is a number based upon standardized testing that purports to assign a value to intelligence.

# 5.0 REFERENCES

American Occupational Therapy Association. (1985). *Standards of practice for occupational therapy.* Rockville, MD: Author.

American Psychiatric Association. (1994). *Diagnostic and statistical manual of mental disorders* (4th ed.). Washington, DC: Author.

Arps, G. F. (1920). Work with KR versus work without KR. *Psychological Monographs, 28.*

Crawley, S. L. (1926). An experimental investigation of recovery from work. *Archives of Psychology, 13, 26.*

Eastwood, E. A., & Fisher, G. A. (1988). Skills acquisition among matched samples of institutionalized and community-based persons with mental retardation. *American Journal of Mental Retardation, 93,* 75–83.

Elwell, J. L., & Grindley, G. S. (1938). The effects of knowledge of results on learning and performance. *British Journal of Psychology, 29,* 39–53.

Firth, H. (1987). A move from hospital to community: Evaluation of community contacts. *Child: Care, Health, and Development, 13,* 341–354.

Flinn, N.A., & Radomski, M.V. (2002). Learning. In C.A. Trombly & M.V. Radomski (Eds.), *Occupational therapy for physical dysfunction* (5th ed.). Baltimore: Lippincott Williams & Wilkins.

Gillespie, M. (2003). Summary versus every-trial knowledge of results for individuals with intellectual disabilities. *Adapted Physical Activity Quarterly, 20,* 46–57.

Law, M. (2002). Assessing roles and competence. In C.A. Trombly & M.V. Radomski (Eds.), *Occupational therapy for physical dysfunction* (5th ed.; pp. 31–45). Baltimore: Lippincott Williams &Wilkins.

Merrill, S.C., & Mulligan, S.E. (2003). Neurological dysfunction in children. In E. B. Crepeau, E. S. Cohn & B. A. Boyt Schell (Eds.), *Willard & Spackman's occupational therapy* (10th ed.; pp. 699–702). Baltimore: Lippincott Williams & Wilkins.

Neistadt, M. E. (1987). An occupational therapy program for adults with developmental disabilities. *The American Journal of Occupational Therapy, 41,* 433–438.

O'Neil, J., Brown, M. Gordon, W., & Schonhern, R. (1985). The impact of deinstitutionalization on activities and skills of severly/profoundly mentally retarded multiply-handicapped adults. *Applied Research in Mental Retardation, 6,* 361–371.

Ottenbacher, K., & York, J. (1984). Strategies for evaluating clinical change: Implications for practice and change. *The American Journal of Occupational Therapy, 38,* 647–659.

Payton, O. (1994). *Research: The validation of clinical research* (3rd ed.). Philadelphia: Davis.

Poole, J., Dunn, W., Schell, B., Tiernam, K., McKay Barnhart, J., Abreu, B., et al. (1991). Statement: Occupational therapy services management of persons with cognitive impairments. *The American Journal of Occupational Therapy, 45,* 1067–1068.

Rice, M. S., & Hernandez, H. G. (2006). Frequency of knowledge of results and motor learning in persons with developmental delay. *Occupational Therapy International, 13,* 35–48.

Salmoni, A. W, Schmidt, R. A, & Walter, C. B. (1984). Knowledge of results and motor learning: A review and critical reappraisal. *Psychological Bulletin, 95,* 355–386.

Schmidt, R. A., Lange, C. J, & Young, D. E. (1990). Optimizing summary knowledge of results for skill learning. *Human Movement Science, 9,* 325–348.

Schmidt, R. A., & Lee, T. D. (2005) *Motor control and learning: A behavioral emphasis* (4th ed.). Champaign, IL: Human Kinetics.

Shea, C. H., & Wulf, G. (2005). Schema theory: A critical appraisal and reevaluation. *Journal of Motor Behavior, 37,* 85–101.

Sidaway, B., Fairweather, M., Powell, J., & Hall, G. (1992). The acquisition and retention of a timing task: Effects of summary KR ad movement time. *Research Quarterly for Exercise and Sport, 63,* 328–334.

The Arc (2004, October). *Introduction to mental retardation.* Retrieved February 13, 2006, from http://www.thearc.org/faqs/intromr.pdf.

The Arc California Edition (1997, January). What causes mental retardation. *Prevention News.* Retrieved March 26, 2006 from http://www.prevention–news.com/1997/causes.htm.

## 6.0 ANNOTATED BIBLIOGRAPHY

Firth, H. (1987). A move from hospital to community: Evaluation of community contacts. *Child: Care, Health, and Development, 13,* 341–354.

*Abstract:* A small-scale evaluation was made of the activities and social contacts of a group of young mentally handicapped people in one project, leaving hospital to a house in the community. The results are consistent with other recent work in suggesting that residential provision in small homes for people with severe or profound intellectual or multiple handicaps is likely to lead to increased family contact, increased participation in activities outside of the residence, and an increased frequency and duration of contact with non-handicapped people. The study suggests that many of these benefits of life in the community are dependent in various ways upon the staff employed. The nature of the young people's social contacts is examined and conclusions are drawn about specific issues, including staff selection and training, and attention to the maintenance as well as the provision of social contact.

Gillespie, M. (2003). Summary versus every-trial knowledge of results for individuals with intellectual disabilities. *Adapted Physical Activity Quarterly, 20,* 46–57.

*Abstract:* The purpose of this study was to examine the effect of a summary knowledge of results (KR) feedback schedule (KR after every fifth trial) versus every-trial KR on the acquisition and retention of a golf putting task for individuals with intellectual disabilities. Thirty-two individuals with mild intellectual disabilities were randomly assigned to either a summary or every-trial KR group. Participants performed 50 acquisition trials, 25 one-day retention trials, and 25 one-week retention trials. Participants in the every-trial KR group scored significantly better during acquisition, while the summary KR group performed significantly better for both retention intervals. Because of the absence of an acquisition block effect, results relative to learning must be viewed with caution. Findings partially support the guidance hypothesis.

Rice, M. S., & Hernandez, H. G. (2006). Frequency of knowledge of results and motor learning in persons with developmental delay. *Occupational Therapy International, 13,* 35–48.

*Abstract:* The purpose of this study was to investigate the effect of high versus low frequency knowledge of results (KR) in a group of 16 individuals with developmental delay and in gender and age-matched average individuals learning a motor skill on a laptop computer. Participants were randomly assigned to either a 100% KR or a 50% KR group. KR was provided during the acquisition phase according to group assignment as participants learned the motor skill, whereas no KR was provided during the retention phase. Results indicated both populations who received 50% KR in the acquisition phase demonstrated better performance in the retention phase than those who received 100% KR. The results of this study suggest that, as has been found in the average population, feedback that is too frequent can interfere with learning and retention of tasks for individuals with developmental disabilities (DD). Limitations involved the small sample size along with the task potentially being artificial in nature. Future research is needed to study further the effects of frequency of KR on skill acquisition, particularly in instrumental activities of daily living in this population.

Shea, C. H., & Wulf, G. (2005). Schema theory: A critical appraisal and reevaluation. *Journal of Motor Behavior, 37,* 85–101.

*Abstract:* The authors critically review a number of the constructs and associated predictions proposed in schema theory (R. A. Schmidt, 1975). The authors propose that new control and learning theories should include a reformulated (a) notion of a generalized motor program that is not based on motor program but still accounts for the strong tendency for responses to maintain their relative characteristics; (b) mechanism or processes whereby an abstract movement structure based on proportional principles (e.g., relative timing, relative force) is developed through practice; and (c) explanation for parameter learning that accounts for the benefits of parameter variability but also considers how variability is scheduled. Furthermore, they also propose that new theories of motor learning must be able to account for the consistent findings spawned as a result of the schema theory proposal and must not be simply discounted because of some disfavor with the motor program notion, in general, or schema theory, more specifically.

## 7.0 INFORMED CONSENT

See Chapter 7 for an example

# Appendix A-1

## Web Addresses of Selected Professional Associations

**World Federation of Acupuncture Association – Moxibustion Societies** http://www.wfas.org.cn/en/

**American Academy of Physician Assistants:** http://www.aapa.org/

**American Association for Respiratory Care Therapy:** http://www.aarc.org/

**American Association on Intellectual and Developmental Disabilities (AAIDD):** http://www.aamr.org/

**The American Chiropractic Association:** http://www.acatoday.org/

**American Dental Association:** http://www.ada.org/

**American Dietetic Association:** http://www.eatright.org/

**American Health Information Management Association (Medical Records):** http://www.ahima.org/

**American Hospital Association:** http://www.aha.org/

**American Medical Association:** http://www.ama-assn.org

**American Nurses Association:** http://www.nursingworld.org/

**American Occupational Therapy Association (AOTA):** http://www.aota.org/

**American Optometric Association:** http://www.aoa.org/

**American Orthotic and Prosthetic Association:** http://www.aopanet.org/

**American Osteopathic Association:** http://www.osteopathic.org/

**American Pharmaceutical Association:** http://www.pharmacyandyou.org/

**American Physical Therapy Association:** http://www.apta.org//AM/Template.cfm?Section=Home

**American Podiatric Medical Association:** http://www.apma.org/

**American Psychiatric Association:** http://www.psych.org/

**American Psychological Association (APA):** http://www.apa.org/

**American Society for Clinical Laboratory Science:** http:// www.ascls.org/

**American Society of Radiologic Technologists:** https://www.asrt.org/

**American Speech-Language-Hearing Association (ASHA):** http://www.asha.org/

**The American Therapeutic Recreation Association (ATRA):** http://www.atra-online.com/

**Council for Exceptional Children (CEC; Special Education):** http://www.cec.sped.org/

**National Association of School Psychologists (NASP):** http://www.nasponline.org/

**National Association of Social Workers:** http://www.naswdc.org/

**National Rehabilitation Association (NRA):** http://www.nationalrehab.org/cwt/external/wcpages/index.aspx

**Rehabilitation Engineering and Assistive Technology Society of North America (RESNA):**
http://www.resna.org/

# Appendix A-2

## Selected List of Consumer Health Organizations

**Alzheimer's Association:** http://www.alz.org/index.asp

**American Cancer Society:** http://www.cancer.org/index

**American Council of the Blind:** http://acb.org/index.html

**American Heart Association:** http://www.heart.org/HEARTORG/

**American Lung Association:** http://www.lungusa.org/

**The Arc (For people with intellectual and developmental disabilities):** http://www.thearc.org/

**Arthritis Foundation:** http://www.arthritis.org/

**The Association for the Severely Handicapped (THE TASH):** http://www.tash.org/index.html

**Autism Society of America:** http://www.autism-society.org/

**Brain Injury Association:** http://www.biausa.org/

**Children with Attention Deficit Disorders (CHADD):** http://chadd.org/

**Cystic Fibrosis Foundation (CFF):** http://www.cff.org/

**Epilepsy Foundation of America:** http://www.epilepsyfoundation.org/

**Learning Disabilities Association (LDA):** http://www.ldanatl.org/

**Muscular Dystrophy Association (MDA):** http://mdausa.org/

**National Alliance for the Mentally Ill (NAMI):** http://www.nami.org/

**National Association of People with AIDS (NAPWA):** http://www.napwa.org/

**National Easter Seal Society (NESS):** http://www.easterseals.com/site/PageServer?pagename=ntl_homepage

**National Multiple Sclerosis Society:** http://www.nationalmssociety.org/index.aspx

**National Stroke Association:** http://www.stroke.org/site/PageNavigator/HOME

**Spina Bifida Association of America (SBAA):** http://www.spinabifidaassociation.org/site/c.liKWL7PLLrF/b.2642297/k.5F7C/Spina_Bifida_Association.htm

**Spinal Injuries Associations (SIA):** http://www.spinal.co.uk/

**United Cerebral Palsy Association (UCP):** http://www.ucp.org/

# Appendix B

## *Commonly Used Medical Abbreviations*

| | |
|---|---|
| **/d** | per day |
| **a** | of each |
| **a.c.** | before a meal |
| **ABI** | acquired brain injury |
| **ACTH** | adrenocorticotropic hormone |
| **ad lib.** | freely |
| **ADA** | Americans with Disabilities Act |
| **ADD** | attention deficit disorder |
| **ADHD** | Attention-Deficit/Hyperactivity Disorder |
| **admov.** | apply |
| **AIDS** | Acquired Immune Deficiency Syndrome |
| **ALS** | amyotrophic lateral sclerosis |
| **alt.dieb** | every other day |
| **AMA** | against medical advice |
| **ap** | before dinner |
| **ASAP** | as soon as possible |
| **b.i.d.** | twice a day |
| **bib.** | drink |
| **bol.** | pill |
| **BP** | blood pressure |
| **BRP** | bathroom privileges |
| **c̄** | with (usually written with a bar on top of the "c") |
| **CA** | cancer |
| **CBC** | complete blood count |
| **Cc** | cubic centimeters |

| | |
|---|---|
| CMC | carpometacarpal joint |
| CNS | central nervous system |
| COPD | chronic obstructive pulmonary disease |
| CP | cerebral palsy |
| CPR | cardio-pulmonary resuscitation |
| CSF | cerebrospinal fluid |
| CT | computed tomography, also referred to as CAT (computer axial tomography) |
| CVA | cerebro vascular accident |
| D and C | dilatation and curettage |
| d | daily |
| DIP | distal interphalangeal |
| DNR | do not resuscitate |
| DO | Doctor of Osteopathic Medicine |
| Dx | diagnosis |
| ECG | electrocardiogram |
| ECT | electroconvulsive therapy |
| ED | emergency departure |
| EEG | electroencephalogram |
| EMG | electromyogram |
| ER | emergency room |
| FAE | Fetal Alcohol Effects |
| FAS | Fetal Alcohol Syndrome |
| FASD | Fetal Alcohol Spectrum Disorder |
| GBS | Guillain-Barre Syndrome |
| GI | gastrointestinal |
| H/A | headache |
| $H_2O$ | water |
| Hct | hematocrit |
| Hgb | hemoglobin |
| HIV | human immunodeficiency virus |
| Hx | history |
| ICU | intensive care unit |
| ID | intellectual disabilities |
| IDEIA | Individuals with Disabilities Education Improvement Act of 2004 (often referred to as "IDEA-2004") |
| IEP | Individualized Education Plan |
| IFSP | Individualized Family Service Plan |
| IM | intramuscular in |
| IQ | intelligence quotient |
| ITP | Individualized Transition Plan |

| | |
|---|---|
| IV | intravenous |
| kg | kilogram |
| KVO | keep vein open |
| lb | pound |
| LOC | loss of consciousness |
| LP | lumbar puncture |
| MCP | metacarpophalangeal |
| MD | muscular dystrophy |
| MED | minimum effective dose |
| MMR | measles-mumps-rubella vaccine |
| MR | mental retardation |
| MRI | magnetic resonance imaging |
| MRSA | methicillin resistant *staphylococcum* aureus |
| MS | multiple sclerosis |
| MVA | motor vehicle accident |
| MVR | mitral valve replacement |
| Nasogastric | a tube that leads from the nose or mouth into the stomach |
| NICU | neonatal intensive care unit |
| NP | nurse practitioner |
| NPO | nothing by mouth; nothing to eat or drink usually within a defined time frame |
| NWB | non-weight bearing |
| OB/GYN | obstetrics and gynecology |
| OD | Doctor of Osteopathic Medicine |
| ODA | operating day admission |
| OR | operating room |
| p | after |
| p.c. | after meals |
| p.o. | by mouth or orally |
| p.r.n. | as needed |
| PA | physician's assistant |
| PAC | premature atrial contraction |
| PE | physical examination |
| per os | by mouth |
| PET Scan | positron emission tomography |
| PICC Line | peripherally inserted central catheter for delivery of medication |
| PIP | proximal interphalangeal |
| PROM | passive range of motion |
| PWB | partial weight bearing |
| q.h. | every hour |
| q.i.d. | four times a day |

| | |
|---|---|
| **q2h, q3h,...** | every two hours, every three hours, etc. |
| **quotid** | every day |
| **R/R** | respiratory rate |
| **RBC** | red blood cells |
| **REM** | rapid eye movement |
| **RESNA** | Rehabilitation Engineering and Assistive Technology Society of North America |
| **ROM** | range of motion |
| **Rx** | prescription, treatment, or therapy |
| **SCI** | spinal cord injury |
| **sine** | without |
| **SNF** | skilled nursing facility |
| **STD** | sexually transmitted disease |
| **Strep** | streptococcus |
| **Sx** | symptoms |
| **t.i.d.** | three times a day |
| **TBI** | traumatic brain injury |
| **TIA** | transient ischemia attacks |
| **U.S.P.** | United States Pharmacopoeia |
| **UTI** | urinary tract infection |
| **VS** | vital signs |
| **VSD** | ventricular septal defect |
| **W/C** | wheel chair |
| **w/o** | without |
| **w/** | with |
| **WB** | weight bearing |
| **WBC** | white blood cells |
| **WNL** | within normal limits |

# Appendix C

## Statistical Tables

## TABLE C-1

**Random Numbers**

| | | | | | | | | | |
|---|---|---|---|---|---|---|---|---|---|
| 8048 | 5782 | 104 | 2930 | 1079 | 5212 | 6344 | 3835 | 5859 | 7803 |
| 688 | 5873 | 2773 | 5633 | 2335 | 9919 | 5097 | 3953 | 1163 | 258 |
| 836 | 1346 | 250 | 1158 | 5479 | 1370 | 9851 | 6226 | 3224 | 3478 |
| 4732 | 5066 | 5419 | 7379 | 297 | 2594 | 9259 | 1864 | 7474 | 1883 |
| 5135 | 9798 | 7122 | 1194 | 5145 | 7622 | 2130 | 8803 | 9948 | 965 |
| 5662 | 9432 | 7273 | 584 | 7814 | 2103 | 1628 | 3232 | 5370 | 6216 |
| 9356 | 7449 | 207 | 976 | 85 | 5398 | 1765 | 6246 | 3856 | 4468 |
| 8734 | 1569 | 5055 | 5941 | 2292 | 7995 | 1819 | 9033 | 6805 | 5923 |
| 376 | 1875 | 8721 | 4270 | 7710 | 5550 | 9743 | 4122 | 9914 | 6382 |
| 8499 | 8513 | 1064 | 2108 | 8233 | 4488 | 5248 | 7441 | 1830 | 5602 |
| 7066 | 7282 | 8452 | 7577 | 9040 | 2685 | 625 | 3600 | 861 | 8673 |
| 198 | 6847 | 9815 | 5220 | 7272 | 1121 | 3742 | 6843 | 9439 | 6061 |
| 149 | 6503 | 1890 | 922 | 2008 | 8392 | 5004 | 2954 | 685 | 7190 |
| 877 | 5967 | 7769 | 8695 | 2721 | 6067 | 8550 | 3078 | 6730 | 9864 |
| 3992 | 3495 | 2656 | 7579 | 5429 | 1245 | 1046 | 7302 | 2359 | 7931 |
| 156 | 1747 | 4822 | 7976 | 2965 | 6451 | 8307 | 5665 | 5025 | 7608 |
| 1670 | 4498 | 6500 | 6383 | 5052 | 9557 | 1948 | 1050 | 2345 | 5574 |
| 4236 | 7918 | 2912 | 222 | 7252 | 9700 | 6223 | 9927 | 4753 | 5302 |
| 9641 | 943 | 5277 | 3556 | 8315 | 229 | 8545 | 7499 | 6283 | 7863 |
| 5137 | 5368 | 5441 | 3761 | 3238 | 731 | 66 | 160 | 4473 | 6029 |
| 1528 | 3007 | 642 | 1378 | 4383 | 934 | 992 | 692 | 6816 | 5306 |
| 425 | 8664 | 2017 | 1299 | 9649 | 2771 | 3105 | 2521 | 1965 | 5257 |
| 4384 | 7408 | 8253 | 3927 | 5933 | 7750 | 3790 | 6984 | 7999 | 3380 |
| 2873 | 7236 | 3901 | 3716 | 2373 | 7686 | 9602 | 8441 | 1959 | 1152 |
| 2028 | 9052 | 598 | 8949 | 2530 | 1249 | 5235 | 6936 | 2477 | 268 |
| 3691 | 5409 | 9324 | 3932 | 1406 | 4374 | 4009 | 6654 | 6317 | 4399 |
| 4402 | 4512 | 2908 | 4492 | 2738 | 7937 | 3826 | 9407 | 7985 | 4648 |
| 8003 | 610 | 3763 | 6781 | 5483 | 925 | 2613 | 310 | 9053 | 6014 |
| 1655 | 6535 | 9428 | 6983 | 2541 | 3450 | 1435 | 4682 | 2618 | 1775 |
| 5653 | 7921 | 8487 | 2254 | 9815 | 9384 | 1552 | 8303 | 4372 | 5489 |
| 7861 | 408 | 7336 | 600 | 314 | 5485 | 3865 | 7556 | 2052 | 9331 |
| 162 | 7528 | 3878 | 6058 | 5872 | 7796 | 1507 | 5602 | 5600 | 3149 |
| 1274 | 8234 | 2569 | 4512 | 2256 | 8250 | 8913 | 9306 | 9282 | 2581 |
| 3970 | 9506 | 5739 | 3526 | 7924 | 7264 | 7257 | 2895 | 3182 | 5030 |
| 8518 | 7756 | 6255 | 3975 | 5281 | 9532 | 2730 | 3948 | 6221 | 614 |

*continues*

## TABLE C-1

**Random Numbers** *continued*

| | | | | | | | | | |
|---|---|---|---|---|---|---|---|---|---|
| 815 | 1089 | 8481 | 9607 | 5469 | 1461 | 9682 | 3443 | 6477 | 8089 |
| 6848 | 4343 | 9849 | 9184 | 4839 | 5819 | 6334 | 4562 | 5155 | 7080 |
| 385 | 4548 | 1925 | 440 | 6420 | 1001 | 5746 | 462 | 7430 | 8009 |
| 3119 | 3552 | 2489 | 6473 | 9350 | 4552 | 1936 | 7793 | 3054 | 351 |
| 7233 | 1284 | 3441 | 3947 | 7953 | 299 | 9964 | 3687 | 3379 | 1242 |

**Source:** The table was generated by Martin S. Rice, Department of Rehabilitation Sciences, The University of Toledo, using Microsoft Office Excel 2007.

## TABLE C-2

**Proportion of Areas under the Normal Curve (Percentile Rank)**

| z | 0.00 | 0.01 | 0.02 | 0.03 | 0.04 | 0.05 | 0.06 | 0.07 | 0.08 | 0.09 |
|---|------|------|------|------|------|------|------|------|------|------|
| 0.0 | .50000 | .50399 | .50798 | .51197 | .51595 | .51994 | .52392 | .52790 | .53188 | .53586 |
| 0.1 | .53983 | .54380 | .54776 | .55172 | .55567 | .55962 | .56356 | .56749 | .57142 | .57535 |
| 0.2 | .57926 | .58317 | .58706 | .59095 | .59483 | .59871 | .60257 | .60642 | .61026 | .61409 |
| 0.3 | .61791 | .62172 | .62552 | .62930 | .63307 | .63683 | .64058 | .64431 | .64803 | .65173 |
| 0.4 | .65542 | .65910 | .66276 | .66640 | .67003 | .67364 | .67724 | .68082 | .68439 | .68793 |
| 0.5 | .69146 | .69497 | .69847 | .70194 | .70540 | .70884 | .71226 | .71566 | .71904 | .72240 |
| 0.6 | .72575 | .72907 | .73237 | .73565 | .73891 | .74215 | .74537 | .74857 | .75175 | .75490 |
| 0.7 | .75804 | .76115 | .76424 | .76730 | .77035 | .77337 | .77637 | .77935 | .78230 | .78524 |
| 0.8 | .78814 | .79103 | .79389 | .79673 | .79955 | .80234 | .80511 | .80785 | .81057 | .81327 |
| 0.9 | .81594 | .81859 | .82121 | .82381 | .82639 | .82894 | .83147 | .83398 | .83646 | .83891 |
| 1.0 | .84134 | .84375 | .84614 | .84849 | .85083 | .85314 | .85543 | .85769 | .85993 | .86214 |
| 1.1 | .86433 | .86650 | .86864 | .87076 | .87286 | .87493 | .87698 | .87900 | .88100 | .88298 |
| 1.2 | .88493 | .88686 | .88877 | .89065 | .89251 | .89435 | .89617 | .89796 | .89973 | .90147 |
| 1.3 | .90320 | .90490 | .90658 | .90824 | .90988 | .91149 | .91309 | .91466 | .91621 | .91774 |
| 1.4 | .91924 | .92073 | .92220 | .92364 | .92507 | .92647 | .92785 | .92922 | .93056 | .93189 |
| 1.5 | .93319 | .93448 | .93574 | .93699 | .93822 | .93943 | .94062 | .94179 | .94295 | .94408 |
| 1.6 | .94520 | .94630 | .94738 | .94845 | .94950 | .95053 | .95154 | .95254 | .95352 | .95449 |
| 1.7 | .95543 | .95637 | .95728 | .95818 | .95907 | .95994 | .96080 | .96164 | .96246 | .96327 |
| 1.8 | .96407 | .96485 | .96562 | .96638 | .96712 | .96784 | .96856 | .96926 | .96995 | .97062 |
| 1.9 | .97128 | .97193 | .97257 | .97320 | .97381 | .97441 | .97500 | .97558 | .97615 | .97670 |
| 2.0 | .97725 | .97778 | .97831 | .97882 | .97932 | .97982 | .98030 | .98077 | .98124 | .98169 |
| 2.1 | .98214 | .98257 | .98300 | .98341 | .98382 | .98422 | .98461 | .98500 | .98537 | .98574 |
| 2.2 | .98610 | .98645 | .98679 | .98713 | .98745 | .98778 | .98809 | .98840 | .98870 | .98899 |
| 2.3 | .98928 | .98956 | .98983 | .99010 | .99036 | .99061 | .99086 | .99111 | .99134 | .99158 |
| 2.4 | .99180 | .99202 | .99224 | .99245 | .99266 | .99286 | .99305 | .99324 | .99343 | .99361 |
| 2.5 | .99379 | .99396 | .99413 | .99430 | .99446 | .99461 | .99477 | .99492 | .99506 | .99520 |
| 2.6 | .99534 | .99547 | .99560 | .99573 | .99585 | .99598 | .99609 | .99621 | .99632 | .99643 |
| 2.7 | .99653 | .99664 | .99674 | .99683 | .99693 | .99702 | .99711 | .99720 | .99728 | .99736 |
| 2.8 | .99744 | .99752 | .99760 | .99767 | .99774 | .99781 | .99788 | .99795 | .99801 | .99807 |
| 2.9 | .99813 | .99819 | .99825 | .99831 | .99836 | .99841 | .99846 | .99851 | .99856 | .99861 |
| 3.0 | .99865 | .99869 | .99874 | .99878 | .99882 | .99886 | .99889 | .99893 | .99896 | .99900 |
| 3.1 | .99903 | .99906 | .99910 | .99913 | .99916 | .99918 | .99921 | .99924 | .99926 | .99929 |
| 3.2 | .99931 | .99934 | .99936 | .99938 | .99940 | .99942 | .99944 | .99946 | .99948 | .99950 |
| 3.3 | .99952 | .99953 | .99955 | .99957 | .99958 | .99960 | .99961 | .99962 | .99964 | .99965 |
| 3.4 | .99966 | .99968 | .99969 | .99970 | .99971 | .99972 | .99973 | .99974 | .99975 | .99976 |

*continues*

**TABLE C-2**

**Proportion of Areas under the Normal Curve (Percentile Rank)** *continued*

| z | 0.00 | 0.01 | 0.02 | 0.03 | 0.04 | 0.05 | 0.06 | 0.07 | 0.08 | 0.09 |
|-----|--------|--------|--------|--------|--------|--------|--------|--------|--------|--------|
| 3.5 | .99977 | .99978 | .99978 | .99979 | .99980 | .99981 | .99981 | .99982 | .99983 | .99983 |
| 3.6 | .99984 | .99985 | .99985 | .99986 | .99986 | .99987 | .99987 | .99988 | .99988 | .99989 |
| 3.7 | .99989 | .99990 | .99990 | .99990 | .99991 | .99991 | .99992 | .99992 | .99992 | .99992 |
| 3.8 | .99993 | .99993 | .99993 | .99994 | .99994 | .99994 | .99994 | .99995 | .99995 | .99995 |
| 3.9 | .99995 | .99995 | .99996 | .99996 | .99996 | .99996 | .99996 | .99996 | .99997 | .99997 |
| 4.0 | .99997 | .99997 | .99997 | .99997 | .99997 | .99997 | .99998 | .99998 | .99998 | .99998 |
| 4.1 | .99998 | .99998 | .99998 | .99998 | .99998 | .99998 | .99998 | .99998 | .99999 | .99999 |
| 4.2 | .99999 | .99999 | .99999 | .99999 | .99999 | .99999 | .99999 | .99999 | .99999 | .99999 |
| 4.3 | .99999 | .99999 | .99999 | .99999 | .99999 | .99999 | .99999 | .99999 | .99999 | .99999 |
| 4.4 | .99999 | .99999 | 1.0000 | 1.0000 | 1.0000 | 1.0000 | 1.0000 | 1.0000 | 1.0000 | 1.0000 |

**Note:** z-score values are provided at two decimal places. For example, a z-score of 1.27 represents .89796 proportion of the normal curve or percentile rank.

**Source:** The table was generated by Martin S. Rice, Department of Rehabilitation Sciences, The University of Toledo, using Microsoft Office Excel 2007.

TABLE C-3

**Critical Values for *t*-Test**

| | Level of significance for one-tailed *t*-test | | | | | |
|---|---|---|---|---|---|---|
| | 0.1 | 0.05 | 0.025 | 0.01 | 0.005 | 0.0005 |
| | Level of significance for two-tailed *t*-test | | | | | |
| *df* | 0.2 | 0.1 | 0.05 | 0.02 | 0.01 | 0.001 |
| 1 | 3.0777 | 6.3138 | 12.7062 | 31.8205 | 63.6567 | 636.6192 |
| 2 | 1.8856 | 2.9200 | 4.3027 | 6.9646 | 9.9248 | 31.5991 |
| 3 | 1.6377 | 2.3534 | 3.1824 | 4.5407 | 5.8409 | 12.9240 |
| 4 | 1.5332 | 2.1318 | 2.7764 | 3.7469 | 4.6041 | 8.6103 |
| 5 | 1.4759 | 2.0150 | 2.5706 | 3.3649 | 4.0321 | 6.8688 |
| 6 | 1.4398 | 1.9432 | 2.4469 | 3.1427 | 3.7074 | 5.9588 |
| 7 | 1.4149 | 1.8946 | 2.3646 | 2.9980 | 3.4995 | 5.4079 |
| 8 | 1.3968 | 1.8595 | 2.3060 | 2.8965 | 3.3554 | 5.0413 |
| 9 | 1.3830 | 1.8331 | 2.2622 | 2.8214 | 3.2498 | 4.7809 |
| 10 | 1.3722 | 1.8125 | 2.2281 | 2.7638 | 3.1693 | 4.5869 |
| 11 | 1.3634 | 1.7959 | 2.2010 | 2.7181 | 3.1058 | 4.4370 |
| 12 | 1.3562 | 1.7823 | 2.1788 | 2.6810 | 3.0545 | 4.3178 |
| 13 | 1.3502 | 1.7709 | 2.1604 | 2.6503 | 3.0123 | 4.2208 |
| 14 | 1.3450 | 1.7613 | 2.1448 | 2.6245 | 2.9768 | 4.1405 |
| 15 | 1.3406 | 1.7531 | 2.1314 | 2.6025 | 2.9467 | 4.0728 |
| 16 | 1.3368 | 1.7459 | 2.1199 | 2.5835 | 2.9208 | 4.0150 |
| 17 | 1.3334 | 1.7396 | 2.1098 | 2.5669 | 2.8982 | 3.9651 |
| 18 | 1.3304 | 1.7341 | 2.1009 | 2.5524 | 2.8784 | 3.9216 |
| 19 | 1.3277 | 1.7291 | 2.0930 | 2.5395 | 2.8609 | 3.8834 |
| 20 | 1.3253 | 1.7247 | 2.0860 | 2.5280 | 2.8453 | 3.8495 |
| 21 | 1.3232 | 1.7207 | 2.0796 | 2.5176 | 2.8314 | 3.8193 |
| 22 | 1.3212 | 1.7171 | 2.0739 | 2.5083 | 2.8188 | 3.7921 |
| 23 | 1.3195 | 1.7139 | 2.0687 | 2.4999 | 2.8073 | 3.7676 |
| 24 | 1.3178 | 1.7109 | 2.0639 | 2.4922 | 2.7969 | 3.7454 |
| 25 | 1.3163 | 1.7081 | 2.0595 | 2.4851 | 2.7874 | 3.7251 |
| 26 | 1.3150 | 1.7056 | 2.0555 | 2.4786 | 2.7787 | 3.7066 |
| 27 | 1.3137 | 1.7033 | 2.0518 | 2.4727 | 2.7707 | 3.6896 |
| 28 | 1.3125 | 1.7011 | 2.0484 | 2.4671 | 2.7633 | 3.6739 |
| 29 | 1.3114 | 1.6991 | 2.0452 | 2.4620 | 2.7564 | 3.6594 |
| 30 | 1.3104 | 1.6973 | 2.0423 | 2.4573 | 2.7500 | 3.6460 |
| 31 | 1.3095 | 1.6955 | 2.0395 | 2.4528 | 2.7440 | 3.6335 |
| 32 | 1.3086 | 1.6939 | 2.0369 | 2.4487 | 2.7385 | 3.6218 |
| 33 | 1.3077 | 1.6924 | 2.0345 | 2.4448 | 2.7333 | 3.6109 |

*continues*

TABLE C-3

**Critical Values for *t*-Test** *continued*

| df | Level of significance for one-tailed *t*-test | | | | | |
|---|---|---|---|---|---|---|
| | 0.1 | 0.05 | 0.025 | 0.01 | 0.005 | 0.0005 |
| | Level of significance for two-tailed *t*-test | | | | | |
| | 0.2 | 0.1 | 0.05 | 0.02 | 0.01 | 0.001 |
| 34 | 1.3070 | 1.6909 | 2.0322 | 2.4411 | 2.7284 | 3.6007 |
| 35 | 1.3062 | 1.6896 | 2.0301 | 2.4377 | 2.7238 | 3.5911 |
| 36 | 1.3055 | 1.6883 | 2.0281 | 2.4345 | 2.7195 | 3.5821 |
| 37 | 1.3049 | 1.6871 | 2.0262 | 2.4314 | 2.7154 | 3.5737 |
| 38 | 1.3042 | 1.6860 | 2.0244 | 2.4286 | 2.7116 | 3.5657 |
| 39 | 1.3036 | 1.6849 | 2.0227 | 2.4258 | 2.7079 | 3.5581 |
| 40 | 1.3031 | 1.6839 | 2.0211 | 2.4233 | 2.7045 | 3.5510 |
| 50 | 1.2987 | 1.6759 | 2.0086 | 2.4033 | 2.6778 | 3.4960 |
| 60 | 1.2958 | 1.6706 | 2.0003 | 2.3901 | 2.6603 | 3.4602 |
| 70 | 1.2938 | 1.6669 | 1.9944 | 2.3808 | 2.6479 | 3.4350 |
| 80 | 1.2922 | 1.6641 | 1.9901 | 2.3739 | 2.6387 | 3.4163 |
| 90 | 1.2910 | 1.6620 | 1.9867 | 2.3685 | 2.6316 | 3.4019 |
| 100 | 1.2901 | 1.6602 | 1.9840 | 2.3642 | 2.6259 | 3.3905 |
| 110 | 1.2893 | 1.6588 | 1.9818 | 2.3607 | 2.6213 | 3.3812 |
| 120 | 1.2886 | 1.6577 | 1.9799 | 2.3578 | 2.6174 | 3.3735 |
| 130 | 1.2881 | 1.6567 | 1.9784 | 2.3554 | 2.6142 | 3.3669 |
| 140 | 1.2876 | 1.6558 | 1.9771 | 2.3533 | 2.6114 | 3.3614 |
| 150 | 1.2872 | 1.6551 | 1.9759 | 2.3515 | 2.6090 | 3.3566 |

**Source:** The table was generated by Martin S. Rice, Department of Rehabilitation Sciences, The University of Toledo, using Microsoft Office Excel 2007.

© Cengage Learning 2013

### Steps in Determining Critical Values for *t* for Table C–3

1. Calculate the degrees of freedom (*df*).

   - In a one-sample *t*-test, it is the number of cases of the sample minus 1.
   - In a paired-data of correlated *t*-test, it is the number of pairs minus 1.
   - In an independent *t*-test, it is the number of cases in $N_1 + N_2$ minus 2.

2. Determine if the hypothesis requires a one-tailed or two-tailed *t*-test.
3. Establish the level of significance ($\alpha$) (e.g., .05, .01).
4. Locate *t*-critical ($t_{crit}$) value. For example, if *df* is 10, using a two-tailed test with $\alpha = .05$, then $t_{crit} = 2.2281$.
5. Note that these critical values are the same for negative or positive numbers.
6. Calculate *t*-observed ($t_{obs}$) using an appropriate *t*-test formula (e.g., one-sample, paired, or independent *t*-test).
7. Decision Rule:

   - If $t_{obs}$ is equal to or above $t_{crit}$, then reject the null hypothesis.
   - If $t_{obs}$ is below $t_{crit}$, then accept the null hypothesis.

## TABLE C-4

### Critical Values for *F* (Analysis of Variance, ANOVA)

| Denominator *df* | | Numerator *df* | | | | | | | | | |
|---|---|---|---|---|---|---|---|---|---|---|---|
| | α | 1 | 2 | 3 | 4 | 5 | 6 | 7 | 8 | 9 | 10 |
| 1 | .05 | 4052 | 4999 | 5403 | 5625 | 5764 | 5859 | 5928 | 5981 | 6022 | 6056 |
| | .01 | 161.4 | 199.5 | 215.7 | 224.6 | 230.2 | 234.0 | 236.8 | 238.9 | 240.5 | 241.9 |
| 2 | .05 | 98.50 | 99.00 | 99.17 | 99.25 | 99.30 | 99.33 | 99.36 | 99.37 | 99.39 | 99.40 |
| | .01 | 18.513 | 19.000 | 19.164 | 19.247 | 19.296 | 19.330 | 19.353 | 19.371 | 19.385 | 19.396 |
| 3 | .05 | 34.116 | 30.817 | 29.457 | 28.710 | 28.237 | 27.911 | 27.672 | 27.489 | 27.345 | 27.229 |
| | .01 | 10.128 | 9.5521 | 9.2766 | 9.1172 | 9.0135 | 8.9406 | 8.8867 | 8.8452 | 8.8123 | 8.7855 |
| 4 | .05 | 21.198 | 18.000 | 16.694 | 15.977 | 15.522 | 15.207 | 14.976 | 14.799 | 14.659 | 14.546 |
| | .01 | 7.7086 | 6.9443 | 6.5914 | 6.3882 | 6.2561 | 6.1631 | 6.0942 | 6.0410 | 5.9988 | 5.9644 |
| 5 | .05 | 16.258 | 13.274 | 12.060 | 11.392 | 10.967 | 10.672 | 10.456 | 10.289 | 10.158 | 10.051 |
| | .01 | 6.6079 | 5.7861 | 5.4095 | 5.1922 | 5.0503 | 4.9503 | 4.8759 | 4.8183 | 4.7725 | 4.7351 |
| 6 | .05 | 13.745 | 10.925 | 9.7795 | 9.1483 | 8.7459 | 8.4661 | 8.2600 | 8.1017 | 7.9761 | 7.8741 |
| | .01 | 5.9874 | 5.1433 | 4.7571 | 4.5337 | 4.3874 | 4.2839 | 4.2067 | 4.1468 | 4.0990 | 4.0600 |
| 7 | .05 | 12.246 | 9.5466 | 8.4513 | 7.8466 | 7.4604 | 7.1914 | 6.9928 | 6.8400 | 6.7188 | 6.6201 |
| | .01 | 5.5914 | 4.7374 | 4.3468 | 4.1203 | 3.9715 | 3.8660 | 3.7870 | 3.7257 | 3.6767 | 3.6365 |
| 8 | .05 | 11.259 | 8.6491 | 7.5910 | 7.0061 | 6.6318 | 6.3707 | 6.1776 | 6.0289 | 5.9106 | 5.8143 |
| | .01 | 5.3177 | 4.4590 | 4.0662 | 3.8379 | 3.6875 | 3.5806 | 3.5005 | 3.4381 | 3.3881 | 3.3472 |
| 9 | .05 | 10.561 | 8.0215 | 6.9919 | 6.4221 | 6.0569 | 5.8018 | 5.6129 | 5.4671 | 5.3511 | 5.2565 |
| | .01 | 5.1174 | 4.2565 | 3.8625 | 3.6331 | 3.4817 | 3.3738 | 3.2927 | 3.2296 | 3.1789 | 3.1373 |
| 10 | .05 | 10.044 | 7.5594 | 6.5523 | 5.9943 | 5.6363 | 5.3858 | 5.2001 | 5.0567 | 4.9424 | 4.8491 |
| | .01 | 4.9646 | 4.1028 | 3.7083 | 3.4780 | 3.3258 | 3.2172 | 3.1355 | 3.0717 | 3.0204 | 2.9782 |
| 11 | .05 | 9.6460 | 7.2057 | 6.2167 | 5.6683 | 5.3160 | 5.0692 | 4.8861 | 4.7445 | 4.6315 | 4.5393 |
| | .01 | 4.8443 | 3.9823 | 3.5874 | 3.3567 | 3.2039 | 3.0946 | 3.0123 | 2.9480 | 2.8962 | 2.8536 |
| 12 | .05 | 9.3302 | 6.9266 | 5.9525 | 5.4120 | 5.0643 | 4.8206 | 4.6395 | 4.4994 | 4.3875 | 4.2961 |
| | .01 | 4.7472 | 3.8853 | 3.4903 | 3.2592 | 3.1059 | 2.9961 | 2.9134 | 2.8486 | 2.7964 | 2.7534 |
| 13 | .05 | 9.0738 | 6.7010 | 5.7394 | 5.2053 | 4.8616 | 4.6204 | 4.4410 | 4.3021 | 4.1911 | 4.1003 |
| | .01 | 4.6672 | 3.8056 | 3.4105 | 3.1791 | 3.0254 | 2.9153 | 2.8321 | 2.7669 | 2.7144 | 2.6710 |
| 14 | .05 | 8.8616 | 6.5149 | 5.5639 | 5.0354 | 4.6950 | 4.4558 | 4.2779 | 4.1399 | 4.0297 | 3.9394 |
| | .01 | 4.6001 | 3.7389 | 3.3439 | 3.1122 | 2.9582 | 2.8477 | 2.7642 | 2.6987 | 2.6458 | 2.6022 |
| 15 | .05 | 8.6831 | 6.3589 | 5.4170 | 4.8932 | 4.5556 | 4.3183 | 4.1415 | 4.0045 | 3.8948 | 3.8049 |
| | .01 | 4.5431 | 3.6823 | 3.2874 | 3.0556 | 2.9013 | 2.7905 | 2.7066 | 2.6408 | 2.5876 | 2.5437 |
| 16 | .05 | 8.5310 | 6.2262 | 5.2922 | 4.7726 | 4.4374 | 4.2016 | 4.0259 | 3.8896 | 3.7804 | 3.6909 |
| | .01 | 4.4940 | 3.6337 | 3.2389 | 3.0069 | 2.8524 | 2.7413 | 2.6572 | 2.5911 | 2.5377 | 2.4935 |
| 17 | .05 | 8.3997 | 6.1121 | 5.1850 | 4.6690 | 4.3359 | 4.1015 | 3.9267 | 3.7910 | 3.6822 | 3.5931 |
| | .01 | 4.4513 | 3.5915 | 3.1968 | 2.9647 | 2.8100 | 2.6987 | 2.6143 | 2.5480 | 2.4943 | 2.4499 |

*continues*

## TABLE C-4

**Critical Values for F (Analysis of Variance, ANOVA)** *continued*

| Denominator df | | | | | | Numerator df | | | | | |
|---|---|---|---|---|---|---|---|---|---|---|---|
| | α | 1 | 2 | 3 | 4 | 5 | 6 | 7 | 8 | 9 | 10 |
| 18 | .05 | 8.2854 | 6.0129 | 5.0919 | 4.5790 | 4.2479 | 4.0146 | 3.8406 | 3.7054 | 3.5971 | 3.5082 |
| | .01 | 4.4139 | 3.5546 | 3.1599 | 2.9277 | 2.7729 | 2.6613 | 2.5767 | 2.5102 | 2.4563 | 2.4117 |
| 19 | .05 | 8.1849 | 5.9259 | 5.0103 | 4.5003 | 4.1708 | 3.9386 | 3.7653 | 3.6305 | 3.5225 | 3.4338 |
| | .01 | 4.3807 | 3.5219 | 3.1274 | 2.8951 | 2.7401 | 2.6283 | 2.5435 | 2.4768 | 2.4227 | 2.3779 |
| 20 | .05 | 8.0960 | 5.8489 | 4.9382 | 4.4307 | 4.1027 | 3.8714 | 3.6987 | 3.5644 | 3.4567 | 3.3682 |
| | .01 | 4.3512 | 3.4928 | 3.0984 | 2.8661 | 2.7109 | 2.5990 | 2.5140 | 2.4471 | 2.3928 | 2.3479 |
| 21 | .05 | 8.0166 | 5.7804 | 4.8740 | 4.3688 | 4.0421 | 3.8117 | 3.6396 | 3.5056 | 3.3981 | 3.3098 |
| | .01 | 4.3248 | 3.4668 | 3.0725 | 2.8401 | 2.6848 | 2.5727 | 2.4876 | 2.4205 | 2.3660 | 2.3210 |
| 22 | .05 | 7.9454 | 5.7190 | 4.8166 | 4.3134 | 3.9880 | 3.7583 | 3.5867 | 3.4530 | 3.3458 | 3.2576 |
| | .01 | 4.3009 | 3.4434 | 3.0491 | 2.8167 | 2.6613 | 2.5491 | 2.4638 | 2.3965 | 2.3419 | 2.2967 |
| 23 | .05 | 7.8811 | 5.6637 | 4.7649 | 4.2636 | 3.9392 | 3.7102 | 3.5390 | 3.4057 | 3.2986 | 3.2106 |
| | .01 | 4.2793 | 3.4221 | 3.0280 | 2.7955 | 2.6400 | 2.5277 | 2.4422 | 2.3748 | 2.3201 | 2.2747 |
| 24 | .05 | 7.8229 | 5.6136 | 4.7181 | 4.2184 | 3.8951 | 3.6667 | 3.4959 | 3.3629 | 3.2560 | 3.1681 |
| | .01 | 4.2597 | 3.4028 | 3.0088 | 2.7763 | 2.6207 | 2.5082 | 2.4226 | 2.3551 | 2.3002 | 2.2547 |
| 25 | .05 | 7.7698 | 5.5680 | 4.6755 | 4.1774 | 3.8550 | 3.6272 | 3.4568 | 3.3239 | 3.2172 | 3.1294 |
| | .01 | 4.2417 | 3.3852 | 2.9912 | 2.7587 | 2.6030 | 2.4904 | 2.4047 | 2.3371 | 2.2821 | 2.2365 |
| 26 | .05 | 7.7213 | 5.5263 | 4.6366 | 4.1400 | 3.8183 | 3.5911 | 3.4210 | 3.2884 | 3.1818 | 3.0941 |
| | .01 | 4.2252 | 3.3690 | 2.9752 | 2.7426 | 2.5868 | 2.4741 | 2.3883 | 2.3205 | 2.2655 | 2.2197 |
| 27 | .05 | 7.6767 | 5.4881 | 4.6009 | 4.1056 | 3.7848 | 3.5580 | 3.3882 | 3.2558 | 3.1494 | 3.0618 |
| | .01 | 4.2100 | 3.3541 | 2.9604 | 2.7278 | 2.5719 | 2.4591 | 2.3732 | 2.3053 | 2.2501 | 2.2043 |
| 28 | .05 | 7.6356 | 5.4529 | 4.5681 | 4.0740 | 3.7539 | 3.5276 | 3.3581 | 3.2259 | 3.1195 | 3.0320 |
| | .01 | 4.1960 | 3.3404 | 2.9467 | 2.7141 | 2.5581 | 2.4453 | 2.3593 | 2.2913 | 2.2360 | 2.1900 |
| 29 | .05 | 7.5977 | 5.4204 | 4.5378 | 4.0449 | 3.7254 | 3.4995 | 3.3303 | 3.1982 | 3.0920 | 3.0045 |
| | .01 | 4.1830 | 3.3277 | 2.9340 | 2.7014 | 2.5454 | 2.4324 | 2.3463 | 2.2783 | 2.2229 | 2.1768 |
| 30 | .05 | 7.5625 | 5.3903 | 4.5097 | 4.0179 | 3.6990 | 3.4735 | 3.3045 | 3.1726 | 3.0665 | 2.9791 |
| | .01 | 4.1709 | 3.3158 | 2.9223 | 2.6896 | 2.5336 | 2.4205 | 2.3343 | 2.2662 | 2.2107 | 2.1646 |
| 35 | .05 | 7.4191 | 5.2679 | 4.3957 | 3.9082 | 3.5919 | 3.3679 | 3.2000 | 3.0687 | 2.9630 | 2.8758 |
| | .01 | 4.1213 | 3.2674 | 2.8742 | 2.6415 | 2.4851 | 2.3718 | 2.2852 | 2.2167 | 2.1608 | 2.1143 |
| 40 | .05 | 7.3141 | 5.1785 | 4.3126 | 3.8283 | 3.5138 | 3.2910 | 3.1238 | 2.9930 | 2.8876 | 2.8005 |
| | .01 | 4.0847 | 3.2317 | 2.8387 | 2.6060 | 2.4495 | 2.3359 | 2.2490 | 2.1802 | 2.1240 | 2.0772 |
| 45 | .05 | 7.2339 | 5.1103 | 4.2492 | 3.7674 | 3.4544 | 3.2325 | 3.0658 | 2.9353 | 2.8301 | 2.7432 |
| | .01 | 4.0566 | 3.2043 | 2.8115 | 2.5787 | 2.4221 | 2.3083 | 2.2212 | 2.1521 | 2.0958 | 2.0487 |

| Denominator df | | Numerator df | | | | | | | | | |
|---|---|---|---|---|---|---|---|---|---|---|---|
| | α | 1 | 2 | 3 | 4 | 5 | 6 | 7 | 8 | 9 | 10 |
| 50 | .05 | 7.1706 | 5.0566 | 4.1993 | 3.7195 | 3.4077 | 3.1864 | 3.0202 | 2.8900 | 2.7850 | 2.6981 |
| | .01 | 4.0343 | 3.1826 | 2.7900 | 2.5572 | 2.4004 | 2.2864 | 2.1992 | 2.1299 | 2.0734 | 2.0261 |
| 55 | .05 | 7.1194 | 5.0132 | 4.1591 | 3.6809 | 3.3700 | 3.1493 | 2.9834 | 2.8534 | 2.7485 | 2.6617 |
| | .01 | 4.0162 | 3.1650 | 2.7725 | 2.5397 | 2.3828 | 2.2687 | 2.1813 | 2.1119 | 2.0552 | 2.0078 |
| 60 | .05 | 7.0771 | 4.9774 | 4.1259 | 3.6490 | 3.3389 | 3.1187 | 2.9530 | 2.8233 | 2.7185 | 2.6318 |
| | .01 | 4.0012 | 3.1504 | 2.7581 | 2.5252 | 2.3683 | 2.2541 | 2.1665 | 2.0970 | 2.0401 | 1.9926 |
| 80 | .05 | 6.9627 | 4.8807 | 4.0363 | 3.5631 | 3.2550 | 3.0361 | 2.8713 | 2.7420 | 2.6374 | 2.5508 |
| | .01 | 3.9604 | 3.1108 | 2.7188 | 2.4859 | 2.3287 | 2.2142 | 2.1263 | 2.0564 | 1.9991 | 1.9512 |
| 100 | .05 | 6.8953 | 4.8239 | 3.9837 | 3.5127 | 3.2059 | 2.9877 | 2.8233 | 2.6943 | 2.5898 | 2.5033 |
| | .01 | 3.9361 | 3.0873 | 2.6955 | 2.4626 | 2.3053 | 2.1906 | 2.1025 | 2.0323 | 1.9748 | 1.9267 |
| 120 | .05 | 6.8509 | 4.7865 | 3.9491 | 3.4795 | 3.1735 | 2.9559 | 2.7918 | 2.6629 | 2.5586 | 2.4721 |
| | .01 | 3.9201 | 3.0718 | 2.6802 | 2.4472 | 2.2899 | 2.1750 | 2.0868 | 2.0164 | 1.9588 | 1.9105 |

**Source:** The table was generated by Martin S. Rice, Department of Rehabilitation Sciences, The University of Toledo, using Microsoft Office Excel 2007.

© Cengage Learning 2013

## Steps in Determining Critical Values for $F$ for Table C–4

1. Calculate the degrees of freedom ($df$) for numerator and denominator.
   - The $df$ for the numerator is derived from the number of groups in the study minus 1. For example, if three treatment methods are being compared, then $df$ equals 3 minus 1, or 2 $df$, for numerator.
   - The df for the denominator is derived from the total number of subjects in all groups being compared minus the number of groups. For example, for three treatment methods with 6 subjects in each group, the $df$ for the denominator will equal 18 minus 3, or 15 $df$.
2. Apply the level of significance ($\alpha$), such as .05 or .01.
3. Locate the critical value of $F$. For example, a numerator $df$ of 2, a denominator $df$ of 15 with $\alpha = .05$, the critical value of $F$ equals 6.3589.
4. Calculate $F_{obs}$ for data.
5. Decision Rule:
   - If $F_{obs}$ is equal to or above $F_{crit}$, then reject the null hypothesis.
   - If $F_{obs}$ is below $F_{crit}$, then accept the null hypothesis.

TABLE C-5

**Critical Values for the Pearson Product-Moment Correlation Coefficient (r)**

| | Level of significance for one-tailed test | | | | | |
| | .25 | .10 | .05 | .025 | .01 | .005 |
| | Level of significance for two-tailed test | | | | | |
| df | .50 | .20 | .10 | .05 | .02 | .01 |
| 1 | 0.7071 | 0.9511 | 0.9877 | 0.9969 | 0.9995 | 0.9999 |
| 2 | 0.5000 | 0.8000 | 0.9000 | 0.9500 | 0.9800 | 0.9900 |
| 3 | 0.4040 | 0.6870 | 0.8054 | 0.8783 | 0.9343 | 0.9587 |
| 4 | 0.3473 | 0.6084 | 0.7293 | 0.8114 | 0.8822 | 0.9172 |
| 5 | 0.3091 | 0.5509 | 0.6694 | 0.7545 | 0.8329 | 0.8745 |
| 6 | 0.2811 | 0.5067 | 0.6215 | 0.7067 | 0.7887 | 0.8343 |
| 7 | 0.2596 | 0.4716 | 0.5822 | 0.6664 | 0.7498 | 0.7977 |
| 8 | 0.2423 | 0.4428 | 0.5493 | 0.6319 | 0.7155 | 0.7646 |
| 9 | 0.2281 | 0.4187 | 0.5214 | 0.6021 | 0.6851 | 0.7348 |
| 10 | 0.2161 | 0.3981 | 0.4973 | 0.5760 | 0.6581 | 0.7079 |
| 11 | 0.2058 | 0.3802 | 0.4762 | 0.5529 | 0.6339 | 0.6835 |
| 12 | 0.1968 | 0.3646 | 0.4575 | 0.5324 | 0.6120 | 0.6614 |
| 13 | 0.1890 | 0.3507 | 0.4409 | 0.5140 | 0.5923 | 0.6411 |
| 14 | 0.1820 | 0.3383 | 0.4259 | 0.4973 | 0.5742 | 0.6226 |
| 15 | 0.1757 | 0.3271 | 0.4124 | 0.4822 | 0.5577 | 0.6055 |
| 16 | 0.1700 | 0.3170 | 0.4000 | 0.4683 | 0.5426 | 0.5897 |
| 17 | 0.1649 | 0.3077 | 0.3887 | 0.4555 | 0.5285 | 0.5751 |
| 18 | 0.1602 | 0.2992 | 0.3783 | 0.4438 | 0.5155 | 0.5614 |
| 19 | 0.1558 | 0.2914 | 0.3687 | 0.4329 | 0.5034 | 0.5487 |
| 20 | 0.1518 | 0.2841 | 0.3598 | 0.4227 | 0.4921 | 0.5368 |
| 21 | 0.1481 | 0.2774 | 0.3515 | 0.4132 | 0.4815 | 0.5256 |
| 22 | 0.1447 | 0.2711 | 0.3438 | 0.4044 | 0.4716 | 0.5151 |
| 23 | 0.1415 | 0.2653 | 0.3365 | 0.3961 | 0.4622 | 0.5052 |
| 28 | 0.1281 | 0.2407 | 0.3061 | 0.3610 | 0.4226 | 0.4629 |
| 33 | 0.1179 | 0.2220 | 0.2826 | 0.3338 | 0.3916 | 0.4296 |
| 38 | 0.1098 | 0.2070 | 0.2638 | 0.3120 | 0.3665 | 0.4026 |
| 43 | 0.1032 | 0.1947 | 0.2483 | 0.2940 | 0.3457 | 0.3801 |
| 48 | 0.0976 | 0.1843 | 0.2353 | 0.2787 | 0.3281 | 0.3610 |
| 58 | 0.0888 | 0.1678 | 0.2144 | 0.2542 | 0.2997 | 0.3301 |
| 68 | 0.0820 | 0.1550 | 0.1982 | 0.2352 | 0.2776 | 0.3060 |

| df | Level of significance for one-tailed test | | | | | |
| --- | --- | --- | --- | --- | --- | --- |
| | .25 | .10 | .05 | .025 | .01 | .005 |
| | Level of significance for two-tailed test | | | | | |
| | .50 | .20 | .10 | .05 | .02 | .01 |
| 78 | 0.0765 | 0.1448 | 0.1852 | 0.2199 | 0.2597 | 0.2864 |
| 88 | 0.0720 | 0.1364 | 0.1745 | 0.2072 | 0.2449 | 0.2702 |
| 98 | 0.0682 | 0.1292 | 0.1654 | 0.1966 | 0.2324 | 0.2565 |

**Source:** Adapted from Table 19.1 Critical Values for the Product-Moment Correlation Coefficient, originally published in Handbook of Statistical Tables, (pp. 509–510), by D. B. Owen, 1962. Reading, MA: Addison-Wesley.

**Steps in Determining Critical Values for Pearson $r$ for Table C–5**

1. Determine the number of variables being correlated. For example if $x = 20$ and $y = 20$, then $n = 20$.
2. Determine if hypothesis calls for a one-tailed or two-tailed test.
3. Apply level of significance, for example, .05 or .01.
4. Locate critical value of $r$ from statistical table. For example, with $n = 20$, two-tailed test, .05 level, then $r_{crit} = .4438$; $df = 18$.
5. Calculate $r_{obs}$ from data.
6. Decision Rule:

   a. If $r_{obs}$ is equal to or greater then $r_{crit}$, then reject null hypothesis.
   b. If $r_{obs}$ is below $r_{crit}$, then accept null hypothesis.

## TABLE C-6

**Spearman Rank Correlation Coefficient (r)**

| n* | Level of significance for one-tailed test | | | |
| | .05 | .025 | .01 | .005 |
| | Level of significance for two-tailed test | | | |
| | .10 | .05 | .02 | .01 |
|---|---|---|---|---|
| 5 | .900 | 1.000 | 1.000 | |
| 6 | .829 | .886 | .943 | 1.000 |
| 7 | .714 | .786 | .893 | .929 |
| 8 | .643 | .738 | .833 | .881 |
| 9 | .600 | .683 | .783 | .833 |
| 10 | .564 | .648 | .746 | .794 |
| 12 | .506 | .591 | .712 | .777 |
| 14 | .456 | .544 | .645 | .715 |
| 16 | .425 | .506 | .601 | .665 |
| 18 | .399 | .475 | .564 | .625 |
| 20 | .377 | .450 | .534 | .591 |
| 22 | .359 | .428 | .508 | .562 |
| 24 | .343 | .409 | .485 | .537 |
| 26 | .329 | .392 | .465 | .515 |
| 28 | .317 | .377 | .448 | .496 |
| 30 | .306 | .364 | .432 | .478 |

*n = number of pairs

**Source:** Adapted from "The 5 percent significance levels of sums of squares of rank differences and a correction," by E. G. Olds, 1949, *Annals of Mathematical Statistics, 20,* pp. 117–118. Reprinted with permission of the Institute of Mathematical Statistics.

## Steps in Determining Critical Values for Spearman $r_s$ (formerly *rho*) for Table C–6

1. Determine the number of pairs of variables being correlated.
2. Determine if hypothesis calls for a one-tailed or two-tailed test.
3. Apply level of significance, .05 or .01.
4. Locate critical value of $r_s$ from statistical table. For example, with $n = 12$, two-tailed test, .05 level, then $r_s$ critical = .591.
5. Calculate $r_{s\text{-obs}}$ from data.
6. Decision Rule:
   a. If $r_{s\text{-obs}}$ is equal to or greater then $r_{s\text{-crit}}$, then reject the null hypothesis.
   b. If $r_{s\text{-obs}}$ is below $r_{s\text{-crit}}$, then accept the null hypothesis.

## TABLE C-7A

### Critical Values for the Mann-Whitney U Test[a]

| $n_B$ \ $n_A$ | 1 | 2 | 3 | 4 | 5 | 6 | 7 | 8 | 9 | 10 | 11 | 12 | 13 | 14 | 15 | 16 | 17 | 18 | 19 | 20 |
|---|---|---|---|---|---|---|---|---|---|---|---|---|---|---|---|---|---|---|---|---|
| 1 | | | | | | | | | | | | | | | | | | | | |
| 2 | | | | | | | | 0 | 0 | 0 | 0 | 1 | 1 | 1 | 1 | 1 | 2 | 2 | 2 | 2 |
|   | | | | | | | | 16 | 18 | 20 | 22 | 23 | 25 | 27 | 29 | 31 | 32 | 34 | 36 | 38 |
| 3 | — | — | — | — | 0 | 1 | 1 | 2 | 2 | 3 | 3 | 4 | 4 | 5 | 5 | 6 | 6 | 7 | 7 | 8 |
|   | | | | | 15 | 17 | 20 | 22 | 25 | 27 | 30 | 32 | 35 | 37 | 40 | 42 | 45 | 47 | 50 | 52 |
| 4 | — | — | — | 0 | 1 | 2 | 3 | 4 | 4 | 5 | 6 | 7 | 8 | 9 | 10 | 11 | 11 | 12 | 13 | 13 |
|   | | | | 16 | 12 | 22 | 25 | 28 | 32 | 35 | 38 | 41 | 44 | 47 | 50 | 53 | 57 | 60 | 63 | 67 |
| 5 | — | — | 0 | 1 | 2 | 3 | 5 | 6 | 7 | 8 | 9 | 11 | 12 | 13 | 14 | 15 | 17 | 18 | 19 | 20 |
|   | | | 15 | 19 | 23 | 27 | 30 | 34 | 38 | 42 | 46 | 49 | 53 | 57 | 61 | 65 | 68 | 72 | 76 | 80 |
| 6 | — | — | 1 | 2 | 3 | 5 | 6 | 8 | 1 | 11 | 13 | 14 | 16 | 17 | 19 | 21 | 22 | 24 | 25 | 27 |
|   | | | 17 | 22 | 27 | 31 | 36 | 40 | 44 | 12 | 53 | 58 | 62 | 67 | 71 | 75 | 80 | 84 | 89 | 93 |
| 7 | — | — | 1 | 3 | 5 | 6 | 8 | 10 | 12 | 14 | 16 | 18 | 20 | 22 | 24 | 26 | 28 | 30 | 32 | 34 |
|   | | | 20 | 25 | 30 | 36 | 11 | 46 | 51 | 56 | 61 | 66 | 71 | 76 | 81 | 86 | 21 | 96 | 101 | 106 |
| 8 | — | 0 | 2 | 4 | 6 | 8 | 10 | 13 | 15 | 17 | 19 | 22 | 24 | 26 | 29 | 31 | 34 | 36 | 38 | 41 |
|   | | 16 | 22 | 28 | 34 | 40 | 46 | 51 | 57 | 63 | 69 | 74 | 80 | 86 | 21 | 97 | 102 | 108 | 111 | 119 |
| 9 | — | 0 | 2 | 4 | 7 | 10 | 12 | 15 | 17 | 20 | 23 | 26 | 28 | 31 | 34 | 37 | 39 | 42 | 45 | 48 |
|   | | 18 | 25 | 32 | 38 | 44 | 51 | 57 | 64 | 70 | 76 | 82 | 89 | 95 | 101 | 107 | 114 | 120 | 126 | 132 |
| 10 | — | 0 | 3 | 5 | 8 | 11 | 14 | 17 | 20 | 23 | 26 | 29 | 33 | 36 | 39 | 42 | 45 | 48 | 52 | 55 |
|   | | 20 | 27 | 35 | 42 | 49 | 56 | 63 | 70 | 77 | 84 | 21 | 97 | 104 | 111 | 118 | 125 | 132 | 138 | 145 |
| 11 | — | 0 | 3 | 6 | 9 | 13 | 16 | 19 | 23 | 26 | 30 | 33 | 37 | 40 | 44 | 47 | 51 | 55 | 58 | 62 |
|   | | 22 | 30 | 38 | 46 | 53 | 61 | 69 | 76 | 84 | 21 | 22 | 106 | 114 | 121 | 129 | 136 | 143 | 151 | 158 |
| 12 | — | 1 | 4 | 7 | 11 | 14 | 18 | 22 | 26 | 29 | 33 | 37 | 41 | 45 | 49 | 53 | 57 | 61 | 65 | 69 |
|   | | 23 | 32 | 41 | 49 | 58 | 66 | 74 | 82 | 91 | 99 | 107 | 115 | 123 | 131 | 139 | 147 | 155 | 163 | 171 |
| 13 | — | 1 | 4 | 8 | 12 | 16 | 20 | 24 | 28 | 33 | 37 | 41 | 45 | 50 | 54 | 59 | 63 | 67 | 72 | 76 |
|   | | 25 | 35 | 44 | 53 | 62 | 71 | 80 | 89 | 97 | 106 | 115 | 124 | 132 | 141 | 149 | 158 | 167 | 175 | 184 |
| 14 | — | 1 | 5 | 9 | 13 | 17 | 22 | 26 | 31 | 36 | 40 | 45 | 50 | 55 | 59 | 64 | 67 | 74 | 78 | 83 |
|   | | 27 | 37 | 47 | 51 | 67 | 76 | 86 | 95 | 104 | 114 | 123 | 132 | 141 | 151 | 160 | 171 | 178 | 188 | 197 |
| 15 | — | 1 | 5 | 10 | 14 | 19 | 24 | 29 | 34 | 39 | 44 | 49 | 54 | 59 | 64 | 70 | 75 | 80 | 85 | 90 |
|   | | 29 | 40 | 50 | 61 | 71 | 81 | 21 | 101 | 111 | 121 | 131 | 141 | 151 | 161 | 170 | 180 | 190 | 200 | 210 |
| 16 | — | 1 | 6 | 11 | 15 | 21 | 26 | 31 | 37 | 42 | 47 | 53 | 59 | 64 | 70 | 75 | 81 | 86 | 92 | 98 |
|   | | 31 | 42 | 53 | 65 | 75 | 86 | 97 | 107 | 118 | 129 | 139 | 149 | 160 | 170 | 181 | 191 | 202 | 212 | 222 |
| 17 | — | 2 | 6 | 11 | 17 | 22 | 28 | 34 | 39 | 45 | 51 | 57 | 63 | 67 | 75 | 81 | 87 | 93 | 99 | 105 |
|   | | 32 | 45 | 57 | 68 | 80 | 91 | 102 | 114 | 125 | 136 | 147 | 158 | 171 | 180 | 191 | 202 | 213 | 224 | 235 |

*continues*

## TABLE C-7A

**Critical Values for the Mann-Whitney *U* Test[a]** *continued*

| $n_B$ \ $n_A$ | 1 | 2 | 3 | 4 | 5 | 6 | 7 | 8 | 9 | 10 | 11 | 12 | 13 | 14 | 15 | 16 | 17 | 18 | 19 | 20 |
|---|---|---|---|---|---|---|---|---|---|---|---|---|---|---|---|---|---|---|---|---|
| 18 | — | 2 | 7 | 12 | 18 | 24 | 30 | 36 | 42 | 48 | 55 | 61 | 67 | 74 | 80 | 86 | 93 | 99 | 106 | 112 |
|  |  | 34 | 47 | 60 | 72 | 84 | 96 | 108 | 120 | 132 | 143 | 155 | 167 | 178 | 190 | 202 | 213 | 225 | 236 | 248 |
| 19 | — | 2 | 7 | 13 | 19 | 25 | 32 | 38 | 45 | 52 | 58 | 65 | 72 | 78 | 85 | 92 | 99 | 106 | 113 | 119 |
|  |  | 36 | 50 | 63 | 76 | 89 | 101 | 114 | 126 | 138 | 151 | 163 | 175 | 188 | 200 | 212 | 224 | 236 | 248 | 261 |
| 20 | — | 2 | 8 | 13 | 20 | 27 | 34 | 41 | 48 | 55 | 62 | 69 | 76 | 83 | 90 | 98 | 105 | 112 | 119 | 127 |
|  |  | 38 | 52 | 67 | 80 | 93 | 106 | 119 | 132 | 145 | 158 | 171 | 184 | 197 | 210 | 222 | 235 | 248 | 261 | 273 |

[a]Test for a one-tailed test at .025 or a two-tailed test at .05. If the $U_{obs}$ value falls within the two values in the table for $n_A$ and $n_B$, do not reject the null hypothesis. If the $U_{obs}$ is less than or equal to the lower value in the table or greater than or equal to the larger value in the table, then reject the null hypothesis.

**Source:** Adapted from "On a test of whether one of two random variables is stochastically larger than the other" by H. B. Mann and D. R. Whitney, 1947, *Annals of Mathematical Statistics*, (pp. 18, 52–54). Permission granted by Institute of Mathematical Statistics; Aubel D. (1953). Extended tables for the Mann-Whitney statistic, *Bulletin of the Institute of Educational Research at Indiana University*, I, No. 2; and *Handbook of Statistical Tables* (pp. 349–353) by D. B. Owen, 1962 originally published by Addison-Wesley Publishing Company, Inc.

## TABLE C-7B

### Critical Values for the Mann-Whitney U Test[b]

| $n_B$ \ $n_A$ | 1 | 2 | 3 | 4 | 5 | 6 | 7 | 8 | 9 | 10 | 11 | 12 | 13 | 14 | 15 | 16 | 17 | 18 | 19 | 20 |
|---|---|---|---|---|---|---|---|---|---|---|---|---|---|---|---|---|---|---|---|---|
| 1 |  |  |  |  |  |  |  |  |  |  |  |  |  |  |  |  |  |  | 0 | 0 |
|   |  |  |  |  |  |  |  |  |  |  |  |  |  |  |  |  |  |  | 19 | 20 |
| 2 |  |  |  |  | 0 | 0 | 0 | 1 | 1 | 1 | 1 | 2 | 2 | 2 | 3 | 3 | 3 | 4 | 4 | 4 |
|   |  |  |  |  | 10 | 12 | 14 | 15 | 17 | 19 | 21 | 22 | 21 | 26 | 27 | 29 | 31 | 32 | 31 | 36 |
| 3 | — | — | 0 | 0 | 1 | 2 | 2 | 3 | 3 | 4 | 5 | 5 | 6 | 7 | 7 | 8 | 9 | 9 | 10 | 11 |
|   |  |  | 9 | 11 | 14 | 16 | 11 | 21 | 21 | 26 | 28 | 31 | 33 | 35 | 38 | 40 | 12 | 15 | 17 | 19 |
| 4 |  | — | 0 | 1 | 2 | 3 | 4 | 5 | 6 | 7 | 8 | 9 | 10 | 11 | 12 | 14 | 15 | 16 | 17 | 18 |
|   |  |  | 11 | 11 | 18 | 21 | 24 | 27 | 30 | 33 | 36 | 39 | 12 | 45 | 18 | 50 | 53 | 56 | 59 | 62 |
| 5 |  | 0 | 1 | 2 | 4 | 5 | 6 | 8 | 9 | 11 | 12 | 13 | 15 | 16 | 18 | 19 | 20 | 22 | 23 | 25 |
|   |  | 10 | 14 | 18 | 21 | 25 | 29 | 32 | 36 | 39 | 43 | 47 | 50 | 51 | 57 | 61 | 65 | 68 | 72 | 75 |
| 6 |  | 0 | 2 | 3 | 5 | 7 | 8 | 10 | 12 | 14 | 16 | 17 | 19 | 21 | 23 | 25 | 26 | 28 | 30 | 32 |
|   |  | 11 | 16 | 21 | 25 | 29 | 34 | 38 | 42 | 46 | 50 | 55 | 59 | 63 | 67 | 71 | 76 | 80 | 81 | 88 |
| 7 |  | 0 | 2 | 4 | 6 | 8 | 11 | 13 | 15 | 17 | 19 | 21 | 24 | 26 | 28 | 30 | 33 | 35 | 37 | 39 |
|   |  | 14 | 19 | 24 | 29 | 34 | 38 | 43 | 48 | 53 | 58 | 63 | 67 | 72 | 77 | 82 | 86 | 91 | 96 | 101 |
| 8 |  | 1 | 3 | 5 | 8 | 10 | 13 | 15 | 18 | 20 | 23 | 26 | 28 | 31 | 33 | 36 | 39 | 41 | 44 | 47 |
|   |  | 15 | 21 | 27 | 32 | 38 | 43 | 49 | 54 | 60 | 65 | 70 | 76 | 81 | 87 | 92 | 97 | 103 | 108 | 113 |
| 9 | — | 1 | 3 | 6 | 9 | 12 | 15 | 18 | 21 | 24 | 27 | 30 | 33 | 36 | 39 | 42 | 45 | 48 | 51 | 54 |
|   |  | 17 | 24 | 30 | 36 | 42 | 48 | 54 | 60 | 66 | 72 | 78 | 81 | 90 | 96 | 102 | 108 | 114 | 120 | 126 |
| 10 | — | 1 | 4 | 7 | 11 | 14 | 17 | 20 | 24 | 27 | 31 | 34 | 37 | 41 | 44 | 48 | 51 | 55 | 58 | 62 |
|   |  | 11 | 26 | 33 | 39 | 46 | 53 | 60 | 66 | 73 | 79 | 86 | 93 | 99 | 106 | 112 | 119 | 125 | 132 | 138 |
| 11 |  | 1 | 5 | 8 | 12 | 16 | 19 | 23 | 27 | 31 | 34 | 38 | 42 | 46 | 50 | 54 | 57 | 61 | 65 | 69 |
|   |  | 21 | 28 | 36 | 43 | 50 | 58 | 65 | 71 | 79 | 87 | 94 | 101 | 108 | 115 | 122 | 130 | 137 | 144 | 151 |
| 12 | — | 2 | 5 | 9 | 13 | 17 | 21 | 26 | 30 | 34 | 38 | 42 | 47 | 51 | 55 | 60 | 64 | 68 | 72 | 77 |
|   |  | 22 | 31 | 39 | 47 | 55 | 63 | 70 | 78 | 86 | 94 | 102 | 109 | 117 | 125 | 132 | 140 | 148 | 156 | 163 |
| 13 |  | 2 | 6 | 10 | 15 | 19 | 24 | 28 | 33 | 37 | 42 | 47 | 51 | 56 | 61 | 65 | 70 | 75 | 80 | 84 |
|   |  | 24 | 33 | 42 | 50 | 59 | 67 | 76 | 84 | 93 | 101 | 109 | 118 | 126 | 134 | 143 | 151 | 159 | 167 | 176 |
| 14 |  | 2 | 7 | 11 | 16 | 21 | 26 | 31 | 36 | 41 | 46 | 51 | 56 | 61 | 66 | 71 | 77 | 82 | 87 | 92 |
|   |  | 26 | 35 | 45 | 54 | 63 | 72 | 81 | 90 | 99 | 108 | 117 | 126 | 135 | 144 | 153 | 161 | 170 | 179 | 188 |
| 15 | — | 3 | 7 | 12 | 18 | 23 | 28 | 33 | 39 | 44 | 50 | 55 | 61 | 66 | 72 | 77 | 83 | 88 | 94 | 100 |
|   |  | 27 | 38 | 48 | 57 | 67 | 77 | 87 | 96 | 106 | 115 | 125 | 134 | 144 | 153 | 163 | 172 | 182 | 191 | 200 |
| 16 | — | 3 | 8 | 14 | 19 | 25 | 30 | 36 | 42 | 48 | 54 | 60 | 65 | 71 | 77 | 83 | 89 | 95 | 101 | 107 |
|   |  | 29 | 40 | 50 | 61 | 71 | 82 | 92 | 102 | 112 | 122 | 132 | 143 | 153 | 163 | 173 | 183 | 193 | 203 | 213 |
| 17 | — | 3 | 9 | 15 | 20 | 26 | 33 | 39 | 45 | 51 | 57 | 64 | 70 | 77 | 83 | 89 | 96 | 102 | 109 | 115 |
|   |  | 31 | 42 | 53 | 65 | 76 | 86 | 97 | 108 | 119 | 130 | 140 | 151 | 161 | 172 | 183 | 193 | 204 | 214 | 225 |

*continues*

## TABLE C-7B

### Critical Values for the Mann-Whitney U Test[b] continued

| $n_A$ / $n_B$ | 1 | 2 | 3 | 4 | 5 | 6 | 7 | 8 | 9 | 10 | 11 | 12 | 13 | 14 | 15 | 16 | 17 | 18 | 19 | 20 |
|---|---|---|---|---|---|---|---|---|---|---|---|---|---|---|---|---|---|---|---|---|
| 18 | — | 4 | 9 | 16 | 22 | 28 | 35 | 41 | 48 | 55 | 61 | 68 | 75 | 82 | 88 | 95 | 102 | 109 | 116 | 123 |
|  |  | <u>32</u> | <u>45</u> | <u>56</u> | <u>68</u> | <u>80</u> | <u>91</u> | <u>103</u> | <u>114</u> | <u>123</u> | <u>137</u> | <u>148</u> | <u>159</u> | <u>170</u> | <u>182</u> | <u>193</u> | <u>204</u> | <u>215</u> | <u>226</u> | <u>237</u> |
| 19 | 0 | 4 | 10 | 17 | 23 | 30 | 37 | 44 | 51 | 58 | 65 | 72 | 80 | 87 | 94 | 101 | 109 | 116 | 123 | 130 |
|  | <u>12</u> | <u>34</u> | <u>47</u> | <u>59</u> | <u>72</u> | <u>84</u> | <u>96</u> | <u>108</u> | <u>120</u> | <u>132</u> | <u>144</u> | <u>156</u> | <u>167</u> | <u>179</u> | <u>191</u> | <u>203</u> | <u>214</u> | <u>226</u> | <u>238</u> | <u>250</u> |
| 20 | 0 | 4 | 11 | 18 | 25 | 32 | 39 | 47 | 54 | 62 | 69 | 77 | 84 | 92 | 100 | 107 | 115 | 123 | 130 | 138 |
|  | <u>20</u> | <u>36</u> | <u>49</u> | <u>62</u> | <u>75</u> | <u>88</u> | <u>101</u> | <u>113</u> | <u>126</u> | <u>138</u> | <u>151</u> | <u>163</u> | <u>176</u> | <u>188</u> | <u>200</u> | <u>213</u> | <u>225</u> | <u>237</u> | <u>250</u> | <u>262</u> |

[b]Test for a one-tailed test at .05 or a two-tailed test at .10. If the $U_{obs}$ value falls within the two values in the table for $n_A$ and $n_B$, do not reject the null hypothesis. If the $U_{obs}$ is less than or equal to the lower value in the table or greater than or equal to the larger value in the table, then reject the null hypothesis.

**Source:** Adapted from "On a test of whether one of two random variables is stochastically larger than the other" by H. B. Mann and D. R. Whitney, 1947, *Annals of Mathematical Statistics*, (pp. 18, 52–54). Permission granted by Institute of Mathematical Statistics; Aubel D. (1953). Extended tables for the Mann-Whitney statistic, *Bulletin of the Institute of Educational Research at Indiana University, I*, No. 2; and *Handbook of Statistical Tables* (pp. 349–353) by D. B. Owen, 1962 originally published by Addison-Wesley Publishing Company, Inc."

## TABLE C-7C

### Critical Values for the Mann-Whitney $U$ Test[c]

| $n_B$ \ $n_A$ | 1 | 2 | 3 | 4 | 5 | 6 | 7 | 8 | 9 | 10 | 11 | 12 | 13 | 14 | 15 | 16 | 17 | 18 | 19 | 20 |
|---|---|---|---|---|---|---|---|---|---|---|---|---|---|---|---|---|---|---|---|---|
| 1 | | | | | | | | | | | | | | | | | | | | |
| 2 | | | | | | | | | | | | | 0 | 0 | 0 | 0 | 0 | 0 | 1 | 1 |
| | | | | | | | | | | | | | 26 | 28 | 30 | 32 | 34 | 36 | 37 | 39 |
| 3 | | | | | | | 0 | 0 | 1 | 1 | 1 | 2 | 2 | 2 | 3 | 3 | 4 | 4 | 4 | 5 |
| | | | | | | | 21 | 24 | 26 | 29 | 32 | 34 | 37 | 40 | 42 | 45 | 47 | 50 | 52 | 55 |
| 4 | | — | — | — | 0 | 1 | 1 | 2 | 3 | 3 | 4 | 5 | 5 | 6 | 7 | 7 | 8 | 9 | 9 | 10 |
| | | | | | 20 | 23 | 27 | 30 | 33 | 37 | 40 | 43 | 47 | 50 | 53 | 57 | 60 | 63 | 67 | 70 |
| 5 | — | — | — | 0 | 1 | 2 | 3 | 4 | 5 | 6 | 7 | 8 | 9 | 10 | 11 | 12 | 13 | 14 | 15 | 16 |
| | | | | 20 | 24 | 28 | 32 | 36 | 40 | 44 | 48 | 52 | 56 | 60 | 64 | 68 | 72 | 76 | 80 | 84 |
| 6 | — | — | — | 1 | 2 | 3 | 4 | 6 | 7 | 8 | 9 | 11 | 12 | 13 | 15 | 16 | 18 | 19 | 20 | 22 |
| | | | | 23 | 28 | 33 | 38 | 42 | 47 | 52 | 57 | 61 | 66 | 71 | 75 | 80 | 84 | 89 | 94 | 93 |
| 7 | — | — | 0 | 1 | 3 | 4 | 6 | 7 | 9 | 11 | 12 | 14 | 16 | 17 | 19 | 21 | 23 | 24 | 26 | 28 |
| | | | 24 | 27 | 32 | 38 | 43 | 49 | 54 | 59 | 65 | 70 | 75 | 81 | 86 | 21 | 96 | 102 | 107 | 112 |
| 8 | — | — | 0 | 2 | 4 | 6 | 7 | 9 | 11 | 13 | 15 | 17 | 20 | 22 | 24 | 26 | 28 | 30 | 32 | 34 |
| | | | 24 | 30 | 36 | 42 | 49 | 55 | 61 | 67 | 73 | 79 | 84 | 90 | 96 | 102 | 108 | 114 | 120 | 126 |
| 9 | — | — | 1 | 3 | 5 | 7 | 9 | 11 | 14 | 16 | 18 | 21 | 23 | 26 | 28 | 31 | 33 | 36 | 38 | 40 |
| | | | 26 | 33 | 40 | 47 | 54 | 61 | 67 | 74 | 81 | 87 | 94 | 100 | 107 | 113 | 120 | 126 | 133 | 140 |
| 10 | — | — | 1 | 3 | 6 | 8 | 11 | 13 | 16 | 19 | 22 | 24 | 27 | 30 | 33 | 36 | 38 | 41 | 44 | 47 |
| | | | 29 | 37 | 44 | 52 | 59 | 67 | 74 | 81 | 88 | 96 | 103 | 110 | 117 | 124 | 132 | 139 | 146 | 153 |
| 11 | — | — | 1 | 4 | 7 | 9 | 12 | 15 | 18 | 22 | 25 | 28 | 31 | 34 | 37 | 41 | 44 | 47 | 50 | 53 |
| | | | 32 | 40 | 48 | 57 | 65 | 73 | 81 | 88 | 96 | 104 | 112 | 120 | 128 | 135 | 143 | 151 | 159 | 167 |
| 12 | — | — | 2 | 5 | 8 | 11 | 14 | 17 | 21 | 24 | 28 | 31 | 35 | 38 | 42 | 46 | 49 | 53 | 56 | 60 |
| | | | 34 | 43 | 52 | 61 | 70 | 79 | 87 | 96 | 104 | 113 | 121 | 130 | 138 | 146 | 155 | 163 | 172 | 180 |
| 13 | — | 0 | 2 | 5 | 9 | 12 | 16 | 20 | 23 | 27 | 31 | 35 | 39 | 43 | 47 | 51 | 55 | 59 | 63 | 67 |
| | | 26 | 37 | 47 | 56 | 66 | 75 | 84 | 94 | 103 | 112 | 121 | 130 | 139 | 148 | 157 | 166 | 175 | 184 | 193 |
| 14 | — | 0 | 2 | 6 | 10 | 13 | 17 | 22 | 26 | 30 | 34 | 38 | 43 | 47 | 51 | 56 | 60 | 65 | 69 | 73 |
| | | 28 | 40 | 50 | 60 | 71 | 81 | 90 | 100 | 110 | 120 | 130 | 139 | 149 | 159 | 168 | 178 | 187 | 197 | 207 |
| 15 | — | 0 | 3 | 7 | 11 | 15 | 19 | 24 | 28 | 33 | 37 | 42 | 47 | 51 | 56 | 61 | 66 | 70 | 75 | 80 |
| | | 30 | 42 | 53 | 64 | 75 | 86 | 96 | 107 | 117 | 128 | 138 | 148 | 159 | 169 | 179 | 189 | 200 | 210 | 220 |
| 16 | — | 0 | 3 | 7 | 12 | 16 | 21 | 26 | 31 | 36 | 41 | 46 | 51 | 56 | 61 | 66 | 71 | 76 | 82 | 87 |
| | | 32 | 45 | 57 | 68 | 80 | 21 | 102 | 113 | 124 | 135 | 146 | 157 | 168 | 179 | 190 | 201 | 212 | 222 | 233 |
| 17 | — | 0 | 4 | 8 | 13 | 18 | 23 | 28 | 33 | 38 | 44 | 49 | 55 | 60 | 66 | 712 | 77 | 82 | 88 | 93 |
| | | 34 | 47 | 60 | 72 | 84 | 96 | 108 | 120 | 132 | 143 | 155 | 166 | 178 | 189 | 201 | 212 | 224 | 234 | 247 |

*continues*

## TABLE C-7C

### Critical Values for the Mann-Whitney U Test[c] continued

| $n_A$ / $n_B$ | 1 | 2 | 3 | 4 | 5 | 6 | 7 | 8 | 9 | 10 | 11 | 12 | 13 | 14 | 15 | 16 | 17 | 18 | 19 | 20 |
|---|---|---|---|---|---|---|---|---|---|---|---|---|---|---|---|---|---|---|---|---|
| 18 | — | 0 | 4 | 9 | 14 | 19 | 24 | 30 | 36 | 41 | 47 | 53 | 59 | 65 | 70 | 76 | 82 | 88 | 94 | 100 |
|  |  | 36 | 50 | 63 | 76 | 89 | 102 | 114 | 126 | 139 | 151 | 163 | 175 | 187 | 200 | 212 | 224 | 236 | 248 | 260 |
| 19 | 1 | 4 | 9 | 15 | 20 | 26 | 32 | 38 | 44 | 50 | 56 | 63 | 69 | 75 | 82 | 88 | 94 | 101 | 107 |
|  |  | 37 | 53 | 67 | 80 | 94 | 107 | 120 | 133 | 146 | 159 | 172 | 184 | 197 | 210 | 222 | 235 | 248 | 260 | 273 |
| 20 | 1 | 5 | 10 | 16 | 22 | 28 | 34 | 40 | 47 | 53 | 60 | 76 | 73 | 80 | 87 | 93 | 100 | 107 | 114 |
|  |  | 39 | 55 | 70 | 84 | 98 | 112 | 126 | 140 | 153 | 167 | 180 | 193 | 207 | 220 | 233 | 247 | 260 | 273 | 286 |

[c]Test for a one-tailed test at .01 or a two-tailed test at .02. If the $U_{obs}$ value falls within the two values in the table for $n_A$ and $n_B$, do not reject the null hypothesis. If the $U_{obs}$ is less than or equal to the lower value in the table or greater than or equal to the larger value in the table, then reject the null hypothesis.

**Source:** Adapted from "On a test of whether one of two random variables is stochastically larger than the other" by H. B. Mann and D. R. Whitney, 1947, *Annals of Mathematical Statistics,* (pp. 18, 52–54). Permission granted by Institute of Mathematical Statistics; Aubel D. (1953). Extended tables for the Mann-Whitney statistic, *Bulletin of the Institute of Educational Research at Indiana University, I,* No. 2; and *Handbook of Statistical Tables* (pp. 349–353) by D. B. Owen, 1962 originally published by Addison-Wesley Publishing Company, Inc.

## TABLE C-8

### Critical Values of $T$ for the Wilcoxon Signed-Rank Test[a]

| | Level of significance for one-tailed test | | | | | Level of significance for one-tailed test | | | |
|---|---|---|---|---|---|---|---|---|---|
| | .05 | .025 | .01 | .005 | | .05 | .025 | .01 | .005 |
| | Level of significance for two-tailed test | | | | | Level of significance for two-tailed test | | | |
| N | .10 | .05 | .02 | .01 | N | .10 | .05 | .02 | .01 |
| 5 | 0 | — | — | — | 28 | 130 | 116 | 101 | 91 |
| 6 | 2 | 0 | — | — | 29 | 140 | 126 | 110 | 100 |
| 7 | 3 | 2 | 0 | — | 30 | 151 | 137 | 120 | 109 |
| 8 | 5 | 3 | 1 | 0 | 31 | 163 | 147 | 130 | 118 |
| 9 | 8 | 5 | 3 | 1 | 32 | 175 | 159 | 140 | 128 |
| 10 | 10 | 8 | 5 | 3 | 33 | 187 | 170 | 151 | 138 |
| 11 | 13 | 10 | 7 | 5 | 34 | 200 | 182 | 162 | 148 |
| 12 | 17 | 13 | 9 | 7 | 35 | 213 | 195 | 173 | 159 |
| 13 | 21 | 17 | 12 | 9 | 36 | 227 | 208 | 185 | 171 |
| 14 | 25 | 21 | 15 | 12 | 37 | 241 | 221 | 198 | 182 |
| 15 | 30 | 25 | 19 | 15 | 38 | 256 | 235 | 211 | 194 |
| 16 | 35 | 29 | 23 | 19 | 39 | 271 | 249 | 224 | 207 |
| 17 | 41 | 34 | 27 | 23 | 40 | 286 | 264 | 238 | 220 |
| 18 | 47 | 40 | 32 | 27 | 41 | 302 | 279 | 252 | 233 |
| 19 | 53 | 46 | 37 | 32 | 42 | 319 | 294 | 266 | 247 |
| 20 | 60 | 52 | 43 | 37 | 43 | 336 | 310 | 281 | 261 |
| 21 | 67 | 58 | 49 | 42 | 44 | 353 | 327 | 296 | 276 |
| 22 | 75 | 65 | 55 | 48 | 45 | 371 | 343 | 312 | 291 |
| 23 | 83 | 73 | 62 | 54 | 46 | 389 | 361 | 328 | 307 |
| 24 | 91 | 81 | 69 | 61 | 47 | 407 | 378 | 345 | 322 |
| 25 | 100 | 89 | 76 | 68 | 48 | 426 | 396 | 362 | 339 |
| 26 | 110 | 98 | 84 | 75 | 49 | 446 | 415 | 379 | 355 |
| 27 | 119 | 107 | 92 | 83 | 50 | 466 | 434 | 397 | 373 |

[a]The $T_{crit}$ value indicates the smaller sum of ranks associated with differences that are all of the same sign. For any given N (number of ranked differences), the $T_{obs}$ is significant at a given level if it is equal to or less than the critical value in the table.

**Source:** Adapted from *New Cambridge Statistical Tables* (p.65), Table 20. Percentage Points of Wilcoxon's Signed-Rank Distribution, by D. V. Lindley and W. F. Scott, 1984, Cambridge, England: Cambridge University Press; and *Handbook of Statistical Tables* (pp. 325-362), by D. B. Owen, 1962, originally published in Reading, MA: Addison-Wesley Publishing.

## TABLE C-9

### Student Range Statistic for Tukey's Honestly Significantly Difference Test (HSD)

| df for Error Term | K = Number of Treatments | | | | | | | | | | |
|---|---|---|---|---|---|---|---|---|---|---|---|
| | 2 | 3 | 4 | 5 | 6 | 7 | 8 | 9 | 10 | 11 | 12 |
| 4 | 3.927[a] | 5.040 | 5.757 | 6.287 | 6.706 | 7.053 | 7.347 | 7.602 | 7.826 | 8.027 | 8.208 |
| | 6.511 | 8.120 | 9.173 | 9.958 | 10.583 | 11.101 | 11.542 | 11.925 | 12.263 | 12.565 | 12.839 |
| 5 | 3.635 | 4.602 | 5.218 | 5.673 | 6.033 | 6.330 | 6.582 | 6.801 | 6.995 | 7.167 | 7.323 |
| | 5.702 | 6.976 | 7.804 | 8.421 | 8.913 | 9.321 | 9.669 | 9.971 | 10.239 | 10.479 | 10.696 |
| 6 | 3.460 | 4.339 | 4.896 | 5.305 | 5.628 | 5.895 | 6.122 | 6.319 | 6.493 | 6.649 | 6.789 |
| | 5.243 | 6.331 | 7.033 | 7.556 | 7.972 | 8.318 | 8.612 | 8.869 | 9.097 | 9.300 | 9.485 |
| 7 | 3.344 | 4.165 | 4.681 | 5.060 | 5.359 | 5.606 | 5.815 | 5.997 | 6.158 | 6.302 | 6.431 |
| | 4.949 | 5.919 | 6.542 | 7.005 | 7.373 | 7.678 | 7.939 | 8.166 | 8.367 | 8.548 | 8.711 |
| 8 | 3.261 | 4.041 | 4.529 | 4.886 | 5.167 | 5.399 | 5.596 | 5.767 | 5.918 | 6.053 | 6.175 |
| | 4.745 | 5.635 | 6.204 | 6.625 | 6.959 | 7.237 | 7.474 | 7.680 | 7.863 | 8.027 | 8.176 |
| 9 | 3.199 | 3.948 | 4.415 | 4.755 | 5.024 | 5.244 | 5.432 | 5.595 | 5.738 | 5.867 | 5.983 |
| | 4.596 | 5.428 | 5.957 | 6.347 | 6.657 | 6.915 | 7.134 | 7.325 | 7.494 | 7.646 | 7.784 |
| 10 | 3.151 | 3.877 | 4.327 | 4.654 | 4.912 | 5.124 | 5.304 | 5.460 | 5.598 | 5.722 | 5.833 |
| | 4.482 | 5.270 | 5.769 | 6.136 | 6.428 | 6.669 | 6.875 | 7.054 | 7.213 | 7.356 | 7.485 |
| 11 | 3.113 | 3.820 | 4.256 | 4.574 | 4.823 | 5.028 | 5.202 | 5.353 | 5.486 | 5.605 | 5.713 |
| | 4.392 | 5.146 | 5.621 | 5.970 | 6.247 | 6.476 | 6.671 | 6.841 | 6.992 | 7.127 | 7.250 |
| 12 | 3.081 | 3.773 | 4.199 | 4.508 | 4.750 | 4.950 | 5.119 | 5.265 | 5.395 | 5.510 | 5.615 |
| | 4.320 | 5.046 | 5.502 | 5.836 | 6.101 | 6.320 | 6.507 | 6.670 | 6.814 | 6.943 | 7.060 |
| 13 | 3.055 | 3.734 | 4.151 | 4.453 | 4.690 | 4.884 | 5.049 | 5.192 | 5.318 | 5.431 | 5.533 |
| | 4.260 | 4.964 | 5.404 | 5.726 | 5.981 | 6.192 | 6.372 | 6.528 | 6.666 | 6.791 | 6.903 |
| 14 | 3.033 | 3.701 | 4.111 | 4.407 | 4.639 | 4.829 | 4.990 | 5.130 | 5.253 | 5.364 | 5.463 |
| | 4.210 | 4.895 | 5.322 | 5.634 | 5.881 | 6.085 | 6.258 | 6.409 | 6.543 | 6.663 | 6.772 |
| 15 | 3.014 | 3.673 | 4.076 | 4.367 | 4.595 | 4.782 | 4.940 | 5.077 | 5.198 | 5.306 | 5.403 |

| df for Error Term | K = Number of Treatments | | | | | | | | | | |
|---|---|---|---|---|---|---|---|---|---|---|---|
| | 2 | 3 | 4 | 5 | 6 | 7 | 8 | 9 | 10 | 11 | 12 |
| 16 | 4.167 | 4.836 | 5.252 | 5.556 | 5.796 | 5.994 | 6.162 | 6.309 | 6.438 | 6.555 | 6.660 |
| | **2.998** | **3.649** | **4.046** | **4.333** | **4.557** | **4.741** | **4.896** | **5.031** | **5.150** | **5.256** | **5.352** |
| 17 | 4.131 | 4.786 | 5.192 | 5.489 | 5.722 | 5.915 | 6.079 | 6.222 | 6.348 | 6.461 | 6.564 |
| | **2.984** | **3.628** | **4.020** | **4.303** | **4.524** | **4.705** | **4.858** | **4.991** | **5.108** | **5.212** | **5.306** |
| 18 | 4.099 | 4.742 | 5.140 | 5.430 | 5.659 | 5.847 | 6.007 | 6.147 | 6.270 | 6.380 | 6.480 |
| | **2.971** | **3.609** | **3.997** | **4.276** | **4.494** | **4.673** | **4.824** | **4.955** | **5.071** | **5.173** | **5.266** |
| 19 | 4.071 | 4.703 | 5.094 | 5.379 | 5.603 | 5.787 | 5.944 | 6.081 | 6.201 | 6.309 | 6.407 |
| | **2.960** | **3.593** | **3.977** | **4.253** | **4.468** | **4.645** | **4.794** | **4.924** | **5.037** | **5.139** | **5.231** |
| 20 | 4.046 | 4.669 | 5.054 | 5.334 | 5.553 | 5.735 | 5.889 | 6.022 | 6.141 | 6.246 | 6.342 |
| | **2.950** | **3.578** | **3.958** | **4.232** | **4.445** | **4.620** | **4.768** | **4.895** | **5.008** | **5.108** | **5.199** |
| 25 | 4.024 | 4.639 | 5.018 | 5.293 | 5.510 | 5.688 | 5.839 | 5.970 | 6.086 | 6.190 | 6.285 |
| | **2.913** | **3.523** | **3.890** | **4.153** | **4.358** | **4.526** | **4.667** | **4.789** | **4.897** | **4.993** | **5.079** |
| 30 | 3.942 | 4.527 | 4.885 | 5.144 | 5.347 | 5.513 | 5.655 | 5.778 | 5.886 | 5.983 | 6.070 |
| | **2.888** | **3.486** | **3.845** | **4.102** | **4.301** | **4.464** | **4.601** | **4.720** | **4.824** | **4.917** | **5.001** |
| 35 | 3.889 | 4.455 | 4.799 | 5.048 | 5.242 | 5.401 | 5.536 | 5.653 | 5.756 | 5.848 | 5.932 |
| | **2.871** | **3.461** | **3.814** | **4.066** | **4.261** | **4.421** | **4.555** | **4.606** | **4.773** | **4.863** | **4.945** |
| 40 | 3.852 | 4.404 | 4.739 | 4.980 | 5.169 | 5.323 | 5.453 | 5.566 | 5.666 | 5.755 | 5.835 |
| | **2.858** | **3.442** | **3.791** | **4.039** | **4.232** | **4.388** | **4.521** | **4.634** | **4.735** | **4.824** | **4.904** |
| 50 | 3.825 | 4.367 | 4.695 | 4.931 | 5.114 | 5.265 | 5.392 | 5.502 | 5.599 | 5.685 | 5.764 |
| | **2.841** | **3.416** | **3.758** | **4.002** | **4.190** | **4.344** | **4.473** | **4.584** | **4.681** | **4.768** | **4.846** |
| 60 | 3.787 | 4.316 | 4.634 | 4.863 | 5.040 | 5.185 | 5.308 | 5.414 | 5.507 | 5.590 | 5.665 |
| | **2.829** | **3.399** | **3.737** | **3.977** | **4.163** | **4.314** | **4.441** | **4.550** | **4.646** | **4.732** | **4.808** |
| | 3.762 | 4.282 | 4.594 | 4.818 | 4.991 | 5.133 | 5.253 | 5.356 | 5.447 | 5.528 | 5.601 |

*continues*

## TABLE C-9

**Student Range Statistic for Tukey's Honestly Significantly Difference Test (HSD)** continued

© Cengage Learning 2013

| df for Error Term | K = Number of Treatments | | | | | | | | | | |
| | 2 | 3 | 4 | 5 | 6 | 7 | 8 | 9 | 10 | 11 | 12 |
|---|---|---|---|---|---|---|---|---|---|---|---|
| 80 | **2.814** | **3.377** | **3.711** | **3.947** | **4.129** | **4.277** | **4.402** | **4.509** | **4.603** | **4.686** | **4.761** |
| | 3.732 | 4.241 | 4.545 | 4.763 | 4.931 | 5.069 | 5.185 | 5.284 | 5.372 | 5.451 | 5.521 |
| 100 | **2.806** | **3.365** | **3.695** | **3.929** | **4.109** | **4.256** | **4.379** | **4.484** | **4.577** | **4.659** | **4.733** |
| | 3.714 | 4.216 | 4.516 | 4.730 | 4.896 | 5.031 | 5.144 | 5.242 | 5.328 | 5.405 | 5.474 |
| 200 | **2.789** | **3.339** | **3.664** | **3.893** | **4.069** | **4.212** | **4.332** | **4.435** | **4.525** | **4.605** | **4.677** |
| | 3.678 | 4.168 | 4.459 | 4.666 | 4.826 | 4.956 | 5.065 | 5.159 | 5.242 | 5.315 | 5.381 |

[a]Bolded critical Q-values are at p = .05. Nonbolded critical Q-values are at p = .01.

**Source:** The table was generated by Martin S. Rice, Department of Rehabilitation Sciences, The University of Toledo, using R version 2.13.0.

## TABLE C-10

**Critical Values for the Chi-Square Distribution ($\chi^2$)**

| df | 0.25 | 0.1 | 0.05 | 0.025 | 0.01 | 0.005 | 0.001 |
|---|---|---|---|---|---|---|---|
| 1 | 1.3233 | 2.7055 | 3.8415 | 5.0239 | 6.6349 | 7.8794 | 10.8276 |
| 2 | 2.7726 | 4.6052 | 5.9915 | 7.3778 | 9.2103 | 10.5966 | 13.8155 |
| 3 | 4.1083 | 6.2514 | 7.8147 | 9.3484 | 11.3449 | 12.8382 | 16.2662 |
| 4 | 5.3853 | 7.7794 | 9.4877 | 11.1433 | 13.2767 | 14.8603 | 18.4668 |
| 5 | 6.6257 | 9.2364 | 11.0705 | 12.8325 | 15.0863 | 16.7496 | 20.5150 |
| 6 | 7.8408 | 10.6446 | 12.5916 | 14.4494 | 16.8119 | 18.5476 | 22.4577 |
| 7 | 9.0371 | 12.0170 | 14.0671 | 16.0128 | 18.4753 | 20.2777 | 24.3219 |
| 8 | 10.2189 | 13.3616 | 15.5073 | 17.5345 | 20.0902 | 21.9550 | 26.1245 |
| 9 | 11.3888 | 14.6837 | 16.9190 | 19.0228 | 21.6660 | 23.5894 | 27.8772 |
| 10 | 12.5489 | 15.9872 | 18.3070 | 20.4832 | 23.2093 | 25.1882 | 29.5883 |
| 11 | 13.7007 | 17.2750 | 19.6751 | 21.9200 | 24.7250 | 26.7568 | 31.2641 |
| 12 | 14.8454 | 18.5493 | 21.0261 | 23.3367 | 26.2170 | 28.2995 | 32.9095 |
| 13 | 15.9839 | 19.8119 | 22.3620 | 24.7356 | 27.6882 | 29.8195 | 34.5282 |
| 14 | 17.1169 | 21.0641 | 23.6848 | 26.1189 | 29.1412 | 31.3193 | 36.1233 |
| 15 | 18.2451 | 22.3071 | 24.9958 | 27.4884 | 30.5779 | 32.8013 | 37.6973 |
| 16 | 19.3689 | 23.5418 | 26.2962 | 28.8454 | 31.9999 | 34.2672 | 39.2524 |
| 17 | 20.4887 | 24.7690 | 27.5871 | 30.1910 | 33.4087 | 35.7185 | 40.7902 |
| 18 | 21.6049 | 25.9894 | 28.8693 | 31.5264 | 34.8053 | 37.1565 | 42.3124 |
| 19 | 22.7178 | 27.2036 | 30.1435 | 32.8523 | 36.1909 | 38.5823 | 43.8202 |
| 20 | 23.8277 | 28.4120 | 31.4104 | 34.1696 | 37.5662 | 39.9968 | 45.3147 |
| 21 | 24.9348 | 29.6151 | 32.6706 | 35.4789 | 38.9322 | 41.4011 | 46.7970 |
| 22 | 26.0393 | 30.8133 | 33.9244 | 36.7807 | 40.2894 | 42.7957 | 48.2679 |
| 23 | 27.1413 | 32.0069 | 35.1725 | 38.0756 | 41.6384 | 44.1813 | 49.7282 |
| 24 | 28.2412 | 33.1962 | 36.4150 | 39.3641 | 42.9798 | 45.5585 | 51.1786 |
| 25 | 29.3389 | 34.3816 | 37.6525 | 40.6465 | 44.3141 | 46.9279 | 52.6197 |
| 26 | 30.4346 | 35.5632 | 38.8851 | 41.9232 | 45.6417 | 48.2899 | 54.0520 |
| 27 | 31.5284 | 36.7412 | 40.1133 | 43.1945 | 46.9629 | 49.6449 | 55.4760 |
| 28 | 32.6205 | 37.9159 | 41.3371 | 44.4608 | 48.2782 | 50.9934 | 56.8923 |
| 29 | 33.7109 | 39.0875 | 42.5570 | 45.7223 | 49.5879 | 52.3356 | 58.3012 |
| 30 | 34.7997 | 40.2560 | 43.7730 | 46.9792 | 50.8922 | 53.6720 | 59.7031 |
| 31 | 35.8871 | 41.4217 | 44.9853 | 48.2319 | 52.1914 | 55.0027 | 61.0983 |
| 32 | 36.9730 | 42.5847 | 46.1943 | 49.4804 | 53.4858 | 56.3281 | 62.4872 |
| 33 | 38.0575 | 43.7452 | 47.3999 | 50.7251 | 54.7755 | 57.6484 | 63.8701 |
| 34 | 39.1408 | 44.9032 | 48.6024 | 51.9660 | 56.0609 | 58.9639 | 65.2472 |

*continues*

TABLE C-10

**Critical Values for the Chi-Square Distribution ($\chi^2$)** *continued*

| df | 0.25 | 0.1 | 0.05 | 0.025 | 0.01 | 0.005 | 0.001 |
|----|------|-----|------|-------|------|-------|-------|
| 35 | 40.2228 | 46.0588 | 49.8018 | 53.2033 | 57.3421 | 60.2748 | 66.6188 |
| 36 | 41.3036 | 47.2122 | 50.9985 | 54.4373 | 58.6192 | 61.5812 | 67.9852 |
| 37 | 42.3833 | 48.3634 | 52.1923 | 55.6680 | 59.8925 | 62.8833 | 69.3465 |
| 38 | 43.4619 | 49.5126 | 53.3835 | 56.8955 | 61.1621 | 64.1814 | 70.7029 |
| 39 | 44.5395 | 50.6598 | 54.5722 | 58.1201 | 62.4281 | 65.4756 | 72.0547 |
| 40 | 45.6160 | 51.8051 | 55.7585 | 59.3417 | 63.6907 | 66.7660 | 73.4020 |
| 41 | 46.6916 | 52.9485 | 56.9424 | 60.5606 | 64.9501 | 68.0527 | 74.7449 |
| 42 | 47.7663 | 54.0902 | 58.1240 | 61.7768 | 66.2062 | 69.3360 | 76.0838 |
| 43 | 48.8400 | 55.2302 | 59.3035 | 62.9904 | 67.4593 | 70.6159 | 77.4186 |
| 44 | 49.9129 | 56.3685 | 60.4809 | 64.2015 | 68.7095 | 71.8926 | 78.7495 |
| 45 | 50.9849 | 57.5053 | 61.6562 | 65.4102 | 69.9568 | 73.1661 | 80.0767 |
| 46 | 52.0562 | 58.6405 | 62.8296 | 66.6165 | 71.2014 | 74.4365 | 81.4003 |
| 47 | 53.1267 | 59.7743 | 64.0011 | 67.8206 | 72.4433 | 75.7041 | 82.7204 |
| 48 | 54.1964 | 60.9066 | 65.1708 | 69.0226 | 73.6826 | 76.9688 | 84.0371 |
| 49 | 55.2653 | 62.0375 | 66.3386 | 70.2224 | 74.9195 | 78.2307 | 85.3506 |
| 50 | 56.3336 | 63.1671 | 67.5048 | 71.4202 | 76.1539 | 79.4900 | 86.6608 |

**Source:** The table was generated by Martin S. Rice, Department of Rehabilitation Sciences, The University of Toledo, using Microsoft Office Excel 2007.

## Steps in Determining Critical Values for Chi-Square ($\chi^2$) for Table C–10

1. Calculate the degrees of freedom (*df*). The formula is $df = (r - 1)(c - 1)$. $r$ = number of rows in the matrix and $c$ = number of columns in the matrix. For example, in a 2 X 3 matrix, 2 rows and 3 columns, $df = (2 - 1)(3 - 1) = 2$ *df*.
2. Apply the level of significance such as .05 or .01.
3. Locate the critical value for $\chi^2$ from the statistical table. For example, $df = 2$, .05 level of significance, $\chi^2_{crit} = 5.9915$.
4. Calculate $\chi^2_{obs}$ from the data.
5. Decision Rule:
   - If $\chi^2_{obs}$ is equal to or above $\chi^2_{crit}$, then reject the null hypothesis.
   - If $\chi^2_{obs}$ is below $\chi^2_{crit}$, then accept the null hypothesis.

# Glossary

## A

**A-B-A research design:** single-subject research where the A phase represents the collection of baseline data and the B phase represents the intervention. For example a participant who has had a stroke is first measured for the ability to do ADL tasks such as measured by the Katz Scale (Katz 1983.) This represents the period of collecting baseline data (A phase of study). The intervention (B) phase is the experimental manipulation such as applying constraint therapy. The outcome measure (A phase) is repeated to determine if the participant improved.

**abscissa:** the horizontal coordinate or $X$ in a Cartesian coordinate system.

**abstract:** a summary of a published article (150 to 300 words) that contains the important points of each section, including purpose of study, literature review, methodology, results, clinical implications, limitations of research design, and recommendations for further research.

**action research:** application of research to a site-specific environment using a problem-solving approach. It is an outgrowth of both qualitative and quantitative research. For example, an occupational therapist is interested in finding the best splint to use with a client who has a cumulative trauma injury. The methodology may be replicated in another setting to test for generalizability of results.

**age-scale:** a scoring format to determine the ratio between an individual's obtained age-score on a developmental test to that individual's chronological age.

**alpha:** the probability of a Type I error in research. It is usually defined as .05 or .01 in the social sciences. It is also referred to as "significance level" and "$p$-value."

**alternative hypothesis ($H_1$):** the hypothesis that is the opposite of the null hypothesis and predicts that there is a treatment effect or differences between the variables. For example the investigator stating an alternative hypothesis states that "Sensory integration therapy is more effective than behavior modification in increasing fine motor activities in children diagnosed with autism." The null hypothesis ($H_0$) predicts no significant differences between the two interventions.

**analysis of covariance (ANCOVA):** a statistical test arising from an analysis of variance that adjusts for a priori differences in comparable groups that may potentially affect the results such as age or intelligence.

**analysis of variance (ANOVA):** an inferential statistical test that is applied to data when comparing two or more independent group means. An $F$ score is derived. The formula for $F$ in a one-way ANOVA is:

$$F = \frac{\textit{Variance between group means}}{\textit{Variance within groups}}$$

**annotated bibliography:** includes the bibliographical citation and the abstract.

**ANOVA:** an acronym for "analysis of variance."

**applied research:** the direct application of research to improving the quality of life in areas such as reduction of work injuries, prevention of alcoholism, and evaluation of clinical treatment methods. *See also* problem-oriented research.

**a priori:** deductive reasoning from cause to effect. *A priori* criteria are criteria that an investigator states before collecting data.

**aptitude:** inherent, natural ability of an individual; underlying capacity to learn or perform in a specific area.

**artifact:** an unexplained result in an experiment not caused by the independent variable.

**associational relationship:** degree of correlation between two variables.

**attitude scale:** a measure of an individual's feeling, belief, or opinion toward a subject or topic.

**average:** There are three different types of average:

**Mean:** what we often think of as "average"— we add all the values and divide by the number of values added.

**Median** (or midpoint): the value in the exact center of the list of responses.

**Mode:** the most selected value.

For example, if nine college students and Bill Gates are in a room, how we determine the "average" annual earnings can present vastly differing results. Let's say each student earns $10k, and Bill Gates earns $10 million. The mean would be $1,009,000 (adding together everyone's earnings and dividing by 10). The mean makes the students appear to be doing rather well. On the other hand, the median (the value in the middle of the list) is $10,000. The mode is also $10,000, since nine people have that response. An example like this makes clear the need to be careful about which measure of central tendency is chosen.

## B

**bar graph:** a histogram with unattached bars.

**baseline data:** the results of initial testing of a subject before intervention.

**basic research:** investigations in areas related to processes, functions, and attributes that can lead to applied research. An example of basic research is examining how serotonin, a neurochemical transmitter, operates in the brain. The results of basic research often have important significance for clinical researchers.

**before-and-after design:** an experimental research design in which performance or characteristics are measured before and after a treatment intervention.

**beta:** the probability of a Type II error in research.

**bias:** any prejudicial factor in the researcher or methodology that may distort results.

**biased sample:** a sample that is not representative of a target population from which it is drawn. It does not reflect the major characteristics of the target population, and therefore results from a biased sample cannot be generalized.

**bibliographical citation:** the exact reference for a journal, book, or article referred to in the research paper or manuscript. The citation includes the author; date of publication; title of article, journal, or book; volume and page numbers; and in books, the place of publication and the publisher.

**bimodal:** a frequency distribution showing two highest points.

**binomial distribution:** probability distribution used to describe dichotomous outcomes in a population.

**bivariate analysis:** statistical analysis in which there is one dependent variable and one independent variable.

**Boolean logic:** the strategy most information retrieval systems use to build search statements with logical operators *and*, *or*, and *not* and sometimes with *with* and *in*.

**box and whisker plots, box plots, box graphs:** type of exploratory data analysis that produces descriptive figures displaying the maximum and minimum scores and the median and quartiles in a rectangular box; useful in demonstrating graphically the degree of skewness of data.

# C

**case study:** intensive study of individual either through an experimental prospective design or through retrospective research.

**central tendency:** a summary measure of a distribution indicated by the mean, median, or mode. Frequently referred to as "measures of central tendency."

**Chi-square:** a nonparametric statistical technique that tests the probability between observed and expected frequencies using nominal level measurement.

**clinical observation research:** the systematic and objective investigation in normal development, course of a disease, cultural ethnography, field studies, and naturalistic observations.

**clinical trial:** in experimental medical research, a clinical trial refers to large-scale research studies exploring the effectiveness of drugs or vaccines on populations. For example, the Salk vaccine was used in a clinical trial during the 1950s to examine its effectiveness in preventing polio.

**closed-ended questions:** questions that can be answered by either *yes* or *no*. This type of question is not considered useful in survey research. The opposite of a closed-ended question is an open-ended question.

**coding:** a term in qualitative research to refer to the systematic categorization of interview responses, focus group conversations, or observed documents with common characteristics (e.g., residents of a community or an occupational group).

**cohort:** a study population.

**concurrent validity:** a measure of a test's correlation with an established instrument to test its accuracy in measuring a variable. For example, a new test for intelligence frequently will be correlated with the Wechsler Intelligence Scales because the Wechsler Scales have a high reliability and established validity. New tests are developed to include updated concepts and improved administration, cost, and time considerations.

**confidence interval:** the area in a distribution that contains a population parameter. The confidence interval is related to the level of statistical confidence in results.

**confounding variable:** the effect of extraneous variables on research results. For example, test anxiety, fatigue, and lack of control are confounding variables.

**construct validity:** highest form of empirical evidence that is sought; assumes a theoretical rationale underlies the test instrument.

**content validity:** the most elementary type of validity. It is determined by a logical analysis of test items to see whether the items are consistent and measure what they purport to measure. Sometimes referred to as "face validity."

**contingency table:** a table of values that includes observed and expected frequencies such as in a Chi-square table.

**continuous variable:** a quantitative value that has infinite number of measures between any two points. Examples of continuous variables are height, weight, and heart rate.

**control group:** a comparative group included in a study to control for the Hawthorne effect and other extraneous variables. Both the experimental and comparative groups should receive equal time or attention.

**convenience sample:** a sample selected that is readily available. For example, a researcher will select participants who are in a hospital where the researcher is employed.

**correlation:** describes a relationship between two or more variables.

**correlation coefficient:** a statistical value that indicates the degree of relationship between two variables. It can range from + 1.00 to 0 to −1.00.

**correlation matrix:** a statistical table describing the degree of correlation between two variables. The correlation matrix indicates the correlation coefficient index for each pair of correlates.

**correlational research:** research in which the investigator compares the relationships between variables. The investigator neither manipulates independent variables nor simulates a cause-effect relationship.

**covariate:** an independent variable in a study.

**Cox proportional hazard regression:** statistical test for assessing time to a dichotomous event where the independent variable(s) are nominal or continuous.

**credibility:** in qualitative research, the authenticity of the results based on acceptance of the conclusions from the phenomenological evidence. Triangulation (e.g., obtaining data from different perspectives) increases the credibility of the research.

**criterion:** standard of performance that is the basis or yardstick for comparisons.

**criterion-referenced test:** a test based on a standard of performance, competence, or mastery, rather than on a comparison with a normative group. For example, for an individual to pass a test in driver competency, he or she would have to demonstrate mastery of a specific set of criteria. The determination of the criteria is not based on the bell-shaped curve, but on minimal standards for performance (e.g., parallel parking).

**critical value:** the statistical value displayed in tables that is used to accept or reject the null hypothesis.

**cross-validation:** a method to measure test validity by extending testing from the initial target population to other groups.

**culture-free test:** a test that is not culturally biased and can be administered across cultures.

## D

**data:** the numerical results of a study. The term is always plural (e.g., data are ...). The singular term is *datum* representing a single measure.

**decile:** a point in a distribution where 10 percent of the cases fall at or below that point.

**deductive reasoning:** inference to particulars from a general principle. For example, proposing a theory and then hypothesizing specific results from an experiment.

**degrees of freedom (*df*):** a mathematically derived value that is used in reading statistical tables.

**demographic variables:** related to the statistical characteristics of a target population such as distribution of ages, gender, income, presence of disease (morbidity), death rates (mortality), occupation, accident and injury rates, health status, and nutritional input.

**demography:** the application of statistical methods to describe human populations regarding, for example, mortality, morbidity, birth and marriage rates, gender differences, physical and intellectual characteristics, socioeconomic status, and religious beliefs. In general, demography can be defined as the statistical study of human populations regarding their size, their structure, and development (United Nations, 1958).

**dependent variable:** resultant effect of the independent variable. In clinical research, the dependent variable represents the desired outcome, such as decrease in anxiety, increase in range of motion, or increase in reading achievement.

**descriptive statistics:** statistical tests or procedures to describe a population, sample, or variable. Examples of descriptive statistics include measures of central tendency, measures of variability, frequency distribution, vital statistics, scatter diagram, polygons, and histograms.

**descriptive statistics (exploratory data analysis):** methods of organizing, summarizing, and displaying data; includes calculating measures of central tendency and measures of dispersion.

**developmental observation research:** research concerned with the rigorous investigations into the process, states, and hierarchical steps in human development.

**developmental test:** a measure of a child's performance in age-related tasks such as language, perceptual-motor, social, emotional, and ambulation.

**Deviation IQ:** normalized standard score that measures how far an individual deviates from the mean; generally assumes that the mean is 100 and the standard deviation is either 15 or 16, depending on the test.

**"devil effect":** a negative prejudgment of a subject's performance based on the rater's bias.

**dichotomous variable:** variable that only has two possible outcomes, (e.g., gender).

**directional hypothesis:** a statement by the researcher predicting that there will be a statistically significant difference or relationship between variables. For example, a clinical researcher states, "Aerobic exercise is more effective than antidepressive medication in reducing anxiety in individuals with clinical depression."

**directory of references:** a book that provides a comprehensive source for locating studies in specified fields; sources include lists and short reviews of available textbooks, journals, bibliographies, dictionaries, atlases, databases, and government documents.

**discourse analysis:** the study of language as communication through the forms and mechanisms of verbal interaction.

**discrete variable:** a variable that is distinct and does not have an infinite number of values between categories. Examples of discrete variables are gender, diagnostic categories, or eye color.

**double-blind control:** a research design in which neither the researcher nor the subjects know whether the subjects are in the experimental or control group.

## E

**effect modification (interaction):** a situation in which two or more independent factors modify the effect of each other with regard to an outcome; thus the outcome differs depending on whether or not an effect modifier is present.

**effect size:** the degree of differences between two means or the degree of relationship between two variables in the results of a study. Effect size index is related to statistical power, which is the probability of not making a Type II error (e.g., accepting the null hypothesis when it should be rejected). (See Cohen, 1988.)

**empirical data:** data based on controlled observation that is observable, measured, verified, and replicated.

**empiricism:** the philosophy that advocates knowledge based on controlled observation and experiment.

**error variance:** the presence of error factors in the subject, researcher, test instrument, and environment that threatens internal validity. These factors include poor motivation, fatigue, and test anxiety in the subject; researcher bias; unreliability of the test instrument; and a distracting or noisy testing environment.

**ethnography:** a field that reconstructs accurately a particular culture and searches for patterns that can be generalized to a specific population; observations occur in a natural setting.

**ethnoscience:** the study of the characteristics of language as culture in terms of lexical or semantic relations.

**evaluation research:** the qualitative and systematic evaluation of systems and organizations such as hospitals and educational programs by applying a priori criteria or standards.

**evidence-based practice (EBP):** the application of research studies to justify and implement treatment or intervention. The occupational therapist uses the results of research to design treatment protocols. In another sense, it is the application of scientific findings to clinical practice. In order for EBP to be effective, the clinical practitioner must be able to retrieve the latest research, to evaluate the study in terms of methodology, and to transfer the knowledge into clinical practice. This represents the "best practice" model.

**exclusion criteria:** factors that should not be present in the subject when screening possible participants for a study.

**experimental group:** the group identified that the researcher manipulates; for example, the experimental group receives an innovative method of intervention in treating individuals with traumatic brain injury.

**experimental research:** a prospective study in which the investigator seeks to discover cause-and-effect relationships by manipulating the independent variable and observing the effects on the dependent variable.

**experimental study:** study that examines groups where an intervention has been allocated.

**ex post facto design:** a retrospective study in which the investigator examines the relationships of variables that have already occurred, such as the relationship between cancer and smoking.

**external validity:** the degree to which the results of a study can be generalized to a target population. External validity depends on the representativeness of a sample and the rigor of an experiment. Replication of a study producing consistent results increases the external validity.

**extraneous historical factors:** threats to internal validity when unexpected events take place during an experiment that affect the results such as an unexpected death in the family of an individual in a study or the effects of medication on depression. These unpredictable events in the subject are extraneous variables.

**extraneous variable:** a variable other than the independent variable that can potentially affect the results of a study. Extraneous variables can include such factors as gender, intelligence, severity of disability, or socioeconomic status. These variables, if they are uncontrolled, can threaten the internal validity of a study.

## F

**F:** "frequency ratio" or "Fisher ratio"—the difference in variances between variables. A larger number is better.

**factor analysis:** a statistical method to categorize data into identifiable factors. The proce-dure is an extension of a correlation matrix where a set of variables are correlated with each other.

**factorial design:** a research study exploring the interaction between variables, such as a two-factor analysis of variance.

**feasible research study:** a study in which the investigator has examined in detail and provided solutions for the practical aspects of implementing a research study, such as costs, time, setting, availability of subjects, human ethics, selection of outcome measures, and procedure for collecting data.

**Fisher's exact test:** statistical test used to compare two unpaired (independent) samples where the outcome is dichotomous or nominal and the sample size is small; alternative to the Chi-square test.

**forced choice test items:** items that require participants to make a choice when completing a questionnaire, rating scale, or attitude inventory. Participants select items generated by the researcher.

**frequency:** the number of times a result occurs; a descriptive statistic summarizing data by showing the number of times each score value occurs in a set category or interval.

**frequency polygon:** a line graph depicting the number of cases that fall into designated categories. It is composed of an $X$ and a $Y$ axis.

**Friedman's test:** statistical test used to compare three or more paired (dependent) samples when the outcome is either ordinal or continuous with a skewed distribution.

**functional capacity evaluation (FCE):** a comprehensive and systematic approach that measures the client's overall physical capacity such as muscle strength and endurance. Examples are the Isernhagen Work Systems and BTE.

## G

**Gaussian distribution:** synonymous with a symmetrical bell-shaped or normal curve distribution.

**generalizable:** the extent to which findings from a study from a sample population can be applied to the entire population.

**grounded theory analysis:** referring to qualitative research, the search for regularities by constantly comparing and contrasting similarities and differences in issues to form categories or themes with distinctive properties and conceptual relationships.

**Guttman scale:** a cumulative attitude scale that indicates an individual's feelings toward a specific issue. The respondent usually answers *yes* or *no* to a statement.

## H

**habilitation:** the development of functions and capacities in individuals with disabilities (e.g., cerebral palsy, autism, or Down Syndrome) occurring at birth or during early childhood.

**halo effect:** a carry-over effect from previous knowledge of an individual, resulting in a bias on the part of a tester or rater. Halo effects typically occur when raters positively prejudge a subject's performance based on the rater's previous experience with him or her. It is a bias in testing.

**Hawthorne effect:** a confounding variable that creates a positive result that is not caused by the independent variable. The Hawthorne effect is eliminated by introducing a control group or by using the subject as one's own control.

**hermeneutics:** the study and interpretation of text in which each event is understood by reference to the whole of which it is a part, especially the broader historical context.

**heterogeneous:** of different origin or characteristic, such as male and female or mixed ages.

**heuristic research:** investigations that seek to discover relationships between variables through pilot studies and factor analysis. The major purpose is to generate further research.

**histogram:** a descriptive statistic describing a frequency distribution using attached bars.

**historical research:** the systematic and objective investigation, through primary sources, into the events and people that shaped history.

**homogeneous:** of like characteristic such as age, gender, or intelligence.

**honeymoon effect:** a confounding variable that produces a short-term beneficial effect. It is created by the initial optimism of the researcher desiring to show the positive effects of a specific treatment method and the patient or subject wanting the treatment method to work. The subject rejects the initial effects of treatment and disregards side effects or negative results. It is controlled by long-term follow-up and reduction of researcher bias.

**hypothesis:** a statement that predicts results and can be testable. An example of a hypothesis is, "Aerobic exercise lowers blood pressure in middle-aged, sedentary men." A hypothesis can be stated in a null or directional form. (*See* alternative hypothesis, null hypothesis.)

## I

**idiographic approach:** intensive study of an individual or dynamic case study.

***if-then* contingency:** a hypothesis as stated in logic; *if* (results positive or negative)... *then* (recommendations and options taken); the initial strategy that the researcher proposes.

**incidence rate:** the rate of the initial occurrence or new cases of a disease over a period of time. For example, the incidence of AIDS in the United States for the year 2012 includes all the new cases of AIDS diagnosed during 2012.

**independent living evaluation:** an assessment tool used to measure a client's ability to perform the activities of daily living. An example is the *Barthel Self-Care Index*.

**independent variable:** a variable manipulated by the researcher. In clinical research, it represents the treatment method, such as sensory-integration therapy or cognitive-behavioral therapy.

**inductive reasoning:** inferences from particulars or experiments to the general (e.g., integrating the results of research studies to a general theory or conclusion).

**inferential statistics:** statistical tests or procedures for making inferences from samples and populations based on objectively derived data from a Gaussian distribution. They include, but are not limited to *t*-tests, analysis of variance (ANOVA), Pearson product-moment correlation, factor analysis, and multiple regression.

**information retrieval systems:** automated system for storing and retrieving information. In the health fields, examples include OT Search, MEDLINE, PubMed®, CINAHL, ERIC, or HealthStar.

**informed consent form:** a voluntary consensual agreement between the investigator and the subject detailing the procedures in the study and the possible psychological and physical risks that could result in harm to the subject.

**institutional review board (IRB):** an interdisciplinary committee established in a university, hospital, or private industry to protect the rights of human subjects from possible harm that could occur by participating in a research study. It is recommended that all research with human subjects be approved for ethical consideration before data are collected or the research is initiated.

**internal validity:** the degree of rigor in an experiment in controlling for extraneous variables and error variance. Potential sources of internal validity have been identified as extraneous historical factors, maturation, instrumentation, and lack of random sampling. Internal validity is an indication of the trustworthiness of the results. Well-designed studies with good control of variables that can potentially distort the results have high internal validity. The quality of a research study is increased by eliminating the threats to internal validity.

**interquartile range (IQR):** measure of spread or dispersion in the data calculated as the difference between the 25th and 75th percentile values.

**interrater reliability:** the degree of agreement and consistency between two independent raters in measuring a variable.

**interval scale:** quantification of a variable in which there are infinite points between each measurement, as well as equal intervals. Examples include the measurement of systolic blood pressure or intelligence scores as measured by the Wechsler scales. An absolute zero is not assumed in measuring a variable, nor are comparative statements such as "$X$ is twice as large as $Y$" assumed.

**intervention protocol:** the operational definition of the independent variable or intervention method. The intervention protocol should have enough detail so that it can be replicated. One purpose of designing a treatment protocol is to evaluate its effectiveness.

**intrarater reliability:** the degree of consistency within a single rater.

## K

**Kappa test (*k*):** a statistical procedure to detect the degree of interrater agreement based on probability.

**Kendall's coefficient of concordance:** statistical test used to quantify the association between two variables when the outcome is ordinal.

**key word:** an important word or concept in a study that is identified by the researcher. It is used to retrieve a study when it is part of a database.

**Kruskal-Wallis test:** nonparametric statistical test used to compare three or more unpaired (independent) samples where the outcome is either ordinal or continuous with a skewed distribution.

## L

**Likert scale:** a measurement scale used in questionnaires to assess a subject's agreement or disagreement with a statement. Likert scales usually include five to seven descriptors (e.g., totally agree, agree, neutral, disagree, or totally disagree).

**linear regression:** regression analysis used to quantify the association between one independent variable and a continuous outcome that is normally distributed.

**logical positivism:** a philosophical approach to verifying reality. Logical positivists assert that reality is a result of sensory data.

**logistic regression:** regression analysis used to quantify the association between one independent variable and a dichotomous outcome.

**longitudinal research:** method of research in which one observes the effects of independent variables on dependent variables over a determined period of time; used to predict an outcome based on the presence of causative factors. For example an investigator may want to observe the effects of hormone replacement therapy (HRT) on breast cancer over a 10 year period with women in menopause. A control group would be used to match the women receiving HRT. After ten years both groups would be tested for breast cancer.

# M

**MANCOVA:** "multiple analysis of covariance" is a statistical technique that is based on the analysis of variance where multiple variables are being analyzed and corrected for differences in initial scores.

**Mann-Whitney *U* test:** a nonparametric test that is an alternative to the independent *t*-test when testing significant differences between two independent means. The normality assumptions and equal variances assumptions need not be satisfied when applying the Mann-Whitney *U* test.

**matched group:** a control group selected to use as a comparable group to experimental group. Variables matched typically include age, gender, intelligence, socioeconomic status, and degree of disability.

**maturation:** a threat to internal validity that occurs when the researcher does not account for the subject's maturity during an experiment. For example, in testing children, the researcher must consider the age variable in measuring changes from pre- to posttest evaluation. Maturation can also refer to a practice effect and development in the subject during the experiment.

**McNemar's test:** statistical test used to compare two paired (dependent) samples when the outcome of interest is dichotomous (or nominal with only two outcomes).

**mean:** the arithmetic average derived from all scores in a distribution. It is a measure of central tendency.

**measures of central tendency:** mean, mode, and median.

**measures of variability or dispersion:** range, variance, and standard deviation.

**median:** the score at the 50th percentile or midpoint where all the cases in a distribution are divided in half. It is a measure of central tendency.

**meta-analysis:** a quantitative or qualitative analysis of a group of related research studies to determine if the results of the study are consistent and therefore lend support to their conclusions. Meta-analysis is based on the effect size estimation. (*See* Rosenthal and Rosnow, 1991, for a detailed discussion of meta-analysis.)

**methodological research:** objective and systematic investigation for designing instruments, tests, procedures, curriculum, software programs, and treatment programs.

**mode:** the most frequent score or numerical value in a frequency distribution. It is a measure of central tendency.

**multinomial logistic regression:** logistic regression used to quantify the association between one or more independent variables and a nominal outcome having more than two levels.

**multiple linear regression:** linear regression used to quantify the association between more than one independent variable and a continuous outcome that is normally distributed.

**multiple logistic regression:** logistic regression used to quantify the association between more than one independent variable and a dichotomous outcome.

**multiple regression:** a statistical method that is used to predict the individual effects of independent variables on a designated dependent variable. Multiple regression has been used in medical research to identify the multiple risk factors in a certain disease such as cardiovascular disease, stroke, or emphysema. For example, multiple regression is used to predict the effect of designated risk factors (presumed independent variables) on a dependent variable (such as heart disease). *See* the Framingham Study (Dawber, Meadors, & Moore, 1951).

**multivariable analysis:** statistical analysis in which there is one dependent variable and more than one independent variable.

# N

***n:*** the number of subject/participants in the sample size.

**nominal scale:** classification of variables into discrete categories, such as diagnostic groups, professions, or gender. There is no specific order in the categories; no category is more important than any other category. Likewise, each category is mutually exclusive from any other category.

**nominal variable:** variable having descriptive categories, such as medical diagnoses.

**nomothetic approach:** research leading to general laws in science or universal knowledge.

**nonparametric regression:** a type of regression used to quantify the association between one or more independent variables and a continuous outcome having a skewed distribution.

**nonparametric statistics:** inferential statistical procedures that calculate data from samples that are distribution-free and not based on the normal curve. These tests include Mann-Whitney $U$ test, Kruskal-Wallis test, Chi-square, Spearman rank correlation, and Wilcoxon signed-rank test.

**normal (bell-shaped) curve:** a symmetrical curve that describes a mathematical probability distribution of a population where most scores cluster around the mean. Also known as *Gaussian distribution.*

**normality:** an ideal state of health without the presence of a disability or disease. The current term used is "typical".

**norm-referenced test:** a test used to assess the degree of achievement, aptitude, capacity, interest, or attitude compared to established norms or standard scores based on population.

**null hypothesis ($H_0$):** a statement by the researcher that predicts no statistically significant differences or relationships between variables. For example, a clinical researcher states, "There is no statistically significant difference between exercise and splinting in reducing spasticity in children with cerebral palsy."

# O

**objective psychological test:** standardized test that contains comparative norms for interpreting individual raw scores.

**observational study:** descriptive study that examines groups at one or more points in time without allocation of an intervention.

**observed statistical value:** the value obtained from applying a statistical formula to statistical results. These values such as $t$ or $F$ observed are compared to the critical value that is derived from a statistical table to accept or reject the null hypothesis.

**one-tailed test of statistical significance:** used when researcher predicts a directional hypothesis and there is prior evidence that there will be a statistically significant difference between the groups or a statistically positive correlation between variables.

**open-ended questions:** used in survey research. The investigator elicits attitudes, beliefs, and emotions from subjects by asking nonobjective questions, or questions that cannot be answered by *yes* or *no*. The opposite of an open-ended question is a closed-ended question.

**operational definition of variable:** specific test, procedure, or set of criteria that defines independent or dependent variables and the target population. This factor is important in replicating a study or in evaluating a group of studies such as through a meta-analysis.

**operations research:** originally developed in Great Britain during World War II; used to analyze production methods and efficiency of operations; has three characteristics: (a) systems orientation, (b) interdisciplinary teams, and (c) adaptation of scientific method.

**ordinal logistic regression:** logistic regression used to quantify the association between one or more independent variables and an ordinal outcome.

**ordinal scale:** classification of variables into rank order, such as the degree of anxiety, or academic achievement, or grade level. The classification defines which group is first, second, third, and so forth; however, it does not define the distance between classifications.

**ordinal variable:** variable having categories with an implicit ranking (e.g., ranking of school performance using whole numbers).

**ordinate:** the vertical coordinate or *Y* axis in a Cartesian coordinate system.

**outcome measure:** the specific test or procedure to measure the dependent variable. For example, an outcome measure for pain is the *McGill-Melzack Pain Inventory*.

**outlier:** a test result or score outside the normal range of values.

# P

**p:** or "probability level"; the probability that the results presented are a result of chance and not an actual difference in variables. Probability level can be, for example, 0.01 or 0.05. If probability value is 0.01, then the probability that the results are not due to chance are .99.

**paired t-test:** or correlated *t*-test, used to compare two paired (dependent) samples where the outcome measure is continuous and normally distributed.

**parameter:** a descriptive value assigned to a condition or population. Parameters are constant, such as the characteristics of a specified population.

**parametric statistics:** inferential statistics that are based on certain assumptions, such as the normally distributed population variable, random selection of subjects, homogeneity of variance, and independence of samples.

**Pearson product-moment correlation:** an inferential parametric test used to test whether there is a statistically significant relationship between two variables. An *r* score is derived: *r* can range from +1.00 (a perfect correlation), to 0.00 (no correlation), to −1.00 (a perfect negative or inverse correlation). A computational formula is used in calculating *r*.

***People First* language:** a convention in writing when all references to disabilities are written with the individual placed first (e.g., *child with autism* rather than *autistic child*).

**percentage:** the number of cases per hundred.

**percentile:** a point in a distribution that defines where a given percentage of the cases fall. For example, the 80th percentile is the point where 80 percent of the cases are at that point or below.

**performance test:** a test of an individual's skill or capacity, such as grip strength, range of motion, manual dexterity, or driving skills.

**personal equation in testing:** the effect of the presence of the tester on the subject's performance. The tester, as the evaluator, is a variable in the test situation, and if uncontrolled, can distort the test results. For example, if the test administrator does not follow the directions as stated in the manual exactly, then the test results may not be valid.

**pilot study:** a research study, usually with a small number of subjects, that is innovative but that does not control for all extraneous variables.

The primary advantage of a pilot study is that it generates further research.

**placebo effect:** a confounding variable that occurs when the subject shows signs of improvement or the reduction of symptoms that is not caused by a treatment effect. It is instead caused by the subject's belief that a treatment method is causing improvement even though the subject is receiving a "dummy" or "sham" treatment. The placebo effect was initially observed in drug studies where an experimental drug was compared to a placebo or nonactive drug. Researchers observed that some of the subjects receiving a placebo improved. The current explanation of the placebo effect is that the subject produces a psychophysiologic response that results in a more relaxed and less stressed state. In a way, the subject wills himself or herself to health in a placebo effect. The placebo effect is controlled by comparing baseline measures with posttreatments in the experimental and control groups.

**plagiarism:** when a researcher deliberately takes another person's ideas and incorporates them into his or her own writing without giving any credit to the original author.

**point-scale:** a scoring format that converts raw scores into standard scores and an overall score.

**population (N):** an entire collection of people (e.g., the entire University of South Dakota student body).

**positive correlation:** a relationship between two variables when scores on both variables tend to be in the same direction such as high values for cholesterol and obesity.

**poster display:** an opportunity for researchers to present their research in an informal environment such as a conference where participants can ask questions related to the research.

**posttesting:** the results of testing after the intervention has taken place.

**postulate:** a principle or hypothesis presented without supporting evidence.

**power:** the ability of a study to detect a difference when one exists; probability of rejecting the null hypothesis when it is false.

**practice effect:** when scores on a test increase consistently as a function of the subject's familiarity with the test's contents and his or her reduced anxiety.

**predictive validity:** the degree to which a test or measuring instrument can predict future performance, functioning, or behavior. For example, the *Scholastic Aptitude Test* (SAT) is tested for predictive validity in its ability to predict academic success in college.

**pre-post group design with control group:** classical experimental design where the investigator compares the results obtained by both groups.

**pretesting:** the results of testing before intervening with an independent variable or treatment.

**prevalence rate:** the number of individuals with a disability or disease divided by the total individuals in a population. For example, the prevalence rate of spinal cord injury in the United States in 2012 is the number of individuals with spinal cord injury living in the United States in 2012 divided by the total population in the United States in 2012.

**primary prevention:** the prevention of the initial onset of a disease, such as the prevention of polio with a vaccination.

**primary source:** published articles or conference proceedings that include original data, such as a research study.

**probability:** the mathematical or statistical likelihood that an event will occur.

**probability distribution:** a description of the probability associated with all possible observed outcomes.

**problem-oriented research:** applied research initiated by the investigator identifying a significant problem, such as a rapid increase in attention deficit disorders in children, or the dramatic rise of homeless men in urban areas. The research design addresses the problem directly.

**"Procrustean bed":** applying a treatment method such as a panacea to all patients, regardless of individual differences and needs. For example, applying a treatment procedure to all patients with arthritis, as well as to all patients with cancer, without regard to the individual and specific needs of the patient. In this method, the patient is fitted to the treatment method, rather than, as in good treatment, being given the best and most effective treatment method. Treatment should be tailored to the individual based on his or her specific needs.

**proportion:** fraction in which the numerator consists of a subset of individuals represented in the denominator.

**prospective research:** research that is future oriented and attempts to discover cause-and-effect relationships between variables. In prospective studies, the investigator manipulates an independent variable that is predicted to affect function or performance and then collects data. Experimental and longitudinal research are examples of prospective designs.

## Q

**qualitative research:** study of people and events in their natural setting. This type of research uses multimodal methods in a naturalistic setting. The researcher using qualitative research methods seeks to explore perceptions and experiences to understand phenomena in terms of the meanings that people bring to them. Methods for this type of study include interviews, open-ended questions, observation, and document analysis.

**qualitative variable:** variable that describes attributes (ordinal or nominal).

**quantitative research:** the application of the scientific method to test hypotheses. The quantitative researcher begins with a testable hypothesis, collects data, and uses statistical analyses to decide whether to accept or reject the hypothesis. Objectivity of the researcher, operational definitions of the variables, and control of extraneous factors are the key points in quantitative research.

**quantitative variable:** variable that describes an amount or quantity (continuous or ratio).

**quartile:** a point in a distribution where 25 percent of the cases fall at or below that point. Quartiles are values that divide a set of data into four equal parts.

**quasi experimental designs:** a term defined by Campbell and Stanley (1963) to identify research studies in which subjects are not randomly assigned to equivalent groups or in which single case studies are employed. In general, most clinical research studies are within the quasi experimental model because it is almost impossible to truly select a random sample from a target population or to have truly equivalent experimental and control groups.

**questionnaire:** a standardized list of objective questions or personal opinions developed to obtain information directly from a sample.

## R

**random assignment:** assigning subjects to experimental or control groups with every subject having an equal chance of being selected.

**random errors:** the effect of uncontrolled variables in an experiment, such as unexpected events, test procedural errors, and anxiety within the subject. These errors are unpredictable and unsystematic.

**random sample/sampling:** an unbiased portion of a target population that has been selected by chance such as through random numbers.

**range:** a measure of variability that is the difference between the highest and lowest values in a distribution of scores.

**rank order variables:** examples of ordinal scale measurement in which ranks are assigned in measuring a variable. Most personality tests such as the *Minnesota Multiphasic Personality Inventory* (MMPI) measure rank order variables.

**Rasch analysis:** a statistical method that is particularly suited for evaluating psychometric concepts such as attitudes, abilities, and personality traits; calculates the likelihood of something being true based on the probabilities of how strong effects are while considering the effectiveness of "control" variables.

**rating scale:** an individual's appraisal regarding such variables as competence, nonacademic qualities in students, or patient behavior in a psychiatric hospital.

**ratio scale:** quantification of a variable that includes equal intervals and an absolute zero point, such as in measuring heart rate, height, and weight. Comparative statements using "twice as" or "half" are possible with ratio scales.

**referral source:** a database that lists journal articles, books (e.g., Index Medicus), and information retrieval systems accessed by computer (e.g., OT Search ERIC, MedLine, e-mail, and news lists).

**regression analysis:** statistical method used to describe the association between one dependent variable and one or more independent variables; used to adjust for confounding variables.

**regression line:** a figure that best describes the linear relationship between the $X$ and $Y$ variables. In a high correlation, the researcher is able to predict the unknown value of $Y$ from the known value of $X$.

**regression to the mean:** the observation by statisticians that outlier scores will affect the value of the mean disproportionately especially when there are small numbers of cases. It is also apparent when one remeasures a variable and finds that the initial score was unexpectedly very high or very low as compared with the group mean. On the second measure, the score usually comes closer to the group mean.

**rehabilitation:** is the restoration of function in an individual with an acquired disability, such as a stroke or amputation. Function relates to the individual's ability to work, carry out activities of daily living, use effective social skills, and engage in leisure activities or occupation.

**relative frequency:** the ratio of the number of observations having a certain characteristic or value divided by the total number of observations.

**reliability:** a measure of the consistency of a test instrument. For example, a test has high reliability if it produces consistent results when measuring a variable. Threats to test reliability include ambiguity in the questions and poor test procedures. Reliability is indicated by the correlation coefficient ($r$). An acceptable test reliability is usually an $r$ of .7 or above.

**repeated measures analysis of variance:** measurements are made repeatedly in each subject (e.g., before, during, and after an intervention). Repeated measures ANOVAs are particularly suited for $2 \times 2$ (or larger) designs where one or both factors are repeated or where there are more than 2 repeated factors in a $1 \times n$ design.

**repeated measures designs:** the replication of observations of the effects of treatment methods over a period of time, for example, measuring the effects of biofeedback in reducing anxiety after meditation or exercise. They are usually made before, during, and after an intervention in an experimental design.

**replicability:** to carry out a research design for the second time by replicating the research methodology. The purpose is to strengthen generalizability of the findings and to ensure external validity.

**representative sample:** an unbiased portion of a target population that is representative in terms of demographic characteristics.

**research:** the systematic and objective investigation into a topic by stating a hypothesis or guiding question and collecting primary data. It includes quantitative and qualitative designs.

**researcher bias:** occurs when the researcher's enthusiasm and desire for the treatment to be effective or when the researcher's knowledge of the study affects the results of the study.

**research hypothesis:** a prediction of results.

**research plan:** the outline of the methodology of a study that includes the number of subjects to be in the study, the criteria for subject inclusion, where the study will take place, the intervention, the outcome measures, the length of the study, the estimated costs of the study, personnel needed to implement the study and statistical tests to be applied in data analysis.

**research question (or "Purpose of the Study"):** the central question that should be answered by the research. A good research article has this labeled clearly, either at the beginning or after reviewing some literature. For example, the researcher states that "the primary purpose of this study is to evaluate the effects of sensory integration therapy in increasing social skills with children who are diagnosed with autism".

**research text:** a construction that integrates and interprets data and researcher understanding of the area of study. The completed product is the public text, which may be delivered either as a research report, journal article, book, or seminar paper.

**response rate:** the number and proportion of responses to a researcher's questionnaire or survey. If a researcher sends surveys to 100 people, and 89 people respond, the response rate is 89 percent.

**retrospective research:** research based on causative factors that have already occurred. For example, in a correlational study the researcher may want to examine the relationship between the onset of emphysema and previous smoking behavior. Both variables have already occurred. The researcher tries to reconstruct events and to hypothesize regarding a presumed cause-and-effect relationship. Retrospective research can be used to generate experimental designs to further investigate cause-and-effect relationships.

**risk-benefit ratio:** the estimation by the investigator of the possible risks to the research subject and the benefits accrued through the study. The researcher reveals the potential risks and benefits to the subject taking part in the study through an informed consent form.

## S

**sample (*n*):** a subset of a population (for example, a random sample of occupational therapy students from the University of Toledo).

**sampling error:** the error that results from estimating a population value from a sample.

**scales of measurement:** the level at which a test or instrument measures a specific variable such as intelligence, behavior, personality, muscle strength, or academic achievement. Traditionally, scales of measurement are classified into four levels: nominal, ordinal, interval, and ratio.

**scattergram, scatter diagram, scatterplot:** a figure describing the relationship between the *X* and *Y* variables.

**scientific law:** consistent and uniform occurrences that are predictable. Mendelian law of genetic determination predicts characteristics of offspring when genetic traits of parents are known.

**scientific method:** objective, systematic investigation into a subject by stating a hypothesis and collecting empirical data.

**screening criteria:** inclusion and exclusion factors that narrow the target population in a study.

**secondary prevention:** the prevention of the recurrence of a disease, such as preventing a second stroke in an individual.

**secondary source:** a published article or book that reviews primary sources, such as a literature review.

**self-evaluation method:** subjects in a clinical research study assess their own progress. Self-evaluation is an important factor in assessing treatment effectiveness. Other factors used in assessing treatment effectiveness include objective tests, psychophysiological measures, and mechanical procedures.

**self-fulfilling prophecy:** the expectation by the researcher or rater that a subject will perform at a certain level based on prejudice or bias toward the group to which the subject belongs.

**semantic differential:** an attitude scale in which the respondent rates concepts such as good-bad, fast-slow, and hard-soft.

**significance:** the probability that the results presented are a result of chance and not an actual difference in variables. Also known as "probability value" or "*p*."

**significance level:** in testing a hypothesis, it is the critical level between accepting or rejecting the null hypothesis.

**simple linear regression:** regression analysis used to quantify the association between one independent variable and a continuous outcome that is normally distributed.

**simple logistic regression:** regression analysis used to quantify the association between one independent variable and a dichotomous outcome.

**single-subject design:** research design that systematically compares the performance of a participant under experimental and control conditions. It may include more than one participant, but comparisons are made only within each participant's performance. Common designs include ABA, ABAB where A is the control condition and B is the experimental condition. *See* case study.

**skewed distribution:** a distribution of values that is not symmetric (i.e., not bell-shaped).

    **positively skewed:** data are distributed such that a greater proportion of the observations have values less than or equal to the mean (i.e., more observations with lower values).

    **negatively skewed:** data are distributed such that a greater proportion of the observations have values greater than or equal to the mean (i.e., more observations with higher values).

**skewness:** an indication in a frequency polygon of the asymmetry of a distribution. A distribution can be skewed to the right side or left side of the polygon.

**slope:** the linear direction and angle of a line. It is calculated in the regression line.

**Spearman rank correlation (formerly *rho* [*p*]):** a nonparametric test measured by ordinal scales or non-Gaussian data used in determining the degree of relationship between two variables. It is an alternative to the Pearson product-moment coefficient (*r*).

**split-half reliability:** a method to estimate the degree of consistency in a test by correlating one half of the test items, such as even number items, with the other half of the test, such as the odd number items.

**standard deviation (*SD*):** a statistical measure of the variability of scores from the mean. This is one measure of dispersion or variability. The larger the standard deviation, the more varied (or potentially skewed) the data.

**standard error of measurement (*SEM* or *SE$_m$*):** a statistical value that indicates the band of error surrounding a test score. For example, a raw score of 90 with a *SEM* of 4 represents a score ranging from 86 to 94.

**standardized test:** a test that has been administered to a target population and for which norms are available.

**statistic:** (a) the number that describes a property of a set of data (Anderson, 1998) or (b) the actual subject included in a study.

**statistical assumptions:** conditions in research required for a specific statistical test. These assumptions relate to randomness, scale of measurement, sample size, and independence of samples.

**statistical pie:** a descriptive statistic using the circumference of a circle to describe the percentage of cases for each category within a frequency distribution.

**statistical power:** the ability of a statistical test to accurately reject the null hypothesis and to detect a difference between groups when one exists; *see also* power.

**statistical sample:** a portion of a target population comprising a specific variable such as gender, age, geographical location, income, or occupation.

**statistical significance:** It is the probability of some result from a statistical test occurring by chance. For example a "*p*" level of 0.01 means that you can be sure that 99 percent of the time the results were not due to chance and are actually true. Most researchers in occupational therapy accept the .05 level of probability.

**statistical tables:** contain critical levels and values of probability for accepting or rejecting a hypothesis.

**statistics:** the application of statistical tests and procedures for organizing, analyzing, and interpreting results and data according to mathematical formulas; *see also* statistic.

**stem and leaf display:** descriptive data analysis that orders and organizes data to display trends and patterns in a distribution. The "stem" contains the first digit or digits of each observation, and the "leaf" contains the remaining digit or digits of each observation.

**stratified sample:** a homogeneous subgroup of a population based on variables such as geography, educational level, and treatment setting (e.g., community vs. hospital or disability group).

**survey research:** a systematic and objective investigation into the characteristics, attitudes, opinions, and behaviors of target populations through questionnaires and interviews.

**systematic variance:** occurs when the researcher fails to control for extraneous variables that could possibly affect the results such as age, gender, intelligence, education, socioeconomic status, or degree of disability.

## T

**target population:** an identified group in which a representative or random sample of subjects are selected.

**tertiary prevention:** the prevention of secondary problems that can result from a disability (e.g., preventing decubiti in individuals with spinal cord injury).

**test administrator bias:** occurs when the individual testing the outcome of treatment method is aware of which subjects are in the experimental group and which are in the control group.

**test battery:** a group of tests selected to comprehensively measure an individual's capacity (e.g., performance, vocational interests, attitudes, and intelligence or cognition).

**test-retest reliability:** a method to estimate the degree of consistency of a test. In this method, a test is administered to the same group of subjects over a short period of time. Maturation and changes in the subjects can affect the results and must be controlled by the investigator.

**theory:** a comprehensive body of writings that attempts to explain, for example, how individuals contract and resist disease, learn motor tasks, and develop cognitive and language functions.

**time series research:** in experimental research, time series research indicates the measurement of the dependent variable over time intervals, such as 2 weeks or 3 months. Its purpose is to evaluate the effect of a number of interventions or treatment techniques with the same subject or group.

**transformational research:** the use of research as a personal-political activity whereby the research participants become empowered by active engagement in the research process.

**treatment effects:** in experimental research, the application of independent variable in producing a desired or predicted outcome (e.g., use of constraint therapy in increasing function in the affected limb).

**treatment protocols:** operational definitions of the methods used by clinicians. The procedure is described in enough detail so that replication is possible. Treatment protocols are generated through research and are used in evidence-based practice.

**triangulation:** the use of multiple approaches in collecting data and measuring variables. For example, in measuring a variable such as functional independence, the investigator would use a standardized ADL scale, use a functional capacity evaluation, and apply a self-report measure where the patient evaluates his or her performance in self-care activities.

**t-tests:** inferential statistics that are used to determine whether the difference between two means are statistically significant or are attributable to chance. They include one-sample *t*-test, independent *t*-test, and correlated or paired-data *t*-test. For testing two independent groups with approximately the same variance, the formula is:

$$t = \frac{mean_1 - mean_2}{standard\ error\ of\ the\ differences\ between\ the\ means}$$

**two-tailed test of significance:** used in analyzing data if the researcher has stated the hypothesis in a nondirectional or null form.

**Type I error:** the error that results when the null hypothesis is rejected when it is really true; stating there is a difference in outcome when none exists (false positive). It is analogous to a false positive in medicine when a physician detects a disease when no disease is present.

**Type II error:** the error that results when the null hypothesis is accepted when it is really false; stating there is no difference in outcome when one actually exists (false negative). It is analogous to a false negative in medicine when a physician fails to detect a disease when a disease is present.

## U

**unobtrusive methodology:** a research method in which the investigator collects data from indirect sources, such as patient records, historical documents, letters, and relics.

**unpaired (independent) sample:** study design that compares the outcome of two groups where the groups are not matched on any characteristic.

## V

**validity:** as pertaining to measurement, it refers to the degree to which a test or measuring instrument actually measures what it purports to measure. Validity can also refer to the rigor of an experiment in controlling extraneous variables and the generalizability of the results of a study to a target population.

**variability:** *see* measures of variability.

**variables:** characteristics, factors, or attributes that can be measured qualitatively or quantitatively. Variables can be homogeneous groups, such as physical therapy students, individuals with stroke, or hospital administrators. Variables can also be treatment methods such as exercise or biofeedback or outcomes such as muscle strength, spasticity, functional capacity, or academic achievement.

**variance:** the average of each score's deviation from the mean. Variance is an intermediate value that is used in calculating the standard deviation. The variance is the square of the standard deviation. It is a measure of variability or dispersion.

**vocational interest test:** a measure of an individual's preferences toward occupation-related tasks or jobs.

**volunteer:** a self-selected research participant who may or may not be representative of a target population.

## W

**Wilcoxon signed-rank test:** a nonparametric test and an alternative to the correlated *t*-test when comparing matched subjects or two sets of scores from the same subjects. Before-and-after studies are examples of correlated groups.

**work samples:** well-defined activities that are similar to an actual job. Examples include Valpar and Micro-Tower.

## Z

**z-score:** a score based on standard deviation units from the mean, for example, a *z*-score of +1 is 1 standard deviation unit above the mean.

# References

## A

AbleData. (n.d.). *About AbleData.* Retrieved from http://www.abledata.com/abledata.cfm?pageid=19329&ksectionid=19329

Abrams, M. (1979). A new work sample battery for vocational assessment of the disadvantaged: VITAS. *Vocational Guidance Quarterly, 28,* 35–43.

Achenbach, T. M. (1991). *Achenbach System of Empirically Based Assessment* (ASEBA). Burlington, VT: University Medical Educational Association. (Available from the University of Vermont College of Education, Room 6436, 1 South Prospect St., Burlington, VT; http://www.uvm.edu/~cbcl/)

Achenbach, T. M., & Rescorla, L. A. (2001). *Manual for the ASEBA school-age forms & profiles.* Burlington, VT: University of Vermont, Research Center for Children, Youth, & Families.

Achenbach, T. M., & Rescorla, L. A. (2007). *Multicultural supplement to the manual for the ASEBA school-age forms & profiles.* Burlington, VT: University of Vermont, Research Center for Children, Youth, & Families.

Achenbach, T. M., & Rescorla, L. A. (2010). *Multicultural supplement to the manual for the ASEBA preschool forms & profiles.* Burlington, VT: University of Vermont, Research Center for Children, Youth, & Families.

Ackoff, R. L., & Rivett, P. (1963). *A manager's guide to operation research.* New York: Wiley.

Adger, C. (1994). *Enhancing the delivery of services to Black special education students from non-standard English backgrounds. Final report.* College Park: Maryland University, College Park Institute for the Study of Exceptional Children and Youth. (ERIC Document Reproduction Service No ED 370–377)

Adler, P. A., & Adler, P. (1994). Observational techniques. In N. K. Denzin & Y. S. Lincoln (Eds.), *Handbook of qualitative research* (pp. 377–392). Thousand Oaks, CA: Sage.

Affleck, J. W., Aitken, R. C, Hunter, J. A., McGuire, R. J., & Roy, C. W. (1988). Rehabilitation status: A measure of medicosocial dysfunction. *The Lancet, 1,* 230–233.

Ahmed, M. B. (2001). Alzheimer's disease: Recent advances in etiology, diagnosis, and management. *Texas Medicine, 9,* 50–58.

Ainsworth, M. D., Blehar, M. C., Waters, E., & Wall, S. (1978). *Patterns of attachment: A psychological study of the strange situation.* Hillsdale, NJ: Lawrence Erlbaum.

Alberg, A. J., & Samet, J. M. (2003). Epidemiology of lung cancer. *Chest, 123*(1 Suppl.), 21S–49S.

Allen, C. K. (1985). *Occupational therapy for psychiatric diseases: Measurement and management of cognitive disabilities.* Boston: Little, Brown.

Allen, C. K., Austin, S. L, David, S. K., Earhart, C. A., McCraith, D. B., & Riska-Williams, L. (2007). *Allen Cognitive Level Screen-5 (ACLS-5)/Large Allen Cognitive Level Screen-5 (LACLS-5).* Camarillo, CA: ACLS and LACLS

Committee. Retrieved from http://www.allen-cognitive-network.org/index.php/allen-model/assessments/72-allen-cognitive-level-screen-5-acls-5-large-allen-cognitive-level-screen-5-lacls-5

Allen, C. K., Earhart, C. A., & Blue, T. (1992). *Occupational therapy treatment goals for the physically and cognitively disabled.* Rockville, MD: American Occupational Therapy Association.

Allen, S., & Donald, M. (1995). The effect of occupational therapy on the motor proficiency of children with motor/ learning difficulties: A pilot study. *British Journal of Occupational Therapy, 58,* 385–391.

Alpern, G. D. (2007). *Developmental Profile 3* (DP-3). Los Angeles: Western Psychological Services.

Als, H. (1984). *Manual for the naturalistic observation of newborn behavior (preterm and full term infants).* Boston: Children's Hospital.

Als, H., Butler, S., Kosta, S., & McAnulty, G. (2005). The Assessment of Preterm Infants' Behavior (APIB): Furthering the understanding and measurement of neurodevelopmental competence in preterm and full-term infants. *Mental Retardation and Developmental Disabilities: Research Reviews, 11,* 94–102.

Als, H., Duffy, F. H., & McAnulty, G. B. (1988a). The APIB: An assessment of functional competence in preterm and full–term newborns regardless of gestational age at birth: II. *Infant Behavior and Development, 11,* 319–331.

Als, H., Duffy, F. H., & McAnulty, G. B. (1988b). Behavioral differences between preterm and full-term newborns as measured with the APIB system scores: I. *Infant Behavior and Development, 11,* 305–318.

American Association of Intellectual and Developmental Disabilities (AAIDD). (2010). *Mission.* Retrieved from http://www.aamr.org/content_443.cfm?navID=129

American College of Healthcare Executives (ACHE). (2008). *About Health Administration Press.* Retrieved from http://www.ache.org/pubs/abouthap.cfm

American Educational Research Association (AERA), American Psychological Association (APA) and National Council on Measurement in Education (NCME). (1999). *The standards for educational and psychological testing.* Washington, DC: Authors.

American Occupational Therapy Association (AOTA). (1999–2009). *About OT Search.* Retrieved from http://www1.aota.org/otsearch/links/about.asp

American Occupational Therapy Association (AOTA). (2002). *Occupational therapy practice framework: Domain and process.* Bethesda, MD: Author.

American Occupational Therapy Association. (2005). Standards of practice for occupational therapy. *American Journal of Occupational Therapy, 59,* 663–665.

American Occupational Therapy Association. (2008). Occupational therapy practice framework: Domain and process (2nd ed.). *American Journal of Occupational Therapy, 62,* 625–683.

American Occupational Therapy Association (AOTA). (2008). *Occupational therapy practice framework: Domain and process* (2nd ed). Bethesda, MD: Author.

American Occupational Therapy Foundation (1998–2011). *Resources & the Wilma L. West (WLW) Library.* Retrieved from http://www.aotf.org/resourceswlwlibrary.aspx

American Physical Therapy Association (2008, October.) *Guidelines: Occupational health physical therapy: Evaluating functional capacity.* Published in the APTA Board Meetings, October 2008, p.1. Retrieved from http://www.apta.org/AM/Template.cfm?Section=Home&Template=/CM/ContentDisplay.cfm&ContentID=68532

American Psychiatric Association (APA). (1994). *Diagnostic and statistical manual* (4th ed.). Washington, DC: Author.

American Psychiatric Association (APA). (2000). *Diagnostic and statistical manual of mental disorders—Text revision* (DSM–IV–TR). Arlington, VA: Author.

American Psychological Association (APA). (2010). *Publication manual of the American*

*Psychological Association* (6th ed.). Washington, DC: Author.

*Americans with Disabilities Act* (ADA) of 1990, Pub. L. No. 101–336, § 2,104 Stat. 328 (1991).

AMPS Project International (2010). *Assessment of motor and process skills.* Retrieved from http://www.ampsintl.com/AMPS/

Anastasi, A. (1988). *Psychological testing* (6th ed.). New York: Macmillan.

Anastasi, A., & Urbina, S. (1997). *Psychological testing* (7th ed.). Englewood Cliffs, NJ: Prentice Hall.

Anderson, K. N. (1998). *Mosby's medical, nursing, and allied health dictionary.* (5th ed.). St. Louis: Mosby.

Anderson, M. H., Bechtol, C. O., & Sollars, R. E. (1959). *Clinical prosthetics for physicians and therapists.* Springfield: IL: Charles C. Thomas.

Annual Reviews. (2010). *Welcome to Annual Reviews.* Retrieved from http://www.annualreviews.org/

Applegate, W., Blass, J., & Williams, F. (1990). Instruments for the functional assessment of older patients. *New England Journal of Medicine, 322,* 1207–1214.

Arias, E. (2010, June 28). United States life tables, 2006. *National Vital Statistics Reports, 58*(10). Retrieved from http://www.cdc.gov/nchs/products/life_tables.htm

Arthur, G. (1949). The Arthur Adaptation of the International Performance Scale. *Journal of Clinical Psychology, 5,* 345–349.

Åsberg, M., Perris, C., Schalling, D., & Sedval, G. (1987). The CPRS—Development and applications of a psychiatric rating scale. *Acta Psychiatrica Scandinavia, 27*(Suppl.), 1–27.

Asher, I. E. (Ed.) (2007). *Occupational therapy assessment tools: An annotated index* (3rd ed.; with CD-ROM). Rockville, MD: American Occupational Therapy Association.

Atalay, A. (2009). Determinants of length of stay in stroke patients: A geriatric rehabilitation unit experience. *International Journal of Rehabilitation Research, 32,* 48–52.

Atwater, E. C. (1973). The medical profession in a new society, Rochester, York (1811–1860).

*Bulletin of the History of Medicine, 47,* 221–235.

Auble, D. (1953). *Extended tables for the Mann-Whitney statistic.* Bulletin of the Institute of Educational Research at Indiana University, 1, No. 2.

Ayres, A. J. (1989). *Sensory Integration and Praxis Tests* (SIPT). Los Angeles: Western Psychological Association.

# B

Babbie, E. R. (2010). *The practice of social research* (12th ed.). Florence, KY: Wadsworth/Cengage.

Baker, J. G., Granger, C. V., & Fiedler, R. C. (1997). A brief outpatient functional assessment measure: Validity using Rasch measures. *American Journal of Physical Medicine and Rehabilitation, 76,* 8–13.

Ball, K. K., & Roenker, D. L. (1998). *UFOV Useful Field of View Manual.* San Antonio: Pearson/PsychCorp.

Baptiste, S., & Rochon, S. (1999). Client–centered assessment: The Canadian Occupational Performance Measure. In B. J. Hemphill-Pearson (Ed.), *Assessments in occupational therapy mental health: An integrative approach* (pp. 41–58). Thorofare, NJ: SLACK.

Barnard, A., McCosker, H., & Gerber, R. (1999). Phenomenography: A qualitative research approach for exploring understanding in health care. *Qualitative Health Research, 9.* 212–226.

Barnes, L. L. (2007). Correlates of life space in a volunteer cohort of older adults. *Experimental Aging Research, 33,* 77-93.

Barnhard, C. L. (Ed.). (1948). *American college dictionary.* New York: Random House.

Barnhart, R. C. (2001). Aging adult children with developmental disabilities and their families: Challenges for occupational therapists and physical therapists. *Physical and Occupational Therapy in Pediatrics, 21*(4), 69–81.

Barrett, A. J., & Murk, P. J. (2006). *Life satisfaction index for the third age (LSITA): A measurement of successful aging.* Retrieved from http://hdl.handle.net/1805/1160 Available at https://scholarworks.iupui.edu/bitstream/handle/1805/1160/Barrett_%26_Murk_Life%20Satisfaction.pdf?sequence=1

Barzun, J. (1974). *Clio and the doctors: Psychohistory, quantohistory and history.* Chicago: University of Chicago Press.

Barzun, J., & Graff, H. (1970). *The modern researcher.* New York: Harcourt, Brace and World.

Baugh, J. B., Hallcom, A. S., & Harrison, M. E. (2010.). Computer assisted qualitative data analysis software: A practical perspective for applied research. *Revista del Instituto Internacional de Costos, 6*(4), 69–81. Available from http://www.revistaiic.org/articulos/num6/articulo4_esp.pdf

Bayley, N. (1993). *Bayley Scales of Infant Development—II* (BSID–II). San Antonio, TX: Pearson/PsychCorp.

Bayley, N. (2005). *Bayley Scales of Infant and Toddler Development®,* (3rd ed.; Bayley-III®). San Antonio, TX: Pearson Assessments.

Beard, J. (2008). "Prosthetics". DARPA's Bio-Revolution. [Online]. Available: http://www.darpa.mil/Docs/Biology- biomedical_services_200807171322092.pdf

Beard, J. G., & Ragheb, M. G. (1980). Measuring leisure satisfaction. *Journal of Leisure Research, 12,* 20–33.

Beck, A. T., Ward, C. H., Mendelson, M., Mock, J., & Erbaugh, J. (1961). An inventory for measuring depression. *Archives of General Psychiatry, 4,* 561–571.

Becker, R. L. (1981). *Reading-Free Vocational Interest Inventory.* Columbus, OH: Elbern.

Becker, R. L. (2000). *Reading-Free Vocational Interest Inventory-Revised* (R-FVII:2). Columbus, OH: Elbern Publications.

Beers, C. A. (1908). *A mind that found itself.* New York: Doubleday.

Beery, K. K., Buktenica, N. A., & Beery, N. A. (2010). *Beery-Buktenica Developmental Test of Visual-Motor Integration* (6th ed.; VMI-6). San Antonio, TX: Pearson.

Bender, L. (1938). A visual motor Gestalt test and its clinical use. *American Orthopsychiatric Association Research Monograph,* No. 3.

Benison, S. (1972). The history of polio research in the United States: Appraisal and lessons. In G. Holton (Ed.), *The twentieth-century sciences: Studies in the biography of ideas* (pp. 308–343). New York: W. W. Norton.

Bennett, A. E., Power, T. J., Eiraldi, R. B., Leff, S. S., & Blum, N. J. (2009). Identifying learning problems in children evaluated for ADHD: The Academic Performance Questionnaire. *Pediatrics, 124,* e633–e639. doi:10.1542/peds.2009–0143

Bennett, G. K. (1946). *Hand Tool Dexterity Test.* San Antonio, TX: Pearson/PsychCorp.

Bennett, G. K. (1994). *Bennett Mechanical Comprehension Test.* San Antonio, TX: Pearson/PsychCorp.

Bergner, M., Bobbitt, R. A., with Carter, W. B., & Gilson, B. S. (1981). The Sickness Impact Profile: Development and final revision of a health status measure. *Medical Care, 19,* 787–805. Retrieved from http://www.jstor.org/stable/3764241

Berinstein, S., & Magalhaes, L. (2009). A study of the essence of play experience to children living in Zanzibar, Tanzania. *Occupational Therapy International, 16,* 89–106.

Bermann, E. (1973). *Scapegoat: The impact of death-fear on an American family.* Ann Arbor: University of Michigan Press.

Bernard, C. (1957). *An introduction to the study of experimental medicine* (H. C. Greene, Trans.). New York: Dover. (Original work published 1865)

Best, J. W. (1977). *Research in education* (3rd ed.). Englewood Cliffs, NJ: Prentice Hall.

Best, J. W., & Kahn, J. V. (2005). *Research in education* (10th ed.). Boston: Allyn & Bacon.

Bettelheim, B. (1967). *The empty fortress: Infantile autism and the birth of the self.* New York: The Free Press.

Betz, N. E., Borgen, F. H., & Harmon, L. W. (2004). *Strong Interest Inventory.* Mountain View, CA: CPP, Inc.

Binet, A. (1899/1912). *The psychology of reasoning: Based on experimental researches in hypnotism* (2nd ed.; A. G. Whyte, Trans.). Chicago: Open Court.

Binet, A., & Simon, T. (1905/1916). *The development of intelligence in children* (E. S. Kite, Trans.). Vineland, NJ: Publications of the Training School at Vineland. (Originally published 1905–1911 in *L'Année Psychologique*). Retrieved from http://books.google.com/books?id=2eIJAAAAMAAJ&ots=hZon-Ycdqa&dq=development%20of%20intelligence%20in%20children&pg=PA1#v=onepage&q&f=false

Black, M. M. (1976). Adolescent role assessment. *American Journal of Occupational Therapy, 30,* 73–79.

Blake, J. B., & Roos, C. (Eds.). (1967). *Medical reference works 1679–1966: A selected bibliography.* Chicago: Medical Library Assoc.

Blue, F. R. (1979). Aerobic running as a treatment for moderate depression. *Perceptual and Motor Skills, 48,* 228.

Blumberg, D. F. (1972). The city as a system. In J. Beishon & G. Peters (Eds.), *Systems behavior.* New York: Harper and Row.

Blumstein, J. F. (1997). The Oregon experiment: The role of cost–benefit analysis in the allocation of Medicaid funds. *Social Science & Medicine, 45,* 545–554.

Bohannon, R. W., Peolsson, A., Massy-Westropp, N., Desrosiers, J., & Bear-Lehman, J. (2006). Reference values for adult grip strength measured with a Jamar dynamometer: A descriptive meta-analysis. *Physiotherapy, 92,* 11–15. doi:10.1016/j.physio.2005.05.003

Bone, C., Cheung, G., & Wade, B. (2010). Evaluating person centred care and dementia care mapping in a psychogeriatric hospital in New Zealand: A pilot study. *New Zealand Journal of Occupational Therapy, 57,* 35–40.

Bootes, K., & Chapparo, C. J. (2002). Cognitive and behavioural assessment of people with traumatic brain injury in the work place: Occupational therapists' perceptions. *Work, 19,* 255–268.

Booth, T., & Booth, W. (1994). The use of depth interviewing with vulnerable subjects: Lessons from a research study of parents with learning difficulties. *Social Science and Medicine, 39,* 415–424.

Borowitz, G. H., Costello, J., & Hirsch, J. G. (1971). Clinical observation of ghetto 4-year-olds: Organization, involvement, interpersonal responsiveness and psychosexual content of play. *Journal of Youth and Adolescence, 1,* 59–71.

Bosscher, R. J. (1993). Running and mixed physical exercises with depressed psychiatric patients. *International Journal of Sport Psychology, 24,* 170–184.

Bowker Company. (2011). *Medical and health care books and serials in print: An index to literature in the health sciences.* New York: Author. Available http://www.greyhouse.com/bowk_med.htm

Bowling, A. (2005). *Measuring health: A review of quality of life measurement scales* (3rd ed.). Buckingham, Great Britain: Open University Press/McGraw Hill.

Bowman, J., & Llewellyn, G. (2002). Clinical outcomes research from the occupational therapist's perspective. *Occupational Therapy International, 9,* 145–166.

Brannigan, G. G., & Decker, S. L. (2003). *Bender visual-motor Gestalt test-II* (2nd ed.). Itasca, IL: Riverside Publishing.

Brayman, S. J. (2008). The Comprehensive Occupational Therapy Evaluation (COTE). In B. J. Hemphill-Pearson, *Assessments in occupational therapy mental health: An integrative approach* (2nd ed., pp. 113–124; 406–412). Thoroughfare, NJ: SLACK.

Brayman, S. J., Kirby, T. F., Meisenheimer, A. M., & Short, M. J. (1976). The comprehensive occupational therapy evaluation scale. *American Journal of Occupational Therapy, 30,* 94–100.

Breines, E. (1988). The Functional Assessment Scale as an instrument for measuring changes in levels of function for nursing home residents following occupational therapy. *Canadian Journal of Occupational Therapy, 55,* 135–140.

Breines, E. B. (1996). A cost effective approach to functional assessment. *Occupational Therapy in Health Care, 10*(3), 15–22.

Broca, P. (1961). Remarks on the seat of the faculty of articulated language, following an observation of aphemia (loss of speech). (Trans. C. D. Green). First published in *Bulletin de la Société Anatomique, 6,* 330–357.

Brollier, C., Hamrick, N., & Jackson, B. (1994). Aerobic exercise: A potential occupational therapy modality for adolescents with depression. *Occupational Therapy in Mental Health, 12,* 19–29.

Bronfenbrenner, U. (1979). *The ecology of human development: Experiments by nature and design.* Cambridge: Harvard University.

Brown, G. T., & Rodger, S. (1999). Research utilization models: Frameworks for implementing evidence–based occupational therapy practice. *Occupational Therapy International, 6,* 1–23.

Brown, K. (2004). *Penicillin man: Alexander Fleming and the antibiotic revolution.* Stroud, Gloucestershire, UK: Sutton.

Bruininks, R. H. (1978). *Bruininks-Oseretsky Test of Motor Proficiency.* Circle Pines, MN: American Guidance Service.

Bruininks, R. H., & Bruininks, B. D. (2005). *Bruininks-Oseretsky Test of Motor Proficiency, Second Edition* (BOT-2). San Antonio, TX: Pearson/PsychCorp.

Brunner, T. M., & Spielberger, C. D. (2009). *State-Trait Anger Expression Inventory-2™ Child and Adolescen*t (STAXI-2™ C/A). Lutz, FL: PAR, Inc.

Bryman, A., & Burgess, R. G. (Eds.). (1994). *Analyzing qualitative data.* London: Routledge.

BTE Technologies. (2010). *Physical therapy equipment, occupational therapy equipment, & athletic training equipment.* Retrieved from http://www.btetech.com/eval_rehab_systems.htm

Bulmer, M. (Ed.). (1982). *Social research ethics.* London: Macmillan.

Bureau of Labor Statistics, U.S. Department of Labor. (2009). *Occupational outlook handbook, 2010–11 Edition*, occupational therapists. Retrieved from http://www.bls.gov/oco/ocos078.htm and ftp://ftp.bls.gov/pub/special.requests/ep/ind-occ.matrix/occ_pdf/occ_29-1122.pdf

Burks, H. F. (1968). *Burks' Behavior Rating Scales.* Los Angeles: Western Psychological Services.

Burks, H. F., & Gruber, C. P. (2006). *Burks' Behavior Rating Scale–2* (BBRS-2). Los Angeles: Western Psychological Services.

Burnett, J., Dyer, C. M., & Naik, A. D. (2009). Convergent validation of the Kohlman Evaluation of Living Skills as a screening tool of older adults' ability to live safely and independently in the community. *Archives of Physical Medicine and Rehabilitation, 90,* 1948-1952.

## C

Callinan, N. J., & Mathiowetz, V. (1996). Soft versus hard resting hand splints in rheumatoid arthritis: Pain relief, preference, and compliance. *American Journal of Occupational Therapy, 50,* 347–353.

Campbell, D. T., & Stanley, J. (1963). *Experimental and quasiexperimental design for research.* Chicago: Rand-McNally.

Campione, J. C., & Brown, A. L. (1978). Toward a theory of intelligence: Contributions from research with retarded children. *Intelligence, 2,* 279–304.

Cannon, W. B. (1932). *The wisdom of the body.* New York: W. W. Norton.

Carey, R. G., & Posavac, E. J. (1980). *Manual for the Level of Rehabilitation Scale II.* Park Ridge, IL: Lutheran General Hospital.

Carey, R. G., & Posavac, E. J. (1982). Rehabilitation program evaluation using a revised level of rehabilitation scale (LORS–II). *Archives of Physical Medicine and Rehabilitation, 63,* 367–370.

Carlsson, A. M. (1983). Assessment of chronic pain. I. Aspects of the reliability and validity of the Visual Analogue Scale. *Pain, 16*, 87–101. doi:10.1016/0304-3959(83)90088-X

Carr, J. H., Shepherd, R. B., Nordholm, L., & Lynne, D. (1985). Investigation of a new motor assessment scale for stroke patients. *Physical Therapy, 65,*175–178.

Cattell, J. M. (1890). Mental tests and measurements. *Mind, 15*, 373–381.

Cattell, R. B. (1950). *Culture Fair Intelligence Test.* Champaign, IL: Institute for Personality and Ability Testing.

Cattell, R. B. (1963). Theory of fluid and crystallized intelligence: A critical experiment. *Journal of Educational Psychology, 54*, 615–618.

Cattell, R. B., Cattell, A. K., & Cattell, H. E. P. (1993). *Sixteen Personality Factor Questionnaire* (5th ed.). San Antonio, TX: Pearson/Psych Corp.

Centers for Disease Control and Prevention. (2008, September). *HIV incidence. Statistics and incidents.* Retrieved from http://www.cdc.gov/hiv/topics/surveillance/incidence.htm

Centers for Disease Control and Prevention. (2008, October). *New estimates of U.S. HIV prevalence, 2006. CDC HIV/AIDS facts.* Retrieved from http://www.cdc.gov/hiv/topics/surveillance/resources/factsheets/pdf/prevalence.pdf

Centers for Disease Control and Prevention. National Center for Health Statistics. (2010). *Vital and Health Statistics Series.* Retrieved from http://www.cdc.gov/nchs/products/series.htm#

Centers for Disease Control and Prevention. (2010, May). Deaths: Final data for 2007. *National vital statistics report, 58*(19). Retrieved from http://www.cdc.gov/nchs/data/nvsr/nvsr58/nvsr58_19.pdf

Centers for Disease Control and Prevention (CDC), National Center for Health Statistics. (2010, July 9). Table I: Provisional cases of infrequently reported notifiable diseases (<1,000 cases reported during the preceding year)—United States, week ending July 3, 2010 (26th week). *Morbidity and Mortality Weekly Report, 59*(26), 820–833. Retrieved from http://www.cdc.gov/mmwr/preview/mmwrhtml/mm5926md.htm?s_cid=mm5926md_w#ab1

Chan, A. S., Tsang, H. W., & Li, S. M. (2009). Case report of integrated supported employment for a person with severe mental illness. *American Journal of Occupational Therapy, 63*, 238–244.

Cheng, T. C. E. (1993). Operations research and high education administration. *Journal of Educational Administration, 31*, 77–99.

Chern, J., Kielhofner, G., de las Heras, C., & Magalhaes, L. (1996). The Volitional Questionnaire: Psychometric development and practical use. *American Journal of Occupational Therapy 50*, 516–525.

Childs, J. D., Piva, S., R., & Fritz, J. M. (2005). Responsiveness of the numeric pain rating scale in patients with low back pain. *Spine, 30*, 1331–1334. doi: 10.1097/01.brs.0000164099.92112.29

Chiu, T., & Oliver, R. (2006). Factor analysis and construct validity of the SAFER-HOME. *OTJR: Occupational Participation and Health, 26*(4). Retrieved from http://www.otjronline.com/view.asp?rID=18612

Chiu, T., Oliver, R., Marshall, L., & Letts, L. (2001). *Safety Assessment of Functional and the Environment of Rehabilitation (SAFER) tool manual.* Toronto, Ontario, Canada: COTA Comprehensive Rehabilitation and Mental Health Services.

Church, J. (Ed.). (1966). *Three babies: Biographies of cognitive development.* New York: Crown Publishing House/Random House.

Cinahl Information Systems. (1997). *Cumulative index to nursing and allied health (CINAHL) database.* Retrieved from http://www.biomedsearch.lib.umn.edu/ovidweb/fldguide/nursing.htm

Clandinin, D. J., & Connelly, F. M. (1994). Personal experience methods. In N. K. Denzin & Y. S. Lincoln (Eds.), *Handbook of qualitative research* (pp. 413–427). Thousand Oaks, CA: Sage.

Clark, E. N. (1999). Build a city: A projective task concept. In B. J. Hemphill-Pearson (Ed.), *Assessments in occupational therapy mental health: An integrative approach* (pp. 155–170). Thorofare, NJ: SLACK.

Clark, F., Azen, S. P., Zemke, R., Jackson, J., Carlson, M., Mandel, D. ... Lipson, L. (1997). Occupational therapy for independent-living older adults. A randomized controlled trial. *The Journal of the American Medical Association, 278,* 1321–1326.

Clark, J., Koch, B. A., & Nichols, R. C. (1965a). A factor analytically derived scale: For rating psychiatric patients in occupational therapy. *American Journal of Occupational Therapy, 19,* 14–18.

Clark, J., Koch, B. A., & Nichols, R. C. (1965b). A factor analytically derived scale: For rating psychiatric patients in occupational therapy. In B. J. Hemphill, 1988, *Mental health assessment in occupational therapy: An integrative approach to the evaluative process* (pp. 264–268). Thorofare, NJ: SLACK.

Clarke, G. N., Rohde, P., Lewinsohn, P. M., Hops, H., & Seeley, J. R. (1999). Cognitive-behavioral treatment of adolescent depression: Efficacy of acute group treatment and booster sessions. *Journal of the American Academy of Child and Adolescent Psychiatry, 38,* 272–279.

Clemson, L., Bundy, A., Unsworth, C., & Fiatarone Singh, M. (2008). *Assessment of Living Skills and Resources–Revised 2* (ALSAR-R2). Sydney, Australia: University of Sydney. Retrieved from http://sydney.edu.au/health_sciences/ageing_work_health/docs/Clemson_ALSAR.pdf

Clifford, C. (1990). *Nursing and health care research: A skills-based introduction* (2nd ed.). London: Prentice Hall.

The Cochrane Library. (2010a). *About the Cochrane library.* New York: Wiley. Retrieved from http://www.thecochranelibrary.com/view/0/AboutTheCochraneLibrary.html

The Cochrane Library. (2010b). *About Cochrane systematic reviews and protocols.* New York: Wiley. Retrieved from http://www.thecochranelibrary.com/view/0/AboutCochraneSystematicReviews.html

Cohen, J. (1960). A coefficient of agreement for nominal scales. *Educational and Psychological Measurement, 20,* 37–46.

Cohen, J. (1977). *Statistical power analysis for the behavioral sciences* (Rev. ed.). New York: Academic Press.

Cohen, J. (1988). *Statistical power analysis for the behavioral sciences* (2nd ed.). Hillsdale, NJ: Lawrence Earlbaum Associates.

Colarusso, R. P., & Hammill, D. D. (1996). *Motor-Free Visual Perception Test-Revised* (MFVPT-R). Novato, CA: Academic Therapy Publications.

Colarusso, R. P., & Hammill, D. D. (2002). *Motor-Free Visual Perceptual Test–3* (MFVPT-3; 3rd ed.). Ann Arbor: Academic Therapy Publications.

Coles, R. (1967). *Children of crisis.* Boston: Little, Brown.

Collen, F. M., Wade, D. T., Robb, G. F., & Bradshaw, C. M. (1991). The Rivermead Mobility Index: A further development of the Rivermead Motor Assessment. *International Disability Studies, 13,* 50–54.

Collin, C., Wade, D. T., Davies, S., & Horne, V. (1988). The Barthel ADL Index: A reliability study. *International Disabilities Studies, 10,* 61–63.

Conant, J. B. (1951). *Science and common sense.* New Haven, CT: Yale University Press.

Conners, C. K. (2008). *Conners-3.* (3rd ed.) North Tonawanda, NY: .Multi-Health Systems.

Copi, I. (1953). *Introduction to logic.* New York: Macmillan.

Cork, R. C., Isaac, I., Elsharydah, A., Saleemi, S., Zavisca, F., & Alexander, L. (2004). A comparison of the Verbal Rating Scale and the Visual Analog Scale for pain assessment. *The Internet Journal of Anesthesiology, 8*(1). Retrieved http://www.ispub.com/ostia/index.php?xmlFilePath=journals/ija/vol8n1/vrs.xml

Corrigan, J. D. (1989). Development of a scale for assessment of agitation following traumatic brain injury. *Journal of Clinical and Experimental Neuropsychology, 11,* 261–277.

Corrigan, J. D., & Deming, R. (1995). Psychometric characteristics of the community integration questionnaire: Replication and extension. *Journal of Head Trauma Rehabilitation, 10,* 41–53.

Cot, C., & Finch, E. (1991). Goal setting in physical therapy practise. *Physiotherapy Canada, 43,* 19–22.

Crawford, J. E., & Crawford, D. M. (1985). *The Crawford Small Parts Dexterity Test.* San Antonio, TX: Pearson/PsychCorp.

Creighton, C., Dijkers, M., Bennett, N., & Brown, K. (1995). Reasoning and the art of therapy for spinal cord injury. *American Journal of Occupational Therapy, 49,* 311–317.

Creswell, J. W. (1998). *Qualitative inquiry and research design: Choosing among five traditions.* Thousand Oaks, CA: Sage.

Crowther, J. G., & Whiddington, R. (1948). *Science at war.* New York: Philosophical Library.

Crump, A. (1997). Room to remember. *Elderly Care, 9,* 8–10.

Cullen, K. A., Hall, M. J., & Golosinskiy, A. (2009, January 28/2009, September 4). *Ambulatory surgery in the United States, 2006.* National Health Statistics Reports, #11. Hyattsville, MD: National Center for Health Statistics.

Cunningham, P. H., & Bartuska, T. (1989). The relationship between stress and leisure satisfaction among therapeutic recreation personnel. *Therapeutic Recreation Journal 23,* 65–70.

Cutler, S. K. (1992). *Executive functioning in middle school students who have learning disabilities.* Unpublished doctoral dissertation. University of New Mexico, Albuquerque.

Cutler, S. K., Keyes, D. W., & Urquhart, M. (1993). [Effects of teaching methods on understanding collaboration concepts.] Unpublished raw data.

## D

Dahlgren, A., Karlsson, A-K., Lundgren, Nilsson Å., Fridén, J., & Claesson, L. (2007). Activity performance and upper extremity function in cervical spinal cord injury patients according to the Klein-Bell ADL Scale. *Spinal Cord, 45,* 475–484.

Daniels, L., Williams, M., & Worthingham, C. (1956). *Muscle testing: Techniques of manual examination* (2nd ed.). Philadelphia: W. B. Saunders.

Daniels, L., & Worthingham, C. (1986). *Muscle testing: Techniques of manual examination* (5th ed.). Philadelphia: W. B. Saunders.

Das, J. P., Kirby, J., & Jarman, R. (1975). An alternative model for cognitive abilities. *Psychological Bulletin, 82,* 87–103.

Davis, F. B. (Chair). (1974). *Standards for education and psychological tests.* Prepared by a joint committee of the American Psychological Association, American Educational Research Association, and National Council on Measurement in Education. Washington, DC: American Psychological Association.

Dawber, T. R., & Kannel, W. B. (1958). An epidemiologic study of heart disease: The Framingham study. *Nutrional Review, 16,* 1–4.

Dawber, T. R., Meaders, G. F., & Moore, F. E. (1951). Epidemiological approaches to heart disease: The Framingham study. *American Journal of Public Health, 41,* 279–286.

Dean, C., & Gadd, E. M. (1990). Home treatment for acute psychiatric illness. *British Medical Journal, 302,* 1021–1023.

Dean, R. S., & Woodcock, R. S. (2003). *Dean-Woodcock Sensory-Motor Battery.* Itasca, IL: Riverside.

de Esquirol, J.-É.-D. (1838). *Des Maladies Mentales* [A treatise on insanity]. Reimpression de l'Edition de 1838 (Broché) (Auteur). Paris: Bailliere. Retrieved from http://books.google.com/books/about/Des_maladies_mentales_consider%C3%A9es_sous.html?id=CuvjtGaG0DcC

Defense Advanced Research Projects Agency (DARPA). (2008, February). *Fact sheet.* Washington, DC: Defense Advanced Research Projects Agency. Retrieved from http://www.darpa.mil/Docs/prosthetics_f_s3_200807180945042.pdf

DeGangi, R. A., & Berk, G. A. (1983). *DeGangi-Berk Test of Sensory Integration.* Los Angeles: Western Psychological Services.

de Jong, G. M., Timmerman, I. G., & Emmelkamp, P. M. (1996). The Survey of Recent Life Experiences: A psychometric evaluation. *Journal of Behavioral Medicine, 19*, 529–542.

Delaney-Black, V., Covington, C., Templin, T., Ager, J., Martier, S., Compton, S., & Sokol, R. (1998). Prenatal coke: What's behind the smoke? Prenatal cocaine/alcohol exposure and school-age outcomes: The SCHOO-BE experience. *Annals of the New York Academy of Science, 846*, 277–288.

de las Heras, C. G., Geist, R., Kielhofner, G., & Li, Y. (2007). The Volitional Questionnaire (VQ; version 4.1). Available from Moho Clearing House. Retrieved from http://www.moho.uic.edu/assess/vq.html

Delis, D., Kaplan, E., & Kramer, J. H. (2001). *Delis–Kaplan executive functioning system: Examiner's manual* (D-KEFS). San Antonio, TX: Pearson/PsychCorp.

DeMatteo, C., Law, M., Russell, D., Pollock, N., Rosenbaum, P., & Walter S. (1992). *QUEST: Quality of Upper Extremity Skills Test manual*. Available from *CanChild* Center for Childhood Disability Research IAHS Bldg, Room 408, McMaster University, 1400 Main Street, West, Hamilton, Ontario, Canada, l8S 1c7. Retrieved from http://www.canchild.ca/en/measures/resources/1992_quest_manual.pdf

DeMatteo, C., Law, M., Russell, D., Pollock, N., Rosenbaum, P., & Walter, S. (1993). The reliability and validity of Quality of Upper Extremity Skills Test. *Physical and Occupational Therapy in Pediatrics 13(2)*, 1–18.

Deno, S. L. (1985). Curriculum-based assessment: The emerging alternative. *Exceptional Children, 52*, 219–232.

Denzin, N. K., & Lincoln, Y. S. (Eds.). (1994a). *Handbook of qualitative research*. Thousand Oaks, CA: Sage.

Denzin, N. K., & Lincoln, Y. S. (1994b). Introduction: Entering the field of qualitative research. In N. K. Denzin & Y. S. Lincoln (Eds.), *Handbook of qualitative research* (pp. 1–17). Thousand Oaks, CA: Sage.

Dewey, J. (1933). *How we think*. Boston: D. C. Heath.

Dewey, J. (1964). *John Dewey on education: Selected writings*. Chicago: University of Chicago.

Dickerson, A. E. (1999). The Role Checklist. In B. Hemphill-Pearson (Ed.), *Assessments in occupational therapy mental health: An integrative approach* (pp. 175–182). Thorofare, NJ: SLACK.

Dickerson, A. E. (2008). The Role Checklist. In B. J. Hemphill-Pearson, Ed., 2008, *Assessments in occupational therapy mental health: An integrative approach* (2nd ed., pp. 252–258, 440–450). Thorofare, NJ: SLACK.

Dickinson, D., Tenhula, W., Morris, S., Brown, C., Peer, J., Spencer, K., ... Bellack, A.S. (2010). A randomized, controlled trial of computer-assisted cognitive remediation for schizophrenia. *American Journal of Psychiatry, 167*, 170–180.

Dittmar, S. S., & Gresham, G. E. (2005). *Functional assessment and outcome measures for the rehabilitation health professional*. Austin, TX: Pro-Ed.

Doarn, C. R., McVeigh, F., & Poropatich, R. (2010). Innovative new technologies to identify and treat traumatic brain injuries: Crossover technologies and approaches between military and civilian applications. *Telemedicine Journal and e-Health,16*, 73–81.

Domínguez-Gerpe, L., & Araújo-Vilar, D. (2008). Prematurely aged children: Molecular alterations leading to Hutchinson-Gilford progeria and Werner syndromes. *Current Ageing Science, 1*, 202–212.

Donaldson, S. W., Wagner, C. C., & Gresham, G. E. (1973). Unified ADL evaluation form. *Archives of Physical Medicine and Rehabilitation, 54,*175–179, 185.

Downer, A. H. (1970). *Physical therapy techniques*. Springfield, IL: Charles C. Thomas.

Doyne, E. J., Chambless, D. L., & Beutler, L. E. (1983). Aerobic exercise as a treatment for depression in women. *Behavior Therapy, 14*, 434–440.

Doyne, E. J., Ossip-Klein, D. J., Bowman, E. D., Osborn, D. M., McDougall-Wilson, I. B., & Neimeyer, R. A. (1987). Running versus weight lifting in the treatment of depression. *Journal of Consulting Clinical Psychology, 55,* 748–754.

Duke University Center for the Study of Aging and Human Development. (1978). *Functional assessment: The OARS methodology.* Durham, NC: Duke University.

Dukes, W. F. (1965). *N* = 1. *Psychological Bulletin, 64,* 73–79.

Dunn, L. M. (1968). Special education for the mildly retarded—Is much of it justifiable? *Exceptional Children, 35,* 5–22.

Dunn, W. (1990). A comparison of service provision models in school-based occupational therapy services: A pilot study. *Occupational Therapy Journal of Research, 10,* 300–320.

Dworkin, R. H., Turk, D. C., Revicki, D. A., Harding, G., Coyne, K. S., Peirce-Sandner, S., ... Melzack, R. (2009). Development and initial validation of an expanded and revised version of the Sort Form McGill Pain Questionnaire (SF-MPQ-2). *Pain, 144,* 35–42. Epub 2009 Apr 7.

**E**

Earhart, C. A., & Allen, C. A. (1988). *Cognitive disabilities: Expanded activity analysis.* Los Angeles County: University of Southern California Medical Center.

Easton, D. (1961). *A framework for political analysis.* Englewood Cliffs, NJ: Prentice-Hall.

Ebbinghaus, H. (1885/1913). *Memory: A contribution to experimental psychology.* (H. A. Ruger & C. E. Bussenius, Trans.). New York: Teachers College, Columbia University. Retrieved from http://psy.ed.asu.edu/~classics/Ebbinghaus/index.htm

Edgerton, R. B., & Langness, L. L. (1978). Observing mentally retarded persons in community settings: An anthropological perspective. In G. P. Sackett (Ed.), *Observing behavior. Theory and applications in mental retardation* (pp. 335–348). Baltimore: University Park Press.

Education for All Handicapped Children Act of 1974 [EAHCA; Pub. L. 94–142] U.S.C., Title 20, Sections 1400 et seq. (1975).

Education for All Handicapped Children Act of 1986 [Pub. L. 101–476] U.S.C., 1988, Title 20, Sections 1400 et seq. (1987).

Edwards, D. R., & Bristol, M. M. (1991). Autism: Early identification and management in family practice. *AFP, 44,* 1755–1764.

Ellis, H. (2001). *History of surgery.* Cambridge, UK: Cambridge University Press.

Emerson, H., Cook, J., Polatajko, H., & Segal, R. (1998). Enjoyment experiences as described by persons with schizophrenia: A qualitative study. *Canadian Journal of Occupational Therapy, 65,*183–192.

*Encyclopedia of Associations: International Organizations: An Associations Unlimited Reference* (Ed. 50; Gale Group, 2011) http://www.gale.cengage.com/servlet/ItemDetailServlet?region=9&imprint=000&cf=p&titleCode=EA4&type=3&dc=null&dewey=null&id=247322

Englehart, M. D. (1972). *Methods of educational research.* Chicago: Rand McNally.

Epps, S., & Tindall, G. (1987). The effectiveness of differential programming in serving students with mild handicaps: Placement options and instructional programming. In M. C. Wang, M. C. Reynolds, & H. J. Walberg (Eds.), *Handbook of special education: Research and practice.* (Vol. 1, pp. 213–248). Oxford, England: Pergamon Press.

Erikson, E. H. (1950). *Childhood and society.* New York: Norton.

Erhardt, R. P. (1994). *Erhardt Developmental Prehension Assessment* (3rd ed). Maplewood, MN: Erhardt Developmental Products.

Ernst, A. A., Houry, D., & Weiss, S. J. (1997). Research funding in the four major emergency medicine journals. *American Journal of Emergency Medicine, 15,* 268–270.

**F**

Fadely, J. L., & Hosler, V. N. (1983). *Case studies in left and right hemispheric functioning.* Springfield, IL: Thomas.

Fairbank, J. C. T., Couper, J., Davies., J. B., & O'Brien, J. B. (1980). The Oswestry low back pain questionnaire. *Physiotherapy, 66*, 271–273.

Fairbank, J. C. T., & Pynsent, P. B. (2000a). The Oswestry disability index. *Spine, 25*, 2940–2953.

Fairbank, J. C. T., & Pynsent, P. B. (2000b). The Oswestry disability questionnaire. From J. C. T. Fairbank and P. B. Pynsent, The Oswestry disability index. *Spine, 25*, 2940–2953. Retrieved from http://www.tac.vic.gov.au/upload/Oswestry.pdf

Falk-Ross, F. (1996, Feb.). *Classroom-based language remediation programs: Roles, routines, and reflections.* Paper presented at the 36th Annual Convention of the Illinois Speech-Language-Hearing Association. (ERIC Document Reproduction Service No. ED 417–539)

Family Center on Technology and Disability (FCTD). (2010). *FCTD Fact Sheets: Assistive Technology Laws.* Washington, DC: U. S. Office of Special Education and Rehabilitation (OCERS). Retrieved from http://www.fctd.info/resources/ATlaws_print.pdf

FedStats. (2007). *About FedStats.* Retrieved from http://www.fedstats.gov/aboutfedstats.html

Feigin, G., An, C., Connors, D., & Crawford, I. (1996, April). Shape up, ship out. *ORMS Today, 23*(2), 1–7. Retrieved from http://www.lionhrtpub.com/orms/orms–4–96/ibm.html

Ferguson, P. M., Ferguson, D. L., & Taylor, S. J. (Eds.). (1992). *Interpreting disability. A qualitative reader.* New York: Teachers College Press.

Festinger, L., & Katz, O. (1953). *Research methods in the behavioral sciences.* New York: Holt, Rinehart and Winston.

Finch, E., Brooks, D., Stratford, P., & Mayo, N. (2002). *Physical rehabilitation outcome measures* (2nd ed.; PROM-II with CD-ROM). Hamilton, ON: BC Decker Inc.

Finley, T. W. (1989). Research in physical medicine and rehabilitation: II. The conceptual review of the literature or how to read more articles than you ever want to see in your entire life.

*American Journal of Physical Medicine & Rehabilitation, 68*, 97–102.

Fischer, J., & Corcoran, K. (2007). *Measures for clinical practice: A sourcebook. Volume 1: Couples, family and children* (4th ed.). New York: Oxford University Press.

Fisher, A. (1994). *Assessment of motor and process skills* (AMPS). Unpublished manual. (Available from A. Fisher, Department of Occupational Therapy, University of Illinois at Chicago)

Fisher, B., Bhavnani, V., & Winfield, M. (2009). How patients use access to their full health records: A qualitative study of patients in general practice. *Journal of the Royal Society of Medicine, 102*, 539–544. doi: 10.1258/jrsm.2009.090328

Fitzgerald, M. H., Mullavey-O'Byrne, C., & Clemson, L. (1997). Cultural issues from practice. *Australian Occupational Therapy Journal, 44*, 1–21. doi:10.1111/j.1440-1630.1997.tb00749.x

Flegal, K. M., Carroll, M. D., Ogden, C. L., & Curtin, L. R. (2010). Prevalence and trends in obesity among U.S. adults, 1999–2008. *JAMA: The Journal of the American Medical Association, 303*, 235–241. doi:10.1001/jama.2009.2014

Fleischman, D. A., & Gabriele, J. D. (1998). Repetition priming in normal aging and Alzheimer's disease: A review of findings and theories. *Psychology and Aging, 13*, 88–119.

Flexner, A. (1910). *Medical education in the United States and Canada: A report to the Carnegie Foundation for the Advancement of Teaching* (Bulletin No. 4). New York City: Carnegie Foundation.

Flinn, N., Smith, J., Tripp, C., & White, M. (2009). Effects of robotic-aided rehabilitation on recovery of upper extremity function in chronic stroke: A single case study. *Occupational Therapy International, 16*, 232–243.

Flood, J. F., & Morley, J. E. (1998). Learning and memory in the SAMP8 mouse. *Neuroscience & Biobehavioral Reviews, 22*, 1–20.

Folio, M. R., & Fewell, R. R. (2000). *Peabody Developmental Motor Scales–2* (2nd ed.; PDMS-2). Austin, TX: Pro-Ed.

Folstein, M. F., & Folstein, S. E. (2010). *Mini-Mental® State Examination, 2nd Edition™* (MMSE®–2™). Lutz, FL: PAR.

Folstein, M. F., Folstein, S. E., White, T., & Messer, M. A. (2010). *Mini-Mental® State Examination: User's manual* (MMSE®–2™; 2nd ed.). Lutz, FL: PAR.

Fontana, A., & Frey, J. H. (1994). Interviewing: The art of science. In N. K. Denzin & Y. S. Lincoln (Eds.), *Handbook of qualitative research* (pp. 361–376). Thousand Oaks, CA: Sage.

Forness, S. R., & Kavale, K. A. (1984). Education of the mentally retarded: A note on policy. *Education and Training of the Mentally Retarded, 19,* 239–245.

Fraenkel, J. R., & Wallen, N. E. (1990). *How to design and evaluate research in education.* New York: McGraw.

Fraga, S. (2010). TABACOPanaceia no Século XVI e Patologia no Século XX [Tobacco: panacea in the XVI century and pathology in the XX century]. [Article in Portuguese]. *Acta Médica Portuguesa, 23,* 243–246. Retrieved from http://www.ncbi.nlm.nih.gov/pubmed/20470472

Frank, G. (1996). Life histories in occupational therapy clinical practice. *American Journal of Occupational Therapy, 50,* 251–264.

Frank, G., Bernardo, C. S., Tropper, S., Noguchi, F., Lipman, C., Maulhardt, B., & Weitze, L. (1997). Jewish spirituality through actions in time: Daily occupations of young Orthodox Jewish couples in Los Angeles. *American Journal of Occupational Therapy, 51,* 199–206.

Frankenburg, W. K., Dodds, J. B., Archer, P., Shapiro, H., & Bresnick, B. (1990). *Denver Developmental Screening Test—II.* Denver: Denver Developmental Materials.

Frankenburg, W. K., Dodds, J. B., Archer, P., Shapiro, H., Bresnick, B. (1992). The Denver II: A Major Revision and Restandardization of the Denver Developmental Screening Test. *Pediatrics, 89,* 91–97.

Frederick, M. (1928). *Thrasher: The gang: A study of 1,313 gangs in Chicago.* Chicago: University of Chicago Press.

Freeman, A. R., MacKinnon, J. R., & Miller, L. T. (2004). Assistive technology and handwriting problems: What do occupational therapists recommend? *Canadian Journal of Occupational Therapy. Revue Canadienne D'ergothérapie, 71,* 150–160.

French, S. (Ed.). (1994). *On equal terms. Working with disabled people.* Oxford: Butterworth/ Heinemann.

Freud, S., & Breuer, J. (1895/1955). *Studies in hysteria* (J. Stratchey, Trans.). London: The Hogarth Press. (Original work published 1895)

Frey, J. J., & Fontana, A. (1995). *The group interview.* Newbury Park, CA: Sage.

Frost, M. H., Reeve, B. B., Liepa, A. M., Stauffer, J. W., Hays, R. D., & Mayo/FDA Patient-Reported Outcomes Consensus Meeting Group. (2007). What is sufficient evidence for the reliability and validity of patient-reported outcome measures? *Value in Health: The Journal for the International Society for Pharmacoeconomics and Outcomes Research, 10*(Suppl. 2), S94–S105.

Fry, P. S. (1984). Development of a geriatric scale of hopelessness: Implications for counseling and intervention with the depressed elderly. *Journal of Counseling Psychology, 31,* 322–331.

Fuchs, D., Fuchs, L. S., & Fernstrom, P. (1993). A conservative approach to special education reform: Mainstreaming through transenvironmental programming and curriculum-based measurement. *American Education Research Journal, 30,* 149–177.

Fugl-Meyer, A. R., Jääskö, L., Leyman, I., Olsson, S., & Steglind, S. (1975). The poststroke hémiplégie patient I. A method for evaluation of physical performance. *Scandinavian Journal of Rehabilitation Medicine, 7,* 13–31.

Fukutani, Y., Sasaki, K., Mukai, M., Matsubara, R, Isaki, K., & Cairns, N. J. (1997). Neurons and extracellular neurofibrillary tangles in the hippocampal subdivisions in early-on-set familial Alzheimer's disease: A case study. *Psychiatry & Clinical Neurosciences, 51,* 227–231.

# G

Gagné, D. E. (2003). The effects of collaborative goal-focused occupational therapy on self-care skills: A pilot study. *American Journal of Occupational Therapy, 57*, 215–219.

Gale Group. (2011). *Encyclopedia of associations: International organizations. An associations unlimited reference* (50th ed.). Detroit: Gale Group.

Galen, C. (1971). *On the natural faculties.* In W. P. D. Wightman (Ed.), *The emergence of scientific medicine.* Edinburgh: Oliver and Boyd. (Original work published ca. 192 AD)

Galton, F. (1865). Hereditary talent and character. *Macmillan's Magazine, 12*, 157–166, 318–327. Retrieved from http://psychclassics.yorku.ca/Galton/talent.htm

Galton, F. (1883/1907/1973). *Inquiries into human faculty and its development.* New York: AMS Press.

Gardner, H. (1983). *Frames of mind: Theories of multiple intelligences.* New York: Basic Books.

Gardner, H. (1999) *Intelligence reframed. Multiple intelligences for the 21st century*, New York: Basic Books.

Gee, W. (1950). *Social science research methods.* New York: Appleton-Century-Crofts.

Geist, H. (1988). *Geist Picture Interest Inventory* (Rev.). Torrance, CA: Western Psychological Services.

Geslani, D. M. (2005). Mild cognitive impairment: An operational definition and its conversion rate to Alzheimer's disease. *Dementia & Geriatric Cognitive Disorders, 19*, 383–389.

George, S., & Crotty, M. (2010). Establishing criterion validity of the useful field of view assessment and stroke drivers' screening assessment; Comparison to the result of on-road assessment. *American Journal of Occupational Therapy, 64,*114–122. doi:10.5014/ajot.64.1.114

Gesell, A. (1929). *Infancy and human growth.* NY: Macmillan.

Gesell, A., & Thompson, H. (1923). *Infant behavior: Its genesis and growth.* New York: McGraw-Hill.

Gewurtz, R., Stergiou-Kita, M., Shaw, L., Kirsh, B., & Rappolt, S. (2008). Qualitative meta-synthesis: Reflections on the utility and challenges in occupational therapy. *Canadian Journal of Occupational Therapy, 75*, 301–308.

Gilliam, J., & Barstow, I. K. (1997). Joint range of motion. In J. Van Deusen & D. Brunt (Eds.), *Assessment in occupational therapy and physical therapy* (pp. 49–77). Philadelphia: W. B. Saunders.

Gilson, B. S., Gilson, J. S., Bergner, M., Bobbitt, R. A., Kressel, S., Pollard, W. E., & Vesselago, M. (1975). The Sickness Impact Profile: Development of an outcome measure of health care. *American Journal of Public Health, 65,* 1304–1310.

Gladstone, D. J., Danells, C. J., & Black, S. E. (2002). The Fugl-Meyer assessment of motor recovery after stroke: A critical review of its measurement properties. *Neurorehabilitation and Neural Repair, 16,* 232–240. doi:10.1177/154596802401105171

Glaser, B. G., & Strauss, A. L. (1967). *The discovery of grounded theory: Strategies for qualitative research.* Chicago: Aldine.

Glaser, R. (1963). Instructional technology and the measurement of learning outcomes. *American Psychologist, 18,* 510–522.

Glasser, O. (1933). *Conrad Roentgen and the early history of the Roentgen rays.* London: John Bale Sons and Danielsson.

Gleason, J. J. (1990). Meaning of play: Interpreting patterns in behavior of persons with severe developmental disabilities. *Anthropology and Education Quarterly, 21,* 59–77.

Glesne, C., & Peshkin, A. (1992). *Becoming qualitative researchers: An introduction.* New York: Longman.

Glutting, J. J., & Wilkinson, G. (2003). *Wide Range Interest and Occupation Test—Second Edition* (WRIOT-2). San Antonio, TX: Pearson Assessments/PsychCorp.

Goddard, H. H. (1920). *Human efficiency and levels of intelligence.* Princeton, NJ: Princeton University Press.

Goffman, E. (1961). *Asylums: Essays on the social situation of mental patients and other inmates.* Garden City, NJ: Anchor Books.

Gold, R. L. (1958). Roles in sociological field observations. *Social Forces, 36,* 217–223.

Goldberg, B., Brintnell, E. S., & Goldberg, J. (2002). The relationship between engagement in meaningful activities and quality of life in persons disabled by mental illness *Occupational Therapy in Mental Health, 18*(2), 17–44. doi: 10.1300/J004v18n02_03

Goldberg, R. T. (1974). Rehabilitation research, new directions. *Journal of Rehabilitation, 40*(3), 12–14.

Golden, C. J., Purisch, A. D., & Hammeke, T. A. (1985). *Luria–Nebraska Neuropsychological Battery: Forms I and II* (Manual). Los Angeles: Western Psychological Services.

Goleman, D. (1995). *Emotional intelligence.* New York: Bantam.

Goleman, D. (2010). *Daniel Goleman: Emotional intelligence.* (Blog). Retrieved from http://danielgoleman.info/topics/emotional-intelligence/

Good-Ellis, M. A. (1999). The Role Activity Performance Scale. In B. Hemphill-Pearson (Ed.), *Assessments in occupational therapy mental health: An integrative approach* (pp. 206–226). Thorofare, NJ: SLACK.

Good-Ellis, M. A., Fine, S. B., Spencer, J. H., & Divittis, A. (1987). Developing a role activity performance scale. *American Journal of Occupational Therapy, 41,* 232–241.

Google Scholar. (2010). *About Google scholar.* Retrieved from http://scholar.google.com/intl/en/scholar/about.html

Gordon, E. E. (1968). A view of the target population. In A. J. Tannenbaum (Ed.), *Special education programs for disadvantaged children and youth* (pp. 5–18). Washington, DC: The Council for Exceptional Children.

Gould, J., & Kolb, J. G. (Eds.). (1964). *A dictionary of the social sciences.* (Compiled under the auspices of the United Nations Educational, Scientific and Cultural Organizations.) New York: The Free Press.

Gould, S. J. (1996). *The mismeasure of man* (Rev. ed.). New York: Norton.

Gracely, R. H., & Kwilosz, D. M. (1988). The Descriptor Differential Scale: Applying psychophysical principles to clinical pain assessment. *Pain, 35,* 279–288.

Gracely, R. H., McGrath, P., & Dubner, R. (1978). Validity and sensitivity of ratio scales of sensory and affective verbal pain descriptors: Manipulation of affect by diazepam. *Pain, 5,* 19–29.

Graf, C. (2007). The Lawton Instrumental Activities of Daily Living (IADL) Scale. *Annals of Long Term Care: Clinical Care and Aging, 15*(7). Retrieved from http://www.annalsoflongtermcare.com/article/745

Grandin, T. (2008). *The way I see it: A personal look at autism and Asperser's.* Arlington, TX: Future Horizons.

Granger, C. V., & Greer, D. S. (1976). Functional status measurement and medical rehabilitation outcomes. *Archives of Physical Medicine and Rehabilitation. 57,* 103–109.

Granger, C. V., Hamilton, B. B., Keith, R. A., Zielesky, M., & Sherwin, F. S. (1986). Advances in functional assessment for medical rehabilitation. *Topics in Geriatric Rehabilitation, 1,* 59–74.

Granger, C. V., Markello, S., Graham, J., Deutsch, A., Reistetter, T., & Ottenbacher, K. (2010). The uniform data system for medical rehabilitation: Report of patients with traumatic brain injury discharged from rehabilitation programs in 2000–2007. *American Journal of Physical Medicine & Rehabilitation, 89,* 265–278.

Granger, C. V., Sherwood, C. C., & Greer, D. S. (1977). Functional status measures in a comprehensive stroke care program. *Archives of Physical Medicine and Rehabilitation, 58,* 555–561.

Granger, C. V., & Wright, B. (1993). Looking ahead to the use of functional assessment in ambulatory physiatric and primary care. *Physical Medicine and Rehabilitation Clinics of North America, 4*(3), 1–11.

Gravetter, F. J., & Wallnau, L. B. (1985). *Statistics for the behavioral sciences.* St. Paul, MN: West.

Greist, J. H., Klein, M. H., Eischens, R. R., Faris, J., Gurman, A. S., & Morgan, W. P. (1979). Running as treatment for depression. *Comprehensive Psychiatry, 20*, 41–54.

Gresham, G. E., Labi, M. L., Dittmar, S. S., Hicks, J. T., Joyce, S. Z., & Phillips-Stehlik, M. A. (1986). The Quadriplegia Index of Function (QIF): Sensitivity and reliability demonstrated in a study of thirty quadriplegic patients. *Paraplegia, 24*, 38–44.

Guba, E. G. (1990). Carrying on the dialog. In E. G. Guba (Ed.), *The paradigm dialog* (pp. 368–378). Newbury Park, CA: Sage.

Guilford, J. P. (1967). *The nature of human intelligence.* New York: McGraw-Hill.

## H

Haavardsholm, E. A., Kvien, T. K., Uhlig, T., Smedstad, L. M., & Guillemin, F. (2000). A comparison of agreement and sensitivity to change between AIMS2 and a short form of AIMS2 (AIMS2-SF) in more than 1,000 rheumatoid arthritis patients. *Journal of Rheumatology, 27*, 2810–2816.

Haeger, K. (1988). *The illustrated history of surgery.* London: Harold Starke.

Haertlein, C. L. (1999). The Milwaukee Evaluation of Daily Living Skills (MEDLS). In B. J. Hemphill-Pearson (Ed.), *Assessments in occupational therapy mental health: An integrative approach* (pp. 245–258). Thorofare, NJ: SLACK.

Hajat, S., Fitzpatrick, R., Morris, R., Reeves, B., Rigge, M., Williams, O., ... Gregg, P. (2002). Does waiting for total hip replacement matter? Prospective cohort study. *Journal of Health Services Research & Policy, 7*, 19–25.

Haley, S. M., Coster, W. J., Ludlow, L. H., Haltiwanger, J. T., & Andreilos, P. J. (1992). *Pediatric Evaluation of Disability Inventory* (PEDI). (Available from PEDI Research Group, Department of Rehabilitation Medicine, New England Medical Center Hospital, #75K/R, 750 Washington Street, Boston, MA 02111-2901)

Hall, E. T. (1966). *The hidden dimension.* New York: Doubleday.

Hallahan, D. P., & Kauffman, J. M. (1993). *Exceptional children: Introduction to special education* (6th ed.). Boston: Allyn and Bacon.

Halstead, L., & Hartley, R. B. (1975). Time Care Profile: An evaluation of a new method of assessing ADL dependence. *Archives of Physical Medicine and Rehabilitation, 56*, 110–115.

Hamilton, M. (1960). A rating scale for depression. *Journal of Neurology, Neurosurgery, and Psychiatry, 23*, 468–477.

Hammer, A. M. (2009). Effects of forced use on arm function in the subacute phase after stroke: A randomized, clinical pilot study... including commentary by J. H. Cauraugh, J. J. Summers and J. Charles with authors' response. *Physical Therapy, 89*, 526–545.

Harper, D. (1989). Visual sociology: Expanding sociological vision. In G. Blank, et al. (Eds.), *New technology in sociology: Practical applications in research and work* (pp. 81–97). New Brunswick, NJ: Transaction Books.

Harvard Medical School. (1991). *Guidelines for investigators in scientific research.* (Available from the Office for Research Issues, Harvard Medical School, 25 Shattuck Street, Boston, MA 02115)

Harvard Medical School. (1996). *Guidelines for investigators in clinical research,* Retrieved from http://www.hms.harvard.edu/integrity/clinical.html

Harvey, W. (1938). *On the motion of the heart and blood in animals* (R. Willis, Trans.). In C. W. Eliot (Ed.), *The Harvard classics scientific papers.* New York: P. E. Collier and Sons. (Original work published 1628).

Harvey, W. (1952). An anatomical disquisition on the motion of the heart and blood in animals. In R. M. Hutchins (Ed.), & R. Willis (Trans.), *Great books of the western world* (Vol. 28, pp. 267–304). Chicago: Encyclopedia Britannica. (Original work published 1628.)

Harvey, R. F., & Jellinek, H. M. (1981). Functional performance assessment: A program approach. *Archives of Physical Medicine and Rehabilitation, 62*, 456–460.

Hasselkus, B. R. (2003). The voices of qualitative researchers: Sharing the conversation. *American Journal of Occupational Therapy, 57,* 7–8.

Hasselkus, B. R., & Dickie, V. A. (1993). Doing occupational therapy: Dimensions of satisfaction and dissatisfaction. *American Journal of Occupational Therapy, 48,* 145–154.

Hathaway, S., & McKinley, C. (1970). *Minnesota Multiphasic Personality Inventory.* Minneapolis, MI: National Computer Systems.

Havighurst, R. J. (1952). *Developmental tasks and education.* New York: Longmans, Green.

Haynes, M. C., & Jenkins, J. R. (1986). Reading instruction in special education resource room. *American Educational Research Journal, 23,* 161–190.

Health Outcomes Institute. (1995). *Health Status Questionnaire* (HSQ–12, version 2.0). San Antonio, TX: Pearson Assessment/PsychCorp.

Hébert, R., Carrier, R., & Bilodeau, A. (1988). The Functional Autonomy Measurement System (SMAF): Description and validation of an instrument for the measurement of handicaps. *Age and Ageing, 17,* 2933–3302.

Heisel, M. J., & Flett, G. L. (2005). A psychometric analysis of the Geriatric Hopelessness Scale (GHS): Towards improving assessment of the construct. *Journal of Affective Disorders, 87,* 211–220. doi:10.1016/j.jad.2005.03.016

Hemphill, B. J. (Ed.). (1988). *Mental health assessment in occupational therapy: An integrative approach to the evaluative process.* Thorofare, NJ: SLACK.

Hemphill-Pearson, B. J. (1999a). How to use the BH Battery. In B. J. Hemphill-Pearson (Ed.), *Assessments in occupational therapy mental health: An integrative approach* (pp. 140–155). Thorofare, NJ: SLACK.

Hemphill-Pearson, B. J. (Ed.). (1999b). *Assessments in occupational therapy mental health: An integrative approach.* Thorofare, NJ: SLACK.

Hemphill-Pearson, B. J. (Ed.). (2008). *Assessments in occupational therapy mental health: An integrative approach* (2nd ed.). Thorofare, NJ: SLACK.

Hemsworth, P. (1986). Effects of social environment on welfare status and sexual behaviour of female pigs. II. Effects of space allowance. *Applied Animal Behaviour Science, 16,* 259–267.

Henry, J. (1965). *Pathways to madness.* New York: Random House.

Hester, P. H. (1994, November). *A contextual analysis of classroom interaction at the university level: An operations research approach.* Paper presented at the Annual Meeting of the Mid–South Educational Research Association, Nashville, TN. (ERIC Document Reproduction Service Number ED 382 139)

Hewitt, N. G. (1997). Manipulating the environment—Intensive care versus specialist neurosurgical care. *Australasian Journal of Neuroscience, 10,* 10–12.

Higgs, J. (Ed.). (1997). *Qualitative research: Discourse on methodologies.* Sydney, Australia: Hampden.

Higgs, J. (Ed.). (1998). *Writing qualitative research.* Sydney, Australia: Hampden.

Hill, A. B. (1971). *Principles of medical statistics.* London: Lancet.

Hinshelwood, J. (1917). *Congenital word blindness.* London: Lewis.

Hinkle, D. E., Wiersma, W., & Jurs, S. G. (2003). *Applied statistics for the behavioral sciences* (5th ed.). Boston: Houghton Mifflin.

Hippocratic writings. (1952). *On the articulations.* In R. M. Hutchins (Ed.), & F. Adams (Trans.), *Great books for the western world* (Vol. 10, pp. 91–121). Chicago: Encyclopedia Britannica. (Original work published ca. 5th century, B.C.E.).

Hislop, H., & Montgomery, J. (2002). *Daniels and Worthingham's muscle testing: Techniques of manual examination* (7th ed.) Philadelphia: WB Saunders.

Hoaglin, C. C., Mosteller, F., & Tukey, J. N. (1991). *Fundamentals of exploratory analysis of variance.* New York: Wiley.

Holbrook, M., & Skilbeck, C. E. (1983). An activities index for use with stroke patients. *Age and Ageing 12,* 166–170.

Holland, J. L. (1994). The self-directed search: Professional users guide. Odessa FL: PAR.

Holm, M. B., & Rogers, J. C. (2008). Performance assessment of self-care skills. In B. Hemphill-Pearson (Ed.), *Assessments in occupational therapy mental health: An integrative approach: Version 3.1* (2nd ed., pp. 101–110). Thorofare, NJ: SLACK. (Available from Holm & Rogers at SPIC # 1237, 3811 O'Hara Street, Pittsburgh, PA 15213)

Holmberg, K., Rosen, D., & Holland, J. L. (1999). *The Leisure Activities Finder™* (LAF). Odessa, FL: PAR.

Holstein, J. A., & Gubrium, J. F. (1995). *The active interview.* Thousand Oaks, CA: Sage.

Hoppes, S. (1997). Can play increase standing tolerance? A pilot-study. *Physical and Occupational Therapy in Geriatrics, 15,* 65–73.

Horn, J. L. (1968). Organization of abilities and the development of intelligence. *Psychological Review, 75,* 242–259.

Howland, D. S., Trusko, S. P., Savage, M. J., Reaume, A. G., Lange, D. M., Hirsch, J. D., … Flood, D. G. (1998). Modulation of secreted beta-amyloid precursor protein and amyloid beta-peptide in brain by cholesterol. *Journal of Biological Chemistry, 273,* 16576–16582.

Huber, J. T., Boorkman, J. A., & Blackwell, J. (2008). *Introduction to reference sources in the health sciences* (5th ed.). New York: Neal-Schuman Publishers.

Huberman, A. M., & Miles, M. B. (1994). Data management and analysis methods. In N. K. Denzin & Y. S. Lincoln (Eds.), *Handbook of qualitative research* (pp. 428–444). Thousand Oaks, CA: Sage.

Huebner, R. A., Emery, L. J., & Shordike, A. (2002). The adolescent role assessment: Psychometric properties and theoretical usefulness. *American Journal of Occupational Therapy, 56,* 202–209.

Huezo, C. (1997). Factors to address when periodic abstinence is offered by multimethod family planning programs. *Advances in Contraception, 13,* 261–267.

Hunt, N., & Marshall, K. (1994). *Exceptional children and youth.* Geneva, IL: Houghton Mifflin.

## I

ICD Rehabilitation and Research Center, NY. (1977). *Micro Tower System of Vocational Evaluation.* New York, NY: Author. (Available from ICD Rehabilitation & Research Center, 340 East 24th St., New York, NY 10010)

Illingworth, W. H. (1910). *History of the education of the blind.* London: Marston.

Individuals with Disabilities Education Act Amendments of 1997 (IDEA; P.L. 105–17). 20 U.S.C. § 1400 *et seq.*

Individuals with Disabilities Education Improvement Act of 2004. (IDEIA; P.L. 108–446). 20 U.S.C. § 1400 *et seq.* Retrieved http://idea.ed.gov/download/statute.html

Internet Stroke Center. (1997–2011). *Stroke scales and clinical assessment tools: Stroke scales overview.* St. Louis, MO: Washington University. Retrieved from http://www.strokecenter.org/trials/scales/scales-overview.htm#l

Iverson, C. (Ed.). (1997). *American Medical Association manual of style: A guide for authors and editors* (8th ed.). Philadelphia: Lippincott, Williams and Wilkins.

Iverson, C. (1997). *Manual of style: A guide for authors and editors* (9th ed.). New York: Lippincott Williams & Wilkins.

## J

Jacob, T., & Shapira, A. (2010). Quality of life and health conditions reported from two post-polio clinics in Israel. *Journal of Rehabilitation Medicine, 42,* 377–379.

Jacobson, N. S., Dobson, K. S., Traux, P. A., Addis, M. E., Koerner, K., Gollan, J. K., … Prince, S. E. (1996). A component analysis of cognitive-behavioral treatment for depression. *Journal of Consulting and Clinical Psychology, 64,* 295–304.

Jahoda, M., Deutsch, M., & Cook, S. W. (1951). *Research methods in social relations.* New York: Dryden Press.

Jebsen, R. H., Taylor, N., Trieschmann, R. B., Trotter, M. J., & Howard, L. A. (1969). An objective and standardized test of hand function. *Archives of Physical Medicine and Rehabilitation, 50,* 311–319.

Jebsen, R. H., Trieschmann, R. B., Mikulic, M. A., Hartley, R. B., McMillan, J. A., & Snook, M.E. (1970). Measurement of time in a standardized test of patient mobility. *Archives of Physical Medicine & Rehabilitation, 51,*170–175.

Jensen, M. (1998). Play behaviour in dairy calves kept in pens: The effect of social contact and space allowance. *Applied Animal Behaviour Science, 56,* 97–108.

Jensen, M. P., Karoly, P., & Braver, S. (1986). The measurement of clinical pain intensity: A comparison of six methods. *Pain, 27,* 117–126.

Jensen, M. P., Karoly, P., & Harris, P. (1991). Assessment of the affective component of chronic pain: Development of the Pain Discomfort Scale. *Journal of Psychosomatic Research, 35,*149–154.

Jessor, R., Colby, A., & Shweder, R. A. (Eds.). (1996). *Ethnography and human development: Context and meaning in social inquiry.* Chicago: University of Chicago.

Jette, A. M. (1980). Functional Status Index: Reliability of a chronic disease evaluation instrument. *Archives of Physical Medicine and Rehabilitation, 61,* 395–401.

Jette, A. M. (1987). The Functional Status Index: Reliability and validity of a self-report functional disability measure. *Journal of Rheumatology: Supplemental*(Suppl. 15), 15–21.

Johnson, K. (1998). *Deinstitutionalising women: An ethnographic study of institutional closure.* Cambridge, England: Cambridge University Press.

Johnson, T. P., Vinnicombe, B. J., & Merrill, G. W. (1981).Independent living skills evaluation. *Occupational Therapy in Mental Health, 1*(2), 5–18. doi: 10.1300/J004v01n02_02

Jonsson, H. (1998). Ernst Westerlund—A Swedish doctor of occupation. *Occupational Therapy International 5*(2), 155–171.

Jung, B., & Tryssenaar, J. (1998). Supervising students: Exploring the experience through reflective journals. *Occupational Therapy International, 5,* 35–48.

Juul, D. (1981). Special education in Europe. In J. M. Kauffman & D. P. Hallahan (Eds.), *Handbook of special education.* Englewood Cliffs, NJ: Prentice Hall.

## K

Kalverboer, A. (1977). A measurement of play: Clinical applications. In B. Tizard & D. Harvey (Eds.), *Biology of play.* Philadelphia: Lippincott.

Kamhi, A., & Catts, H. (Eds.). (1998). *Language and reading disabilities.* Boston: Allyn & Bacon.

Kaplan, K., Mendelson, L. B., & Dubroff, M. P. (1983). The effect of a jogging program on psychiatric inpatients with symptoms of depression. *The Occupational Therapy Journal of Research, 3,* 173–175.

Katz, S., Downs, T. D., Cash, H .R., & Grotz, R. C. (1970). Progress in the development of the index of ADL. *The Gerontologist, 10,* 20–30.

Katz, S., Ford, R. Q., Moskowitz, R. W., Jackson, B. A., & Jaffe, M. W. (1963). Studies of illness in the aged, the index of ADL: A standardized measure of biological and psychosocial functions. *Journal of the American Medical Association, 185,* 914–918.

Kaufman, A. S., & Kaufman, N. L. (1993). *Kaufman Adolescent and Adult Intelligence Test.* Circle Pines, MN: American Guidance Service.

Kawaguchi, H., Murakami, B., & Kawai, M. (2010). Behavioral characteristics of children with high functioning pervasive developmental disorders during a game. *Journal of Epidemiology, 20*(Suppl. 2), S490–S497.

Keith, R. A. (1984). Functional assessment measures in medical rehabilitation: Current status. *Archives of Physical Medicine and Rehabilitation, 65,* 74–78.

Keith, R. A., Granger, C. V., Hamilton, B. B., & Sherwin, F. S. (1987). The Functional Independence Measure: A new tool for rehabilitation. *Advances in Clinical Rehabilitation, 1,* 6–18.

Kendall, F. P., McCreary, E. K., & Provance, P. G. (1993). *Muscle testing and function* (4th ed.). Baltimore: Williams and Wilkins.

Kendall, H. O., & Kendall, F. M. P. (1949). *Muscles, testing and function.* Baltimore: Williams and Wilkins.

Kenig, S. (1992). *Who plays? Who pays? Who cares? A case study in applied sociology, political economy and the community mental health centers movement.* Amityville, NY: Baywood.

Kerlinger, F. N. (1973). *Foundations of behavioral research* (2nd ed.). New York: Holt, Rinehart and Winston.

Kerlinger, F. N. (1986). *Foundations of behavioral research* (3rd ed.). New York: Holt, Rinehart, and Winston.

Key, G. (Ed.). (1996). *Industrial therapy.* St. Louis, MO: Mosby.

Key Functional Assessments. (2010). *Key Functional Assessments, Inc.* Retrieved from http://www.keymethod.com/

Kielhofner, G., Henry, A. D., & Walens, D. (1989). *A user's guide to the Occupational Performance History Interview.* Rockville, MD: American Occupational Therapy Association.

Kielhofner, G., Mallinson, T., Crawfold, C., Nowak, M., Rigby, M., Henry, A., & Walens, D. (2004). *Occupational Performance History Interview II* (OPHI-II; ver. 2.1). Available from http://www.moho.uic.edu/assess/ophi%202.1.html

Kipfer, B. A. (2010). *Roget's international thesaurus* (7th ed.), New York: Collins References.

Kirk, J., & Miller, M. L. (1986). *Reliability and validity in qualitative research.* Thousand Oaks, CA: Sage.

Kirk, S. A. (April, 1963). Behavioral diagnosis and remediation of learning disabilities. In *Proceedings of the Conference on Exploration into the Problems of the Perceptually Handicapped Child: First Annual Meeting, Vol. 1.* Chicago, IL: Association for Children with Learning Disabilities.

Kirk, S. A., & Gallagher, J. J. (1989). *Educating exceptional children* (5th ed.). Boston: Houghton Mifflin.

Klein, R. M., & Bell, B. (1982). Self-care skills: Behavior measurements with the Klein-Bell ADL Scale. *Archives of Physical Medicine and Rehabilitation, 63,* 335–338.

Klein, R. M., & Bell, B. (1993). *Klein-Bell Activities of Daily Living Scales.* (Available from Health Sciences Center for Educational Resources, University of Washington, T–281 Health Sciences Building, Box 357161, Seattle, WA)

Kliebsch, U., Sturmer, T., Siebert, H., & Brenner, H. (1998). Risk factors of institutionalization in an elderly disabled population. *European Journal of Public Health, 8,* 106–112.

Klimidis, S., Minas, H., & Kokanovic, R. (2006). Ethnic minority community patients and the Better Outcomes in Mental Health Care initiative. *Australasian Psychiatry: Bulletin Of Royal Australian and New Zealand College of Psychiatrists, 14,* 212–215.

Klyczek, J. P. (1999). The Bay Area Functional Performance Evaluation. In B. J. Hemphill-Pearson (Ed.), *Assessments in occupational therapy mental health: An integrative approach* (pp. 87–109). Thorofare, NJ: SLACK.

Klyczek, J. P., & Stanton, E. (2008). The Bay area functional performance evaluation. In B. J. Hemphill-Pearson, *Assessments in occupational therapy mental health: An integrative approach* (2nd ed.; pp. 217–237). Thoroughfare, NJ: SLACK.

Knapp, L. F., & Knapp, R. R. (1982). *CAPS.* San Diego: Educational & Industrial Testing Service.

Knapp, R. B., & Knapp-Lee, L. (1995). *COPSystem Interest Inventory* (Rev. ed.). San Diego: Educational & Industrial Testing Service.

Knapp-Lee, L., Knapp, R. R., & Knapp, L. F. (1982). *COPES.* San Diego: Educational & Industrial Testing Service.

Knox, S. H. (1974). In M. Reilly (Ed.), *Play as exploratory learning* (pp. 247–266). Thorofare, NJ: SLACK.

Knox, S. H. (1997). Knox Preschool Play Scale (Rev. ed.). Developmental and current use of the Knox Preschool Play Scale. In L. D. Parham & L. S. Fanzio (Eds.), *Play in occupational therapy for children* (pp. 35–51). St. Louis, MO: Mosby-Year Book.

Koch, R. (1878/1880). Investigations into the etiology of traumatic infectious diseases. [W. W. Cheyne, Trans.] London: New Sydenham Society. Retrieved http://pds.lib.harvard.edu/pds/view/7027406

Kohlberg, L. (1981). *Essays on moral development, Vol. I: The philosophy of moral development.* San Francisco: Harper & Row.

Kohn, P. M., & MacDonald, J. E. (1992). A survey of recent life experiences: A decontaminated hassles scale for adults. *Journal of Behavioral Medicine, 15,* 221–236.

Kohs, S. (1923). *Intelligence measurements.* New York: Macmillan.

Kopolow, M. S., & Jensen, B. M. (1975). *Psychosocial adjustment to quadriplegia: A double case study.* Unpublished master's thesis, Sargent College, Boston University, Massachusetts.

Koppitz, E. M. (1963). *The Bender Gestalt test for young children.* New York: Grune & Stratton.

Koppitz, E. M. (1975). *The Bender Gestalt Test for young children: Volume II: Research and application, 1963–1973.* New York: Grune & Stratton.

Korkman, M., Kirk, U., & Kemp, S. (2007*). NEPSY-II: A developmental neuropsychological assessment.* San Antonio, TX: Pearson/ Psych Corp.

Kovacs, M. (2011). *Children's Depression Inventory–2nd edition (CDI-2).* San Antonio: Peasron/ PsychCorp.

Koyano, W., & Shibata, H. (1994). Development of a measure of subjective well-being in Japan: Construct validity and reliability of the Life Satisfaction K. *Facts and Research in Gerontology; Suppl. 2,*181–187.

Kozol, J. (2005). *The shame of the nation: The restoration of apartheid schooling in America.* New York: Crown/Random House.

Kraepelin, E. (1919). *Dementia praecox and paraphrenia* (R. M. Barclay, Trans. & G. M. Robertson, Ed.). Chicago: Chicago Medical Book Co. Retrieved from http://openlibrary.org/books/OL7130267M/Dementia_praecox_and_paraphrenia

Kramer, J., Kielhofner, G., & Forsyth, K. (2008). Assessments used with the Model of Human Occupation. In B. J. Hemphill-Pearson, 2008, *Assessments in occupational therapy mental health: An integrative approach* (2nd ed., pp. 159–184). Thorofare, NJ: SLACK.

Krathwohl, D. R. (1988). *How to prepare a research proposal: Guidelines for funding and dissertations in the social and behavioral sciences* (3rd ed.). Syracuse, NY: Syracuse University Press.

Kuder, F. (1979). *Kuder Occupational Interest Survey—Form DD* (Rev.). Chicago: Science Research Associates.

Kuder, F., & Zytowski, D.G. (1991). *Kuder occupational interest survey,* General manual (3rd ed.). Adel, IA: National Career Assessment Services, Inc.

Kuhaneck, H. M., Henry, D. A., & Glennon, T. J. (2007). *Sensory Processing Measure (SPM), Main Classroom and School Environments Forms.* Los Angeles: Western Psychological Services.

Kunz, K. R., & Brayman, S. J. (1999). The comprehensive occupational therapy evaluation. In B. J. Hemphill-Pearson (Ed.), *Assessments in occupational therapy mental health: An integrative approach* (pp. 259–274). Thorofare, NJ: SLACK.

# L

Lachar, D. (1982). *Personality inventory for children—Revised.* Los Angeles: Western Psychological Services.

Lachar, D., & Gruber, C. P. (2001). *Personality inventory for children (2nd ed.; PIC-2).* Los Angeles: Western Psychological Services.

Lane, H. (1976). *The wild boy of Aveyron.* Cambridge, MA: Harvard University Press.

Larson, R. J. (1975). *Statistics for the allied health sciences.* Columbus, OH: Merrill.

Lau, A., Chi, I., & McKenna, K. (1998). Self-perceived quality of life of Chinese elderly people in Hong Kong. *Occupational Therapy International, 5,*118–139.

Law, M., Baptiste, S., Carswell-Opzoomer, A., McColl, M., Polatajko, H., & Pollock, N. (1991). *Canadian Occupational Performance Measure manual.* Toronto, Ontario: Canadian Association of Occupational Therapists.

Law, M., Baptiste, S., Carswell, A., McColl, M., Polatajko, H., & Pollock, N. (1994). *Canadian Occupational Performance Measure* (COPM; 2nd ed.). Toronto, Ontario: Canadian Association of Occupational Therapists.

Law, M., Baptiste, S., Carswell, A., McColl, M. A., Polatajko, H., & Pollock, N. (2004). *Canadian Occupational Performance Measure* (4th ed.) Ottawa, ON: CAOT Publications ACE.

Lawton, E. B. (1956). *Activities of daily living.* New York: New York Institute of Physical Medicine and Rehabilitation, NYU-Bellevue Medical Center.

Lawton, M. P., & Brody, E. M. (1969). Assessment of older people: Self-maintaining and instrumental activities of daily living. *Gerontologist, 9,* 179–186.

Lawton, M. P., Moss, M., Fulcomer, M., & Kleban, M. H. (1982). A research and service orientated multilevel assessment instrument. *Journal of Gerontology, 37,* 91–99.

Lechner, D. E., Page, J. J., & Sheffield, G. (2008). Predictive validity of a functional capacity evaluation: The physical work performance evaluation. *Work, 31,* 21–25.

Lechner, D. E., Roth, D., & Straaton, K. (1991). Functional capacity evaluation in work disability. *Work, 1,* 37–47.

Lehman, A. F. (1988). A quality of life interview for the chronically mentally ill. *Evaluation and Program Planning, 11,* 51–62.

Lehman, L. A., Sindhu, B. S., Shechtman, O., Romero, S., & Velozo, C. A. (2010). A comparison of the ability of two upper extremity assessments to measure change in function. *Journal of Hand Therapy, 23,* 31–40.

Lehr, R. (1992). Sixteen s squared over d squared: A relation for crude sample size estimates. *Statistics in Medicine, 11,* 1099–1102.

Leiter, R. G. (1948). *Leiter International Performance Scale.* Chicago: Stoelting.

Leonardelli, C. A. (1988a). The Milwaukee Evaluation of Daily Living Skills: Evaluation in long-term psychiatric care. In B. J. Hemphill (Ed.), *Mental health assessment in occupational therapy: A integrative approach to the evaluative process* (pp. 151–162). Thorofare, NJ: SLACK.

Leonardelli, C. A. (1988b). *The Milwaukee Evaluation of Daily Living Skills* (MEDLS). Thorofare, NJ: SLACK.

Lewin, K. (1939). Field theory and experiment in social psychology: Concepts and methods. *American Journal of Sociology, 44,* 868–897.

Lewis, C. B., & McNerney, T. (1994). *The functional tool box: Clinical measures of functional outcomes.* Washington, DC: Learn.

Lewis, O. (1965). *La vida.* New York: Random House.

Lezak, M. D., Howieson, D. B., & Loring, D. W. (2004). *Neuropsychological assessment* (4th ed.). New York: Oxford University Press.

Li, Y., & Kielhofner, G. (2004). Psychometric properties of the volitional questionnaire. *The Israel Journal of Occupational Therapy, 13,* E85–E98.

Liberman, I. Y. (1973). Segmentation of the spoken word and reading acquisition. *Bulletin of the Orton Dyslexia Society, 23,* 65–77.

Lincoln, Y. S., & Guba, E. G. (1985). *Naturalistic inquiry.* Beverly Hills, CA: Sage.

Linder, T. W. (2008). *Transdisciplinary Play-Based Assessment-2* (TPBA2). Baltimore, MD: P. H. Brookes.

Lindley, D. V., & Scott, W. F. (1984). *New Cambridge statistical tables.* Cambridge, England: Cambridge University Press.

Linkenhoker, D., & McCarron, L. T. (1979). *Adaptive behaviors: Street Survival Skills Questionnaire* (SSSQ). (Available from McCarron-Dial Systems, P.O. Box 45628, Dallas, TX 75245)

Linkenhoker, D., & McCarron, L. T. (1993). *Adaptive behaviors: Street Survival Skills Questionnaire* (SSSQ; Rev. ed.). (Available from McCarron-Dial Systems, P.O. Box 45628, Dallas, TX 75245)

Linkov, I., Loney, D., Cormier, S., Satterstrom, F. K., & Bridges, T. (2009). Weight-of-evidence evaluation in environmental assessment: Review of qualitative and quantitative approaches. *The Science of the Total Environment, 407,* 5199–5205.

Linn, M. W. (1967). A rapid disability rating scale. *Journal of the American Geriatrics Society, 15,* 211–214.

Linn, M. W., & Linn, B. S. (1982). The Rapid Disability Rating Scale–2. *Journal of the American Geriatrics Society, 30,* 378–382.

Lipton, R. J. (2000). *The Nazi doctors: Medical killing and the psychology of genocide.* New York: Basic Books.

Liu, L., Gauthier, L., & Gauthier, S. (1991). Spatial disorientation in persons with early senile dementia of the Alzheimer type. *The American Journal of Occupational Therapy, 45,* 67–74.

Llewellyn, G. (1995). Qualitative research with people with intellectual disability. *Occupational Therapy International, 2,*108–127.

Llewellyn, G., Sullivan, G., & Minichiello, V. (1999). Sampling in qualitative research. In V. Minichiello, R. Axford, K. Greenwood, & G. Sullivan (Eds.), *Handbook of research methods in health.* Melbourne, Australia: Addison, Wesley, Longman.

Lloyd, C. (1995). Trends in forensic psychiatry. *British Journal of Occupational Therapy, 58,* 209–213.

Lloyd, C. (2007). The association between leisure motivation and recovery: A pilot study. *Australian Occupational Therapy Journal, 54,* 33–41.

Lo, J., & Zemke, R. (1997). The relationship between affective experiences during daily occupations and subjective well-being measures: A pilot study. *Occupational Therapy in Mental Health, 13,* 1–21.

Locke, L. F., Spirduso, W. W., & Silverman, S. J. (1987). *Proposals that work: A guide for planning dissertations and grant proposals* (2nd ed.). Newbury Park, CA: Sage.

Locke, L. F., Spirduso, W. W., & Silverman, S.J. (1997). *Proposals that work: A guide for planning dissertations and grant proposals* (3rd ed.). Newbury Park, CA: Sage.

Lofquist, L. H. (1957). *Vocational counseling with the physically handicapped.* New York: Appleton-Century-Crofts.

Longmore, D. (1970). *Machines in medicine.* New York: Doubleday.

Lorenz, K. Z. (1937/1957). The nature of instinct. In C.H. Schiller (Ed. and Trans.), *Instinctive behavior: The development of a modern concept* (pp. 129–175). New York: International Universities Press.

Lubin, B. (1981). Additional data on the reliability and validity of the brief lists of the depression adjective check lists. *Journal of Clinical Psychology, 37,* 809–811.

Luera, M. (1994). *Understanding family uniqueness through cultural diversity. Project TAKOS.* Albuquerque, NM: Alta Mira Specialized Family Services, Inc. (ERIC Document Reproduction Service No. ED 379–839)

Lundquist, T. S., & Ready, R. E. (2008). Young adult attitudes about Alzheimer's disease. *American Journal of Alzheimer's Disease and Other Dementias, 23,* 267–273.

Luria, A. R. (1961). *The role of speech in the regulation of normal and abnormal behavior.* London: Pergaman.

Luria, A. R. (1980). *Higher cortical functions in man* (2nd ed.; B. Haigh, Trans.). New York: Basic Books.

## M

Macdonald, K. C., Epstein, C. F., & Vastano, S. (1986). Roles and functions of occupational therapy in adult daycare. *American Journal of Occupational Therapy, 40,* 817–821.

Maguire, G. H. (1995). Activities of daily living. In C. B. Lewis (Ed.), *Aging, the health care challenge: An interdisciplinary approach to assessment and rehabilitative management of the elderly* (3rd ed., pp. 61–71). Philadelphia: F. A. Davis Company.

Maher, B. A. (1978). A reader's, writer's, and reviewer's guide to assessing research reports in clinical psychology. *Journal of Consulting and Clinical Psychology, 46,* 835–838.

Mahoney, F. I., & Barthel, D. W. (1965). Functional evaluation: Barthel Index. *Maryland State Medical Journal, 14,* 61–65.

Mahurin, R. K., DeBettignies, B. H., & Pirozzolo, F. J. (1991). Structured Assessment of Independent Living Skills: Preliminary report of performance measure of functional abilities in dementia. *Journal of Gerontology, 46,* 58–66.

Maitra, K., Philips, K., & Rice, M. (2010). Grasping naturally versus grasping with a reacher in people without disability: Motor control and muscle activation differences. *American Journal of Occupational Therapy, 64,* 95–104.

Malave, L. M., & Duquette, G. (1991). *Language, culture and cognition: A collection of studies in first and second language acquisition* (Vol. 69, Multilingual Matters). (Available from Multilingual Matters Ltd., 1900 Frost Road, Suite 101, Bristol, PA 19007). (ERIC Document Reproduction Service No. ED 386–929)

Mann, H. B., & Whitney, D. R. (1947). On a test of whether one of two random variables is stochastically larger than the other. *Annals of Mathematical Statistics, 18,* 52–54.

MAPI Research Institute. (2001–2011). *ProPatient reported outcome and quality of life instruments databases* (ProQoild). Available at http://www.proqolid.org/

Margolis, R. B., Chibnall, J. T., & Tait, R. C. (1988). Test-retest reliability of the pain drawing instrument. *Pain, 33,* 49–51.

Margolis, R. B., Tait, R. C., & Krause, S. J. (1986). A rating system for use with patient pain drawings. *Pain, 3,* 49–51.

Marino, R. J., & Goin, J. E. (1999). Development of a short form Quadriplegia Index of Function scale. *Spinal Cord, 37,* 289–296.

Markowitz, J. D. (2007). Post-traumatic stress disorder in an elderly combat veteran: A case report. *Military Medicine, 172,* 659–662.

Marks, S. R. (1986). *Three corners: Exploring marriage and the self.* Lexington, MA: Lexington Books.

Marshall, S. C., Heisel, B., & Grinnell, D. (1999). Validity of the PULSES profile compared with the Functional Independence Measure for measuring disability in a stroke rehabilitation setting. *Archives of Physical Medicine and Rehabilitation, 80,* 760–765.

Marston, D. (1987–1988). The effectiveness of special education: A time-series analysis of reading performance in regular and special education settings. *Journal of Special Education, 27,* 466–480.

Marti-Ibanez, F. (1962). *The epic of medicine.* New York: Bramhall House.

Martin, N. A. (2006). *Test of Visual-Perceptual Skills* (nonmotor)—3 (3rd ed.). Ann Arbor: Academic Therapy Publications.

Martin, R. P., Hooper, S., & Snow, J. (1986). Behavior rating scale approaches to personality assessment in children and adolescents. In H. M. Knoff (Ed.), *The assessment of child and adolescent personality* (pp. 309–351). New York: Guilford.

Martinsen, E. W., Medhus, A., & Sandvik, L. (1985). Effects of aerobic exercise on depression: A controlled study. *British Medical Journal, 291,*109.

Martinsen, E. W., Medhus, A., & Solberg, O. (1989). Comparing aerobic with nonaerobic forms of exercise in the treatment of clinical depression: A randomized trial. *Comprehensive Psychiatry, 30,* 324–331.

Masagatani, G. N. (1994). *Cognitive Adaptive Skills Evaluation manual* (Rev. ed.). Unpublished manuscript. (Available from Gladys Masagatani, Eastern Kentucky University, Department of Occupational Therapy, Dizney 103, Richmond, KY 40475–3135)

Masagatani, G. N. (1999). The Cognitive Adaptive Skills Evaluation. In B. J. Hemphill-Pearson (Ed.), *Assessments in occupational therapy mental health: An integrative approach* (pp. 279–288). Thorofare, NJ: SLACK.

Maslow, A. H. (1954). *Motivation and personality.* New York: Harper.

Matheson, L. (1988). *Work Capacity Evaluation* (procedure manual). Anaheim, CA:

Employment and Rehabilitation Institute of California.

Matheson, L., & Ogden, L. (1987). *Work Capacity Evaluation*. Anaheim, CA: Employment and Rehabilitation Institute of Southern California.

May-Benson, T. A. (2007). Identifying gravitational insecurity in children: A pilot study. *American Journal of Occupational Therapy, 61*, 142–147.

Mayer, J. D., Salovey, P., & Caruso, D. R. (2008). Emotional intelligence: New ability or eclectic traits. *American Psychologist, 63*, 503–517.

McBride, M. R., & Lewis, I. D. (2004). African American and Asian American elders: An ethnogeriatric perspective. *Annual Review of Nursing Research, 22*, 161–214.

McCall, R. B. (1986). *Fundamental statistics for behavioral sciences* (4th ed.). San Diego: Harcourt Brace Jovanovich.

McCarney, S. B., & Arthaud, T. J. (2004). *The Attention Deficit Disorders Evaluation Scale* (3rd ed., ADDES-3). Columbia: MO: Hawthorne Educational Services.

McCarron-Dial Systems, Inc. (n.d.). *Home–page,* Retrieved from http://www.mccarrondial.com

McCarron, L. T., & Dial, J. G. (1973). McCarron-Dial Evaluation System. Dallas, TX: McCarron-Dial Systems.

McColl, M. A., & Peterson, J. (1997). A descriptive framework for community-based rehabilitation. *Canadian Journal of Rehabilitation, 10*, 297–306.

McDermott, D. E. (1994). Jean Itard: The first child and youth counselor. *Journal of Child and Youth Care, 9*, 59–71.

McFall, S. A., Deitz, J. C., & Crowe, T. K. (1993). Test-retest reliability of the test of visual perceptual skills with children with learning disabilities. *The American Journal of Occupational Therapy, 47*, 819–824.

McGourty, L. K. (1988). Kohlman Evaluation of Living Skills (KELS). In B. J. Hemphill (Ed.), *Mental health assessment in occupational therapy: A integrative approach to the evaluative process* (pp. 133–146). Thorofare, NJ: SLACK.

McGowan, J. F. (Ed.). (1960). *An introduction to the vocational rehabilitation services* (Series no. 555; guidance, training and placement bulletin no. 3). Washington, DC: Office of Vocational Rehabilitation, U.S. Government Printing Office.

McGrew, K. S. (2005). The Catell-Horn-Carroll theory of cognitive abilities: Past, present and future. In D. P. Flanagan & P. L. Harrison (Eds.), *Contemporary intellectual assessment: Theories, tests and issues* (2nd ed., pp. 136–181). New York: Guilford.

McGrew, K. S., Flanagan, D. P., Keith, T. Z., & Vanderwood, M. (1997). Beyond *g*: The impact of *Gf-Gc* specific cognitive abilities research on the future use and interpretation of intelligence tests in the schools. *School Psychology Review, 26*, 189–210.

McIntosh, V. V., Carter, F. A., Bulik, C. M., Frampton, C. M., & Joyce, P. R. (2010). Five-year outcome of cognitive behavioral therapy and exposure with response prevention for bulimia nervosa. *Psychological Medicine, 2*, 1–11.

Mead, M. (1928). *Coming of age in Samoa.* New York: Blue Ribbon Books.

Meckler, L., & Hitt, G. (2010, March 24). Obama signs landmark health bill. *Wall Street Journal,* p. A4.

Meenan, R. B., Mason, J. H., Anderson, J. J., Guccione, A. A., & Kazis, L. E. (1992). AIMS-2: The content and properties of a revised and expanded Arthritis Impact Measurement Scales Health Questionnaire. *Arthritis and Rheumatism, 35*, 1–10.

Meenan, R. F., Gertman, P. M., & Mason, J. H. (1980). Measuring health status in arthritis: The Arthritis Impact Measurement Scales. *Arthritis Rheumatism, 23*,146–152. Available https://www.rheumatology.org/practice/clinical/clinicianresearchers/outcomes-instrumentation/AIMS.asp

Mellor, C. M. (2006). Louis Braille: A touch of genius. Boston, MA: National Braille Press.

Melzack, R. (1975). The McGill Pain Questionnaire: Major properties and scoring methods. *Pain, 1*, 277–299.

Melzack, R. (1987). The short-form McGill Pain Questionnaire. *Pain, 30,* 191–197. doi:10.1016/0304-3959(87)91074-8

*Mental measurements yearbook (MMY), Mental measurements supplement, or Tests in print,* published by The University of Nebraska Press. Retrieved from http://www.unl.edu/buros/

Mercer, C. (1983). *Students with learning disabilities* (2nd ed.). Columbus, OH: Merrill.

Mercer, C. D., Mercer, A. R., & Pullen, P. C. (2011). *Teaching students with learning problems* (8th ed.). Upper Saddle River, NJ: Pearson/Merrill.

*Merriam-Webster's Collegiate Dictionary.* (11th ed.). (2003). Springfield, MA: Merriam-Webster.

Merrington, M., & Thompson, C. M. (1943). Tables of percentage points of the inverted beta *(F)* distribution. *Biometrika, 33,* 73–88.

Meta-OT/Occupation-Matters. (2009). *OT assessments and outcome measures.* Available at http://metaot.com/ot-assessments-outcome-measures

Meyen, E. L., & Skrtic, T. M. (1988). *Exceptional children and youth* (3rd ed.). Aspen, CO: Love.

Mikulic, M. A., Griffith, E. R., & Jebsen, R. H. (1976). Clinical applications of a standardized mobility test. *Archives of Physical Medicine & Rehabilitation, 57,* 143–146.

Milberg, W. P., Hebben, N., & Kaplan, E. (1996). The Boston process approach to neuropsychological assessments. In I. Grant & K. M. Adams, (Ed.). *Neuropsychological assessment of neuropsychiatric disorders* (2nd ed., pp. 58–80). New York: Oxford University Press.

Miles, M. B., & Huberman, A. M. (1994). *Qualitative data analysis. An expanded sourcebook* (2nd ed.). Thousand Oaks, CA: Sage.

Miller, D. C. (Ed.). (2010). *Best practices in school neuropsychology: Guidelines for effective practice, assessment, and evidence-based intervention.* Hoboken, NJ: Wiley.

Miller, L. H., & Smith, A. D. (1983). Stress Audit Questionnaire. *Your Life and Health, 98,* 20–30.

Miller, L. H., Smith, A. D., & Mehler, B. L. (1988). *The Stress Audit manual.* Brookline, MA: Biobehavioral Institute.

Miller, L. J. (1988). *Miller Assessment for Preschoolers.* San Antonio, TX: Pearson/PsychCorp.

Miller, L. J. (2007). Lessons learned: A pilot study on occupational therapy effectiveness for children with sensory modulation disorder. *American Journal of Occupational Therapy, 61,* 161–169.

Miller, L. J., & Roid, G. H. (1994). The T.I.M.E.® Toddler and Infant Motor Evaluation A Standardized Assessment. San Antonio, TX: Pearson/PsychCorp.

Miller, M. (1990). Ethnographic interviews for information about classrooms: An invitation. *Teacher Education and Special Education, 13,* 233–234.

Miller, N. E. (1969). Learning of visceral and glandular responses. *Science, 163,* 434–445.

Million, T., Green, C. J., & Meagher, R. B. (1982). *Million Adolescent Personality Inventory.* Minneapolis, MN: National Computer Services, Inc.

*Mills v. Board of Education of the District of Columbia, 348 F. Supp. 866 (1972).*

Minichiello, V., Aroni, R., Timewell, E., & Alexander, L. (1995). *In-depth interviewing: Principles, techniques, & analysis* (2nd ed.). Melbourne, Australia: Longman Cheshire.

Mitchell, P. (2009). Mental health care roles of non-medical primary health and social care services. *Health and Social Care in the Community, 17,* 71–82.

Modern Language Association of America. (2009). *MLA handbook for writers of research papers* (7th ed.). New York: Author.

Montessori, M. (1912). *The Montessori method* (A. E. George, Trans.). New York: Frederick A. Stokes.

Montgomery, S. A., & Asberg, M. (1979). A new depression scale designed to be sensitive to change. *British Journal of Psychiatry, 134,* 382–389.

Morris, W. (Ed.). (1973). *The American Heritage dictionary of the English language.* Boston: Houghton Mifflin.

Morse, J. M. (Ed.). (1994). *Critical issues in qualitative research methods.* Thousand Oaks, CA: Sage.

Moskowitz, E., & McCann, C. B. (1957). Classification of disability in the chronically ill and aging. *Journal of Chronic Disease, 5,* 342–346.

Moustakas, C. (1994). *Phenomenological research methods.* Thousand Oaks, CA: Sage.

Muhr, T. (1991). ATLAS/Ti. A prototype for the support of text interpretation. *Qualitative Sociology, 14,* 349–371.

Mullen, E. M. (1995). *Mullen Scales of Early Learning.* Circle Pines, MN: American Guidance Service.

## N

Nadolsky, J. M. (1974). The work sample in vocational evaluation: A consistent rationale. *Vocational Evaluation and Work Adjustment Bulletin, 7,* 2–5.

Naglieri, J. A., LeBuffe, P. A., & Pfeiffer, S. I. (1992). *Devereaux behavior rating scales—School form.* San Antonio, TX: Pearson/PsychCorp.

Naglieri, J. A., LeBuffe, P. A., & Pfeiffer, S. I. (1994). *Devereaux scales of mental disorders.* San Antonio, TX: Pearson/PsychCorp.

National Institute on Disability and Rehabilitation Data. (n.d.). *What is ABLEDATA?* Retrieved from http://www.abledata.com/Site2/project.htm

National Institutes of Health Pain Consortium. (2007). *Pain intensity scales.* Bethesda, MD: NIH Pain Consortium, National Institutes of Health. Retrieved from http://painconsortium.nih.gov/pain_scales/

National Library of Medicine. (NLM). (2010a). *Medical subject headings (MeSH®:)* Fact sheet. Retrieved from http://www.nlm.nih.gov/pubs/factsheets/mesh.html

National Library of Medicine. (NLM). (2010b). *National Information Center on Health Services Research and Health Care Technology (NICHSR). Fact sheet.* Retrieved from http://www.nlm.nih.gov/pubs/factsheets/nichsr_fs.html

National Library of Medicine. (NLM). (2010c). *What's the difference between MEDLINE® and PubMed®? Fact sheet.* Retrieved from http://www.nlm.nih.gov/pubs/factsheets/dif_med_pub.html

National Rehabilitation Information Center, (n.d.). *Welcome to NARIC,* Retrieved from http://www.naric.com/

Neistadt, M. E. (1992a). *The Rabideau Kitchen Evaluation—Revised* (RKE–R). (Available from University of New Hampshire Departments of Occupational Therapy, School of Health and Human Services, Durham, NH)

Neistadt, M. E. (1992b). The Rabideau Kitchen Evaluation, Revised: An assessment of meal preparation skill. *Occupational Therapy Journal of Research, 12,* 242–255.

Neistadt, M. E. (2000). The Rabideau Kitchen Evaluation–Revised: An assessment of meal preparation skill. In M. E. Neistadt, *Occupational therapy evaluation for adults: A pocket guide* (pp. 136–137).Baltimore: Lippincott.

Neistadt, M. E. (1993). The relationship between constructional and meal preparation skills. *Archives of Physical Medicine and Rehabilitation, 74,* 144–148.

Neistadt, M. E. (1994). A meal preparation treatment protocol for adults with brain injury. *American Journal of Occupational Therapy, 48,* 431–438.

Neugarten, B. L., Havighurst, R. J., & Tobin, S. S. (1961). The Measurement of Life Satisfaction. *Journal of Gerontolology, 16 ,* 134–143. doi: 10.1093/geronj/16.2.134

Nighswonger, W. E. (1981). *Talent Assessment Programs.* Jacksonville, FL: Talent Assessment, Inc. (Available from Talent Assessment, Inc.; P.O. Box 5087; Jacksonville, FL 32207)

Nobel, L. M., Nobel, A., & Hand, I. L. (2009). Cultural competence of healthcare professionals caring for breastfeeding mothers in urban areas. *Breastfeeding Medicine: The Official Journal of the Academy of Breastfeeding Medicine, 4,* 221–224.

No Child Left Behind Act of 2001, 20 USC 6301 xxx 115 STAT. 1425 Pub. L. 107–110–JAN. 8, 2002. Retrieved from http://www2.ed.gov/policy/elsec/leg/esea02/107-110.pdf

No Child Left Behind. (2002). Pub. L. 107-110, 115 Stat. 1425, enacted January 8, 2002.

Northrop, F. S. C. (1931). *Science and first principles.* New York: Macmillan.

Nouri, F. M., & Lincoln, N. B. (1993). Predicting driving performance after stroke. *BMJ (Clinical Research Ed.), 307,* 482–483. doi:10.1136/bmj.307.6902.482

## O

Oakley, F. M. (1988). *Role Checklist–Revised.* (Available from Frances Oakley, Occupational Therapy Service, National Institutes of Health, Building 10, Room 6S–235, 10 Center Drive MSC 1604, Bethesda, MD, 20892–1604)

Oakley, F. M., Kielhofner, G., Barris, R., & Reichler, R. K. (1986). The Role Checklist: Development and empirical assessment of reliability. *Occupational Therapy Journal of Research, 6,* 157–170.

O'Connor, J. (circa 1920a). *O'Connor Finger Dexterity Test.* Wood Dale, IL: Stoelting Company.

O'Connor, J. (circa 1920b). *O'Connor Tweezer Dexterity Test.* Wood Dale, IL: Stoelting Company.

Okkema, K. A., & Culler, K. H. (1998). Functional evaluation of upper extremity use following stroke: A literature review. *Topics in Stroke Rehabilitation, 4*(4), 54–75. doi: 10.1310/710M-W1QQ-83PP-E08H

Okuma, Y., & Nomura, Y. (1998). Senescence-accelerated mouse (SAM) as an animal model of senile dementia: Pharmacological, neurochemical and molecular biological approach. *Japanese Journal of Pharmacology, 78,* 399–404.

Olds, E. G. (1938). Distribution of the sums of squares of rank differences for small numbers of individuals. *Annals of Mathematical Statistics, 9,* 133–148.

Olds, E. G. (1949). The 5 percent significant levels of sums of squares of rank differences and a correction. *Annals of Mathematical Statistics, 20,* 117–118.

Oliver, M. (Ed.). (1991). *Social work: Disabled people and disabling environments.* London: Jessica Kingsley.

Oliver, R., Blathwayt, J., Brackley, C., & Tamaki, T. (1993). Development of the safety assessment of function in the environment for rehabilitation (SAFER tool). *Canadian Journal of Occupational Therapy, 60,* 78–82.

Oliver, R., Chiu, T., Marshall, L., & Goldsilver, P. (2003). Home safety assessment and intervention practice. *International Journal of Therapy and Rehabilitation, 10,* 144–150.

Osipow, S. H., & Spokane, A. R. (1987). *Occupational Stress Inventory manual: Research version.* Odessa, FL: PAR.

OTseeker. (n.d.). *Welcome to OTseeker.* Retrieved http://www.otseeker.com/default.aspx

Ottenbacher, K. J., & Barrett, K. A. (1990). Statistical conclusion validity in rehabilitation research. *American Journal of Physical Medicine and Rehabilitation, 69,*102–107.

Ottenbacher, K. J., & Cusick, A. (1990). Goal attainment scaling as a method of clinical service evaluation. *American Journal of Occupational Therapy, 44,* 519–525.

Owen, D. B. (1962). *Handbook of statistical tables.* Reading, MA: Addison-Wesley.

## P

*Pain Treatment Topics.* (2005–2011). Available at http://pain-topics.org/

Palmer, M. (1989). Mobilization following lumbar discectomy: A comparison of two methods of bed transfer. *Physiotherapy Canada, 41,* 146–152.

Paracelsus. (1971). *Paragranum.* In W. P. D. Wightman (Ed.), *The emergence of scientific medicine.* Edinburgh, Scotland: Oliver and Boyd. (Original work published 1528)

Parachek, J. F., & King, L. J. (1986). *Parachek Geriatric Rating Scale* (3rd ed.). (Available from Center for Neurodevelopmental Studies, 5340 West Glenn Drive, Glendale, AZ 85301)

Parsons, T. (1939). The professions and social structure. *Social Forces, 17,* 457–467.

Parsons, T. (Ed.). (1964). *Max Weber: The theory of social and economic organization.* New York: Free Press.

Pasteur, L., Jourbert, J.-F., & Chamberland, C. (1878). The germ theory and its applications to medicine and surgery. [H. C. Ernst, Trans.]. Read before the French Academy of Sciences, April 29th, 1878. *Comptes Rendus de l' Academie des Sciences, 86,* 1037–1043. Retrieved from http://biotech.law.lsu.edu/cphl/history/articles/pasteur.htm#paperII

Patterson, C. H. (1958). *Counseling the emotionally disturbed.* New York: Harper and Brothers.

Patton, M. Q. (1990). *Qualitative evaluation and research methods* (2nd ed.). Newbury Park, CA: Sage.

Patton, M. Q. (2001). *Qualitative research and evaluation methods* (3rd ed.) Thousand Oaks, CA: Sage.

Paul, S., & Orchanian, D. (2003). *Pocketguide to assessment in occupational therapy* (1st ed.). Clifton Park, NY: Delmar, Cengage Learning.

Pavlov, I. P. (1927). *Conditioned reflexes.* London: Oxford University Press.

Pearson Assessments. (2010). *Qualification levels.* Retrieved from http://psychcorp.pearsonassessments.com/haiweb/Cultures/en-US/Site/ProductsAndServices/HowToOrder/Qualifications.htm

Pearson, E., & Hartley, H. (1966) *Biometrika tables for statisticians* (3rd ed.). New York: Cambridge University Press.

Pearson, K. (1911). *The grammar of science* (3rd ed.). London: Adam & Charles Black.

*Pennsylvania Association of Retarded Citizens (PARC) v. Commonwealth of Pennsylvania,* 343 F. Suppl. 279 (E. D. Pa., 1972).

Perls, F. (1969). *Gestalt therapy verbatim.* Lafayette, CA: Real People Press.

Pfeiffer, E. (1975). A short portable mental status questionnaire for the assessment of organic brain deficit in elderly patients. *Journal of the American Geriatrics Society, 23,* 433–441.

Piaget, J. (1926). *The language and thought of the child* (M. Gabain & R. Gabain, Trans.). London: K. Paul, Trench, Trubner.

Piaget, J. (1950). *The psychology of intelligence* (M. Piercy & D. E. Berlyne, Trans.). New York: Routledge & Kegan Paul. (Original work published 1947)

Piaget, J. (1977). *Equilibration of cognitive structures.* New York: Viking.

Pickens, S., Naik, A. D., Burnett, J., Kelly, P.A., Gleason, M., & Dyer, C. B. (2007). The utility of the KELS test in substantiated cases of elder self-neglect. *Journal of the American Academy of Nurse Practitioners, 19,* 137–142. doi: 10.1111/j.1745-7599.2007.00205.x

Pinker, S. (2002). *The blank slate.* New York: Viking/Penguin.

Pinninti, N. R., Rissmiller, D. J., & Steer, R. A. (2010). Cognitive-behavioral therapy as an adjunct to second-generation antipsychotics in the treatment of schizophrenia. *Psychiatric Services, 61,* 940–943.

Piper, M. C., & Darrah, J. (1994). *Alberta Infant Motor Scales* (AIMS). Philadelphia: W. W. Saunders.

Piper, M. C., Pinnell, L. E., Darrah, J., Macquire, T., & Byrne, P. M. (1992). Construction and validation of the Alberta Infant Motor Scale (AIMS). *Canadian Journal of Public Health, 83*(Suppl. 2), 46–50.

Pleis, J. R., Lucas, J. W., & Ward, B.W. (2009) Summary health statistics for U.S. adults: National Health Interview Survey, 2008. Provisional report. *Vital Health Statistics, 10*(242). Retrieved from http://www.cdc.gov/nchs/data/series/sr_10/sr10_242.pdf

Plutchik, R., Conte, H., Lieberman, M., Baker, M., Grossman, J., & Lehrman, N. (1970). Reliability and validity of a scale for assessing the functioning of geriatric patients. *Journal of the Geriatric Society, 18,* 491–500.

Plutchik, R., Conte, H., Lieberman, M., Baker, M., Grossman, J., & Lehrman, N. (1970, 1972). Geriatric rating scale (GRS). In L. Israel, D. Kozarevic, & N. Sartorius (1984). *Source book of geriatric assessment.* (Vol. 1, pp. 277–278; Vol. 2, p. 160). Basel: S. Karger.

Poole, J. L., & Whitney, S. L. (1988). Motor assessment scale for stroke patients: Concurrent validity and interrater reliability. *Archives of Physical Medicine and Rehabilitation, 69* (3 Pt. 1), 195–197.

Post, S. G. (Ed.). (2004). *Encyclopedia of bioethics: Volumes 1-5* (3rd ed.). New York: Gale Cengage Learning/Macmillan Reference USA.

Power, P. (2000). *A guide to vocational assessment* (3rd ed.). Austin, TX: Pro-Ed.

Power, P. (2006). *A guide to vocational assessment* (4th ed.). Austin, TX: Pro-Ed.

Poynter, N. (1971). *Medicine and man.* Middlesex, England: Penguin Books.

Pribram, K. (1958). Comparative neurology and the evolution of behavior. In A. Roe & G. G. Simpson (Eds.), *Behavior and evolution* (pp. 140–164). New Haven, CT: Yale University.

Prince, F., Winter, D. A., Sjonnensen, G., Powell, C., & Wheeldon, R. K. (1998). Mechanical efficiency during gait of adults with transtibial amputation: A pilot study comparing the SACH, Seattle, and Golden-Ankle. *Journal of Rehabilitation Research & Development, 35,* 177–185.

Proquest Information and Learning (2009). *Dissertation abstracts online.* Retrieved from http://library.dialog.com/bluesheets/pdf/bl0035.pdf

## R

Rabadi, M. H. (2008). A pilot study of activity-based therapy in the arm motor recovery post stroke: A randomized controlled trial. *Clinical Rehabilitation, 22,* 1071–1082.

Rabadi, M., Galgano, M., Lynch, D., Akerman, M., Lesser, M., & Volpe, B. (2008). A pilot study of activity-based therapy in the arm motor recovery post stroke: A randomized controlled trial. *Clinical Rehabilitation, 22,* 1071–1082.

Raison, C. L., Klein, H. M., & Steckler, M. (1999). The moon and madness reconsidered. *Journal of Affective Disorders, 53,* 99–106.

Ransford, A. O., Cairnes, D., & Mooney, V. (1976). The pain drawing as an aid to the psychologic evaluation of patients with low-back pain. *Spine, 1,* 127–134.

Rape, R. N. (1987). Running and depression. *Perceptual Motor Skills, 64,* 1303–1310.

Rappaport, M. (2005). The Disability Rating Scale and Coma/Near Coma scales in evaluating severe head injury. *Neuropsychological Rehabilitation 15,* 442–453.

Rappaport, M., Hall, K. M., Hopkins, K., Belleza, T., & Cope, D. N. (1982). Disability Rating Scale for severe head trauma patients: Coma to community. *Archives of Physical Medicine and Rehabilitation, 63,* 118–123.

*Rasch Analysis.* (2005–2010). Retrieved from http://www.rasch-analysis.com

Reason, P. (Ed.). (1988). *Human inquiry in action: Developments in new paradigm research.* London: Sage.

Reid, D. T., & Jutai, J. (1997). A pilot study of perceived clinical usefulness of a new computer-based tool for assessment of visual perception in occupational therapy practice. *Occupational Therapy International, 4,* 81–98.

Reid, W. M., Seavor, C., & Taylor, R. G. (1991). Application of a computer-based zero-one methodology to the assignment of nurses to a clinical rotation schedule. *Computers in Nursing, 9,* 219–223.

Reitan, R. M., & Wolfson, D. (1985). *The Halstead-Reitan Neuropsychological Test Battery: Theory and clinical interpretation.* Tuscon, AZ: Neuropsychological Press.

Reitan, R. M., & Wolfson, D. (1993). *The Halstead-Reitan Neuropsychological Test Battery: Theory and clinical interpretation* (2nd ed.). Tuscon, AZ: Neuropsychological Press.

Remsburg, R. E., Bennett, R. G., Inez Wendel, V., & Durso, S. C. (2002). Demographic and health characteristics of residents choosing to use on-site medical care in a newly opened continuing care retirement community (CCRC). *Journal of the American Medical Directors Association, 3,* 297–301.

Ren, X. S., Kazis, L., & Meenan, R. F. (1999). Short-form Arthritis Impact Measurement Scales: Tests of reliability and validity among patients with osteoarthritis. *Arthritis Care Research, 12,* 163–171.

Reynolds, C. R. (2007). *Koppitz developmental scoring system for the Bender Gestalt test* (2nd ed). Austin, TX: Pro–Ed.

Reynolds, C. R. (2008). RTI, neuroscience, and sense: Chaos in the diagnosis and treatment of learning disabilities. In E. Fletcher-Janzen & C. R. Reynolds, *Neuropsychological perspectives on learning disabilities in the era of RTI* (pp. 14–53). Hoboken, NJ: Wiley.

Reynolds, C. R., & Kamphaus, R. W. (2004a). *BASC–2: Behavioral assessment system for children manual* (2nd ed.). Circle Pines, MN: American Guidance System.

Reynolds, C. R., & Kamphaus, R. W. (2004b). *Behavior Assessment System for Children* (2nd ed.; BASC-2). San Antonio, TX: Pearson Assessments/PsychCorp.

Reynolds, C. R., & Voress, J. K. (2007). *Test of Memory and Learning–II*. Austin, TX: Pro-Ed.

Reynolds, W. M., & Kobak, K. A. (1995). *Hamilton Depression Inventory (HDI), professional manual*. Odessa, FL: PAR.

Rice, M. S., & Newell, K. M. (2004). Bimanual upper extremity movements in persons with left hemiplegia due to stroke. *Archives of Physical Medicine and Rehabilitation, 85,* 629–634.

Richards, T., & Richards, L. (1999). *NVivo*. Melbourne, Australia: QSR.

Richardson, G. A. (1998). Prenatal cocaine exposure. A longitudinal study of development. *Annals of the New York Academic of Science, 846,* 144–152.

Rockwood, K., Joyce, B., & Stolee, P. (1997). Use of goal attainment scaling in measuring clinically important change in cognitive rehabilitation patients. *Journal of Clinical Epidemiology, 50,* 581–588.

Roeder, E. W. (1970). *Roeder Manipulative Aptitude Test*. Lafayette. IN: Lafayette Instruments.

*Roget's International Thesaurus*. (1993). New York: HarperCollins.

Roid, G. H. (2003). *Stanford Binet Intelligence Test* (SB5; 5th ed.). Itasca, IL: Riverside Publishing.

Roley, S. S., DeLany, J. V., Barrows, C. J., Brownrigg, S., Honaker, D., Sava, D. I., ... American Occupational Therapy Association Commission on Practice (2008). Occupational therapy practice framework: Domain & practice, Second edition. *American Journal of Occupational Therapy, 62,* 625–683.

Ronald and Nancy Reagan Research Institute of the Alzheimer's Association and the National Institute on Aging Working Group. (1998). Consensus report of the Working Group on "Molecular and biochemical markers of Alzheimer's disease." *Neurobiology of Aging, 19,* 109–116.

Rosenblatt, R. A. (1991). Summary and reactions: Rural health manpower research. In H. Hibbard et al. (Eds.), *Primary care research: Theory and methods. Conference proceedings.* Washington DC: United States Department of Health & Human Services Publications.

Rosenthal, R., & Rosnow, R. (1991). *Essentials of behavioral research: Methods and data analysis* (2nd ed.). New York: McGraw-Hill.

Ross, R. G., & LaStayo, P. C. (1997). Clinical assessment of pain. In J. Van Deusen & D. Brunt (Eds.), *Assessment in occupational therapy and physical therapy* (pp. 123–133). Philadephia: W. B. Saunders.

Rousseau, J. J. (1883). *Emile: Or, concerning education* (J. Steeg, Ed.; E. Worthington, Trans.) Boston: D. C. Heath & Co. (Original work published 1762)

Royeen, C. B. (1987a). Test-retest reliability of a touch scale for tactile defensiveness. *Physical and Occupational Therapy in Pediatrics, 7*(3), 45–52.

Royeen, C. B. (1987b). TIP-Touch inventory for preschoolers: A pilot study. *Physical and Occupational Therapy in Preschoolers, 7,* 29–40. doi:10.1080/J006v07n01_04

Royeen, C. B., & Fortune, J. C. (1990). Touch inventory for elementary-school-aged children. *American Journal of Occupational Therapy, 44,* 155–159.

Runyon, R. (1977). *Nonparametric statistics*. Reading, MA: Addison-Wesley.

Runyon, R. P., & Haber, A. (1967). *Fundamentals of behavioral statistics*. Reading, MA: Addison-Wesley.

Rushmer, R. F. (1972). *Medical engineering: Projections for health care delivery*. New York: Academic Press.

Rusk, H. A. (1971). *Rehabilitation medicine.* St. Louis, MO: Mosby.

Russell, B. (1928). *Sceptical essays.* London: Allen and Unwin.

## S

Sachs, D., & Linn, R. (1997). Client advocacy in action: Professional and environmental factors affecting Israeli occupational therapists' behaviour. *Canadian Journal of Occupational Therapy, 64,* 207–215.

Sachs, D., & Sussman, N. (1995). Historical research: The first decade of occupational therapy in Israel: 1946–1956. *Occupational Therapy International, 2,* 241–256.

Sackett, D. L., Rosenberg, W. M. C., Gray, J. A. M., Haynes, R. B., & Richardson, W. S. (1996). Evidence-based medicine: What it is and what it isn't. *BMJ 312,* 71–72. Retrieved from http://www.bmj.com/content/312/7023/71.full

Sacks, O. (2007). *Musicophilia: Tales of music and the brain.* New York: Knopf.

Sailor, W. (1991). Special education in the restructured school. *Remedial and Special Education, 12*(6), 8–22.

Sainsbury, A., Seebass, G., Bansal, A., & Young, J. B. (2005). Reliability of the Barthel Index when used with older people. *Age Ageing, 34,* 228–232. doi: 10.1093/ageing/afi063

Salovey, P., & Mayer, J. (1990). Emotional intelligence. *Imagination, Cognition, and Personality, 9,* 185–211.

Sand, R. (1952). *The advance to social medicine.* London: Staples Press.

Sarno, J. E., Sarno, M. R, & Levita, E. (1973). Functional Life Scale. *Archives of Physical Medicine and Rehabilitation, 54,* 214–220.

Sapountzi-Krepia, D., Soumilas, A., Papadakis, N., Sapkas, G., Nomicos, J., Theodossopoulou, E., & Dimitriadou, A. (1998). Post traumatic paraplegics living in Athens: The impact of pressure sores and UTIs on everyday life activities. *Spinal Cord, 36,* 432–437.

SAS Institute Inc. (n.d.). *Software and solutions for health care providers: SAS.* Retrieved from http://www.sas.com/industry/healthcare/provider/

Sattler, J. M. (1988). *Assessment of children* (3rd ed.). San Diego: Sattler.

Sattler, J. M. (2008). *Assessment of children: Cognitive foundations* (5th ed.). San Diego: Sattler.

Schatzman, L., & Strauss, A. L. (1973). *Field research. Strategies for a natural sociology.* Englewood Cliffs, NJ: Prentice-Hall.

Schinka, J. A., Raj, A., Loewenstein, D. A., Small, B. J., Duara, R., & Potter, H. (2010). Cross-validation of the Florida Cognitive Activities Scale (FCAS) in an Alzheimer's disease research center sample. *Journal of Geriatric Psychiatry and Neurology, 23,* 9–14.

Schoening, H. A., Anderegg, L., Bergstrom, D., Fonda, M., Steinke, N., & Ulrich, P. (1964). Numerical scoring of self-care status of patients. *Archives of Physical Medicine and Rehabilitation, 46,* 689–697.

Schoening, H. A., & Iversen, I. (1968). Numerical scoring of self-care status: A study of the Kenny Self-care Evaluation. *Archives of Physical Medicine and Rehabilitation, 49,* 221–229.

Scholtz, J., Mannion, R. J., Hord, D. E., Griffin, R. S., Rawal, B., Zheng, H. ... Woolf, C. J. (2009). A novel tool for the assessment of pain: Validation in low back pain. *PLoS Med, 6,* e1000047. doi:10.1371/journal.pmed.1000047

Schrader, C. R. (2006). *History of operations research in the United States Army. Volume I: 1942–62.* Washington, DC: Office of the Deputy Undersecretary for the Army for Operations Research, U.S. Army.

Schuling, J., deHaan, R., Limburg, M., & Groenier, K. (1993). The Frenchay Activities Index: Assessment of functional status in stroke patients. *Stroke, 24,* 1173–1177.

Schwandt, T. A., & Halpern, E. S. (1988). *Linking auditing and meta-evaluation: Enhancing quality in applied research.* Newbury Park, CA: Sage.

Schwartz, D. P., & DeGood, D. E. (1984). Global appropriateness of pain drawings. Blind ratings predict patterns of psychological distress and litigation status. *Pain, 19,* 383–388.

Scrank, F. A., Miller, D. C., Wendling, B., & Woodcock, R. W. (2010). *Essentials of WJIII cognitive abilities assessment* (2nd ed). Hoboken, NJ: Wiley.

Seidel, J. (1989). *The ethnograph.* Littleton, CO: Qualis Research Associates.

Seidman, L. J., Biederman, J., Faraone, S. V., Weber, W., Mennin, D., & Jones, J. (1997). A pilot study of neuropsychological function in girls with ADHD. *Journal of the American Academic of Child & Adolescent Psychiatry, 36,* 366–373.

Selye, H. (1956). *Stress of life.* New York: McGraw-Hill Book.

Sendroy-Terrill, M., Whiteneck, G. G., & Brooks, C. A. (2010). Aging with traumatic brain injury: Cross-sectional follow-up of people receiving inpatient rehabilitation over more than 3 decades. *Archives of Physical Medicine and Rehabilitation, 91,* 489–497.

Séquin, E. (1846/1997). *Traitement moral, hygiène et éducation des idiots.* [Moral treatment, hygiene and education of idiots] Paris: Association pour l'étude de l'histoire de la sécurité sociale.

Shaffir, W. B., & Stebbins, R. A. (Eds.). (1991). *Experiencing fieldwork. An inside view of qualitative research.* Newbury Park, CA: Sage.

Shalik, L. D. (1990). The level 1 fieldwork process. *American Journal of Occupational Therapy, 44,* 700–707.

Shaywitz, S. E., & Shaywitz, B. A. (2008). Paying attention to reading: The neurobiology of reading and dyslexia. *Developmental Psychopathology, 20,* 1329–1349.

Shea, T. M., & Bauer, A. M. (1994). *Learners with disabilities: A social systems perspective of special education.* Madison, WI: Brown and Benchmark.

Sheikh J. I., & Yesavage, J. A. (1986). Geriatric Depression Scale (GDS): Recent evidence and development of a shorter version. *Gerontology, 5,* 165–173.

Sheikh, J. I., Yesavage, J. A., Brooks, J. O., Friedman, L. F., Gratzinger, P., Hill, R. D., ... Crook,

T. (1991). Proposed factor structure of the Geriatric Depression Scale. *International Psychogeriatrics, 3,* 23–28.

Sheslow, D., & Adams, W. (2003). *Wide-Range Assessment of Memory and Learning–II (WRAML-II).* Wilmington, DE: Wide Range.

Sibley, L., & Armbruster, D. (1997). Public health perspectives. Obstetric first aid in the community—Partners in safe motherhood: A strategy for reducing material mortality. *Journal of Nurse-Midwifery, 42,* 117–121.

Sigmon, S. B. (1987). *Radical analysis of special education: Focus on historical development and learning disabilities.* London: Falmer Press.

Simmonds, M. J. (1997). Muscle strength. In J. Van Deusen & D. Brunt (Eds.), *Assessment in occupational therapy and physical therapy* (pp. 27–48). Philadelphia: W. B. Saunders.

Simon, S. (2005). *What is a Kappa coefficient. (Cohen's kappa).* Retrieved from http://www.childrens-mercy.org/stats/definitions/kappa.htm

Sinclair, W. J. (1909). *Semmelweiss: His life and his doctrine.* Manchester, UK: The University Press.

Skinner, B. F. (1953). *Science and human behavior.* New York: Macmillan.

Slade, C., Campbell, W. G., & Ballou, S. V. (1997). *Form and style: Research papers, reports, theses* (10th ed.). Boston: Houghton Mifflin.

Slade, C., & Perrin, R. (2007). *Form and style: Research papers, reports, theses* (13th ed.). Florence, KY: Cengage Learning/Watsworth.

Smith, D. D., & Tyler, N. C. (2010). *Introduction to special education: Making a difference* (7th ed.) Upper Saddle River, NJ: Merrill/Pearson.

Smith, L. M. (1994). Biographical method. In N. K. Denzin & Y. S. Lincoln (Eds.), *Handbook of qualitative research* (pp. 286–305). Thousand Oaks, CA: Sage.

Snow, C. R. (1964). *The two cultures and a second look.* Cambridge, England: Cambridge University Press.

Söderback, I., & Paulsson, E. H. (1997). A needs assessment for referral to occupational therapy: Nurses' judgment in acute cancer care. *Cancer Nursing, 20,* 267–273.

Spearman, C. E. (1927). *The abilities of man.* New York: Macmillan.

Spence, K. V. (1948). The postulates and methods of "behaviorism." *Psychological Review, 55,* 67–68.

Spielberger, C. D. (1983). *Manual for the State-Trait Anxiety Inventory.* Palo Alto, CA: Consulting Psychologists Press.

Spielberger, C. D. (with Edwards, C. D., Lushene, R. E., Montuori, J., & Platzek, D.) (1973). *State-trait Anxiety Inventory for Children* (STAIC). Menlo Park, CA: Mind Gardens Inc.

Spies, R. A., Carlson, J. F., & Geisinger, K. F. (Ed.). (2010). *The Eighteenth Mental Measurements Yearbook.* Lincoln: University of Nebraska Press. Available from http://www.nebraskapress.unl.edu

Spinal Cord Injury Rehabilitation Evidence (SCIRE). (2010). *Jepson Hand Function Test.* Retrieved from http://www.scireproject.com/outcome-measures/jebsen-hand-function-test

Spitz, R. A. (1965). *The first year of life: A psychoanalytic study of normal and deviant development of object relations.* New York: International Universities Press.

Spitzer, S. L. (2003). Using participation observation to study the meaning of occupations of young children with autism and other developmental disabilities. *American Journal of Occupational Therapy, 57,* 66–76

Spradley, J. P. (1979). *The ethnographic interview.* Fort Worth, TX: Holt, Rinehart and Winston.

SPSS Inc., an IBM Company Headquarter. (2010). SPSS industry solutions: Healthcare. Retrieved from http://www.spss.com/vertical_markets/healthcare/

Staff of the Benjamin Rose Hospital. (1959). Multidisciplinary studies of illness in aged persons: II. A new classification of functional status in activities of daily living. *Journal of Chronic Disability, 9,* 55–62.

Stainback, S., & Stainback, W. (Eds.). (1992). *Controversial issues confronting special education.* Boston: Allyn & Bacon.

Stake, R. E. (2010). *Qualitative research: Studying how things work.* New York: Guilford.

Stamm, T., Geyh, S., Cieza, A., Machold, K., Kollerits, B., Kloppenburg, M., ... Stucki, G. (2006). Measuring functioning in patients with hand osteoarthritis—Content comparison of questionnaires based on the International Classification of Functioning, Disability and Health (ICF). *Rheumatology, 45,*1534–1541. Full text available at: http://rheumatology.oxfordjournals.org/content/45/12/1534.full.pdf+html?sid=1c5f5fb4-52d6-4f0c-bbcb-13871810d105

Stanton, A. H., & Schwartz, M. S. (1954). *The mental hospital: A study of institutional participation in psychiatric illness and treatment.* New York: Basic Books.

Stefanyshyn, D. J., Engsberg, J. R., Tedford, K. G., & Harder, J. A. (1994). A pilot study to test the influence of specific prosthetic features in preventing transtibial amputees from walking like able-bodied subjects. *Prosthetics & Orthotics International, 18,* 180–190.

Steffe, L. P., & Gale, J. (Eds.) (1995). *Constructivism in education.* Hillsdale, NJ: Lawrence Erlbaum.

Stein, F. (1987). *Stress Management Questionnaire.* Unpublished questionnaire. (Available from F. Stein, Department of Occupational Therapy, University of South Dakota, 414 E. Clark Street, Vermillion, SD 57069)

Stein, F. (1988). Research analysis of O.T. assessments used in mental health. In B. J. Hemphill (Ed.), *The mental health assessment in occupational therapy: An integrative approach to the evaluative process* (pp. 225–247). Thorofare, NJ: SLACK.

Stein, F., Bentley, D. E., & Natz, M. (1999). Computerized assessment: The Stress Management Questionnaire. In B. J. Hemphill-Pearson (Ed.), *Assessments in occupational therapy mental health: An integrative approach* (pp. 321–337). Thorofare, NJ: SLACK.

Stein, F., & Cutler, S. K. (2002). *Psychosocial occupational therapy: A holistic approach* (2nd ed.). Clifton Park, NY: Delmar, Cengage Learning.

Stein, F., Grueschow, D., Hoffman, M., Taylor, S., & Tronback, R. (2003). The Sorting Out Stress Cards—A version of the SMQ: A reliability study. *Occupational Therapy In Mental Health, 19,* 41-59.

Stein, F., & Smith, J. (1989). Short-term stress management programme with acutely depressed in-patients. *Canadian Journal of Occupational Therapy, 56,* 185–192.

Sternberg, R. J. (1985): *Beyond IQ: A triarchic theory of human intelligence.* Cambridge: Cambridge University Press.

Stevens, S. (1951). *Measurement and psychophysics.* New York: Wiley.

Stolee, P., Rockwood, K., Fox, R. A., & Streiner, D. L. (1992). The use of goal attainment scaling in a geriatric care setting. *Journal of the American Geriatrics Society, 4,* 575–578.

Stratton, M. (1981). Behavioral assessment of oral functions in feeding. *The American Journal of Occupational Therapy, 35,* 719–721.

Strauss, A. A., & Kephart, N. C. (1940). Behavior differences in mentally retarded children measured by a new behavior rating scale. *American Journal of Psychiatry, 96,* 1117–1123.

Strauss, A. A., & Lehtinen, L. L. (1947). *Psychopathology of the brain-injured child.* New York: Grune & Stratton.

Strauss, A. A., & Werner, H. (1941). The mental organization of the brain-injured mentally defective child. *American Journal of Psychiatry, 97,* 1194–1202.

Strauss, A. A., & Werner, H. (1943). Comparative psychopathology of the brain-injured child and the traumatic brain-injured adult. *American Journal of Psychiatry, 99,* 835.

Strauss, A. L., & Corbin, J. (1994). Grounded theory methodology: An overview. In N. K. Denzin & Y. S. Lincoln (Eds.), *Handbook of qualitative research* (pp. 273–285). Thousand Oaks, CA: Sage.

Strauss, A. L., & Corbin, J. (1998). *Basics of qualitative research: Techniques and procedures for developing grounded theory.* Newbury Park, CA: Sage.

Stromberg, E. L. (1947). *The Stromberg Dexterity Test.* San Antonio, TX: Pearson/PsychCorp.

Strong, K. E., Campbell, D. P., & Hansen, J. (1985). *The Strong-Campbell Interest Inventory.* Minneapolis, MN: National Computer Systems.

Strunk, W., & White, E. B. (1979). *The elements of style* (3rd ed.). New York: Macmillan.

Strunk, W., & White, E. B. (1999). *The elements of style* (4th ed.). Boston: Allyn & Bacon.

Suchman, E. A. (1967). *Evaluative research: Principles and practice in public service and social action programs.* New York: Russell Sage Foundation.

Swanson, H. L., & Watson, B. L. (1989). *Educational and psychological assessment of exceptional children: Theories, strategies, and applications* (2nd ed.). Columbus, OH: Merrill.

# T

Takata, N. (1969). The play history. *American Journal of Occupational Therapy, 23,* 314–318.

Takata, N. (1974). Play as a prescription. In M. Reilly (Ed.), *Play as exploratory learning* (pp. 209–246). Beverly Hills, CA: Sage.

Taylor M. L., & Marks, M. (1955). *Aphasic rehabilitation: Manual and workbook.* New York: Rehabilitation, NYU–Bellevue Medical Center.

Têng, S-y. (1943). Chinese influence on the western examination system. *Harvard Journal of Asiatic Studies, 7,* 267–312. Retrieved from http://www.jstor.org/stable/2717830

Terman, L. (1916). *The measurement of intelligence.* Boston: Houghton Mifflin.

Terman, L., & Merrill, M. (1973). *Stanford-Binet Intelligence Scale.* Boston: Houghton Mifflin.

Tesch, R. (1990). *Qualitative research: Analysis types and software tools.* New York: Falmer.

Thomson, L. K. (1992). *The Kohlman Evaluation of Living Skills* (3rd ed.). Rockland, MD: American Occupational Therapy Association.

Thomson, L. K. (1999). The Kohlman Evaluation of Living Skills. In B. J. Hemphill-Pearson (Ed.), *Assessment in occupational therapy mental health: An integrative approach* (pp. 231–244). Thorofare, NJ: SLACK.

Thomson Reuters (2011d). *Science Citation Index Expanded.* Retrieved from http://thomsonreuters.com/products_services/

science/science_products/a-z/science_
citation_index_expanded/

Thorndike, E. L. (1920, January). Intelligence and its uses. *Harper's Magazine, 140,* 227–235.

Thorndike, E. L. (1927). *The measurement of intelligence.* New York: Teachers College Press.

Thornwald, J. (1963). *Science and secrets of early medicine.* New York: Harcourt, Brace and World.

Thurstone, L. L. (1938). Primary mental abilities. *Psychometric Monographs, No. 1.*

Tiffin, J. (1948). *Purdue Pegboard.* Rosemont, IL: London House.

Timpka, T., Leijon, M., Karlsson, G., Svensson, L., & Bjurulf, P. (1997). Long-term economic effects of team-based clinical case management of patients with chronic minor disease and long-term absence from working life. *Scandinavian Journal of Social Medicine, 25,* 229–237.

Tona, J. L., & Schneck, C. M. (1993). The efficacy of upper extremity inhibiting casting: A single subject pilot study. *The American Journal of Occupational Therapy, 47,* 901–910.

Townsend, E. (1996). Institutional ethnography: A method for showing how the context shapes practice. *Occupational Therapy Journal of Research, 16,* 179–199.

Tukey, J. W. (1977). *Exploratory data analysis.* Reading, MA: Addison–Wesley.

Turabian, K. L. (1996). *A manual for writers of term papers, theses, and dissertations* (6th ed.; Revised by J. Grossman & A. Bennett). Chicago: University of Chicago Press.

Turnbull, H. R., III. (1998). *Free appropriate public education: The law and children with disabilities* (5th ed.). Aspen, CO: Love.

Twisk, F. N., & Maes, M. (2009) A review on cognitive behavorial therapy (CBT) and graded exercise therapy (GET) in myalgic encephalomyelitis (ME)/chronic fatigue syndrome (CFS): CBT/GET is not only ineffective and not evidence-based, but also potentially harmful for many patients with ME/CFS. *Neuro Endocrinology Letters, 30,* 284–299.

Tyson, P. (2009). Research in child psychoanalysis: Twenty-five-year follow-up of a severely disturbed child. *Journal of American Psychoanalysis Association, 57,* 919–945.

## U

Uhlig, T., Fongen, C., Steen, E., Christie, A., & Ødegård, S. ( 2010). Exploring Tai Chi in rheumatoid arthritis: A quantitative and qualitative study. *BMC Musculoskeletal Disorders, 11,* 43. doi: 10.1186/1471-2474-11-43

*Unistat for Windows: Key Features.* (1999). Retrieved from http://www.unistat.com/features.htm

United Nations. (1958). *Population studies* (Number 29). New York: Author.

United States Department of Defense, Joint Services Steering Committee. (1963). *Human engineering guide to equipment design.* (Morgan, C. T., et al., Eds.). New York: McGraw-Hill.

United States Department of Education. (1990). *Individuals with Disabilities Education Act.* Washington, DC: Office of Special Education and Rehabilitation Services.

United States Department of Education. (1993). *To assure the free appropriate public education of all children with disabilities: Fifteenth Annual Report to Congress on the Implementation of the Education of the Handicapped Act.* Washington, DC: U.S. Government Printing Office.

United States Department of Education. (1998). *To assure the free appropriate public education of all children with disabilities: Twentieth annual report to Congress on the implementation of the Individuals With Disabilities Education Act.* Washington, DC: U.S. Government Printing Office.

United States Department of Education, Office of Special Education and Rehabilitative Services, Office of Special Education Programs. (2009). *2007 annual report to Congress on the Individuals with Disabilities Education Act, Part D,* Washington, DC: Author. Retrieved from http://www2.ed.gov/about/reports/annual/osep/2007/part-d/idea-part-d-2007.pdf

United States Department of Education, Office of Special Education and Rehabilitative Services, Office of Special Education Programs. (2009). *28th annual report to Congress on the implementation of the Individuals with Disabilities Education Act, 2006,* vol. 1. Washington, DC: Author. Retrieved from http://www2.ed.gov/about/reports/annual/osep/2006/parts-b-c/28th-vol-1.pdf

United States Department of Health and Human Services.(2009). *Code of federal regulations (CFR): Basic HHS policy for protection of human research subjects.* (45 CFR 46 Subpart D, Section 46.402) Retrieved from http://www.hhs.gov/ohrp/humansubjects/guidance/45cfr46.htm

United States Department of Labor. (1951, 1972–73, 1988–89, 1992–93, 1998–99). *Occupational outlook handbook.* Washington, DC: U.S. Government Printing Office. Retrieved from http://stats.bls.gov/ocohome.htm

United States Department of Labor. (1991). *Dictionary of occupational titles* (4th ed.). Washington, DC: U.S. Government Printing Office. Retrieved from http://www.wave.net/upg/immigration/dot index.html

United States Department of Labor, Bureau of Labor Statistics. (1951, 1972–73, 1988–89, 1992–93, 1998–99, 2010–2011). *Occupational outlook handbook.* Washington, DC: U.S. Government Printing Office. Retrieved from http://stats.bls.gov/oco/

University of Chicago Staff. (Ed.). (2010). *The Chicago manual of style: The essential guide for writers, editors, and publishers.* (16th ed.). Chicago: University of Chicago Press.

Uomoto, J. M., & Williams, R. M. (2009). Post-acute polytrauma rehabilitation and integrated care of returning veterans: Toward a holistic approach. *Rehabilitation Psychology, 54,* 259–269.

## V

Vahabzadeh, M., Lin, J. L., Mezghanni, M., Epstein, D. H., & Preston, K. L. (2009). Automation in an addiction treatment research clinic: Computerised contingency management, ecological momentary assessment and a protocol workflow system. *Drug and Alcohol Review, 28,* 3–11.

Valpar International Corporation. (1973). *Valpar component work samples.* Tucson, AZ: Author. (Available from Valpar International Corporation, P. O. Box 5767 Tucson, AZ 85703; http://www.valparint.com/)

Van Boven, L., Kane, J., McGraw, A. P., & Dale, J. (1998). Feeling close: Emotional intensity reduces perceived psychological distance. *Journal of Personality and Social Psychology, 98,* 872–885.

Van Deusen, J., & Brunk, D. (1997). *Assessment in occupational therapy and physical therapy.* Philadelphia: Saunders.

Van Manen, M. (1990). *Researching lived experience: Human science for an action sensitive pedagogy.* London, Ontario: State University of New York.

Velozo, C. A., Kielhofner, G., & Lai, J. (1999). The use of Rasch analysis to produce scale-free measurement of functional ability. *American Journal of Occupational Therapy, 53,* 83–90.

Venes, D. (Ed.). (2009). *Taber's cyclopedic medical dictionary* (21st ed.). Philadelphia: F. A. Davis.

Ventegodt, S., Clausen, B., & Merrick, J. (2006). Clinical holistic medicine: The case story of Anna. II. Patient diary as a tool in treatment. *Scientific World Journal, 10,* 2006–2034.

Vergason, G. A., & Anderegg, M. L. (1992). Preserving the least restrictive environment. In S. Stainback & W. Stainback (Eds.), *Controversial issues confronting special education* (pp. 45–54). Boston: Allyn & Bacon.

Videler, A. C., van Royen, R .J., & van Alphen, S. P. (2010). [Treatment of personality disorders in older adults. Three case studies]. [Article in Dutch]. *Tijdschrift Voor Gerontologie en Geriatrie, 41,* 96–103.

Vidich, A. J., & Lyman, S. M. (1994). Qualitative methods: Their history in sociology and anthropology. In N. K. Denzin & Y. S. Lincoln (Eds.), *Handbook of qualitative research* (pp. 23–59). Thousand Oaks, CA: Sage.

Vissing, K., Brink, M., Lønbro, S., Sørensen, H., Overgaard, K., Danborg, K., ... Aagaard, P. (2008) Muscle adaptations to plyometric vs. resistance training in untrained young men. *Journal of Strength Conditioning Research, 22,* 1799–1810.

Vocational Rehabilitation Act of 1973, 29 U.S.C. § 794 (§504).

Vocational Research Institute. (1980). *VITAS: Vocational Interest, Temperament and Aptitude System.* (Available from Vocational Research Institute, 1528 Walnut Street, Suite 1502; Philadelphia, PA 19102; http://www.vri.org/)

Vygotsky, L. (1962/1986) *Thought and language.* Cambridge: MIT. (Original work published in 1962)

Vygotsky, L. S. (1962). *Thought and language.* (E. Hanfmann & G. Vaka, Eds. & Trans.). Cambridge, MA: MIT Press. (Original work published 1934)

## W

Wade, D. T., Collen, F. M., Robb, G. P., & Warlow, C. P.(1992). Physiotherapy intervention late after stroke and mobility. *BMJ, 304,* 609–613.

Walker, J. E., & Howland, J. (1991). Falls and fear of falling among elderly persons living in the community. *American Journal of Occupational Therapy, 45,* 119–122.

Wallace, M., & Shelkey, M. (2006). Katz Index of Independence in Activities of Daily Living (ADL). *Annals of Long Term Care, 14*(11). Retrieved from http://www.annalsoflongtermcare.com/article/6412

Wallas, G. (1926). *The art of thought.* New York: Harcourt, Brace.

Wallis, W. A., & Roberts, H. V. (1962). *The nature of statistics.* New York: Free Press.

Walls, R. T., Zane, T., & Thveldt, J. E. (1979). *Independent Living Behavior Checklist.* Dunbar: West Virginia Research and Training Center.

Walters, L., Kahn, T. J., & Goldstein, D. M. (Eds.). (2009). *Bibliography of bioethics* (Vol. 35).

Washington, DC: Georgetown University, Kennedy Institute.

Wang, J., Kane, R. L., Eberly, L. E., Virnig, B. A., & Chang, L. H. (2009). The effects of resident and nursing home characteristics on activities of daily living. *Journal of Gerontology Series A: Biological Sciences and Medical Sciences, 64,* 473–580.

Watson, J. D. (1968). *The double helix.* New York: Atheneum.

Weaver, W. (1947). *The scientists speak.* New York: Boni and Gaar.

Wechsler, D. (1939). *The measurement of adult intelligence.* Baltimore: Williams & Wilkins.

Wechsler, D. (2004). *Wechsler Intelligence Scale for Children–Fourth Edition Integrated* (WISC-IV, Integrated). San Antonio, TX: Harcourt Assessment Inc.

Wechsler, D. (2008). *Wechsler Adult Intelligence Scale–Fourth Edition Integrated* (WISC-IV, Integrated). San Antonio, TX: Harcourt Assessment Inc.

Weiner, D., Pieper, C., McConnell, E., Martinez, S., & Keefe, F. (1996). Pain measurement in elders with chronic low back pain: Traditional and alternative approaches. *Pain, 67,* 461–467.

Weiss, C. H. (1972). *Evaluation research: Methods for assessing program effectiveness.* Englewood Cliffs, NJ: Prentice-Hall.

Welkowitz, J., Ewen, R. B., & Cohen, J. (1971). *Introductory statistics for the behavioral sciences.* New York: Academic Press.

Wernicke, K. (1994). The aphasia symptom-complex: A psychological study on an anatomical basis. In P. Eling (Ed.), *Reader in the history of aphasia: From Franz Gall to Norman Geshwin.* (Vol. 4, pp. 69–89). Amsterdam: John Benjamin's. (Original work published 1875)

Westby, C. E. (1991). A scale for assessing children's pretend play. In C. E. Schafer, K. Gitlin, & A. Sandgrund (Eds.), *Play diagnosis and assessment* (pp. 131–161). New York: Wiley.

Westby, C. E. (2000). A scale for assessing development of children's play. In K. Gitlin-Weiner, A. Sandgrund, & C. Schaefer (Eds.), *Play diagnosis and assessment* (pp. 15–57) New York: Wiley.

Westby, M. D., & Backman, C. L. (2010). Patient and health professional views on rehabilitation practices and outcomes following total hip and knee arthroplasty for osteoarthritis: A focus group study. *BMC Health Service Research, 10*, 119. Published online 2010 May 11. doi: 10.1186/1472-6963-10-119 (Retrieved from http://www.ncbi.nlm.nih.gov/pmc/articles/PMC2887446/pdf/1472-6963-10-119.pdf)

White, R. W. (1952). *Lives in progress.* New York: Rinehart and Winston.

Whiteford, G. E. (1995). Other worlds and other lives: A study of occupational therapy student perceptions of cultural difference. *Occupational Therapy International, 2*, 291–313.

Whiting, S., Lincoln, N., Bhavnani, G., & Cockburn, J. (1985). *Rivermead Perceptual Assessment Battery* (RPAB). United Kingdom: NFER-Nelson.

Wiener, N. (1948). *Cybernetics: Or, control and communication in the animal and the machine.* New York: Wiley.

Wightman, W. P. D. (1971). *The emergence of scientific medicine.* Edinburgh, Scotland: Oliver and Boyd.

Will, M. (1986). Educating children with learning problems: A shared responsibility. *Exceptional Children, 52*, 411–415.

Willard, H. S., & Spackman, C. S. (1971). *Occupational therapy* (4th ed.). Philadelphia: J. B. Lippincott.

Wille, D. (2009). Virtual reality-based paediatric interactive therapy system (PITS) for improvement of arm and hand function in children with motor impairment—A pilot study. *Developmental NeuroRehabilitation, 12*, 44–52.

Willer, B., Ottenbacher, K. J., & Coad, M. L. (1994). The community integration questionnaire: A comparative examination. *American Journal of Physical Medicine & Rehabilitation, 73*, 103–111.

Williams, J. H., Drinka, T. J., Greenberg, J. R., Farrell-Holtan, J., Euhardy, R., & Schräm, M. (1991). Development and testing of the assessment of living skills and resources (ALSAR) in elderly community-dwelling veterans. *Gerontologisit, 31*, 84–91.

Williams, S., & Bloomer, J. (1987). *Bay Area Functional Performance Evaluation* (2nd ed.). Palo Alto, CA: Consulting Psychologists Press.

Wilson, B. A., Baddley, A., Cockburn, J., & Hiorns, R. (n.d.). *The Rivermead Behavioural Memory Test. Supplement 2: Validation study.* Titchfield Hants, England: Thames Valley Test Company.

Wilson, B. A., Cockburn, J., & Baddley, A. (1991). *The Rivermead Behavioural Memory Test.* Edmunds, England: Thames Valley Test Company.

Wilson, B. A., Greenfield, E., Clare, L., Baddeley, A., Cockburn, J., Watson, P., ... & Nannery, R. (2008). *Rivermead Behavioural Memory Test—Third Edition* (RBMT-3). San Antonio, TX: Pearson/PsychCorp.

Wilson, D. J., Baker, L. L., & Craddock, J. A. (1984). Functional test for the hemiparetic upper extremity. *American Journal of Occupational Therapy, 38,* 159–164.

Winkler, A. C., & McCuen, J. R. (1998). *Writing the research paper: A handbook* (5th ed.). New York: Harcourt, Brace, & Jovanovich.

Winnie, A. J. (1912). *History and handbook of day schools for the deaf and blind.* Madison, WI: State Department of Education.

Wolfensberger, W. (1972). *The principle of normalization in human services.* Toronto, Ontario: National Institution on Mental Retardation.

Wolpe, J. (1969). *The practice of behavior therapy.* New York: Pergamon.

Woodcock, R. W., McGrew, K. S., & Mather, N. (2001). *Woodcock-Johnson III.* Itasca, IL: Riverside Publishing.

Woods, K., Karrison, T., Koshy, M., Patel, A., Friedmann, P., & Cassel, C. (1997). Hospital utilization patterns and costs for adult sickle cell patients in Illinois. *Public Health Reports, 112*, 44–51.

World Health Organization. (WHO). (1998). *Fifty facts from the world health report 1998: Global health situation and trends 1955–2025,* Retrieved from http://www.who.int/whr/1998/factse.htm

World Health Organization. (WHO). (2010). *Global health observatory (GHO).* Retrieved from http://www.who.int/gho/en/

World Medical Association. (1997). *Handbook of declarations.* Ferney-Voltaire, France: Author. Retrieved from http://bioscience.igh.cnrs.fr/guides/declhels.htm

## X

Xakellis, G. C., Frantz, R. A., Lewis, A., & Harvey, R. (1998). Cost-effectiveness of an intensive pressure ulcer prevention protocol in long-term care. *Advances in Wound Care: The Journal for Prevention & Healing, 11,* 22–29.

## Y

Yerkes, R. M. (1930). Autobiography of Robert M. Yerkes. In C. Murchison (Ed.), *History of psychology in autobiography* (Vol. 2, pp. 381–407). Worcester, MA: Clark University Press. [The great comparative psychologist's own summary of his life's work.]

Yerkes, R. M. (Ed.) (1921). Psychological examining in the United States Army. *Memoirs of the National Academy of Sciences, 15,* 1–890.

Yesavage, J. A., Brink, T. A., Rose, T. L., Lum, O., Huang, V., Adey, M., & Leire, V. O. (1983). Development and validation of a geriatric depression screening scale: A preliminary report. *Journal of Psychiatric Research, 17,* 37–49.

## Z

Zinsser, W. (1990). *On writing well: An informal guide to writing nonfiction* (4th ed.). New York: HarperCollins.

Zinzi, P. (2007). Effects of an intensive rehabilitation programme on patients with Huntington's disease: A pilot study. *Clinical Rehabilitation, 21,* 603–613.

Zung, W. K. (1965). A self-rating depression scale. *Archives of General Psychiatry, 12,* 63–75.

Zytowski, D. G. (n.d.). *Kuder®* career search with person match: Technical manual (ver. 1.2). Adel, IA: Kuder Inc.

Zytowski, D. G. (2001) *Super's Work Values Inventory, Revised, User's manual.* Adel, IA: National Career Assessment Services, Inc.

Zytowski, D. G., & Luzzo, D. A. (2002). Developing the Kuder Skills Assessment. *Journal of Career Assessment, 10,* 190–199. doi: 10.1177/1069072702010002004

# Index

## M

## N

# Q

## S

## Z